Textbook of

Endovascular

Procedures

Textbook of
Endovascular
Procedures

John F. Dyet, FRCP, FRCR
Medical Director,
Consultant Cardiovascular Radiologist
Royal Hull Hospitals
Kingston Upon Hull, East Yorkshire
United Kingdom

Anthony A. Nicholson, MSc, FRCR
Consultant Cardiovascular Radiologist,
President,
British Society of Interventional Radiologists
Royal Hull Hospitals
Kingston Upon Hull, East Yorkshire
United Kingdom

Duncan F. Ettles, MD, MRCP, FRCR
Consultant Cardiovascular Radiologist
and Honorary Senior Lecturer in Radiology,
Head of Vascular Radiology
Royal Hull Hospitals
Kingston Upon Hull, East Yorkshire
United Kingdom

Samuel Eric Wilson, MD
Professor and Chair
Department of Surgery
University of California, Irvine, Medical Center
Orange, California

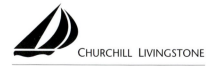

CHURCHILL LIVINGSTONE

A Harcourt Health Sciences Company
New York, Edinburgh, London, Philadelphia

CHURCHILL LIVINGSTONE
A Harcourt Health Sciences Company

The Curtis Center
Independence Square West
Philadelphia, Pennsylvania 19106

Library of Congress Cataloging-in-Publication Data

Textbook of endovascular procedures / John F. Dyet, Duncan F. Ettles, Anthony A. Nicholson, and Samuel Eric Wilson—1st ed.

p.   cm.

ISBN 0–443–06541–1

1. Blood-vessels—Surgery.   I. Dyet, John F. [DNLM: 1. Vascular Surgical
    Procedures.   WG 170 T355 2000]

RD598.5.T48 2000   617.4′13 21—dc21

DNLM/DLC   99–040814

TEXTBOOK OF ENDOVASCULAR PROCEDURES   ISBN 0–443–06541–1

Printed in the United States of America.

Last digit is the print number: 9   8   7   6   5   4   3   2   1

Contributors

Bruce M. Achauer, MC, FACS
Adjunct Professor of Surgery, Division of Plastic
Surgery, University of California, Irvine, Medical
Center, Orange, California
Embolization of Congenital Lesions

Samuel S. Ahn, MD
Associate Professor of Surgery, University of
California, Los Angeles, California
Atherectomy

Jeffrey L. Ballard, MD, FACS
Associate Professor of Surgery, Division of Vascular
Surgery, Loma Linda University Medical Center,
Loma Linda, California
Interventions in the Subclavian and Axillary Arteries

Jonathan D. Beard, ChM, FRCS
Consultant Vascular Surgeon, Northern General
Hospital, Sheffield, United Kingdom
*Endoluminal Treatment of Carotid and Vertebral Artery
Stenosis*

Jill Belch, MB, ChB, MD(Hons), FRCP
Professor and Head of Section, Vascular Medicine
and Biology, Ninewells Hospital and Medical School,
Dundee, Scotland, United Kingdom
*The Basic Science of Angioplasty and Restenosis: Cellular
Mechanisms and Interventional Pharmacotherapy*

Peter R.F. Bell, FRCS
Professor of Surgery, Faculty of Medicine, Leicester
Royal Infirmary, Leicester, United Kingdom
Subintimal Angioplasty

Anna-Marie Belli, FRCR
Consultant Radiologist, Department of Radiology,
St. George's Hospital, London, United Kingdom
Atherectomy

Bernard Beyssen, MD
Radiologie Vasculaire, Diagnostique, et
Interventionelle, Clinique Saint-Gatien, Tours, France
Interventions in Dialysis Fistulas

Kiran Bhirangi, MS, FRCS
Research Instructor, Division of Vascular Surgery,
University of Utah Medical Center, Salt Lake City,
Utah
Interventions in the Femoropopliteal Arteries

José I. Bilbao, MD
Department of Radiology, Clinica Universitaria,
Facultad de Medicina, Universidad de Navarra,
Pamplona, Spain
Venous Access

Ulrich Blum, MD
Head of Interventional Radiology, University
Hospital, Zurich, Switzerland
Endovascular Repair of Abdominal Aortic Aneurysms

Amman Bolia, FRCR
Consultant Radiologist, Radiology Department,
Leicester Royal Infirmary, Leicester, United Kingdom
Subintimal Angioplasty

David P. Brophy, FRCR, FFR, RCSI
Department of Radiology, Beth Israel Deaconess
Medical Center and Harvard Medical School,
Boston, Massachusetts
Chemoembolization

Tim M. Buckenham, FRCR
Professor of Radiology, Edinburgh Royal Infirmary,
Edinburgh, Scotland, United Kingdom
Atherectomy

Teresa J. Chan, MD
Department of Surgery, University of California,
Irvine, Medical Center, Orange, California
Interventions in the Aorta and Iliac Arteries

Melvin E. Clouse, MD
Department of Radiology, Beth Israel Deaconess
Medical Center and Harvard Medical School,
Boston, Massachusetts
Chemoembolization

John Craig Collins, MD
Department of Surgery, University of California,
Irvine, Medical Center, Orange, California
Transjugular Intrahepatic Portosystemic Shunts

Michael D. Dake, MD
Chief of Cardiovascular and Interventional
Radiology and Associate Professor of Radiology,
Stanford University Medical Center, Stanford,
California
*Endovascular Repair of Thoracic and Dissecting Aneurysms
and Aortic Coarctation*

Eric J. Daniels, MS
Division of Vascular Surgery, University of
California, Los Angeles, Center for the Health
Sciences, Los Angeles, California
Atherectomy

Michael R.E. Dean, FRCR
Consultant Radiologist, Royal Shrewsbury Hospital,
Shrewsbury, United Kingdom
*Medicolegal Aspects of Endovascular Procedures and the
Obligations of the Clinical Investigator*

**Gerry Dorros, MD, FACC, FESC, FASCI, FACP,
FCCP**
Interventional Cardiologist, Cardiovascular
Interventionist, and President, Arizona Heart
Institute Foundation, Phoenix, Arizona
*Medicolegal Aspects of Endovascular Procedures and the
Obligations of the Clinical Investigator; Interventions in the
Subclavian and Axillary Arteries*

John F. Dyet, FRCP, FRCR
Consultant Cardiovascular Radiologist, Royal Hull
Hospitals, Kingston Upon Hull, East Yorkshire,
United Kingdom
*The Physical and Biological Properties of Metallic Stents;
Endovascular Repair of Iliac and Other Aneurysms*

Jonothan J. Earnshaw, DM, FRCS
Consultant Vascular Surgeon, Gloucestershire Royal
Hospital, Gloucester, United Kingdom
*Peripheral Arterial Thrombolysis; Lower Limb Venous
Interventions*

Richard D. Edwards, FRCR
Consultant Interventional Radiologist, Radiology
Department, Gartnavel General Hospital, Glasgow,
Scotland, United Kingdom
Pulmonary Embolism

Beatriz Elduayen, MD
Department of Radiology, Clinica Universitaria,
Facultad de Medicina, Universidad de Navarra,
Pamplona, Spain
Venous Access

Duncan F. Ettles, MD, MRCP, FRCR
Consultant Cardiovascular Radiologist, Royal Hull
Hospitals, Kingston Upon Hull, East Yorkshire,
United Kingdom
*Complications of Endovascular Procedures; Endovascular
Repair of Iliac and Other Aneurysms*

Thomas J. Fogarty, MD
Professor of Surgery, Division of Vascular Surgery,
Stanford University Medical Center, Stanford,
California
Future Developments in Endovascular Therapy

Peter Gaines, MRCP, FRCR
Consultant Vascular Radiologist, Northern General
Hospital, Sheffield, United Kingdom
Upper Limb Venous and Superior Vena Cava Intervention

Ian Galloway, FRCS
Consultant Vascular Surgeon, Royal Hull Infirmary,
Royal Hull Hospitals, Kingston Upon Hull, East
Yorkshire, United Kingdom
Lower Limb Venous Interventions

Melissa Graule, MD
Department of Cardiovascular and Interventional
Radiology, Brigham and Women's Hospital and
Harvard Medical School, Boston, Massachusetts
Peripheral Arterial Thrombolysis

James Gunn, FRCS
Department of Vascular Surgery, Royal Hull
Hospitals, Kingston Upon Hull, East Yorkshire,
United Kingdom
Endovascular Repair of Abdominal Aortic Aneurysms

George Hamilton, MB, ChB, FRCS
Consultant Vascular Surgeon and Honorary Senior
Lecturer, University Department of Surgery, Royal
Free Hospital, London, United Kingdom
Renal and Visceral Artery Intervention

Peter Harris, MD, FRCS
Consultant Vascular Surgery, Royal Liverpool
University Hospital, Liverpool, United Kingdom
Endovascular Repair of Abdominal Aortic Aneurysms

George G. Hartnell, MRCP, FRCR
Consultant Radiologist, Beth Israel Deaconess
Medical Center and Harvard Medical School,
Boston, Massachusetts
Intravascular Foreign Body Retrieval

Martin Hauer, MD
Department of Radiology, University Hospital
Freiburg, Freiburg, Germany
Endovascular Repair of Abdominal Aortic Aneurysms

William F. Hendry, MD, ChM, FRCS
Consultant Genitourinary Surgeon, St.
Bartholomew's Hospital, London, United Kingdom
Varicocele Embolization

Brian R. Hopkinson, ChM, FRCS
Professor of Surgery, Division of Vascular Surgery,
University Hospital, Queen's Medical Centre,
Nottingham, United Kingdom
Endovascular Repair of Abdominal Aortic Aneurysms

James E. Jackson, MRCP, FRCR
Consultant in Charge of Vascular and Nonvascular
Interventional Radiology, Hammersmith Hospital,
London, United Kingdom
Visceral Embolization; Embolization of Congenital Lesions

H. Jäger, MD
Städische Kliniken Dortmund, Dortmund, Germany
*Endoluminal Treatment of Carotid and Vertebral Artery
Stenosis*

Brian F. Johnson, MD, FRCS
Consultant Vascular Surgeon, Royal Hull Hospitals,
Kingston Upon Hull, East Yorkshire, United
Kingdom
*Interventions in the Crural Arteries; Peroperative
Transluminal Angioplasty*

Fernando E. Kafie, MD
Department of Surgery, University of California,
Irvine, Medical Center, Orange, California
Upper Limb Venous and Superior Vena Cava Intervention

Erwan Kamboj
Cardiology Fellow, Arizona Heart Institute
Foundation, Phoenix, Arizona
Interventions in the Subclavian and Axillary Arteries

Krishna Kandarpa, MD, PhD
Associate Professor of Radiology, Department of
Cardiovascular and Interventional Radiology,
Brigham and Women's Hospital, Harvard Medical
School, Boston, Massachusetts
Peripheral Arterial Thrombolysis

Stephen T. Kee, MD
Assistant Professor of Radiology, Stanford University
Medical Center, Stanford, California
*Endovascular Repair of Thoracic and Dissecting Aneurysms
and Aortic Coarctation*

David D. Kidney, MB, MRCPI, FFR, FRCR, MSc
Assistant Professor of Radiology, Department of
Radiological Sciences, University of California,
Irvine, Medical Center, Orange, California
The Endovascular Approach to Trauma

Stephen Killick, MD, FRCOG
Professor and Head of Academic Department of
Obstetrics and Gynaecology, Princess Royal
Hospital, Kingston Upon Hull, East Yorkshire,
United Kingdom
Embolization in the Female Pelvis

Jörg Lahann, Dipl Chem
Department of Textile and Macromolecular
Chemistry, University of Technology Aachen,
Aachen, Germany
The Physical and Biological Properties of Metallic Stents

Peter F. Lawrence, MD
Professor of Surgery and Associate Dean, University
of California, Irvine, College of Medicine, Irvine,
California
Interventions in the Femoropopliteal Arteries

Henry W. Loose, FRCR
Consultant Radiologist, The Freeman Hospital,
Newcastle Upon Tyne, United Kingdom
Endovascular Repair of Iliac and Other Aneurysms

Lindsay Machan, MD
Joachim Burhenne Scholar in Abdominal Radiology,
University of British Columbia, Vancouver General
Hospital, Vancouver, British Columbia, Canada
*Embolization in the Female Pelvis; Future Developments in
Endovascular Therapy*

J. Macierewicz, FRCS
Division of Vascular Surgery, University Hospital,
Queen's Medical Centre, Nottingham, United
Kingdom
Endovascular Repair of Abdominal Aortic Aneurysms

Antonio Martínez-Cuesta, FRCR
Department of Radiology, Clinica Universitaria,
Facultad de Medicina, Universidad de Navarra,
Pamplona, Spain
Venous Access

Lynne M. Mathiak, RN
Assistant Medical Director, Dorros Feuer
Interventional Cardiovascular Disease Foundation,
Phoenix, Arizona
Interventions in the Subclavian and Axillary Arteries

Kurt Mathias
Professor, Direktor der Radiologischen Klinik,
Städische Kliniken Dortmund, Dortmund, Germany
Endoluminal Treatment of Carotid and Vertebral Artery Stenosis

James May, MS, FRACS, FACS
Department of Vascular Surgery, Royal Prince Alfred
Hospital, University of Sydney, Sydney, New South
Wales, Australia
Endovascular Repair of Abdominal Aortic Aneurysms

Peter McCollum, MCh, FRCS
Professor of Vascular Surgery, Department of
Vascular Surgery, Royal Hull Hospitals, Kingston
Upon Hull, East Yorkshire, United Kingdom
Endovascular Repair of Abdominal Aortic Aneurysms

Jeffrey C. Milliken, MD
Division of Cardiovascular Surgery, University of
California, Irvine, Medical Center, Orange, California
*Pulmonary Embolism; Endovascular Repair of Thoracic and
Dissecting Aneurysms and Aortic Coarctation*

Jon G. Moss, MB, ChB, FRCS, FRCR
Consultant Interventional Radiologist, Radiology
Department, Gartnavel General Hospital, Glasgow
Scotland, United Kingdom
Renal and Visceral Artery Intervention

Anthony A. Nicholson, MSc, FRCR
Consultant Cardiovascular Radiologist, Royal Hull
Hospitals, Kingston Upon Hull, East Yorkshire,
United Kingdom
*Inferior Vena Cava Filters; Endovascular Repair of Iliac and
Other Aneurysms*

Inge B. Nockler, FRCR
Department of Radiology, Central Middlesex
Hospital, London, United Kindgon
Varicocele Embolization

Gustavo Oderich, MD
Research Associate, University of Utah Medical
Center, Division of Vascular Surgery, Salt Lake City,
Utah
Interventions in the Femoropopliteal Arteries

Takao Ohki, MD
Division of Vascular Surgery, Montefiore Medical
Center, Bronx, New York
*Endovascular Grafting for Occlusive Aortoiliac Disease;
Endovascular Repair of Iliac and Other Aneurysms*

Alex J. Paddon, FRCR
Radiologist, Royal Hull Hospitals, Kingston Upon
Hull, East Yorkshire, United Kingdom
*Endovascular Repair of Thoracic and Dissecting Aneurysms
and Aortic Coarctation*

Paul Petrosek, MD
Department of Surgery, The University of Sydney,
Sydney, New South Wales, Australia
Endovascular Repair of Abdominal Aortic Aneurysms

Alain Raynaud, MD
Radiologie Vasculaire, Diagnostique, et
Interventionelle, Clinique Saint-Gatien, Tours, France
Interventions in Dialysis Fistulas

Jim A. Reekers, MD, PhD
Department of Radiology, Academic Medical Center,
Amsterdam, The Netherlands
Interventions in the Crural Arteries

John Reidy, FRCR
Consultant Radiologist, Radiology Department,
Guy's Hospital, London, United Kingdom
Embolization in the Female Pelvis

Luis A. Sanchez, MD
Division of Vascular Surgery, Montefiore Medical
Center, Bronx, New York
Endovascular Grafting for Occlusive Aortoiliac Disease

Marc Sapoval, MD
Radiologie Vasculaire, Diagnostique, et
Interventionelle, Clinique Saint-Gatien, Tours, France
Interventions in Dialysis Fistulas

I. James Sarfeh, MD
Department of Surgery, University of California,
Irvine, Medical Center, Orange, California
Transjugular Intraheptic Portosystemic Shunts

Karl Schürmann, MD
Klinik für Radiologische Diagnostik, Aachen,
Germany
*The Physical and Biological Properties of Metallic Stents;
Interventions in the Aorta and Iliac Arteries*

Charles P. Semba, MD
Associate Professor, Cardiovascular-Interventional
Radiology, Stanford University School of Medicine,
Stanford, California
Lower Limb Venous Interventions

Dan L. Serna, MD
Department of Surgery, University of California,
Irvine, Medical Center, Orange, California
*Interventions in the Aorta and Iliac Arteries; Pulmonary
Embolism; Endovascular Repair of Thoracic and Dissecting
Aneurysms and Aortic Coarctation*

Bruce Stabile, MD
Professor and Chairman, Department of Surgery,
University of California, Los Angeles, Harbor
Medical Center, Torrance, California
Visceral Embolization

Arthur Stanton, FRACS
Department of Vascular Surgery, Royal Prince Alfred
Hospital, University of Sydney, Sydney, Australia
Endovascular Repair of Iliac and Other Aneurysms

Luc Stockx, MD
Department of Radiology, University Hospitals,
Leuven, Belgium
Interventions in the Femoropopliteal Arteries

Peter R. Taylor, MA, MChir, FRCS
Consultant Vascular Surgeon, Guy's Hospital,
London, United Kingdom
Complications of Endovascular Procedures

Jonathan Tibballs, FRCR
Consultant Radiologist and Honorary Senior
Lecturer, Radiology Department, The Royal Free
Hospital, London, United Kingdom
Transjugular Intrahepatic Portosystemic Shunts

Luc A.E. Turmel-Rodrigues, MD
Radiologie Vasculaire, Diagnostique, et
Interventionelle, Clinique Saint-Gatien, Tours, France
Interventions in Dialysis Fistulas

Mordechai F. Twena, MD
Vascular Surgery Resident, Division of Vascular
Surgery, Loma Linda University Medical Center,
Loma Linda, California
Interventions in the Subclavian and Axillary Arteries

Fermin Urtasun, MD
Department of Radiology, Clinica Universitaria,
Facultad de Medicina, Universidad de Navarra,
Pamplona, Spain
Venous Access

Frank J. Veith, MD
Professor of Surgery, Division of Vascular Surgery,
Montefiore Medical Center, Bronx, New York
Endovascular Grafting for Occlusive Aortoiliac Disease;
Endovascular Repair of Iliac and Other Aneurysms

R. Verhaeghe, MD
Center for Molecular and Vascular Biology,
University of Leuven, Leuven, Belgium
The Principles of Thrombolysis

J. Vermylen, MD
Professor, Center for Molecular and Vascular
Biology, University of Leuven, Leuven, Belgium
The Principles of Thrombolysis

Isabel Vivas, MD
Department of Radiology, Clinica Universitaria,
Facultad de Medicina, Universidad de Navarra,
Pamplona, Spain
Venous Access

Dierk Vorwerk, MD
Professor, Department of Diagnostic and
Interventional Radiology, Klinikum Ingolstadt,
Ingolstadt, Germany
Interventions in the Aorta and Iliac Arteries

Götz Voshage, MD
Department of Radiology, Henriettenstiftung,
Hanover, Germany
Endovascular Repair of Abdominal Aortic Aneurysms

Reese A. Wain, MD
Division of Vascular Surgery, Montefiore Medical
Center, Bronx, New York
Endovascular Grafting for Occlusive Aortoiliac Disease

Anthony Watkinson, FRCR
Consultant and Honorary Senior Lecturer in
Radiology, Radiology Department, The Royal Free
Hospital, London, United Kingdom
Transjugular Intrahepatic Portosystemic Shunts

Irving P. Wells, FRCP, FRCR
Consultant Radiologist, Department of Radiology,
Derriford Hospital, Plymouth, United Kingdom
Varicocele Embolization

Geoffrey White, FRACS
Professor, Department of Surgery, The University of
Sydney, Sydney, New South Wales, Australia
Endovascular Repair of Abdominal Aortic Aneurysms;
Endovascular Repair of Iliac and Other Aneurysms

Alan R. Wilkinson, FRCS
Consultant Vascular Surgeon, Royal Hull Hospitals,
Kingston Upon Hull, East Yorkshire, United
Kingdom
Peroperative Transluminal Angioplasty

Samuel Eric Wilson, MD
Professor and Chair, Department of Surgery,
University of California, Irvine, Medical Center,
Orange, California
Interventions in the Aorta and Iliac Arteries; Upper Limb
Venous and Superior Vena Cava Intervention

S.W. Yusuf, DM, FRCS
Division of Vascular Surgery, University Hospital,
Queen's Medical Centre, Nottingham, United
Kingdom
Endovascular Repair of Abdominal Aortic Aneurysms

Preface

At the beginning of the 21st century, cardiovascular disease remains the principal cause of death in the developed world, and the potential impact of preventive medicine on vascular disease has yet to be realized. Until the mid-1960s, interventional treatment of vascular disease was the preserve of the vascular surgeon, but following the introduction of balloon angioplasty, radiologic vascular intervention came of age.

Rapid developments in imaging technology, device construction, and pharmacologic treatments have allowed the scope and efficacy of vascular intervention to increase dramatically. Endovascular therapy has continued to develop to the point where it is regarded as a specialty in its own right, with specific training and accreditation requirements for doctors undertaking these procedures. Concurrently, there have been major changes in the role of the vascular surgeon, and some traditional revascularization procedures are now rarely performed. Inevitably, this has led to some conflicts, but for the most part, cooperation between endovascular therapists of different specialties has ensured the best and most appropriate treatment for the individual patient and has fostered new technical approaches to vascular disease.

It is hoped that the structure and authorship of this textbook reflect this collaborative, multidisciplinary approach to the treatment of patients with vascular disease. Radiologists, vascular surgeons, and physicians from across Europe, Australia, and the United States have combined to provide a summary of state-of-the-art endovascular and surgical approaches to the management of arterial and venous disease as it exists at the beginning of the new millennium. The distinction between these various subspecialties is to some extent artificial and has already become blurred as more crossover techniques come into existence.

The list of contributing authors includes many eminent authorities in the subject, and we are grateful to all our contributors for the hard work and enthusiasm shown in completing this project. Most chapters are divided into a first section dealing with the endovascular approach to treatment followed by a short commentary on the surgical alternatives and perspectives. References have deliberately been restricted to the most recent and most relevant to each section.

JOHN DYET
DUNCAN ETTLES
TONY NICHOLSON
ERIC WILSON

Acknowledgments

All of us involved in the treatment of patients with vascular disease lead busy lives, and we are grateful for the precious time set aside by all our contributors to produce this work.

We are indebted to Fiona Bennett, Chris Whatling and Helen Willson for their secretarial and typing skills in the preparation of this textbook.

Last, but far from least, we wish to express our gratitude to our wives and families for their tolerance and support throughout the project.

Contents

Section 1

The Principles of Endovascular Treatment

The Basic Science of Angioplasty and Restenosis: Cellular Mechanisms and Interventional Pharmacotherapy

Chapter *1*

Jill Belch

Symptomatic peripheral arterial occlusive disease (PAOD) affects 5% of men who are older than 50 years of age.[1] Its most common manifestation, intermittent claudication, can produce disabling leg pain on exercise, resulting in severely limited mobility. Nevertheless, claudication symptoms seem to stabilize in the majority of patients,[2] and few progress to limb-threatening ischemia.[3] The initial enthusiasm for surgical intervention has thus been attenuated, and bypass surgery is usually reserved for patients with critical limb ischemia or very disabling short-distance claudication. In contrast, percutaneous transluminal angioplasty (PTA) has gained increasing acceptance as a safe and effective therapy for both intermittent claudication and critical limb ischemia.[4] Nevertheless, the longer term benefits of angioplasty have been limited in some patients by the recurrence of the stenotic lesion. The restenosis rate depends on many factors, including length of occlusion, occlusion vs. stenosis,[5] and distribution of disease. In most series, the restenosis rate is between 30 and 60% from 6 months to 1 year after performance of initial angioplasty.[6–8] Acute closure immediately after angioplasty is usually caused by dissection, spasm,[9] or embolism and is frequently complicated by thrombosis.[10] This occurs in 1 to 4% of PTAs.[11] More commonly, restenosis occurs between 1 and 2 months or 9 months and 1 year after angioplasty and includes an intimal proliferation response to the vascular injury induced by the procedure.[12]

ATHEROSCLEROSIS

Atherosclerosis is the most commonly detected underlying pathology in a vessel requiring angioplasty. However, stenoses from other causes do occur, such as those that appear after vascular trauma (e.g., road traffic accidents, radiation therapy), particularly in the upper limb after lung and breast irradiation. Healing vasculitis is another cause of nonatherosclerotic stenoses. Nevertheless, atherosclerotic vascular disease is by far the most frequent underlying disorder, and this review is, therefore, restricted to the cellular responses occurring in the atherosclerotic vessel.

Atherosclerosis is often thought of as a disease of the 20th century, but evidence of atherosclerosis has been found in Egyptian mummies (3rd millennium BC) and in Peruvian remains (1st millennium BC). In the 20th century, however, it has reached epidemic proportions, and cardiovascular disease (CVD) is the leading cause of death in Western Europe and the United States of America, principally resulting from myocardial infarction (MI) and stroke.[13]

Pathogenesis of Atherosclerosis

Currently, there are two favored hypotheses concerning the etiology of atherogenesis, and each of these interacts directly with the other: tissue response to injury,[14] and lipid infiltration and modification.[15] The injury allows the vascular endothelium to increase uptake of plasma lipids, and this injury in turn may be caused by increased plasma lipid or the altered presence of oxidized forms (Fig. 1–1).

The three broad phases of human atherosclerosis are as follows:

1. Lesion initiation
2. Lesion development and growth
3. Complex and advanced lesion formation
   1. Lesion Initiation
      This results from the infiltration of circulating monocytes through the vessel wall into the subendothelial space and from proliferation of smooth muscle cells (SMCs). In order to migrate and multiply, the cells must cross major extracellular barriers, such as the basal lamina and a fibrous mesh made up of collagen and interstitial proteoglycans. For cell migration, therefore, degradation of extracellular matrix (ECM) is required.
   2. Lesion Development and Growth
      In the intima, the proliferating SMCs synthesize ECM components, accumulation of which increases the size of the lesion and alters intimal

structure. Plaque growth is intraluminal, which, in the latter stages, causes arterial stenosis.[16]

3. Complex and Advanced Lesion Formation
Excess breakdown of ECM can occur at vulnerable sites, such as at the "shoulders" of the plaque. It is in these vulnerable regions that plaque rupture most frequently occurs. The plaque becomes less resistant to the mechanical stresses of blood flow pressure. Plaque rupture can completely occlude the vessel, or it can partially occlude the vessel but trigger formation of occlusive thrombus and cause major CV events. If only partial occlusion occurs, and the organ or limb survives, the repair process begins when organization of the thrombus occurs. SMCs migrate to the clot, where they lay down more ECM, further increasing the bulk of the lesion[17] (Fig. 1–2). Clinically, such lesions may be amenable to the procedure of angioplasty (Fig. 1–3).

VASCULAR INJURY SECONDARY TO ANGIOPLASTY

Angioplasty induces a complex process that is analogous to generalized wound healing. As with plaque formation, there are three phases (Fig. 1–4). The first is the thrombotic phrase. In the second phase, granulation occurs, and in the third phase, remodeling takes place. The success of balloon angioplasty was initially thought to be the result of compression of the athero-

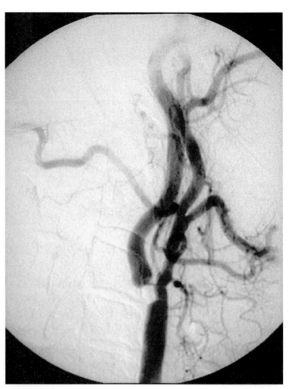

Figure 1–2. Critical internal carotid artery stenosis demonstrated angiographically.

sclerotic lesion followed by remodeling of the plaque. However, this accounts for only a small proportion of the increase in lumen size. Balloon angioplasty principally enlarges the vessel by stretching the elastic components of the vessel wall. Inelastic parts of the plaque fracture or tear, resulting in small, discrete vessel wall dissections. In eccentric lesions, the less diseased part of the wall may stretch without resulting in serious or significant dissection, but some degree of histologic dissection is a feature of nearly all angioplasty procedures.[18]

Healing After Angioplasty

During the angioplasty process, the vascular endothelium is removed, with exposure of the subendothelial plaque to circulating blood. Platelet aggregation and adhesion occur immediately, and platelet clumps form on the exposed lipid and collagen matrix. This platelet binding is mediated through von Willebrand's factor (vWF) and the cell adhesion molecule (CAM) P-selectin.[19] Over the next few hours thrombus forms, most commonly over the fissures created by the procedure. After 24 to 48 hours, the surface becomes less thrombogenic through a process known as passivation.[20] However, although thrombogenicity is decreased, the inflammatory response is stimulated. This is caused in part by release of growth factors

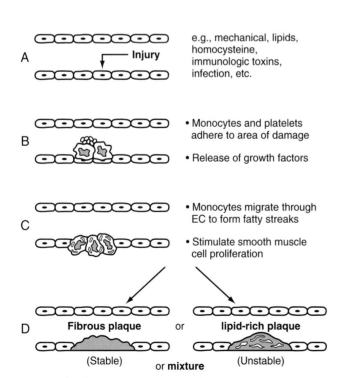

Figure 1–1. Response to injury hypothesis of atherogenesis. EC = endothelial cell.

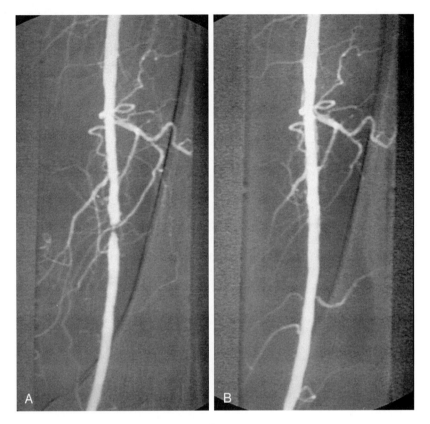

Figure 1–3. Angioplasty of the superficial femoral artery *A*, before treatment, and *B*, appearance on an angiogram after treatment.

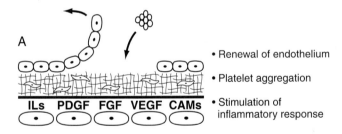

- Renewal of endothelium
- Platelet aggregation
- Stimulation of inflammatory response

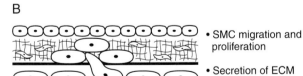

- SMC migration and proliferation
- Secretion of ECM

Figure 1–4. Vascular healing after angioplasty. ILs = interleukins; PDGF = platelet-derived growth factor; FGF = fibroblast growth factor; CAMs = cell adhesion molecules; SMCs = smooth muscle cells; ECM = extracellular matrix. VEGF = vascular endothelial growth factor.

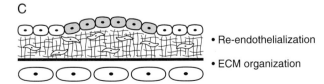

- Re-endothelialization
- ECM organization

(GFs) but also by the reperfusion injury afforded by the angioplasty process. Occlusion of blood flow and return of flow after balloon deflation generate oxidative stress.[21] This inflammatory response continues for several days and is initially characterized by invasion of polymorphonuclear leukocytes (PMNs). This is followed by infiltration of T-lymphocytes and monocyte–macrophage cells.[22]

Granulation results from migration of cells into the damaged vessel area. Normally, vascular SMCs are located in a resting phase in the vessel wall. GFs, cytokines, and CAMs stimulate the SMCs to become mobile, and they then migrate toward the injured site. Various enzymes, such as the metalloproteinases (MMPs), digest the ECM, easing the process of cell migration. The presence of clot provides scaffolding that enhances migration of SMCs as well as providing the stimulus for their proliferation through release of chemicals, such as platelet-derived growth factor (PDGF) from platelets and cytokines from PMNs. Once in the damaged area, the SMCs proliferate further and secrete their own ECM.

The final part of vessel wound healing is vascular remodeling. In this phase, SMCs no longer proliferate but secrete and organize ECM. More than 50% of intimal hyperplasia is made up of ECM,[33] which is principally composed of collagen. Other important components of ECM are fibronectin, laminin, and glycosaminoglycans. If complete healing is obtained, the endothelium regrows over the healed area between 4 and 12 weeks after angioplasty. If this healing response is uncontrolled and does not terminate, restenosis may occur.

CELLULAR MECHANISMS OF RESTENOSIS AFTER ANGIOPLASTY

Restenosis is the consequence of an uncontrolled reparative response to vascular injury. Two principal mechanisms contribute to the restenotic process: neointimal hyperplasia and vascular (geometric) remodeling. Changes in the deposition and turnover of vessel ECM play an important role in both these processes.

Neointimal Hyperplasia in Restenosis

Vascular SMCs in the media proliferate within hours after angioplasty. Migration to the intima occurs by day 4. SMCs multiply three- to five-fold over the next 2 weeks, accounting for 90% of the final intimal cell population. Intimal thickening secondary to ECM expansion plateaus after 3 months.

The stimuli for neointimal hyperplasia are plentiful. Fibroblast growth factor α (FGF-α), for example,

can initiate proliferation, and PDGF induces subsequent SMC migration into the intima. ECM accumulation is increased by PDGF, tumor growth factor β (TGF-β), angiotensin II, and probably also by insulin-like growth factor-1 (IGF-I).[23] Clearly, this process is merely an exaggeration or failure in control of the healing process shown in Figure 1–3. Enhanced production of GFs may contribute to this stimulus as may loss of growth inhibitory factors, such as endothelial cell (EC) secretion of nitric oxide (NO) and heparin sulfate proteoglycan.[24] This loss of production of endothelial inhibitory factors is most likely to occur when complete denudation of endothelium has occurred, or in the presence of extensive atherosclerosis, in which there is little functioning endothelium present. Furthermore, severe reperfusion injury during the angioplasty procedure may also augment endothelial damage (Fig. 1–5).

Interestingly, however, histopathologic analyses of coronary vessel restenotic lesions during postmortem procedures have shown that between 20 and 50% of patients have no evidence of intimal hyperplasia despite their having angiographic and clinical evidence of restenosis.[25] Several studies have suggested that the area of occluded lumen typically exceeds that which can be attributed to neointimal hyperplasia. Instead, it appears to correlate more closely with the loss of area within the external elastic lamina.[26] In atherectomy specimens collected after angioplasty, proliferating cell nuclear antigen staining showed a proliferation rate of less than 1%. On the basis of these observations, it has been suggested that vascular remodeling may be a more critical process in incidence of restenosis.

Vascular Remodeling

Vascular or geometric remodeling may be a greater contributor to restenosis than neointimal formation.[27] Remodeling as applied to the arterial wall can mean a chronic change in diameter (not secondary to spasm) or a change in the constituents of the vessel wall, either with or without a change in vessel shape. Changes in the size of the vessel have the greatest impact on restenosis; therefore, the term vascular remodeling is usually used in reference to either dilatation or constriction of the total vessel area. Because the events in wound healing involve changes in vessel wall constituents and caliber, the entire healing and restenotic process could be viewed as remodeling. For the purpose of this chapter, however, the term remodeling refers to the change in vessel size rather than change in its constituents, and, thus, the term adaptive, or geometric, remodeling is probably most appropriate.[18]

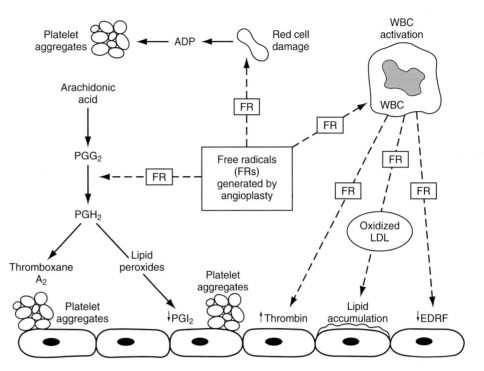

Figure 1–5. Oxidative stress (free-radical generation) secondary to reperfusion may augment vascular damage.

REMODELING IN ATHEROSCLEROSIS

Remodeling is a process that has been recognized for over 40 years. The association between arterial size and exercise is also well known. It has been suggested that exercise-stimulated remodeling enlarges atherosclerotic vessels, and there is certainly some experimental work to suggest this.[28] Support for this hypothesis comes from the clinical findings that exercise improves the condition of patients with claudication symptoms.[29] Early studies of remodeling, however, relate to the coronary arteries,[30] in which coronary artery remodeling during early atherosclerosis allows enlargement of the vessel such that the lumen area is preserved until approximately 40% of the total vessel area is occupied by atherosclerosis. Thereafter, the lesion progressively narrows the lumen as the atherosclerosis worsens. Subsequently, pathologic and intravascular studies of human coronary arteries and carotid and peripheral vessels have shown that this process is ubiquitous, with a positive correlation between compensatory enlargement of the vessel and the extent of the atherosclerotic plaque.[31] Just as exercise promotes improved remodeling, vascular risk factors impair it. For example, the degree of compensatory change in vessel diameter is inversely correlated with low-density lipoprotein (LDL) cholesterol.[32] It is important to note that this vascular remodeling may impinge on formal measurements of restenosis after angioplasty. Because vessel size can change as atherosclerosis progresses, the use of reference segments in determining progression of disease and percent of stenosis can be inaccurate. Compensatory remodeling of the reference segment can significantly alter the apparent severity of the disease.

REMODELING IN RESTENOSIS

The role of remodeling in restenosis has been evaluated. It appears that in some cases, vascular remodeling enlarges the vessel lumen, whereas in other cases remodeling decreases it. In the latter group, there is an increased likelihood of return of clinical symptoms after angioplasty.[34] The importance of remodeling is that relatively small changes in arterial diameter can result in major lumen changes. After angioplasty, there appears to be a close relationship between intimal area and remodeling, with a parallel increase in vessel size as intimal thickening occurs. In restenosis, the amount of remodeling appears to be less for any given degree of intimal thickness. Interestingly, certain forms of vessel injury are more likely to result in constriction than others (e.g., thermal angioplasty).[35]

MECHANISMS OF REMODELING

The factors that are most frequently linked to remodeling are hemodynamic changes in blood pressure, flow rates, patterns of sheer stress, and changes in ECM composition. Table 1–1 lists blood and clinical factors that contribute to remodeling. However, changes in ECM composition are likely to be among the most important determinants. The most important ECM in terms of restenosis appears to be collagen. Total collagen content is significantly less in nonreste-

Table 1–1. Factors That Influence Type of Vascular Remodeling

Dilation Promoted	Constriction Promoted
Nitric oxide	Endothelin-1
Prostacyclin	Blood cell rigidity
Endothelium-derived hyperpolarizing factor	Dyslipidemia
	Hyperviscosity (e.g., elevated fibrinogen)
Exercise	Hypertension
	Cigarette smoking

nosed than in restenosed vessels.[36] The amount of collagen depends on either decreased production or increased collagen degradation. Collagen degradation is mediated by the matrix metalloproteinases. MMP-1 (interstitial collagenase) and MMP-2 (basal membrane collagenase) appear to be the most important components. Increased MMP activity is likely to be responsible for the decreased amount of collagen seen in nonrestenotic vessels. Furthermore, organization of collagen is also important, and there is a lower level of organization in vessels that restenose. SMCs are the prime source of ECM proteins. Vascular SMC production of GF and cytokines stimulates production of ECM by autocrine and paracrine pathways. TGF-β may be the most important GF in this process.

Cellular Mechanisms of Restenosis

In restenosis after angioplasty, the available evidence suggests that both neointimal proliferation and vascular remodeling play important roles. In both processes, changes take place within the vascular cells in terms of migration and proliferation, with an increase in ECM synthesis. The clarification of these mechanisms of restenosis has opened up novel therapeutic strategies in both the treatment and prevention of restenosis.

PHARMACOTHERAPY FOR PREVENTION OF RESTENOSIS AFTER ANGIOPLASTY

The majority of work in evaluating prevention of restenosis after angioplasty has been undertaken in the coronary vessels. The author believes that this does not reflect any less concern on the part of the peripheral operator for optimal results; rather, it highlights the pharmaceutical industry's[7] focus on cardiologic factors. Nevertheless, a number of worthwhile studies have been, and continue to be, carried out in peripheral vessels.

Antiplatelet Drugs

Antithrombotic management before, during, and after balloon angioplasty includes blockade of platelet aggregation and, thus, thrombus formation at the angioplasty site. The efficacy of aspirin in preventing CV events in patients with PAOD is now established,[37] and all patients who are prone to thrombus formation should be on such agents for this reason. Certainly, such patients should take aspirin before undergoing angioplasty. If aspirin is not tolerated (even with the addition of a proton pump inhibitor–H$_2$ blocker), it seems logical to use an alternative antiplatelet agent, such as clopidogrel. Ticlopidine (a related compound but with neutropenic effects) has been shown to prevent restenosis in coronary vessels[38] and graft occlusion in PAOD.[39] A study of clopidogrel in peripheral vessels undergoing angioplasty is warranted.

The IIb–IIIa receptor sites in platelets allow binding of fibrin to the platelets and platelet aggregation. IIb/IIIa receptor site antagonists have been evaluated in coronary vessels,[40] and studies in peripheral vessels are under way. These compounds are efficacious in preventing restenosis in patients after coronary angioplasty, and the advent of the new orally active antagonists will make this therapy more attractive.

Other Antiplatelet Mechanisms Promoted Through Arachidonic Acid Metabolism

Figure 1–6 shows the metabolism of arachidonic acid (AA) to various vasoactive chemicals. Aspirin inhibits the cyclooxygenase enzyme and causes a decrease in thromboxane A$_2$ (TXA$_2$) formation. TXA$_2$ is a potent platelet aggregate and vasoconstrictor. Nevertheless, as can be seen from Figure 1–6, aspirin also has the potential to decrease prostacyclin (PGI$_2$). PGI$_2$ is a potent antiplatelet agent and vasodilator, although aspirin taken at a low dose is reported to affect platelet TXA$_2$ synthesis rather than endothelial PGI$_2$ formation. This, however, has never been proved conclusively. Alternative approaches to modifying AA metabolism are, therefore, being studied in an attempt to promote more effective antiplatelet activity.

ESSENTIAL FATTY ACIDS

Essential fatty acids (EFAs) have unique roles as precursor molecules for the chemical regulators of cell function, the prostaglandins (PGs) and leukotrienes (LTs). These compounds are synthesized and released by almost every tissue in the body and participate in many biological functions. Depending on the EFA predominant in the diet, different antiplatelet and vasodilator effects can be obtained. Evening primrose

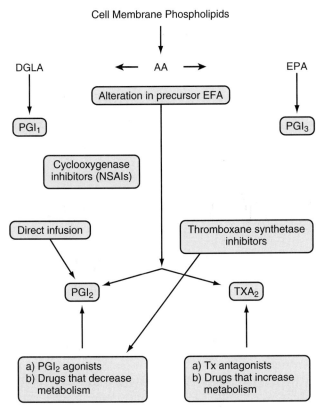

Figure 1–6. Different therapeutic approaches to increasing antiplatelet effects are shown. DGLA = dihomo-gamma-linoleic acid; AA = arachidonic acid; EPA = eicosapentanoic acid; EFA = essential fatty acid.

oil, for example, contains gamma linoleic acid which, when metabolized to dihomogamma linolenic acid, is the precursor for one series of PGs (i.e., PGE_1). Theoretically, the desired antiplatelet vasodilator effect is maintained by PGE_1 without the opposing effects of TXA_2. In restenosis after angioplasty, work has been carried out using other EFAs (i.e., those derived from fish oil). Both eicosapentanoic acid (EPA) and docosahexanoic acid (DHA) produce antiplatelet vasodilator effects via the production of PGI_3. PGI_3 is equipotent to PGI_2, whereas the TXA_3 produced by metabolism of these EFAs is a much less effective platelet aggregate than that of TXA_2.[41] In addition to antiplatelet effects, these EFAs may attenuate free radical generation and can modify the body's inflammatory response to tissue injury.[42]

As stated earlier, the majority of studies have been carried out in relation to the coronary arteries. There are a number of studies in the literature that report evaluation of EFAs. In two of these studies,[43, 44] the restenosis rate appeared to be lower in the treated groups, although this was not confirmed by a third study.[45] However, it should be noted that in this latter study, not all patients received pretreatment for 1 week. Incorporation into the cell membrane may be necessary for some EFAs to produce therapeutic effects; therefore, late start of medication may have

caused a negative result. It is interesting to note that the meta-analysis of seven studies of coronary artery restenosis rates with use of EPA[46] showed a clear, if moderate, beneficial effect on the restenosis rate. In the periphery, we carried out an early pilot study that did, indeed, seem to suggest that a benefit could be derived from fish oil therapy. The results of the large multicenter study evaluating restenosis rates in peripheral vessels of patients after treatment with fish oil or placebo have not yet been reported. Because this study concluded some time ago, it appears unlikely that a positive result was obtained. Further clarification of alteration of essential fatty acids in the diet as a treatment strategy to prevent restenosis is required.

DIRECT INFUSION OF PROSTACYCLIN–PROSTACYCLIN ANALOGS

One of the main objectives of pharmaceutical research is to supply synthetic compounds that overcome the inherent drawbacks of indigenous compounds. A number of synthetic PGI_2 analogues have been developed. Although they are reported to retain PGI_2 antiplatelet effect, they are chemically stable, a distinct advantage over natural PGI_2. There have been at least two multicenter studies of synthetic prostacyclins that have taken place to evaluate restenosis after angioplasty in peripheral vessels. Results of these trials have not been reported, although the work was completed many years ago. Again, it appears unlikely that positive results were obtained.

THROMBOXANE SYNTHETASE INHIBITORS–THROMBOXANE RECEPTOR SITE ANTAGONISTS

Thromboxane synthetase inhibitors should selectively block the transformation of PG endoperoxides into TXA_2 without inhibiting PGI_2 formation. A number of orally active thromboxane synthetase inhibitors have been evaluated in the study of vascular diseases. Disappointingly few have achieved success in any clinical situation. Initially, it was hoped that the extra endoperoxides available after thromboxane synthesis inhibition would be diverted to form extra PGI_2. Unfortunately, it became apparent that endoperoxides themselves could cause vasoconstriction. This could explain the lack of response seen with use of these compounds. Studies in which the newer thromboxane receptor site antagonists are used may prove more fruitful. The results of early studies of these compounds should be available soon. To the author's knowledge, there is one multicenter study of a thromboxane receptor blocker used for treatment of patients who experienced restenosis after peripheral angioplasty. This study terminated a number of years ago and again, disappointingly, the results have not been published. Once more, one could assume that the results were not of immense clinical significance.

SUMMARY

Given that aspirin or another antiplatelet agent is required in this group of patients for protection from cardiovascular events, the discussion regarding aspirin is perhaps academic. Nevertheless, historically, the use of aspirin for prevention of (re)thrombosis in the early phase of balloon angioplasty is based on a number of observations. These data have been accepted widely as evidence for the efficacy of administering periprocedural aspirin to patients undergoing percutaneous procedures. Although we know that platelet activation and adherence to a de-endothelialized surface are thought to contribute to restenosis, perhaps through release of PDGF, various antiplatelet agents fail to prevent the appearance of restenotic lesions.[47] It is, therefore, believed that antiplatelet agents decrease the incidence of acute thrombosis after PTA but not the longer term restenosis rate, possibly because they interfere with platelet-platelet interaction rather than platelet-vessel wall adhesion. The issue of low- vs. high-dose aspirin has been specifically addressed in two trials.[48] These two studies reported less serious gastrointestinal side effects with the lower dose of aspirin, although the 2-year cumulative patency rates were similar at both doses.

Other antiplatelet agents have also been evaluated. Multicenter aspirin-controlled studies have been carried out, but most have not been published. This is disappointing, especially in a field in which there is a lack of good published study data. More success may be obtained by the newer agents, such as clopidogrel and the IIb/IIIa inhibitors. There is plenty of scope for further investigative work in this field.

Anticoagulants and Thrombolytics

ANTICOAGULANTS

The suggestion that heparin should be given to the patient at some point during an angioplasty procedure has gained wide acceptance. There are two reasons for this. First, heparin is thought to prevent the periangioplasty thrombosis previously described, and second, heparin may have anti-SMC proliferation effects. No clinical multicenter, double-blind, controlled trials of angioplasty with or without heparin have been reported for peripheral vessels. There is, however, a universal consensus regarding the need for use of heparin therapy during angioplasty, both in the coronary and the peripheral circulation. The current practice of periprocedural administration of heparin

and oral pretreatment with aspirin is not seriously challenged, even if it is not strictly followed in all centers.

Warfarin has also been assessed and compared with low-dose aspirin (50 mg/day) and dipyridamole, another antiplatelet agent. Interestingly, the patency rate in patients after 1 year of treatment was 69% with aspirin and dipyridamole and 53% with oral anticoagulant. Despite the apparent trend in favor of antiplatelet agents, the result was not statistically significant. Because warfarin has a higher profile of side effects than antiplatelet agents, aspirin or another tolerated antiplatelet agent must be the treatment of choice.

HIRUDIN–HIRULOG

The HELVETICA trial[49] was designed to study hirudin, a specific inhibitor of thrombin, to see if hirudin was able to reduce restenosis in the coronary circulation. The comparator was intravenous heparin given periprocedurally. There was no improved effect on the restenosis rate with use of hirudin. However, it did show an impressive reduction rate in major cardiac events in the first 96 hours after angioplasty compared with that of heparin. The relevance of this finding to the peripheral vessels is unclear.

Hirulog was compared with heparin in a randomized trial in North America and Europe.[50] There was no significant reduction in the endpoints when results with hirulog were compared with those of heparin.

THROMBOLYTIC AGENTS

The role of thrombolytic therapy in the prevention of abrupt thrombosis after angioplasty is controversial. In the coronary circulation, infusion of thrombolytic agents has been used to clear periprocedural clot in patients with recent myocardial infarction. However, pretreatment with thrombolytic agents followed by angioplasty has a deleterious effect, with more immediate complications and a higher rate of bleeding. The HELVETICA study clearly demonstrated that prophylactic thrombolytic therapy should not be used routinely before performance of percutaneous transluminal coronary angioplasty. Nevertheless, clinical experience has prompted some workers to suggest that once occlusive clot has developed over an angioplasty site or embolized to the periphery, judicious use of a small amount of local thrombolytic therapy can produce an encouraging clinical response. More work, however, is required in this area before formal recommendations can be made. Because of the infrequent nature of this complication, multicenter studies will be necessary.

Drugs for the Future

ANIMAL WORK

A wide range of antiproliferative drugs has been tested as a means of preventing restenosis and neointimal formation in animals. These agents include angiotensin-converting enzyme (ACE) inhibitors; antagonists of growth factors, such as turbinafine or trapidil (inhibitory to PDGF); angiopeptin (a peptide analog of simvastatin); cytostatic agents, such as etoposide, calcium-calmodulin antagonists, or the microtubulin inhibiting drug, colchicine.[51] However, clinical trials (again, mainly in the coronary circulation) have generally failed to recapitulate the efficacy documented in animal studies. Failure of these human trials could reflect species differences in relation to the biological response to vascular injury, or they may have resulted from differences in dosing schedules.

More recently, the focus has been on blockade of the proliferative cell cycle. The immunosuppressant sirolimus[52] is a cell cycle inhibitor that is one of a family that can prevent restenosis through systemic administration. It may mediate its beneficial effect through inhibition of cell proliferation. A new class of cell cycle targeting agents with antimitotic and antitumor potency are the purite derivatives olomoucine and roscovitine.[51] These drugs also have an antiproliferative effect. Cellular cyclic guanosine monophosphate (cGMP) levels, promoted by nitrous oxide (NO) donors or stable cGMP analogues, inhibit vascular cell SMC proliferation.[53] Supplementation of L-arginine, the body's precursor of NO, has also been shown to inhibit neointimal formation.[54]

ANTIOXIDANTS AS TREATMENT AGAINST RESTENOSIS

Despite the good theoretical rationale for such treatment (there is generation of free radicals during the angioplasty procedure[21]), little work in evaluating antioxidant therapy has been carried out. Vitamin E has been studied in an animal model.[55] In this study, serotonin-induced vasoconstriction was attenuated. This is an area that may be fruitfully studied further.

GENE THERAPY

Gene therapy has been mooted as the most promising therapy for the future. It can involve either overexpression of genes that may ameliorate the process of restenosis or blockade of the expression of genes that are critical to the pathogenesis of the disorder. Gene blockade can be achieved through the use of nucleic acids known as antisense oligodeoxynucleotides (ODN), which are complementary to a specific segment of the target gene. Hybridization of the ODN with the target messenger ribonucleic acid (mRNA) can inhibit its translation. Antisense ODNs designed to inhibit the expression of some cell cycle regulatory genes are available for study in animal models.[56] In early animal work, a combination of an antisense ODN against more than one cycloregulatory gene was shown to be more effective than a single gene strategy.[57]

Transduction of cells with genes, encoding novel cell-cycle inhibitory proteins, or local overexpression of endogenous inhibitors may reduce neointimal hyperplasia. Infection of animal arteries with an adenovirus vector significantly reduced neointimal formation.[56] As described earlier, NO may have a significant effect on vascular remodeling, and in vivo transfer of endothelial cell NO synthase gene into animal arteries inhibited injury-induced neointimal formation by 70%.[58]

There is increasing evidence that in addition to inhibiting cellular proliferation, cell-cycle inhibitors may influence processes such as cell migration, inflammatory cell recruitment, and thrombus and ECM formation, and these are exciting potential therapies for the future.

RADIATION THERAPY AS A MECHANISM FOR PREVENTING RESTENOSIS

The potential role of radiation in the prevention of coronary artery restenosis after angioplasty has generated much interest, and workers in the peripheral field are following this closely. Animal research and pilot clinical efforts have focused primarily on delivering radiation through intraluminal techniques.[59] The inhibition of neointimal hyperplasia by external-beam radiation has also been studied. These initial small uncontrolled trials must act as stimuli for further work, and indeed intraluminal irradiation has been applied to patients with femoral[60] and coronary artery occlusions as well as narrowed arterial venous dialysis fistulas.

Short-term side effects associated with use of these techniques appear to be few, but there is, of course, the potential for late toxicity. This is particularly pertinent to radiation-induced heart disease as applied to the coronary arteries. This may be less of a problem for the periphery. If validated through rigorous clinical testing, this approach may eventually be applied as a preventive measure against restenosis to patients undergoing peripheral angioplasty.

ENDOVASCULAR TECHNIQUES TO RESTRICT RESTENOSIS

Because a number of the drugs currently being investigated as antistenotic agents have a significant profile of side effects, local drug delivery is an attractive concept. The potential advantages of delivering the required agent locally to the angioplasty area are that agents can be used that might be toxic when given systemically, and drugs can be given in doses that do not produce side effects but do have a local high concentration. This attractive concept has necessitated the development of various delivery devices. Much of this work has been undertaken by industry. Device type can be categorized according to its mechanism of action.[61] Delivery may be effected through apposition (e.g., as is done by the hydrogel balloon). A balloon is coated with a hydrophilic substance that expands when wet, absorbs agents, and then is dried before use on the angioplasty catheter. During inflation, the chemicals are delivered by apposition to the vessel wall when they come in contact with moisture. This device has been used to deliver thrombolytic and genetic material.[62, 63] One disadvantage of this system is the loss of compound from an unprotected balloon as it is inserted into the bloodstream, and use of such devices is often poorly efficient. Other devices are designed to deliver the drug in a chamber produced by the inflation of two small balloons, one above the other. The drug is delivered to the lumen of the vessel and is held in place by the two inflated balloons. The chemical then bathes the endothelial surface after angioplasty is performed. Some systemic spread of the chemical is likely to occur once the balloons have been deflated, and this may limit the effective use of such a technique. Newer catheters allow removal of more toxic agents, such as viral vectors, by aspiration from the chamber before balloon deflation. There are a number of other bathing devices that have been developed, and each has its strengths and weaknesses. Clinical studies are currently being undertaken to determine optimal designs.

The devices described depend on passive delivery of the agent to the vessel wall. Active delivery can be achieved by the use of iontophoresis, whereby an electric current having the same charge as the chemical drives the chemical into the vessel wall.[64] This device has been extensively investigated and may be relevant in the future.[65]

DRUG TARGETING

Although both passive and active local drug delivery are interesting concepts, attention is also often focused on ways of fixing the agent to the target site rather than delivering it temporarily to the endothelial surface. Some researchers have explored the possibility of delivering drug contained in microspheres.[66] Most of these microspheres, however, are lipid macromolecules, and side effects have included microvascular clumping of the spheres with consequent ische-

mia. Specific drug targeting to areas of vascular damage may also be achieved with use of designer drugs. For example, certain monoclonal antibodies directed against proteins expressed on damaged endothelial cells can be conjugated with antiplatelet or thrombolytic agents. The compound is then given through the balloon catheter and localizes to the area of damaged endothelium thanks to its monoclonal antibody component. This work has led to exploration of other localizing agents, such as expressed P-selectin and antitissue factor antibody. Such targeting may allow greater drug retention and prolonged efficacy.

CONCLUSION

The success of PTA is limited by the development of restenosis, which occurs in 30 to 60% of all cases, chiefly within the first 6 to 12 months after intervention. Restenosis is caused by the proliferation of smooth muscle cell with neointimal formation, and to vascular remodeling. Both processes are affected by the overproduction of extracellular matrix in the arterial wall. Our greater understanding of the process of restenosis has led to the development of therapeutic strategies for its prevention. The current mainstay of therapy is an antiplatelet drug combined with periprocedural heparin. Although most pharmacologic interventions into the restenosis process have been undertaken in the coronary vessel, there are a number of good studies that have been conducted in the periphery. The development of novel pharmacotherapeutics in this area, combined with better angioplasty procedures, such as stenting and local drug delivery, have contributed to a rapid expansion in potential therapeutic strategies. The apparent success of several therapies in animal models of restenosis suggests that molecular therapies should be evaluated in human disease.

REFERENCES

1. Dormandy J, Mahir M, Ascady G, et al: Fate of a patient with chronic leg ischemia. J Cardiovasc Surg 30:50–57, 1989.
2. Dormandy JA: Natural history of intermittent claudication. Hosp Update 17:314–320, 1991.
3. Cronenwett JL, Warner KG, Zelenock JB, et al: Intermittent claudication: Current results of non-operative management. Arch Surg 119:430–436, 1984.
4. Jorgensen B: Percutaneous transluminal angioplasty for distal iliac artery stenosis. Crit Ischaem 5:28–32, 1995.
5. Pentecost MJ, Criqui MD, Dorros G, et al: Guidelines for peripheral percutaneous transluminal angioplasty of the abdominal aorta and lower extremity vessels: A statement for health professionals from a special writing group of the councils on cardiovascular radiology, arteriosclerosis, cardio-thoracic and vascular surgery, clinical cardiology, and epidemiology and prevention, the American Heart Association. AHA Medical/ Scientific Statement. Special Report, 1993, pp 511–531.

6. Morin JF, Johnston WK, Wasserman L: Factors that determine the long term results of percutaneous transluminal dilatation for peripheral arterial occlusive disease. J Vasc Surg 4:68–72, 1986.
7. El-Bayar H, Roberts A, Hye R, et al: Determinants of failure in superficial femoral artery angioplasty. J Vasc Surg 28:539–547, 1994.
8. Wilson SE, Wolf GL, Cross AP: Percutaneous transluminal angioplasty versus operation for peripheral arterial sclerosis: Report of a randomised trial in a selected group of patients. J Vasc Surg 9:1–9, 1989.
9. Rooke TW, Stanson AW, Johnson CM: Percutaneous transluminal angioplasty in the lower extremities: A 5 year experience. Mayo Clin Proc 62:85–91, 1987.
10. Mattson E, Jansen I, Edvinsson L, et al: Endothelial influence on vessel wall induced vasospasm after balloon angioplasty. Acta Radiol 34:156–161, 1993.
11. Minar E, Ehringer H, Ahmadi R, et al: Platelet deposition at angioplasty sites and its relation to restenosis in human iliac and femoropopliteal arteries. Radiology 170:767–772, 1989.
12. Gardener GA, Meyerobitz MF, Stokes KR, et al: Complications of transluminal angioplasty. Radiology 159:201–208, 1986.
13. Report of the Working Group of Arteriosclerosis of the National Heart, Lung and Blood Institute, Vol 2: DHEW publication No. (NIH) 82-2035. Washington, DC, US Government Printing Office, 1981.
14. Ross R: The pathogenesis of atherosclerosis—an update. N Engl J Med 314:488–500, 1986.
15. Steinberg D: Lipoproteins and the pathogenesis of atherosclerosis. Circulation 76:508–514, 1987.
16. Libby P: Molecular bases of the acute coronary syndromes. Circulation 91:2844–50, 1995.
17. Fuster V, Badimon L, Badimon JJ: The pathogenesis of coronary artery disease and the acute coronary syndromes (first of two parts). New Engl J Med 326:242–250, 1992.
18. Faxon DP, Coats W, Currier J: Remodeling of the coronary artery after vascular injury. Prog Cardiovasc Dis 40:129–140, 1997.
19. Kirk G, Maple C, McLaren M, et al: A circadian rhythm exists in healthy controls for soluble P-Selectin and platelet count. Platelets 6:414–415, 1995.
20. Marcus AJ: Platelet activation. In Fuster V, Ross R, Topan EJ (eds): Atherosclerosis and Coronary Artery Disease. Philadelphia, Lippincott-Raven, 1996, pp 607–633.
21. Lau CS, Scott N, Brown JE, et al: Increased activity of oxygen free radicals during reperfusion in patients undergoing percutaneous peripheral artery balloon angioplasty. Int Angiol 10:244–246, 1991.
22. Raines EW, Rosenfeld ME, Ross R: The role of macrophages. In Fuster V, Ross R, Topal EJ (eds): Atherosclerosis and Coronary Artery Disease. Philadelphia, Lippincott-Raven, 1996, pp 539–557.
23. Grant MB, Wargovich TJ, Ellis EA, et al: Localization of insulin-like growth factor I and inhibition of coronary smooth muscle cell growth by somatostatin analogues in human coronary smooth muscle cells: A potential treatment for restenosis? Circulation 89:1511–1517, 1994.
24. Kinsella MG, Wight TN: Modulation of sulfated proteoglycan synthesis by bovine aortic endothelial cells during migration. J Cell Biol 102:678–687, 1986.
25. Waller BF, Pinkerton CA, Orr CM, et al: Restenosis 1 to 24 months after clinically successful coronary balloon angioplasty: A necropsy study of 20 patients. J Am Coll Cardiol 17:58B–70B, 1991.
26. Katuka T, Currier JW, Haudenschild CC, et al: Differences in compensatory vessel enlargement, not intimal formation, account for restenosis after angioplasty in the hypercholesterolaemic rabbit model. Circulation 89:2809–2815, 1994.
27. Mintz GS, Popma JJ, Pichard AD, et al: Arterial remodelling after coronary angioplasty—a serial intravascular ultrasound study. Circulation 94:35–43, 1996.
28. Kaplan JR, Manuck SB, Adams MR, et al: Plaque changes and arterial enlargement in atherosclerotic monkeys after manipulation of diet and social environment. Arterioscler Thromb 13:254–263, 1993.
29. Hiatt WR, Wolfel EE, Regensteiner JG: Exercise in the treatment of intermittent claudication due to peripheral arterial disease. Vasc Med Rev 2:61–70, 1991.
30. Glagov S, Weisenberg E, Zarins CK, et al: Compensatory enlargement of human atherosclerotic coronary arteries. N Engl J Med 316:1371–1375, 1987.
31. Pasterkamp G, Wensin PJW, Post MJ et al: Paradoxical arterial wall shrinkage may contribute to luminal narrowing of human atherosclerotic femoral arteries. Circulation 91:1449–1459, 1995.
32. Shicore A, Mack W, Selzer R, et al: Compensatory vascular changes of remote coronary segments in response to lesion progression as observed by sequential angiography from a controlled clinical trial. Circulation 92:2411–2418, 1995.
33. Wight TN, Potter-Perigo S, Aulinskas T: Proteoglycans and vascular cell proliferation. Am Rev Respir Dis 140:1132–1135, 1989.
34. Guzman LA, Mrek MJ, Arnolg AM, et al: Role of intimal hyperplasia and arterial remodelling after balloon angioplasty: An experimental study in the atherosclerotic animal model. Art Thromb Vasc Biol 16:479–487, 1996.
35. Staab ME, Edwards WD, Srivatsa SS, et al: Adventitial injury and cellular response markedly affect arterial remodeling and neointimal formation. Circulation 92:1–93, 1995.
36. Coats WD, Whittaker P, Cheung DT, et al: Collagen content is significantly lower in restenotic versus nonstenotic vessels following balloon angioplasty in the atherosclerotic rabbit model. Circulation 95:1293–1300, 1997.
37. Antiplatelet Trialists' Collaboration. Collaborative overview of randomized trials of antiplatelet therapy. I. Prevention of death, myocardial infarction and stroke by prolonged antiplatelet therapy in various categories of patients. Br Med J 308:81–101, 1994.
38. Bertrand ME, Allain H, Lablanche JM: Results of a randomized trial of ticlopidine versus placebo for prevention of acute closure and restenosis after coronary angioplasty. The TACT study [Abstract]. Circulation 82:III–90, 1990.
39. Blanchard J, Carreras LO, Kindermans M, and the EMATAP group: Results of EMATAP: A double-blind placebo-controlled multicentre trial of ticlopidine in patients with peripheral arterial disease. Nouv Rev Fr Haematol 35:523–528, 1993.
40. EPILOG investigators. Platelet glycoprotein IIB/IIIA receptor blockade and low-dose heparin during percutaneous coronary revascularization. N Engl J Med 336:1689–1696, 1997.
41. Dyerberg J, Bang HO, Stoffersen E, et al: Eicosapentanoic acid and prevention of thrombosis and atherosclerosis. Lancet 2:117, 1978.
42. Belch JJF: Eicosanoids and Rheumatology: Inflammatory and Vascular Aspects. Prostaglandins Leukotrienes and Essential Fatty Acids: Reviews 36:219–234, 1989.
43. Dehmer GJ, Popma JJ, Van den Berg EK, et al: Reduction in the rate of early restenosis after coronary angioplasty by a diet supplemented with n-3 fatty acids. N Engl J Med 319:733–740, 1988.
44. Grigg LE, Kay TWH, Valentine PA, et al: Determinants of restenosis and lack of effect of dietary supplementation with eicosapentoenoic acid on the incidence of coronary artery restenosis after angioplasty. J Am Coll Cardiol 13:665–672, 1989.
45. Reis GJ, Boucher TM, Sipperly ME, et al: Randomised trial of fish oil for prevention of restenosis after coronary angioplasty. Lancet 2:177–181, 1989.
46. O'Connor GT, Malenka DJ, Olmstead EM, et al: A meta-analysis of randomised trials of fish oil in prevention of restenosis following coronary angioplasty. Am J Prev Med 8:186–192, 1992.
47. Schwartz L, Bowassa MG, Lesperance J, et al: Failure of antiplatelet agents to reduce restenosis after PCTA in a double-blind placebo controlled trial. J Am Coll Cardiol 11:236, 1988.
48. Verhaeghe R, Bounameaux H: Peripheral arterial occlusion: Thromboembolism and antithrombotic therapy. In Verstraete M, Fuster V, Topol EJ (eds): Cardiovascular Thrombosis: Thrombocardiology and Thromboneurology, 2nd ed, Philadelphia, Lippincott-Raven, 1998.
49. Serruys PW, Herman JP, Simon R, et al: A comparison of hirudin with heparin in the prevention of restenosis after coronary angioplasty. Helvetica Investigators. N Engl J Med 333:757–763, 1995.
50. Bittl J, Strony J, Brinker JA, et al: Treatment with bivalirudin (hirulog) as compared with heparin during coronary angio-

plasty for unstable or post infarction angina. N Engl J Med 333:764–769, 1995.

51. Braun-Dullaeus RC, Mann MJ, Dzau VJ: Cell cycle progression: New therapeutic target for vascular proliferative disease. Circulation 98:82–89, 1998.

52. Brazelton TR, Morris RE: Molecular mechanisms of action of new xenobiotic immunosuppressive drugs. Curr Opin Immunol 8:710–720, 1996.

53. Sarkar R, Gordon D, Stanley JC, et al: Cell cycle effects of nitric oxide on vascular smooth muscle cells. Am J Physiol 272: H1810–H1818, 1997.

54. Tarry WC, Makhoul RG: L-Arginine improves endothelium-dependent vasorelaxation and reduces intimal hyperplasia after balloon angioplasty. Arterioscler Thromb 14:938–943, 1994.

55. Cartier R, Bouchard D, Buluran J: Effect of vitamin E on the endothelial function of the regenerated aorta in rats following direct arterial injury. Ann-Chir 50:673–681, 1996.

56. Feldman LJ, Tahlil O, Steg G: Perspectives of arterial gene therapy for the prevention of restenosis. Cardiovasc Res 32:194–207, 1996.

57. Morishita R, Gibbons GH, Ellison KE, et al: Single intraluminal delivery of antisense cdc2 kinase and proliferating-cell nuclear antigen oligonucleotides results in chronic inhibition of neointimal hyperplasia. Proc Natl Acad Sci U S A 90:8474–8478, 1993.

58. Chang MW, Barr E, Lu MM, et al: Adenovirus-mediated over-expression of the cyclin-cyclin-dependent kinase inhibitor, p21 inhibits vascular smooth muscle cell proliferation and neoin-tima formation in the rat carotid artery model of balloon angioplasty. J Clin Invest 96: 2260–2268, 1995.

59. Koh W-J, Mayberg MR, Chambers J, et al: The potential role of external beam radiation in preventing restenosis after coronary angioplasty. Int J Radiat Oncol Biol Phys 36:829–834, 1996.

60. Bottcher HD, Schopohl B, Liermann D, et al: Endovascular irradiation—a new method to avoid recurrent stenosis after stent implantation in peripheral arteries: Technique and preliminary results. Int J Radiat Oncol Biol Phys 29:183–186, 1994.

61. Gershlick AH: Endovascular manipulation to restrict restenosis. Vasc Med 3:177–188, 1998.

62. Mitchel JF, Azrin MA, Fram DB, et al: Inhibition of platelet deposition and lysis of intracoronary thrombus during balloon angioplasty using urokinase-coated hydrogel balloons. Circulation 90:1979–1988, 1994.

63. Reissen R, Rahimizadah H, Blessing E, et al: Arterial gene transfer using pure DNA applied directly to a hydrogel-coated angioplasty balloon. Hum Gene Ther 4:749–758, 1993.

64. Khan F, Davidson NC, Littleford RC, et al: Cutaneous vascular responses to acetylcholine are mediated by prostanoid-dependent mechanism in man. Vasc Med 2:82–86, 1997.

65. Gonschior P, Pahl C, Huens TY, et al: Comparison of local intravascular drug-delivery catheter systems. Am Heart J 130: 1174–1181, 1995.

66. Wilensky RL, March KL, Hathaway DR: Direct intra-arterial wall injection of microspheres via a catheter: A potential drug delivery strategy following angioplasty. Am Heart J 122:1136–1140, 1991.

Chapter 2

The Physical and Biological Properties of Metallic Stents

John F. Dyet and Karl Schürmann

This chapter deals with the basic properties of metallic stents and how they influence stent choice for specific lesions. There are now a large number of commercially available stents manufactured from different metals and with differing characteristics. The ideal endovascular stent would be easy to introduce and deliver to its site of deployment (trackability). It would be easy to place accurately (radio-opacity and delivery system), and, once deployed, would take up the contour of the vessel, allow flexion and extension (flexibility), and resistance to elastic recoil and external deforming forces (radial force). Such a stent would not be thrombogenic and would rapidly become endothelialized without promoting significant intimal hyperplasia. At present, there is no ideal stent available; therefore, stent choice has to be based on compromise. This means assessing lesion characteristics and selecting the most appropriate stent.

METALLURGY

The most common metals used for stent manufacture are stainless steel 316L and nitinol. Choice of metal depends on two basic properties: biofunctionality and biocompatibility. Biofunctionality is the degree to which the metal can be adapted to perform the required function: Can the metal be easily manufactured into the required device, and is it resistant to corrosion, metal fatigue, and deformity? Biocompatibility is the degree to which the metal remains inert once implanted and does not promote foreign body reaction or release toxic ions.

Metals used at present for stent manufacture do exhibit satisfactory biofunctionality, as would several other metals. The limiting factor that determines which metals are suitable, therefore, depends much more on biocompatibility. The body provides a hostile environment for foreign bodies and stents, leading to degradation or, in the case of metals, corrosion.[1] Once a metal begins to corrode, it releases ions into the surrounding tissues, where a toxic reaction may be triggered. Thus, any metal susceptible to corrosion

is unsuitable for implantation. In current practice, stainless steel (an alloy of iron, nickel, and chromium plus trace elements), nitinol (nickel-titanium alloy), chromium cobalt alloys, and tantalum are the only metals that show the necessary combination of biofunctionality and biocompatibility required for stent manufacture.

Stainless Steel

Stainless steel is an alloy of iron, chromium, and nickel, that also contains traces of other elements, including molybdenum, manganese, carbon, and copper. Although they constitute only a small percentage of the total, these other elements are important because they can affect the crystalline structure of the metal, thus altering the properties of the alloy. In stainless steel for use in implantable medical devices, the most important constituent is chromium. A concentration of at least 12% is required for chromium oxide to form on the metal surface. All implantable metals rely on formation of an oxidized layer on the metal surface to render them passive in situ. Once a stainless steel stent has been electrochemically polished and sterilized, a very thin layer of chromium oxide forms on its surface. If too much carbon is present in the alloy, chromium carbide forms instead of the oxide, and this makes steel liable to corrosion. Similarly, if abrasive polishing is used, the stent surface becomes microscopically pitted, allowing other elements as well as chromium to react at surface level and reduce the metal's passivity.

The chromium oxide layer is thus essential, and damage to that layer results in corrosion. This can be a significant problem, particularly with stainless steel 316L, because its resting potential of 0.3 to 0.5 volts in saline solution is virtually the same as the potential at which breakdown begins to take place (0.4 to 0.48 volts). Any damage to the oxide layer, therefore, leads to corrosion.[2]

Nitinol

Nitinol is an alloy composed chiefly of nickel and titanium, which contains traces of cobalt, chromium, magnesium, and iron. The name nitinol derives from its original place of manufacture, the Nickel Titanium Naval Ordinance Laboratory. Typically, nickel forms 54 to 60% of the composition of nitinol by weight; changes in this range can be used to affect the metal's characteristics. Nitinol has two very distinct properties that make it particularly suitable for stent manufacture. These are thermal memory and superelasticity.

A thermal memory metal can exist in two distinct forms: a low-temperature form, or martensitic, and a high-temperature form, or austenitic,[3] in which the device assumes its required shape. The austenitic temperature at which the alloy attains its required shape can be modified by changes made to the ratio of nickel to titanium and by heat treatment. Using a thermal memory metal in vivo requires that its austenitic temperature be approximately 30°C. When the metal is cooled, it undergoes a reversible change in its crystalline structure to a martensitic state. In this form, the metal is flexible and can be deformed to allow loading into a delivery device. On release at body temperature (37°C), it regains its original shape and stiffness.

Superelasticity occurs when the metal is at a temperature above that of its austenitic transformation[4] (i.e., in its austenitic form). In its superelastic state, the metal is rubber-like but it has the ability to return to its original state after undergoing substantial deformity (see later section on stent construction). This is a complex reaction; when austenitic nitinol is stressed, it develops a stress-induced martensitic reaction, which is unstable at the higher austenitic temperature. When stress is removed, the metal returns to its original shape by transformation from the martensitic to the austenitic state. This shape recovery occurs not because of temperature change but because of reduction in stress: pseudo- or superelasticity.

As with stainless steel, the implanted device is covered by a thin oxide layer, in this case titanium oxide, which stabilizes the surface layer and, in particular, prevents reaction between nickel ions and body tissues. Nickel tends to promote a hyperallergenic reaction in vivo and is the most common cause of such reactions, particularly on the skin surface. There have, however, been no reports of nickel hypersensitivity in conjunction with nitinol implants.[4] In saline solution, nitinol has a higher corrosion resistance than stainless steel, with a resting potential of approximately 0.3 to 0.4 volts and a breakdown potential betwen 14 and 20 volts. Nevertheless, corrosion can occur if the titanium oxide film is breached, particularly in a strong saline environment.

Tantalum

The only current generation stent using tantalum is the (drawn filled tube) DFT wallstent. This stent has an inner core of tantalum covered by an outer tube of Elgiloy. The exact composition of Elgiloy has not been disclosed, but it is a cobalt-chromium based alloy. Because tantalum does not come in contact with body tissues, it is the cobalt-chromium alloy whose characteristics are important.

Cobalt-Chromium Alloys

These alloys are principally composed of cobalt and chromium but may also contain small quantities of iron, nickel, molybdenum, and other trace elements. Because of their high chromium content, they have a high corrosion resistance[1] and also a high wear resistance that makes them suitable for the articular surfaces of joint prostheses.

THROMBOGENICITY

This is a very important consideration in stenting because early stent thrombosis is a frequent occurrence in the coronary arteries and the superficial femoral artery.

Factors contributing to stent thrombogenicity are:

• Constituent metal
• Stent surface
• Intact oxide layer
• Method of stent deployment

Constituent Metal

The intraluminal surface of blood vessels has electronegative potential and is thromboresistant. Therefore, the ideal metal for stent construction would have electronegative surface potential, because the greater the electronegativity, the greater the thromboresistance.[1] Unfortunately, stainless steel 316L and nitinol have electropositive charges in saline solution. Tantalum in its polished state does have electronegative potential, but on exposure to saline, it soon becomes electropositive. Palmaz,[5] however, points out that this is not entirely undesirable, because the electropositive charge does encourage attraction of plasma proteins, with subsequent deposition of a thin fibrinogen layer that counteracts the electropositive charge. In addition, this layer exhibits surface tension within the thromboresistant range. Another problem in choosing metals for stent construction is that the more electronegative a metal is, the more susceptible it is to corrosion, and at the point that it corrodes, it becomes more thrombogenic.[1]

Stent Surface

The smoother the surface of the polished stent, the more resistant it is to thrombosis.[6] As has been mentioned previously, electropolishing provides a smoother surface than mechanical polishing and hence a more thromboresistant surface.

Oxide Layer

An intact oxide layer is also important because a breach in this layer leads to corrosion, which in turn causes thrombosis.

Stent Deployment

The work of Colombo[7] has documented the importance of stent apposition against the vessel wall during deployment. If craters are left under the stent struts, they can lead to a focus of thrombus that accumulates further and causes intrastent thrombosis. The stent should be thoroughly embedded, with no gaps left between the struts and the vessel wall. Embedding also has the added advantage of promoting more rapid stent endothelialization, because the islands of vessel wall between the struts act as a source of endothelial cell spread. With the stent firmly embedded, maximum luminal diameter is obtained, and this also reduces shear stress.

STENT CONSTRUCTION

The construction of the stent determines many of its basic properties. The original Palmaz stent[8] consists of a tube of stainless steel with eight rows of staggered offset slots cut into it. Balloon expansion of the slotted tube produces a stent with a diamond-shaped configuration (Fig. 2–1). The stent has good radial force, and if the length of the stent and the slots is adjusted; it is possible to produce a device suitable for different vessel diameters that does not shorten significantly on balloon expansion unless an oversized balloon is used. These first-generation stents have stood the test of time and are still very much in use. However, they have certain deficiencies, and modifications in design have been made to improve flexibility and trackability. Flexibility has been improved by linking one or more short stents with a single-filament bridge (Palmaz-Shatz stent). This pro-

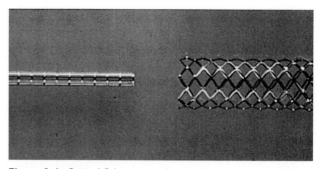

Figure 2–1. Original Palmaz stent showing slotted tube and expanded stent showing diamonds.

duces the desired effect, but, particularly when the stents are flexed, a gap is left between the stent bodies into which tissue can protrude.

As laser technology and computer capacity have improved, it has become possible to conceive and execute much more complex designs that enhance the stent flexibility, avoid shortening, and retain radial force. The AVE Iliac Bridge Stent (Fig. 2–2) achieves this by severing points at which diamonds are joined along opposing sides of the stent, thus making it flexible in one plane. In practice, if the stent is in a tortuous vessel, it tends to align itself and allow this flexibility to come into play. The VIP model (Medtronic) has the most complex design of any stent (Fig. 2–3). The construction produces no shortening on deployment, and the stent exhibits reasonable flexibility and well-maintained radial strength.

All the designs and constructions that have been mentioned are intended for balloon-expandable stents. This type of construction gives the stent a high radial force. Stress-strain analysis measures the force required to cause a predetermined loss of luminal diameter. Figure 2–4 shows the stress-strain curve for an AVE stainless steel stent. The points on the curve

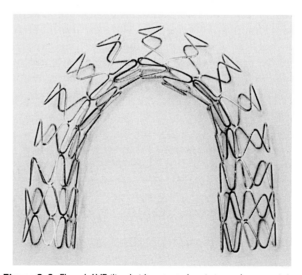

Figure 2–2. Flexed AVE iliac bridge stent showing cuts between joints.

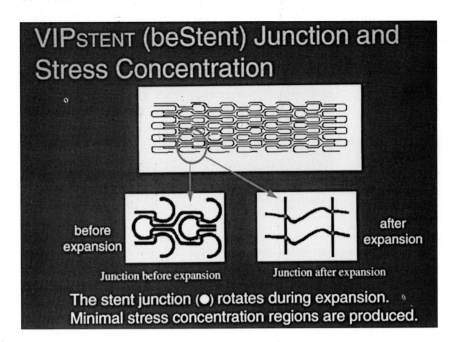

Figure 2–3. Medtronic VIP stent showing complex laser cutting.

show the force in newtons required to deform the stent up to a maximum of 50% luminal loss. The method used is documented by Lossef and associates.[9]

As the force increases, the stent resists deformity in a relatively uniform manner (Fig. 2–4) as shown by the straight line on the graph. At this stage, the stent performs elastically, but as the force increases, the yield point is reached and the stent begins to exhibit plastic deformation. It has less resistance as shown by the curved portion of the graph and requires less additional force to cause further deformity. On removal of the force, the stent shows slight recoil but remains permanently deformed.

Self-expanding stents owe this property either to their method of construction (i.e., Wallstent) or to the metal from which they are constructed (nitinol).

The Wallstent is a woven tube of 24 monofilaments of Elgiloy. The method of weaving and the crossing angles (140 degrees) between the filaments give the stent its self-expanding capabilities and radial strength. Because the crossing points are not welded or fixed, the stent can be elongated to reduce its diameter. The absence of welding also makes the

stent extremely flexible. Elongating the stent allows it to be mounted on a 7 French (F) delivery system. Initially, the stent was constrained under a membrane that could be rolled back to release it.[10] On release, however, the stent shortened by up to one third of its length. The updated version of this stent is now made with a core of tantalum. By changing the crossing angles of the filaments to 120 degrees, it is possible to reduce the amount of shortening, this reduction occurs at the expense of radial strength. To maintain radial force, the number of wires was increased to 30 and the delivery system was replaced by a coaxial one. The stress-strain curve for the Wallstent appears to show elastic behavior because of its construction and is similar to that shown in Figure 2–8.

Other self-expanding stents make use of the thermal memory characteristics of nitinol. The Memotherm (Bard) stent is manufactured from a tube of nitinol with laser-cut slots similar to those of stainless steel balloon-expandable stents. Flexibility is obtained by selectively cutting joining points of the diamonds (Fig. 2–5). The Cragg stent (Boston Scientific) is formed by a single zigzag nitinol wire wound into a tube, with zigs and zags sutured together with Prolene (Fig. 2–6). The Instent Vascucoil (Medtronic) is composed of a single nitinol wire wound into a simple spiral (Fig. 2–7).

Nitinol self-expanding stents all have similar stress-strain curves (Fig. 2–8). As force is applied and increased, the stress-strain relationship is more linear, without the tendency to plateau at higher force. The force required to obtain 50% luminal narrowing is, however, less than that required for balloon-expandable stents of the same diameter.[11] As the force is gradually decreased, the stent exhibits elastic recoil

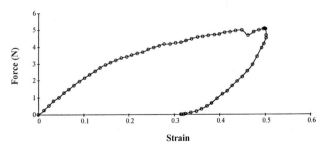

Figure 2–4. Stress-strain curve for AVE iliac bridge stent.

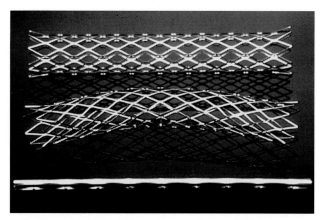

Figure 2–5. Memotherm stent (Bard) showing slotted tube and expanded stent.

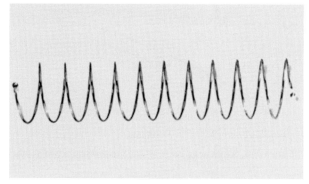

Figure 2–7. Instent Vascucoil (Medtronic).

and at zero force is effectively returned to its original diameter.

From the aforementioned description, it can be ascertained that balloon-expandable stents are of most value in situations in which there may be a constant and fairly high deforming force (i.e., in a vessel with calcified plaque), but they should not be placed where there is danger of repeated high force that may deform them (i.e., over a joint) as they do not re-expand and the lumen remains compromised.

Self-expanding stents are ideally placed where moderate but repeated deforming may be expected (i.e., in the vicinity of a joint).

FLEXIBILITY

Stent flexibility is obtained in a variety of ways as previously outlined. The most flexible stents are the Wallstent and Instent Vascucoil, which can both be flexed through 180 degrees without luminal narrowing or kinking. Other stents have varying levels of flexibility.[11] Some stents can theoretically be placed over joints because of their elastic recoil and flexibility, but other factors, such as metal fatigue, have to be taken into account, and there are reported incidences of stents breaking when placed over joints (particularly the knee) with resultant vessel occlusion.

RADIO-OPACITY

All metallic stents are radio-opaque to a greater or lesser extent. Radio-opacity is a product of the metal used, the thickness of the stent, and how closely the stent struts or wires lie together. As a rule, stainless steel stents are more radio-opaque than those made of nitinol.[11] Radio-opacity is most important for achieving accurate deployment of a stent where an artery overlies a bone (iliac stents). Most manufacturers have to balance increased metal thickness, size of delivery system, and crossing profile.

DELIVERY SYSTEMS

The most frequently used delivery systems are either balloon mounts for balloon-expandable stents or coaxial systems with the stent contained within an outer sheath for self-expanding stents. Ideally the delivery systems should be very flexible, but they should have good pushability and a low crossing profile. Smaller French (F) sized systems are preferred (5 or 6 F rather than 7 or 8 F). Balloon-expandable stents are positioned between balloon markers on the shaft and can usually be placed accurately. Self-expanding stents have markers identifying the position of the stent within its coaxial system, but movement of the stent on release can cause malpositioning, particularly where there is shortening of the stent.

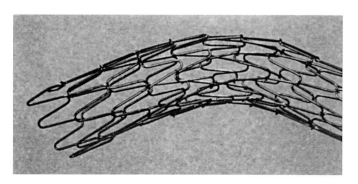
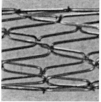

Figure 2–6. Cragg stent with individual zigzag rings held together by Prolene sutures.

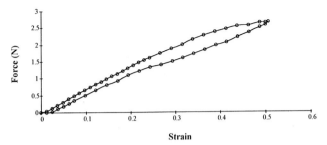

Figure 2–8. Stress-strain curve for the Memotherm nitinol stent.

TRACKABILITY

The ability of the stent on its delivery system to track to its site of deployment is a function of its construction and flexibility as well as its delivery system. It is important to know which stents track easily in a very tortuous vessel or which stents can be delivered from the contralateral limb.[11]

BIOENGINEERING

The focus of research has shifted away from questions of stent mechanics and metallurgy to questions of how to improve the biocompatibility of stents by bioengineering (surface coating, covering).

Bioengineering of endovascular devices is based on the increase in knowledge of the cellular, subcellular, and molecular mechanisms that influence stent patency and restenosis. There is increasing evidence that most cell-cell interactions, such as those that occur among platelets, thrombocytes, leucocytes, monocytes, and endothelial and smooth muscle cells are mediated through so-called cellular adhesion molecules (CAMs).[12] Cell-extracellular matrix interactions, such as between platelets and endothelial cells or smooth muscle cells and fibronectin, collagen, laminin, vitronectin, or von Willebrand factor are similarly mediated. CAMs are surface proteins or glycoproteins working like receptor-counter-receptor or receptor-ligand pairs and playing a key role in such different areas as thrombosis and endothelialization of stents. With reference to their molecular composition, several families of adhesion molecules have been designated, among them integrins, selectins, and the immunoglobulin superfamily. Different types of CAMs may be present on the same cell, and the same CAM may be able to bind different counter-receptors or ligands. Because only certain sites (amino acid sequences) of a ligand molecule (e.g., vitronectin, fibronectin) are necessary to bind a receptor, the same ligand may have several different sites for binding different CAMs.

Probably the best known CAM and a good example to demonstrate briefly the mechanisms of action of CAMs is glycoprotein II 3 (IIb/IIIa), an integrin in humans solely present on platelets.[13] Activation of this integrin is the final common pathway of platelet aggregation. In a randomized prospective clinical study (Evaluation of IIb/IIIa platelet receptor antagonist 7E3 in Preventing Ischemic Complications [EPIC] trial), systemic administration of the monoclonal IIb/IIIa receptor blocker c7E3 (abciximab) not only reduced acute thrombosis after coronary interventions but also caused a significant reduction in the rate of restenosis 6 months after intervention. Interestingly, abciximab blocks not only the receptor II3 but also the vitronectin receptor V3, another integrin, which is expressed on activated human smooth muscle cells and also on endothelial cells. Therefore, the effect of abciximab therapy on restensis may well be the result of a combined effect.

ENDOTHELIALIZATION OF ENDOVASCULAR PROSTHESES

Stents

Without CAMs, endothelial cells are not able to adhere and grow on a bare metal surface. Subendothelial extracellular matrix components may be produced by endothelial cells, such as fibronectin, vitronectin, laminin, or collagen, and are necessary to allow endothelial growth and migration.

Complete endothelialization of the metal stent surface eliminates stent thrombogenicity. Although new drugs, such as ticlopidine, abciximab, and hirudin, or a combination of new and established drugs, such as ticlopidine and aspirin, have made antithrombotic therapy after stent insertion more effective, acute thrombosis still remains a critical point in stent therapy.

Endothelialization of stents starts from patches of remaining viable endothelial cells lodged between the stent struts and from endothelial cells found in the vascular segments adjacent to the ends of the stents. It was also suggested that endothelial cells may derive from blood sources.

The speed of endothelialization or re-endothelialization may differ depending on the degree of vascular damage, the vascular territory, the local flow conditions, and the type of stent used. In addition, there are very limited autopsy data, and, therefore, it is not possible to give a definite time interval for stent endothelialization in humans. The time interval is probably at least in the range of several weeks. Even for experimental animal models, time intervals in the literature for complete arterial stent endothelialization are not consistent. They range from 1 to 3 weeks in swine and sheep to 1 to 2 months in rabbits and 3 weeks to 8 months in dogs. While some investigators reported complete endothelialization 3 weeks after placement of Palmaz stents in healthy and stenosed renal arteries in dogs and swine, others found complete endothelialization of Palmaz stents inserted in aortic stenoses of dogs only after 8 months.[14] Differences within breeds of the same species and between species in their ability to endothelialize a metal surface, differences in the vascular trauma before and during stent insertion, and technical difficulties in reliably preserving and detecting endothelium on a metal stent in histopathologic specimens may account for the divergent results. Moreover, it has not been evaluated whether certain physicochemical surface properties or wire mesh designs of metal stents affect endothelialization.

The importance of flow conditions on endothelialization of a metal surface was demonstrated in an in vitro study.[15] Human aortic endothelial cell migration onto a flat piece of 316 stainless steel 1 cm^2 in width was assessed under static conditions as well as under high-stress (15 dynes/cm^2) and low-stress (2 dynes/cm^2) laminar flow, comparable to conditions in straight segments of normal elastic major arteries (high shear) and areas near arterial branch points (low shear), respectively. Under static conditions, endothelialization of the metal surface occurred with similar speed from all four edges of the metal piece and was completed after 14 days. Laminar flow with high shear stress significantly accelerated endothelialization in the direction of flow by an enhanced speed of endothelial cell migration. There was no relevant difference in the endothelialized surface area between low shear flow and static conditions. In contrast, in an experimental study in rats, acute induction of a 75 to 80% area of stenosis in the abdominal aorta led to loss of most of the endothelium in the stenotic area within 3 minutes as a result of massive shear stress and turbulent flow.[16] Both studies clearly show the importance of maintaining or restoring laminar flow for endothelialization or re-endothelialization.

There is increasing evidence that stent endothelialization and neointimal hyperplasia are inversely related. In an experiment in nonatherosclerotic rabbits, endothelialization of Palmaz stents placed into the iliac arteries was accelerated from 28 days (control group) to 7 days by local channel catheter delivery of human recombinant vascular endothelial growth factor (VEGF). Local administration of VEGF decreased not only acute stent thrombosis but also instent neointima formation. However, reproducibility of these effects and species specificity have to be clarified. Although a similar positive effect of local administration of VEGF was reported in a model of balloon-injured rat carotid artery, another group using a rat and a mouse model of arterial injury could not confirm this effect of VEGF.[17]

Stent Grafts

Most stent grafts in clinical use have a nonbiodegradable synthetic cover of polyester (PET, Dacron), polytetrafluoroethylene (PTFE), or, less frequently, polyurethane (PU).[18] Dacron and PTFE prostheses have been used successfully as a replacement for large-caliber vessels (aorta, iliac arteries) for approximately 30 to 40 years. However, up to now, there have been no synthetic prostheses that reach the long-term patency of natural vessel replacements, such as autologous vein or artery grafts. Compared with the latter, polymeric materials in use are burdened with enhanced thrombogenicity, reduced elasticity, kinking, degeneration, induction of an inflammatory response, and increased neointimal hyperplasia, mainly at the anastomotic site. Though PTFE is less thrombogenic than Dacron, it is a widely accepted fact that even PTFE grafts should be avoided in vessels with a diameter of less than 5 to 6 mm, because graft failure is frequent as a result of acute thrombosis and late neointimal hyperplasia at the anastomotic site.[19] Compared with bare metal stents, currently used stent grafts are less biocompatible, a fact also underlined by the frequent use of bare metal stents and the very limited use of stent grafts in the coronary arteries.

In the past, there was general agreement that as a result of differences in the potential for graft healing, endothelialization of human PTFE or Dacron grafts does not occur except in the perianastomotic region. In contrast, complete endothelialization was regularly observed in various experimental animals, such as baboons, dogs, swine, sheep, and calves.[19] Luminal surfaces of human vascular grafts were found to be covered mainly with impacted, cross-linked fibrin. However, reports now indicate that endothelialization of Dacron and PTFE grafts and stent grafts in humans occur more frequently than previously assumed. Of 7 PTFE aortoiliac or femoropopliteal stent grafts explanted between 0.5 and 7 months after endovascular insertion in patients with limb-threatening ischemia, 4 demonstrated endothelium up to 8 cm from the anastomotic region between 1.5 and 7 months after implantation.[20] Endothelium was also detected on the luminal surface of 3 of 11 aortic Dacron prostheses explanted several years after implantation in humans.[21] Improved identification of endothelium was attributed to very rapid fixation of the specimens. Nevertheless, for unknown reasons, the capability of humans to endothelialize a luminal polymer graft surface appears to be reduced compared with that of experimental animals.

Endothelial cells are the main source of endothelialization in stent grafts in the vascular segments adjacent to the graft. Depending on the porosity of the cover, endothelium may also originate from capillary ingrowth through interstices in the cover material. In baboons, all PTFE grafts with a 60-μm internodal distance endothelialized within 2 weeks, whereas after 12 weeks, less than 20% of grafts with a 30-μm internodal distance were completely covered with endothelium.[22] However, although several animal studies revealed a positive correlation between the rapidity of endothelialization and the porosity of the graft material, this has not yet been verified clinically.

If the healing characteristics of surgically placed Dacron or PTFE grafts, endovascularly placed Dacron-covered stent grafts or PTFE-covered stent grafts, and bare metal stents, in regard to rapid endothelialization and neointimal hyperplasia, are compared, results from experimental animal studies indicate that bare metal stents are superior to endovascularly placed stent grafts, and the latter are superior to conventional surgically placed grafts.[23, 24] In an experimental study, 30-μm PTFE stent grafts endovascularly placed in the infrarenal aortas of dogs demonstrated significantly enhanced endothelialization and attenuated neointimal hyperplasia compared with surgically interposed PTFE grafts of the same type.[23] Improved results of endovascularly placed stent grafts may result from reduction in trauma to the vascular wall and the endothelium adjacent to the implantation site or close contact with the porous stent graft cover (with the underlying vessel wall allowing capillary ingrowth and accelerated endothelialization, or both.

Improved healing characteristics of bare metal stents in animal studies may be explained by several points. The small foreign surface of a metal stent endothelializes easier and faster than the relatively large foreign surface of a stent graft. Bare metal stents are less thrombogenic than stent grafts. For unknown causes, Dacron particularly, and to a lesser extent PTFE and PU, may cause a local inflammatory reaction of the vascular wall[24] (Fig. 2–9A to 2–9D). Activated inflammatory cells are known to release various smooth muscle cell cytokines and mitogens, which may increase neointimal hyperplasia.

However, it may not be advisable to simply transfer these results to the clinical situation. In experimental animals, the vascular wall at the site of the inserted prosthesis is usually healthy, whereas it is severely degenerated and diseased in most patients. Healthy vessels are likely to support and accelerate healing, whereas the ability of severely diseased vessels to do so may be limited or even abolished. Therefore, it was hypothesized that a bare metal stent, leaving large areas of the irregular vascular flow surface of a diseased vessel uncovered and in direct contact with flowing blood may be less favourable under certain circumstances than complete exclusion of the diseased vascular segment from flowing blood and provision of a new smooth flow surface by the tight polymer cover of a stent graft.[18, 20] A prospective randomized study would be necessary to verify this hypothesis.

STENT DESIGN AND NEOINTIMA

There are no prospective randomized clinical studies comparing different types of stents in the peripheral arteries. Clinical studies evaluating a single type of stent are frequently limited in comparability because study designs are nonuniform. Therefore, animal studies were performed to compare the patency and the propensity of different types of stents for inducing neointima. Thereby, parameters of stent design that may be relevant to stent patency and neointima formation were assessed.

Parameters that may have influence on neointimal formation are surface area, rigidity or flexibility (high or low hoop strength), wire material, wire profile, wire thickness, wire mesh geometry, and the method of stent delivery (self-expandability vs. balloon expandability).

Two different surface areas of stents may be calculated. First, the outer surface area that is occupied by wires and comes into contact with the wall vessel, and, second, that area of the stent surface that comes into contact with flowing blood. Both may be expressed as a percentage of the total surface area of the cylinder formed by the expanded stent. One should bear in mind that even in healthy vessels with a smooth luminal surface, both areas may vary considerably depending on the relationship of the stent diameter to the vessel diameter. Oversizing a stent may increase the portion of the stent surface exposed to the vessel wall and decrease the portion exposed to flowing blood by embedding the stent struts more deeply into the vessel wall. A certain extent of oversizing (10 to 15%) may be useful,[25] whereas undersizing should be avoided.

Most types of clinical stents differ in more than one parameter. Therefore, some investigators constructed prototype stents that differed in only a single parameter.[26–28]

Barth and associates evaluated Palmaz stents, Strecker stents, and Wallstents in healthy iliac and femoral arteries of dogs and found that Strecker stents were afflicted with significantly decreased patency and increased neointimal formation.[29] Palmaz stents and Wallstents did not differ from one another. Differences observed were related to the reduced hoop strength and the special wire mesh geometry of Strecker stents. Inhomogenous distribution of the wires along the circumference of the Strecker stent was supposed to cause a more irregular flow surface and induce flow disturbences, thereby enhancing neointimal formation. In another study, Memotherm nitinol stents, Wallstents and the rigid Palmaz stents

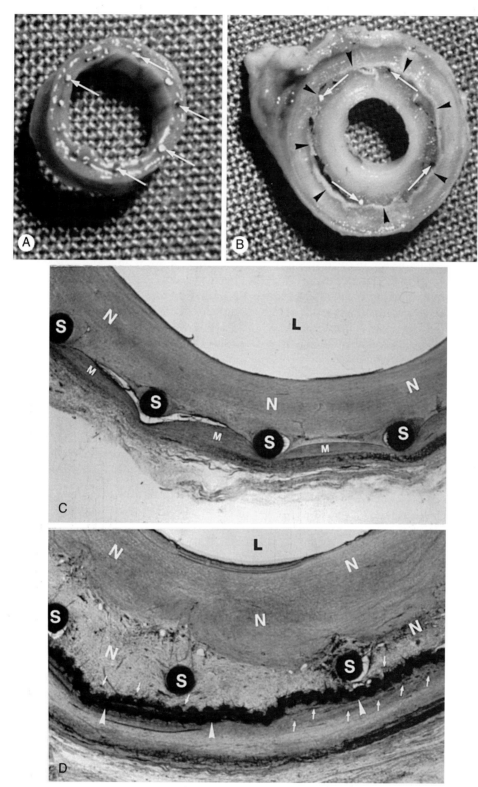

Figure 2–9. *A,* Macroscopic cross-sectional specimen of a bare nitinol stent and *B,* a heparin-coated Dacron covered nitinol stent graft 6 months after insertion into the iliac arteries of the same sheep. The nominal diameter of both prostheses was 8 mm. The stent graft shows markedly increased periprosthetic thickening of the vascular wall and enhanced neointimal formation with more than 50% diameter reduction compared with the patent bare nitinol stent. Arrows = stent struts; arrowheads = Dacron fabric. *C,* Photomicrograph of a cross-sectional histologic slice from a bare nitinol stent (another animal) 6 months after stent placement depicts a clearly delineated medial layer (M) that is compressed by the stent struts, a small adventitia and moderate homogenous neointimal formation (N). *D,* Conversely, in the heparin-coated Dacron covered stentgraft, clear delineation of the medial layer is not possible, the adventitia is thickened, and there is marked inhomogenous neointimal formation (N). At higher magnifications, the greyish spotty areas (small arrows) near the Dacron fabric (arrowheads) corresponded to numerous inflammatory cells. L = lumen, S = stent struts. Methylmethacrylate embedding, Giemsa stains, original magnification x8.75.

implanted in healthy iliac arteries of sheep showed similar patency and neointimal formation.[30]

There is no doubt that a certain amount of hoop strength is required for a stent to minimize recoil of the vascular wall. The hoop strength of Palmaz stents is markedly higher than that of Wallstents. However, similar results of the above experimental studies for Palmaz stents and Wallstents indicate that limited differences in hoop strength are irrelevant to stent patency, at least in noncalcified animal vessels. This is supported by a study of Vorwerk and associates who compared two types of Wallstents, one with half the hoop strength of the other, and observed no difference in neointimal formation in a dog model.[27] Fontaine and associates compared flexible (low hoop strength) and rigid stents (high hoop strength) that were otherwise identical in design in overdilated iliac arteries of swine and found that the rigid stents caused significantly more neointima than the flexible stents; however, rigid stents maintained a significantly larger total vessel diameter.[28] The residual patent arterial diameter was thus almost identical for both types of stents.

The relevance of wire mesh geometry and stent surface area to neointima formation was demonstrated by Tominaga and associates who compared two types of nitinol stents differing only in metal surface area in the infrarenal aorta of healthy rabbits.[26] Neointimal formation was significantly increased in stents with greater surface area. And, finally, the metal surface area of Strecker stents was reported to be about 30%, and that of Palmaz stents to be about 13%.[28] This may be a further explanation for the enhanced neointimal formation of Strecker stents in the aforementioned studies.

Increasing wire thickness also increases surface area. Whether or not the profile of a stent wire (round, square, rectangular) influences neointimal formation is unclear. However, given the same diameter, a wire with a round profile has the smallest surface area.

The results of the studies discussed earlier suggest that it is probably irrelevant to stent patency if a stent is balloon expandable or self-expanding.

Main surface properties (roughness, surface tension), surface area, and wire mesh geometry of a stent may affect neointimal formation and stent patency through the local thrombosis and perhaps the flow changes they induce.

In animal experiments, the amount of acute thrombus formed in response to balloon angioplasty and stent implantation correlated with the degree of late neointimal formation.[31] Thrombin not only plays a pivotal role in acute thrombosis but may also contribute to restenosis by induction of smooth muscle cell proliferation. The mitogenic effect of thrombin is mediated through a special receptor that is detected on platelets, smooth muscle cells, endothelial cells, and various other cells. Thrombin may incite smooth muscle cell proliferation indirectly through stimulating secretion of mitogens from platelets and endothelial cells as well as directly through activation of the smooth muscle cell receptor.

However, though several antithombotic drugs successfully prevented neointimal hyperplasia in animal studies, in prospective clinical trials of coronary interventions, except for the previously mentioned abciximab in the EPIC study, other anticoagulative agents, such as aspirin, dipyridamole, ticlopidine, thromboxane A_2 receptor blocker, heparin or hirudin, failed to reduce restenosis.[13]

There are several possible explanations for this divergent outcome. In many clinical studies, the dosage has been smaller than in experimental studies. The local dose at the site of intervention may have been too small to be effective. Susceptibility to drug therapy of mostly healthy animal arteries may be enhanced compared with severely diseased human arteries. Positive effects of a drug may have been concealed because only one of several sources of restenosis present in diseased human arteries was effectively targeted. For example, besides platelets, there are several other cell types, such as injured endothelial cells, smooth muscle cells, or white blood cells, which may also release smooth muscle cell growth factors. Proved clinical effectiveness of abciximab that targets a different receptor on platelets and smooth muscle cells (see earlier discussion) indicates that a combined effect may be a major factor of successful restenosis therapy.

IMPROVING THE BIOCOMPATIBILITY OF ENDOVASCULAR PROSTHESES

Surface bioengineering techniques have been introduced to vascular stenting. These techniques allow creation of biological surfaces on nonbiological medical implants, such as vascular stents and stent grafts, with the intention of enhancing the long-term efficacy of these devices.[32] Inherent in these techniques is the potential for local drug delivery.

The exceptional properties of metal bonding make it difficult to bind a drug directly to a metal surface. A polymer coating may serve as an interface for bonding a bioactive agent. The coating may be nonbiodegradable or biodegradable. Requirements for a high quality polymer coating are homogenety of the coating, nontoxicity, and mechanical strength, and also elasticity, because stents may abruptly change their shape during delivery. Nonbiodegradable polymer coatings should also be chemically resistant. The thickness of the polymer layer should be as small as possible.

For chemical bonding of bioactive agents, the

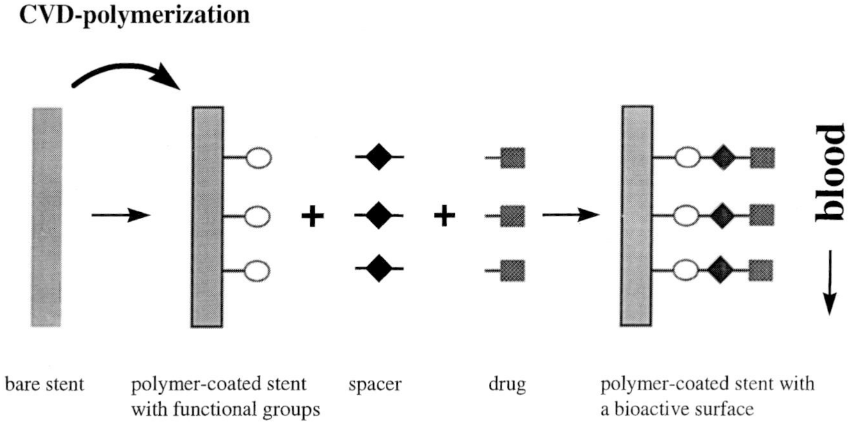

CVD-polymerization

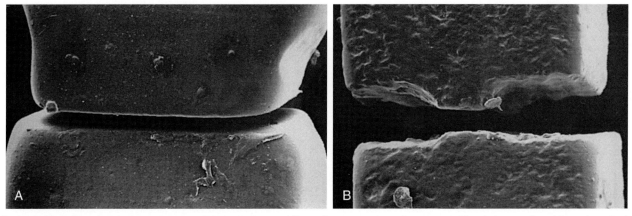

Figure 2–10. Schematic drawing illustrating how a bioactive agent (drug) may be bound to a metal surface by chemical vapor deposition (CVD), polymerization, and spacer techniques.

bare stent   polymer-coated stent with functional groups   spacer   drug   polymer-coated stent with a bioactive surface

polymer surface needs to have chemical functional groups, such as amino, carboxy, or hydroxy groups. The techniques required to achieve a polymer coating, including such a coating for functional groups, are demanding. Depending on the chemical structures of the bioactive agent and the polymer, both may be bound to one another directly or through a so-called spacer (Fig. 2–10). A spacer is a bivalent molecule that serves as a link between polymer and bioactive agent. Care must be taken to maintain the bioactive site or sites of the agent after immobilization to the polymer. Sustained activity of the bioactive agent after sterilization has to be verified as well.

Several coating techniques are available, such as dipping procedures, plasma polymerization, or the chemical vapor deposition (CVD) treatment (Fig. 2–11A, B). Covalent bonding stably connects the bioactive agent to the polymer surface, whereas a drug-releasing stent results if the drug-polymer bonding is less strong, as in ion bonding, mere adsorption of the drug to a polymer, or incorporation into a biodegradable polymer. In the latter case, the time course of the

degradation of the polymer determines the release of the agent.

Among the nonbiodegradable polymers evaluated in animal studies are polyurethane, silicone, polyethylene terephthalate, cellulose, and polyethylene imine; some biodegradable polymers that have already been tested are poly-L-lactic acid, polyhydroxybuturate valerate and polycaprolactone.[33] Biodegradable and nonbiodegradable polymers may lead to a severe local inflammation with subsequent neointimal formation that may counteract the effect of the bioactive agent. Therefore, in vitro and in vivo testing of the biocompatibility of a polymer coating is mandatory.

Most drugs considered suitable for stent coating act either as anticoagulants, such as heparin, hirudin, glycoproten IIb/IIIa receptor antibodies, and nitric oxide donors; or as antiproliferative agents, such as angiopeptin; cytostatics, including corticosteroids and taxol; or as promotors of endothelial cell growth, such as VEGF. Results of comparative animal studies of drug polymer coated and noncoated stents are pre-

Figure 2–11. *A,* Scanning electron microscopy image of a bare and *B,* a polymer-coated metal stent strut. Chemical vapor deposition polymerization was employed to apply the polymer polyparaxylylene to the metal surface. Depending on the source substances used, paraxylylene may have, for example, hydroxy, amino, or carboxy groups to which a bioactive agent may be bound. Smoothness of the polymer-coated metal surface is considerably improved compared with the surface of the bare metal stent.

liminary and divergent. However, a trend is detectable from several studies suggesting that heparin-coated stents may reduce the incidence of acute stent thrombosis but do not decrease neointimal formation during short-term follow-up (4 to 6 weeks).

There is one major prospective clinical study in which Palmaz stents coated with polyethylene imine with covalently bound heparin were inserted into the coronary arteries (Benestent II trial). However, the primary purpose of the study was not to compare the long-term patency of coated and noncoated stents but to evaluate the safety of minimizing peri-interventional anticoagulative therapy in patients receiving a heparin-coated stent. This goal was achieved; however, further conclusions, particularly with regard to prevention of restenosis, have no valid basis.

Finally, coating techniques compete with other procedures and devices, such as local drug delivery via special catheters, radioactive stents, or purely polymeric stents, in the attempt to improve the patency of vascular stents.

CONCLUSION

Because there is no ideal stent, the interventionist require a stock of both balloon-expandable and self-expanding stents if all types of lesions are to be treated in different arteries.

REFERENCES

1. Gotman I: Characteristics of metals used in implants. J Endourol 11:383, 1997.
2. Hoar TP, Mears DC: Corrosion-resistant alloys in chloride solution: Materials for surgical implants. Proc R Soc London 294:486, 1996.
3. Ryhanen J, Niami E, Serlo W, et al: Biocompatibility of nickel-titanium shape memory metal and its corrosion behaviour in human cell cultures. J Biomed Mater Res 35:451, 1997.
4. Shabalovskaya S: On the nature of the biocompatibility and on medical applications of NiTi shape memory and superelastic alloys. Biomed Mater Eng 6:267, 1996.
5. Palmaz JC, Tio FO, Shatz RA, et al: Early endothelialisation of balloon-expandable stents: Experimental observations. J Intervent Radiol 3:119, 1998.
6. Ratner BD, Johnston AB, Lenk TJ: Biomaterial Surfaces. J Biomed Mater Res 21:59, 1987.
7. Colombo A, Hall P, Nakamura S, et al: Intracoronary stenting with intravascular ultrasound guidance. Circulation 91:1676, 1995.
8. Palmaz JC, Windeler SA, Garcia F, et al: Atherosclerotic rabbit aortas: Expandable intraluminal grafting. Radiology 160:723, 1986.
9. Lossef SV, Lutz RJ, Mundorf J, et al: Comparison of mechanical deformation properties of metallic stents with use of stress-strain analysis. J Vasc Interv Radiol 5:341, 1994.
10. Dyet JF, Shaw JW, Cook AM, et al: The use of the Wallstent in aorto-iliac vascular disease. Clin Radiol 48:227, 1993.
11. Dyet JF: New stent developments (Abstract). Cardiovasc Intervent Radiol 20:1:544, 1997.
12. Jang Y, Lincoff M, Plow EF, et al: Cell adhesion molecules in coronary artery disease. J Am Coll Cardiol 24:1591, 1994.
13. Le Breton H, Plow EF, Topol EJ: Role of platelets in restenosis after percutaneous revascularization. J Am Coll Cardiol 28:1643, 1996.
14. Pisco JM, Correla M, Esperanca-Pina JA, et al: Vasa vasorum changes following stent placement in experimental arterial stenoses. J Vasc Interv Radiol 4:269, 1993.
15. Sprague E, Luo M, Palmaz JC: Human aortic endothelial cell migration onto stent surfaces under static and flow conditions. J Vasc Interv Radiol 8:83, 1997.
16. Joris I, Zand T, Majno G: Hydrodynamic injury of the endothelium in acute aortic stenosis. Am J Pathol 106:394, 1982.
17. Schneider DB, Dichek DA: Intravascular stent endothelialization. A goal worth pursuing? Circulation 95:308, 1997.
18. Cragg AH, Dake MD: Treatment of peripheral vascular disease with stent-grafts. Radiology 205:307, 1997.
19. Pasquinelli G, Freyrie A, Preda P, et al: Healing of prosthetic arterial grafts. Scanning Microsc 4:351, 1990.
20. Marin LM, Veith FJ, Cynamon J, et al: Human transluminally placed endovascular stented grafts: Preliminary histopathologic analysis of healing grafts in aortoiliac and femoral artery occlusive disease. J Vasc Surg 21:595, 1995.
21. Shi Q, De Wu MH, Onuki Y, et al: Endothelium on the flow surface of human aortic Dacron vascular grafts. J Vasc Surg 25:736, 1997.
22. Clowes AW, Zacharias RK, Kirkman TR: Early endothelial coverage of synthetic arterial grafts: Porosity revisited. Am J Surg 153:501, 1987.
23. Ombrellaro MP, Stevens SL, Kerstetter K, et al: Healing characteristics of intraarterial stented grafts: Effect of intraluminal position on prosthetic graft healing. Surgery 120:60, 1996.
24. Schürmann K, Vorwerk D, Uppenkamp R, et al: Iliac arteries: Plain and heparin-coated Dacron-covered stent-grafts compared with noncovered metal stents. An experimental study. Radiology 203:55, 1997.
25. Palmaz JC: Intravascular stents: Tissue-stent interactions and design considerations. AJR 160:613, 1993.
26. Tominaga R, Kambic HE, Emoto H, et al: Effects of design geometry of intravascular endoprostheses on stenosis rate in normal rabbits. Am Heart J 123:21, 1992.
27. Vorwerk D, Redha F, Neuerburg J, et al: Neointima formation following placement of self-expanding stents of different radial force: Experimental results. Cardiovasc Interv Radiol 17:27, 1994.
28. Fontaine AB, Spigos DG, Eaton G, et al: Stent-induced intimal hyperplasia: Are there fundamental differences between flexible and rigid stent designs? J Vasc Interv Radiol 5:739, 1994.
29. Barth KH, Virmani R, Froelich J, et al: Paired comparison of vascular wall reactions to Palmaz stents, Strecker tantalum stents, and Wallstents in canine iliac and femoral arteries. Circulation 93:2161, 1996.
30. Schürmann K, Vorwerk D, Kulisch A, et al: Neointimal hyperplasia in low-profile Nitinol stents, Palmaz stents and Wallstents: A comparative experimental study. Cardiovasc Intervent Radiol 19:248, 1996.
31. Unterberg C, Sandrock D, Nebendahl K, et al: Reduced acute thrombus formation results in decreased neointimal proliferation after coronary angioplasty. J Am Coll Cardiol 26:1747, 1995.
32. Ratner BD: New ideas in biomaterials science—a path to engineered biomaterials. J Biomed Mater Res 27:837, 1993.
33. Fischell TA: Polymer coatings for stents. Can we judge a stent by its cover? Circulation 94:1494, 1996.

Chapter 3

The Principles of Thrombolysis

R. Verhaeghe and J. Vermylen

HISTORICAL ASPECTS

The phenomenon of spontaneous fibrinolysis was recognized at the end of the 19th century, and soon afterward, the concept that coagulation and fibrinolysis constituted distinct stages of a continuing proteolytic process was proposed. Early in the present century, it was suggested that a proteolytic enzyme was responsible for fibrinolysis, and subsequently, an enzyme with similarities to trypsin was shown to develop in serum treated with chloroform, which removed the inhibition to proteolytic enzymes. Important progress was made in the 1930s with the demonstration that certain strains of beta-hemolytic streptococci produce a substance that induces rapid lysis of plasma clots. Initially, this agent was called *streptococcal fibrinolysin*, but it was renamed *streptokinase* after this streptococcal product was shown to behave as an activator rather than as a direct fibrinolysin. By the mid 1940s, it became clear that the proteolytic enzyme responsible for fibrinolysis existed in plasma as an inactive precursor that could be activated rapidly by streptokinase. The precursor was referred to as *plasminogen* and the activation product as *plasmin*. These terms were preferred to profibrinolysin and fibrinolysin because the activity of plasmin is not restricted to the digestion of fibrin (Fig. 3–1).

The first clinical use of streptokinase involved local instillation into patients with hemorrhagic or fibrinous pleural effusions.[1] Additional purification and animal experiments preceded its introduction for intravascular infusion in volunteers and in patients with myocardial infarction in the late 1950s. Further delay in the development of thrombolytic therapy was mainly the result of a high incidence of pyrogenic reactions with some preparations of streptokinase, and it took another 10 years before consistently high-quality preparations were produced such as to make them available for general use in the management of arterial and venous thromboembolism. In the meantime, purification of urokinase had started. As a naturally occurring plasminogen activator produced by kidney cells and excreted in urine, it was devoid of antigenic properties and pyrogenic complications.

THE FIBRINOLYTIC SYSTEM AND ITS CONTROL

Fibrin is cleared primarily from the circulation by the fibrinolytic system acting as an antithrombotic defense mechanism. Plasmin is the effector enzyme of this system and is formed from an inactive precursor, plasminogen, under the action of a plasminogen activator. Plasmin cleaves fibrin and produces progressively smaller degradation products that typically contain the D-domain of two fibrin-monomers that are cross-linked (D-dimer).

Physiologic fibrinolysis is regulated by specific molecular interactions between plasminogen activators and their inhibitors, plasminogen, plasmin and its inhibitors, as well as by the interaction of these molecules with fibrin and with cellular and extracellular binding sites[2, 3] (Fig. 3–2). The liver metabolizes and eliminates most of the components of the fibrinolytic system and contributes toward modulating their plasma levels. The important role of the fibrinolytic system in maintaining the patency of blood vessels is illustrated by the augmented risk of thrombosis in patients with hypofibrinolysis (either congenital or acquired) and by gene deletion studies in mice.[4]

Human plasminogen is a glycoprotein (92,000 dalton) with four functional domains: (1) the carboxyl terminal serine-protease domain, (2) the amino-terminal finger domain, (3) the growth factor domain, and (4) the domain with the five triple-looped kringle structures that contain the binding sites. Plasminogen contains an aminoterminal glutamic acid in its native form (glu-plasminogen), but native plasminogen is converted easily by limited plasmic digestion to modified forms with aminoterminal lysine, valine, or methionine, commonly designated as lys-plasminogen. Plasminogen is converted to plasmin by cleavage of a single peptide bond. Plasmin is a two-chain molecule. Its heavy A-chain contains structures that medi-

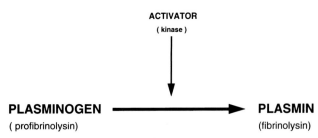

Figure 3–1. Early scheme of the fibrinolytic system.

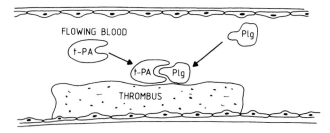

Figure 3–3. Surface assembly of plasminogen (Plg) and tissue plasminogen activator (t-PA) on the fibrin clot enhances the interaction between Plg and t-PA.

ate the interaction with fibrin and antiplasmin, the so-called lysine-binding sites that may play a crucial role in the endogenous regulation of fibrinolysis. The active site contains serine and is located on the light B-chain.

The most important physiologic activator is tissue plasminogen activator (t-PA), a 70,000-dalton molecule with a carboxyl-terminal serine protease domain, an amino-terminal finger domain, a growth factor domain, and two kringle domains. It is synthesized continuously and is secreted by endothelial cells as a one-chain molecule that is converted to a two-chain molecule in the presence of plasmin or kallikrein, but the activity of both forms is roughly comparable. Control of the release of t-PA represents a primary mechanism in regulating the fibrinolytic activity of blood. However, an increase in the plasma level of t-PA, as induced, for example, by physical exercise, produces only a slight increase in plasmin activity that is neutralized rapidly by circulating α_2-antiplasmin.

t-PA has a low affinity for plasminogen in the absence of fibrin, but the presence of a fibrin surface strikingly enhances the activation rate of plasminogen by a factor of approximately 1000-fold. This increased affinity results from surface assembly of plasminogen and plasminogen activator on the fibrin clot (Fig. 3–3). Plasminogen binds specifically but weakly with fibrin through the structures called *lysine-binding sites*. t-PA also has a specific affinity for fibrin, and the presence

of t-PA enhances the binding of plasminogen to fibrin. Thus, fibrin provides a surface onto which t-PA and plasminogen absorb in a sequential and ordered way to yield a ternary complex. In this way, fibrin essentially facilitates the interaction between t-PA and its substrate. Efficient activation of plasminogen by t-PA, therefore, is limited to the fibrin surface, whereas no efficient activation occurs in plasma. The restriction of efficient activation to the fibrin clot is another means by which fibrinolysis is controlled. In addition, plasmin generated on the fibrin surface has both its lysine-binding sites and active site occupied and is thus only slowly inactivated by α_2-antiplasmin.

The second physiologic activator of plasminogen is produced by kidney cells and found in urine (urokinase-type plasminogen activator [u-PA]), and its primary role is to keep the ureters patent. It is a 54,000-dalton protein with a carboxyl-terminal catalytic domain, an amino-terminal growth factor domain, and a single kringle domain. It activates plasminogen to plasmin as well in the presence as in the absence of fibrin. u-PA is a two-chain molecule (tcu-PA) but is present in plasma under the form of a single-chain inactive precursor (scu-PA or pro-urokinase). Pro-urokinase is converted to two-chain urokinase by hydrolysis of a single peptide bond in the presence of plasmin.

Further regulation of fibrinolytic activity occurs at the level of the interaction of plasmin and the plasminogen activators with specific inhibitors. α_2-antiplasmin (a 70,000-dalton protein) is a very rapid and potent inhibitor of all unbound plasmin. Plasminogen activator inhibitor-1 (PAI-1) is synthesized in endothelial cells and also is found in platelets, from which it is released during aggregation. Interaction of t-PA with PAI-1 results in a decreased activity of the activator, but t-PA bound to fibrin is protected largely from inactivation. Clinical studies support a role for an elevated plasma level of PAI-1 in the genesis of thrombotic events. A second inhibitor, PAI-2, is detected only in pregnant women.

Thus, plasmin is formed locally in the thrombus because of the local release of the activator from the adjacent endothelial cells and the special assembly

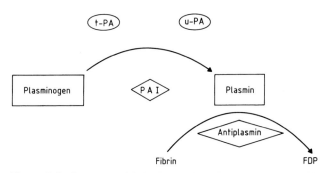

Figure 3–2. Current simplified scheme of the fibrinolytic system. t-PA = tissue plasminogen activator; u-PA = urokinase type plasminogen activator; PAI = plasminogen activator inhibitors; FDP = fibrin degradation products.

of plasminogen and t-PA on fibrin. Free plasmin is prevented from escaping into the circulation by antiplasmin that inactivates it; activator inhibitors help to confine the activation to the vicinity of the thrombotic mass.

THROMBOLYTIC AGENTS

Five thrombolytic agents have been in clinical use for several years. These are:

1. Streptokinase
2. Anistreplase (anisoylated plasminogen–streptokinase activator complex [APSAC])
3. Urokinase (tcu-PA)
4. Saruplase (scu-PA or pro-urokinase)
5. Alteplase (t-PA)

Alteplase and saruplase exhibit fibrin specificity, whereas the remaining three are non–fibrin-specific.[5, 6] In addition, several new agents currently are being introduced or evaluated.[7]

Non–Fibrin-Specific Agents

STREPTOKINASE AND ANISTREPLASE

Streptokinase is produced by several strains of beta-hemolytic streptococci and consists of a single polypeptide chain. It has no active site and thus cannot directly cleave peptide bonds. It activates plasminogen to plasmin indirectly after the formation of an equimolar complex with plasminogen.

Anistreplase is an equimolar complex between human lys-plasminogen and streptokinase. It was developed with the aim of controlling the enzymatic activity of the complex by a specific reversible chemical protection (acylation) of its catalytic center that does not affect the weak fibrin-binding capacity of the plasminogen moiety in the complex. De-acylation occurs both in the circulation and at the fibrin surface and regenerates the catalytic center. Streptokinase activates plasminogen by means of a three-step mechanism. In the first step, streptokinase forms an equimolar complex with plasminogen, which undergoes a conformational change, resulting in the exposure of an active site in the plasminogen moiety. In the second step, this active site catalyzes the activation of plasminogen to plasmin. In the third step, plasminogen–streptokinase molecules are converted to plasmin–streptokinase complexes. The potential of the plasminogen–streptokinase complex to activate plasminogen is two- to threefold higher than that of the plasmin–streptokinase complex. Thus, the equimolar plasminogen–streptokinase complex converts rapidly to the plasmin–streptokinase complex by proteolytic cleavage in the two moieties. The active site residues in the plasmin–streptokinase complex are the same as those in the plasmin molecule. However, there are also differences: Plasmin is unable to activate plasminogen and is neutralized rapidly by α_2-antiplasmin; plasmin complexed with streptokinase activates plasminogen and escapes inhibition by antiplasmin. Because streptokinase generates free-circulating plasmin, its use is associated with generation of a systemic lytic state.

Streptokinase is eliminated from the circulation with a half-life of approximately 20 minutes (initial half-life of 4 minutes and terminal half-life of 30 minutes). The level of antistreptokinase antibodies, which result from previous infections with beta-hemolytic streptococci, varies widely among individuals. These antibodies inactivate streptokinase, and therefore, sufficient streptokinase must be infused to neutralize the antibodies. Roughly 350,000 units of streptokinase are required to neutralize 95% of the circulating antibodies in 95% of a healthy population, with individual requirements ranging from 25,000 to 3 million units. A few days after streptokinase administration, the antistreptokinase titer rises rapidly to 50 to 100 times the preinfusion value and remains high for 4 to 6 months, during which period a new thrombolytic therapy with streptokinase becomes impracticable because exceedingly high doses are needed to overcome the antibodies.

Anistreplase has a de-acylation half-life of approximately 1.5 to 2 hours; its plasma elimination half-life in humans is approximately 1 hour. The plasma clearance of fibrinolytic activity in patients treated with anistreplase was reported to have a half-life of 1.5 hours. Anistreplase causes a 60-fold increase in the streptokinase antibody titer after 2 to 3 weeks, which persists after 3 months.

UROKINASE

Urokinase is the naturally occurring plasminogen activator excreted in human urine. It is produced from tissue cultures of human embryonic kidney cells and with recombinant techniques. It has two polypeptide chains, a heavy chain with 253 amino acids and a light chain with 158 amino acids. The two-chain molecule is obtained by proteolytic cleavage of its single-chain precursor. Urokinase is available in high and low molecular weight forms. It is a direct activator of human plasminogen but does not distinguish between freely circulating and fibrin-bound plasminogen. Extensive plasminogen activation with urokinase and depletion of antiplasmin may lead to a systemic lytic state with low fibrinogen levels.

Urokinase is cleared rapidly from the plasma by the liver with an initial plasma half-life of 3 minutes.

Fibrin-Specific Agents

ALTEPLASE

Alteplase is the generic name of recombinant human tissue-type plasminogen activator (rt-PA). It is a serine proteinase that consists of a single polypeptide chain. Hydrolysis of a single peptide bond yields a two-chain activator linked together by one disulfide bond. The mechanism of action of t-PA is discussed in the previous section.

Alteplase is cleared rapidly from the circulation with an initial half-life of 6 minutes and a terminal half-life of 1 hour. Both hepatocytes and endothelial cells in the liver have a recognition system for removal of t-PA.

SARUPLASE

Saruplase is the generic name for nonglycosylated human recombinant single-chain urokinase-type plasminogen activator (scu-PA or pro-urokinase). It is a glycoprotein (54,000 dalton) with 411 amino acids. Limited hydrolysis by plasmin or kallikrein of a single peptide bond converts the molecule to the two-chain derivative (tcu-PA or urokinase).

In the absence of fibrin, scu-PA is stable in plasma and does not activate plasminogen; in the presence of a fibrin clot, scu-PA induces fibrin-specific clot lysis. Several hypotheses for the mechanism of plasminogen activation and fibrin specificity of clot lysis with scu-PA in plasma have been proposed. The first claims that scu-PA does not activate glu-plasminogen but only lys-plasminogen bound to partially degraded fibrin. An alternative proposal is that the intrinsic plasminogen-activating potential of scu-PA is counteracted by a competitive inhibitory mechanism in plasma, which is reversed by fibrin. A third view is that scu-PA is a genuine proenzyme with negligible activating potential toward fibrinogen, unless tcu-PA is generated. Studies in vitro suggest that conversion of scu-PA to tcu-PA during clot lysis constitutes a primary positive feedback system for accelerating lysis, but mutants of scu-PA that are resistant to conversion to tcu-PA exhibit only moderately reduced thrombolytic potency in vivo.

Animal studies on turnover of recombinant and natural scu-PA, as well as of tcu-PA, point toward a two-compartment model of metabolism with central and peripheral compartments and rapid hepatic clearance from the central compartment. An initial half-life of approximately 3 minutes was observed experimentally. In patients with myocardial infarction, intravenous infusion of scu-PA resulted in a biphasic disappearance rate with an initial postinfusion half-life in plasma of approximately 4 minutes.

Newer Agents

Several mutants and variants of rt-PA currently are being evaluated in animal and clinical studies. These agents are produced by deletion or substitution of functional domains, by site-specific point mutations, and/or by altering the carbohydrate composition of rt-PA. They are designed to augment activity and fibrin specificity, to prolong plasma half-life, and to resist inhibition by PAI. Examples are reteplase and TNK-rt-PA, both of which have been tested in patients with myocardial infarction. Reteplase is a single-chain nonglycosylated deletion variant of rt-PA. In TNK-rt-PA, two single amino acids are substituted, and another short sequence is altered. The two products have a slower plasma clearance; TNK-rt-PA also exhibits marked resistance to PAI-1 and enhanced fibrin specificity.

Staphylokinase is a plasminogen activator originally made by certain strains of *Staphylococcus aureus* but currently is produced by recombinant techniques. Its profibrinolytic activity first was demonstrated half a century ago. The staphylokinase gene has been cloned and encodes a protein of 163 amino acids. Amino acid 28 corresponds to the amino-terminal residue of the mature protein that consists of 136 amino acids in a single polypeptide chain.

Animal and human studies reveal that recombinant staphylokinase is an efficient and highly fibrin-specific plasminogen activator. Whereas streptokinase produces a complex with plasminogen that exposes the active site in the plasminogen moiety without proteolytic cleavage, staphylokinase behaves differently. It forms a complex with plasminogen and with plasmin. The former complex, however, is inactive; the plasmin staphylokinase complex is the active enzyme. Trace amounts of plasmin appear to initiate the reaction sequence, which is amplified by generation of a plasmin–staphylokinase complex, which in turn converts excess plasminogen to plasmin.[8] Binding studies indicate that staphylokinase has a much higher affinity for plasmin than for circulating plasminogen and support the view that activation of plasminogen by the plasmin–staphylokinase complex is the main pathway for generation of plasmin rather than conversion of the plasminogen–staphylokinase complex. The high fibrin specificity of staphylokinase is explained by the finding that in the absence of fibrin, alpha-2-antiplasmin inhibits all trace amounts of plasmin. In the presence of fibrin, generation of the plasmin–staphylokinase complex is facilitated because traces of plasmin bound to fibrin are protected from inhibition by antiplasmin. In addition, antiplasmin neutralizes the plasmin–staphylokinase complex at the clot surface extremely slowly. Thus, this complex can efficiently convert excess plasminogen to plasmin (and plasminogen–staphylokinase complex to plasmin–staphylokinase complex). Furthermore, staphylokinase dissociates from neutralized complex and is recycled to other plasmin and plasminogen molecules.

The postinfusion disappearance rate of staphylokinase-related antigen from plasma occurs in a biphasic way with an initial half-life of 6 minutes and a terminal half-life of 30 to 40 minutes. In most patients who receive recombinant staphylokinase, neutralizing antibodies develop after about 7 to 12 days; titers remain high for several months. No cross-reactivity has been found between antibodies to streptokinase and those to staphylokinase. Variants of recombinant staphylokinase obtained by protein engineering induce significantly less antibody formation in patients, although the thrombolytic potency remains intact.

CLINICAL INDICATIONS

The main clinical use of thrombolytic agents is in the setting of acute myocardial infarction. Megatrials with thousands of patients have identified unequivocally thrombolytic therapy as the mainstay of acute management in most patients with suspected acute myocardial infarction. In thrombotic stroke, major efforts have been spent over the past few years to investigate the feasibility and efficacy of thrombolytic agents, infused within the early hours of neurologic symptoms. However, the use of thrombolytic therapy in this condition remains a contentious issue. These two clinical indications of thrombolysis are beyond the scope of the present chapter, which now deals with thrombolytic therapy in arterial and venous thromboembolic disease.

Peripheral Arterial Occlusion

Peripheral venous administration of streptokinase and urokinase was investigated 3 decades ago as a treatment for acute arterial occlusion of the lower limbs. Infusion of high doses of streptokinase was shown to restore patency in almost two thirds of recently (< 72 hours) occluded arteries.[9] In longer standing occlusions, the success rate was lower, and almost no lysis was obtained in iliac or femoral thrombi older than 3 months.[10] This therapeutic effect was obtained at significant expense, and the incidence of major hemorrhagic complications was considerable, with fatal bleeding in 1% to 3% of the patients.

With few exceptions,[11] the systemic use of thrombolytic agents for peripheral arterial occlusion largely was abandoned in the 1980s in favor of intra-arterial infusion. Chesterman and colleagues[12] and Dotter and associates[13] were the first to report lysis of thrombi in peripheral arteries with a low dose of locally delivered streptokinase. The intra-arterial infusion technique gradually gained acceptance after the publication of the large experience of Hess and colleagues.[14] Over the past 15 years, a number of catheter techniques and infusion methods have been developed, and these are discussed further in Chapter 12.

DOSE AND CHOICE OF THROMBOLYTIC AGENT

In the early days of catheter thrombolysis, streptokinase was the most widely used agent, but in recent years urokinase and alteplase (rt-PA) largely have superseded streptokinase as preferred agents. For urokinase, dosage schemes varied initially, but the low-dose concept gradually was abandoned in favor of higher doses with progressive tapering. For instance, a popular therapeutic regimen is 240,000 IU/h for 2 hours or until restoration of antegrade flow, reduced to 120,000 IU/h for another 2 hours and 60,000 IU/h until lysis is complete.[15] With alteplase, the dosage schemes applied varied from 0.025 mg/kg/h to 0.1 mg/kg/h and from 0.25 mg/h to 10 mg/h. In general, no obvious benefit was found when using the higher doses.

Analysis of retrospective and nonrandomized reports suggests that alteplase may achieve the optimal combination of thrombolytic success and safety. However, randomized studies that directly compare different agents are few. In fact, there currently is no scientific proof of definite superiority of any thrombolytic agent for peripheral arterial thrombolysis in terms of efficacy and safety, but despite this, clinical practice has moved away from the use of streptokinase in many countries. Table 3–1 lists acceptable dosage regimens for intra-arterial catheter thrombolysis. With delivery systems that pursue accelerated lysis, initial bolus injections may be used.

Clinical studies in leg arterial occlusion also have been reported for recombinant glycosylated pro-urokinase[16] and recombinant staphylokinase.[17–19] These

Table 3–1. Frequently Used Dosage Schemes in Catheter Thrombolysis for Leg Ischemia

Agent	Infusion	Initial "Bolus" Dose
SK	5000 U/h continuous infusion	
UK	4000 U/min till antegrade flow	
	1000 U/min till complete lysis	120,000–240,000 U
rt-PA	Either 1 mg/h or 0.05 mg/kg/h continuous infusion	5 mg (may be repeated twice at 5- to 10-min intervals)
STAR	1 mg/h	2 mg

SK = streptokinase; UK = urokinase; rt-PA = alteplase; STAR = staphylokinase.

two agents appear to exhibit at least similar efficacy as currently available agents but without inducing fibrinogen depletion. Superior fibrin specificity may raise hope for a lower bleeding complication rate, but severe hemorrhage did occur in the early studies with these agents. Staphylokinase is antigenic and induces antibody formation (see previous section). A discussion of the published trials comparing thrombolysis with surgical treatment is included in Chapter 12.

Deep Vein Thrombosis

Heparin followed by warfarin is the conventional therapy for deep vein thrombosis. Thrombolytic agents might be an ideal treatment if they produced rapid lysis of all thrombi with rapid resolution of the clinical symptoms of acute thrombosis and complete elimination of all pulmonary embolism risk. In addition, they would have to preserve the normal valve function to avoid development of late post-thrombotic sequelae. Both streptokinase and urokinase have been used extensively to treat venous thrombosis, whereas clinical experience with alteplase is more limited. Most results have been obtained with systemic rather than local administration.

LYSIS OF VENOUS THROMBI

In 13 controlled trials, 48% of patients had a complete or significant clearing of their obstructed veins on a post-treatment venogram, and an additional 20% had partial clearing; the corresponding figures with heparin were 6% and 12%, respectively.[20] When the analysis is limited to trials with strict criteria for randomization, it appears that thrombolysis is achieved 3.7 times more often with streptokinase than with heparin.[21] This possible advantage must be weighed against an incidence of major bleeding of 20.2% with streptokinase vs. 6.6% with heparin. In the 1980s, ultra-high doses of streptokinase (1.5 million units over 6 hours; repeated if necessary for up to 5 days) were advocated in some countries, with reportedly similar success rates as with standard dosage schemes (250,000 units over first hour followed by 100,000 units per hour).

An appreciation of the efficacy of urokinase in venous thrombosis is hampered by the enormous variation in infusion schedules used. The overall impression is that the rate of venographic lysis is roughly similar to that achieved with streptokinase. Published experience with alteplase is limited, and there is no consensus on the dosage scheme: some advocate short infusions with a fairly high dose (50–100 mg over 3–4 hours), whereas others study lower doses over extended periods (0.25 or 0.5 mg/kg/d for 3–7 days). Preliminary data suggest that the rate

of lysis achieved with the short dosage schemes using alteplase is similar to that reported previously with streptokinase, but experience with lower doses over several days was disappointing.[22]

INFLUENCE ON CLINICAL EVOLUTION

Pain and leg swelling subside rapidly in most patients treated with heparin and leg elevation. There is no evidence that symptomatic improvement occurs more rapidly with thrombolytic agents than with heparin alone. The incidence of pulmonary embolism is rather low under full heparinization, and it probably would require a megatrial to investigate whether thrombolytic therapy influences the frequency of this complication. The initial fear that thrombolytic agents may augment the risk of embolism has never been substantiated in clinical studies.

EFFECT ON POST-THROMBOTIC SEQUELAE

Proponents of thrombolysis hope that vascular incompetence can be avoided by timely lysis of venous thrombi and that this will lead to a decrease in the occurrence of the postphlebitic syndrome. The late results of clinical trials comparing thrombolysis with conventional heparin treatment are equivocal. When patients are evaluated based on therapeutic response in the acute phase (lysis or no lysis) rather than on assigned treatment group, there is some evidence that successful lysis may lead to less late sequelae, with the exception of very extensive thrombosis from the calf veins to the pelvic veins. Thus, the early results of thrombolysis may be more important than the nature of the treatment.

PROCEDURE

Thrombolytic therapy may be considered in patients with proximal deep vein thrombosis of recent onset (< 5 days) causing severe pain and discomfort, provided that no increased risk of bleeding is present. Until recently, the thrombolytic agent was infused via a peripheral vein. A rarely applied procedure is so-called regional thrombolysis either via the femoral artery or via a foot vein with a tourniquet around the ankle. In recent years, catheters have been advanced in the obstructing thrombus for local thrombolysis as in peripheral arterial occlusion.[23–25] The catheter is introduced via the contralateral femoral vein, the ipsilateral popliteal vein, or the jugular vein. Urokinase, alteplase, and staphylokinase have been infused (Table 3–2). In the authors' center, local thrombolysis has been the usual procedure over the past 4 years for patients with leg thrombosis of recent onset extending into the iliac vein and causing severe pain and swelling. The same general contraindications as for cathe-

Table 3–2. Dosage Schemes in Catheter Thrombolysis for Deep Vein Thrombosis

Agent	Infusion	Reference
UK	250,000 IU/h (after bolus of 500,000 IU)	Bounameaux et al[22]
	150,000–200,000 IU/h	Comerota et al[23]
	2000–2500 IU/h	Semba and Dake[24]
rt-PA	3 mg/h	Bjarnason et al[25]
STAR	0.5–1 mg/h (after bolus of 2 mg)	Verhaeghe et al[26]

UK = urokinase; rt-PA = alteplase; STAR = staphylokinase.

ter-directed arterial thrombolysis are observed, in particular a 10-day delay after a surgical intervention is respected. With this protocol, a 75% recanalization rate can be obtained. An unexpected finding was the considerable number of patients with underlying anatomical venous anomalies and lesions, many of which are amenable to simultaneous correction with percutaneous interventional techniques.[26, 27] Infusion of thrombolytic drugs also may be considered in patients with severe symptoms from upper limb venous thrombosis or organ vein thrombosis.

More detailed discussion of clinical approaches and techniques used in venous thrombolysis is included in Chapters 17 and 18.

Pulmonary Embolism

Many physicians consider thrombolytic treatment a worthwhile option in patients with massive pulmonary embolism leading to overt hemodynamic instability and cardiogenic shock if no other facilities for aggressive intervention are immediately available. Although this approach may be lifesaving for individual patients, scientific proof of a decreased mortality in controlled trials appears hard to obtain. The use of thrombolytic therapy in patients with stable hemodynamic parameters and echocardiographic evidence of right ventricular dysfunction is more controversial.[28]

Over the years, a tendency to use shorter dosage regimens followed the evolution in myocardial infarction (Table 3–3). One study suggests that infusion of the thrombolytic agent into the pulmonary artery

Table 3–3. Thrombolysis Dosage Schemes in Pulmonary Embolism

Agent	Bolus	Infusion	Total Duration
rt-PA		50 mg/h	2 h
SK	250,000 IU	100,000 IU/h	24 h
UK	4400 IU/kg	4400 IU/kg/h	12 h

rt-PA, alteplase; SK, streptokinase; UK, urokinase.

is not superior to systemic infusion into a peripheral vein.[29] Nevertheless, if pulmonary angiography is the diagnostic technique, it appears almost natural to position the catheter into the embolus for local delivery (Fig. 3–4).

ADJUNCTIVE ANTITHROMBOTIC THERAPY

Heparin usually is given when a patient initially presents with acute limb ischemia. Well-managed anticoagulation does not hinder the start of catheter thrombolysis. Nevertheless, little scientific data exist that specifically address the potential advantages of heparinization during thrombolysis. In vitro and animal studies suggest that heparin may enhance fibrinolysis, but this has not been demonstrated for peripheral thrombolysis in humans. Concomitant heparin administrated either systemically or around the catheter through a proximal sheath may reduce the incidence of pericatheter thrombosis. After thrombolysis, there is a hypercoagulable state, and heparin can be expected to be of value in limiting rethrombosis after successful lysis. Physicians then may choose to continue anticoagulation orally, at least for a while, but current practice favors the use of aspirin to slow the progression of atherosclerosis and the occurrence of thrombotic complications.

In patients with venous thromboembolism, conventional anticoagulation is the mainstay of management, and this approach is unaltered even if systemic thrombolysis is used in the initial phase. Anticoagulation typically is started after termination of thrombolysis with streptokinase and urokinase; however, with alteplase, heparin frequently is given simultaneously. With local delivery via a catheter advanced into the thrombus or embolus, heparin also is infused concomitantly. No formal study that addresses the question of concomitant need and optimal dosage of heparin is available.

LABORATORY MONITORING

Repeated laboratory monitoring was common practice in the early days of systemic thrombolysis. Coagulation and fibrinolytic tests were advocated to detect and monitor the presence of a fibrinolytic state and to predict clinical outcome and the occurrence of complications. There is, however, no clear association between the result of any single coagulation or fibrinolytic test and reperfusion, reocclusion, or bleeding. With the use of lower dosage schemes or of shorter infusion times, much of the need for laboratory control has disappeared. Expert clinical and nursing care and hemodynamic surveillance may be more im-

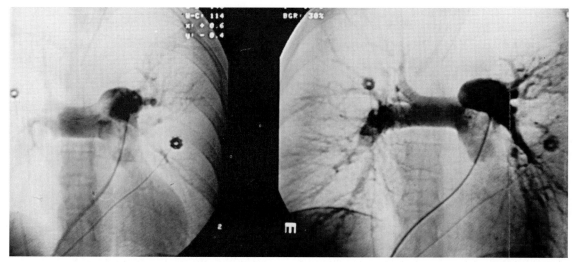

Figure 3–4. Massive pulmonary embolism in 35-year-old woman (left). Infusion of 100 mg alteplase over 2 hours via the catheter in the pulmonary artery results in a marked improvement of the perfusion (right).

portant. Daily estimation of hemoglobin, hematocrit, and renal function is considered prudent.

CONTRAINDICATIONS

Thrombolysis should not be started in any patient who has a bleeding disorder or an anatomic lesion that is expected to bleed. The usual contraindications are listed in Table 3–4. Patients with important or minor contraindications for systemic thrombolysis still may be considered for catheter-directed thrombolysis. However, these conditions still may increase the risk of bleeding during and after local thrombolysis and, as always, the potential risks should be weighed on an individual basis against the anticipated benefits. Additional minor risk factors for

Table 3–4. Contraindications to Thrombolysis

Major	Established cerebrovascular event (within last 2 mo)
	Bleeding diathesis or active bleeding
	Recent gastrointestinal bleeding (<10 d)
	Neurosurgery or intracranial trauma within last 3 mo
Relative Major	Cardiopulmonary resuscitation within last 10 d
	Surgery or trauma within last 10 d
	Uncontrolled hypertension
	Puncture of noncompressible vessel
	Intracranial tumor
Minor	Hepatic failure, particularly if coagulopathy
	Bacterial endocarditis
	Diabetic hemorrhagic retinopathy

From Working Party on Thrombolysis in the Management of Limb Ischemia: Thrombolysis in the management of limb peripheral arterial occlusion—A consensus document. Am J Cardiol 81:207–218, 1998.

bleeding include older age, female sex, and lower body weight.

COMPLICATIONS

Bleeding

The most feared complication with infusion of all thrombolytic agents is severe bleeding. It can be local (e.g., puncture site) or systemic, and results from lysis of a pre-existing hemostatic plug (thus, it also occurs with fibrin-specific agents), from the induced fibrinolytic or anticoagulated state, or from loss of the integrity of blood vessels (e.g., previous puncture).

Most of the data on the frequency of bleeding with thrombolysis are derived from large cardiologic trials. Patient selection, dosage of thrombolytic agents, and concomitant drugs often differ with thrombolysis for peripheral vascular disease. Berridge and colleagues[30] reviewed 19 prospective series of patients undergoing peripheral thrombolysis and found that the incidence of hemorrhagic stroke was 1%, whereas major hemorrhage (causing hypotension or requiring transfusion or other specific treatment) and minor hemorrhage occurred in 5.1% and 14.8% of patients, respectively. The British Thrombolysis Study Group reported an incidence of (hemorrhagic and ischemic) stroke of 2.3% (27/1157), half of which occurred during the thrombolytic procedure.[31] In prospective randomized trials comparing surgery to thrombolysis, intracranial bleeding rates with thrombolysis of between 1.2% and 2.1% were recorded.[32, 33, 34] In general, the bleeding risk with thrombolysis increases with the duration of the lytic therapy.

Most bleeding during catheter thrombolysis is local and occurs at sites of venous or arterial puncture.

Pericatheter bleeding is particularly common but is usually minor and can be controlled with prolonged local pressure. Bleeding into the retroperitoneal space from inadvertent posterior wall puncture frequently is overlooked until hypotension develops. Retroperitoneal or intra-abdominal bleeding also may occur spontaneously. Renal tract bleeding causing macroscopic hematuria is rare and may be the first sign of an anatomic bladder or kidney lesion. Gastrointestinal bleeding is equally rare and may be overt or occult. Early overt gastrointestinal blood loss frequently results from an undiagnosed peptic ulcer.

Management of severe bleeding follows a standard pattern: stop the thrombolytic agent and anticoagulants, replenish coagulation factors and fibrinolysis inhibitors by giving fresh frozen plasma or/and blood, and intervene surgically only to evacuate hematoma causing pressure phenomena on adjacent tissues or to repair a vascular injury that continues to bleed.[35] When a neurologic deficit occurs, an emergency computed tomography scan should determine whether the stroke is thrombotic or hemorrhagic.

Fragmentation and Embolization

The use of thrombolytic agents may cause fragmentation of thrombus and embolization of partially lysed thrombus. Small emboli may be clinically silent, but larger fragments are potentially more harmful and frequently lead to clinical symptoms. Transient acute deterioration of limb ischemia is fairly common during thrombolysis for arterial occlusion. Thrombolysis should be continued; thrombus aspiration may be an alternative if thrombolysis fails to improve the clinical condition.

Pulmonary embolism is rarely a significant problem during thrombolysis for venous thrombosis and does not justify routine prophylactic insertion of a vena cava filter.

Anaphylaxis

Anaphylaxis is rare with any of the thrombolytic agents, but early flushing, vasodilatation, rash, and hypotension are frequent with streptokinase. This so-called allergic reaction usually responds to discontinuation of the infusion and administration of hydrocortisone and antihistamines. Serum sickness-like illness is a rare late complication of streptokinase administration.

REFERENCES

1. Tillett WS, Sherry S: The effect in patients of streptococcal fibrinolysin (streptokinase) and streptococcal desoxyribo-nuclease on fibrous purulent and sanguinous pleural exsudations. J Clin Invest 28:173–179, 1949.
2. Collen D: On the regulation and control of fibrinolysis. Thromb Haemost 43:77–89, 1981.
3. Collen D, Lijnen HR: Molecular basis of fibrinolysis as relevant for thrombolytic therapy. Thromb Haemost 74:167–171, 1995.
4. Carmeliet P, Schoonjans L, Kieckens L, et al: Physiological consequences of loss of plasminogen activator gene function in mice. Nature 368:419–424, 1994.
5. Verstraete M, Verhaeghe R, Peerlinck K, et al: Haematological disorders. In Speight TM, Holfold NHG (eds): Avery's Drug Treatment. Auckland, Adis International, 1997, pp 1163–1251.
6. Lijnen HR, Collen D, Verstraete M: Thrombolytic agents. In Verstraete M, Fuster V, Topol EJ (eds): Cardiovascular Thrombosis: Thrombocardiology and Thromboneurology. Philadelphia, Lippincott-Raven, 1998, pp 301–320.
7. Verstraete M, Lijnen HR, Collen D: Thrombolytic agents in development. Drugs 50:29–42, 1995.
8. Collen D: Staphylokinase: A potent, uniquely fibrin-selective thrombolytic agent. Nature Med 4:279–284, 1998.
9. Amery A, Deloof W, Vermylen J, et al: Outcome of recent thromboembolic occlusions of limb arteries treated with streptokinase. Br Med J 4:639–644, 1970.
10. Verstraete M, Vermylen J, Donati MB: The effect of streptokinase infusion on chronic arterial occlusions and stenoses. Ann Intern Med 74:377–382, 1971.
11. Pilger E, Decrinis M, Stark G, et al: Thrombolytic treatment and balloon angioplasty in chronic occlusion of the aortic bifurcation. Ann Intern Med 120:40–44, 1994.
12. Chesterman CN, Nash T, Biggs JC: Small vessel thrombosis following vascular injury: Successful treatment with a low-dose intra-arterial infusion of streptokinase. Br J Surg 58:582–583, 1971.
13. Dotter CT, Rösch J, Seaman AJ: Selective clot lysis with low-dose streptokinase. Radiology 111:31–37, 1974.
14. Hess H, Ingrisch H, Mietaschk A, et al: Local low-dose thrombolytic therapy of peripheral arterial occlusions. N Engl J Med 307:1627–1630, 1982.
15. McNamara TO, Fischer JR: Thrombolysis of peripheral arterial and graft occlusions: Improved results using high-dose urokinase. AJR Am J Roentgenol 144:769–775, 1985.
16. Hartmann JR, Enger EL, Villiard EM, et al: Dose ranging trial of intraarterial r-prourokinase (A-74187) for thrombolysis of total peripheral arterial occlusions. J Am Coll Cardiol 23(Suppl):95A (Abstract 869–65), 1994.
17. Vanderschueren S, Stockx L, Wilms G, et al: Thrombolytic therapy of peripheral arterial occlusion with recombinant staphylokinase. Circulation 92:2050–2057, 1995.
18. Collen D, Moreau H, Stockx L, et al: Recombinant staphylokinase variants with altered reactivity: II, Thrombolytic properties and antibody induction. Circulation 84:1216–1234, 1996.
19. Collen D, Stockx L, Lacroix H, et al: Recombinant staphylokinase variants with altered reactivity: IV, Identification of variants with reduced antibody induction but intact potency. Circulation 95:463–472, 1997.
20. Comerota AJ, Aldridge SE: Thrombolytic therapy for deep venous thrombosis: A clinical review. Can J Surg 36:359–364, 1993.
21. Goldhaber SZ, Buring JE, Lipnick RJ, et al: Pooled analyses of randomized trials of streptokinase and heparin in phlebographically documented acute deep venous thrombosis. Am J Med 76:393–397, 1984.
22. Bounameaux H, Banga JA, Bluhmki E, et al: Double-blind, randomized comparison of systemic continuous infusion of 0.25 versus 0.50 mg/kg/24h of alteplase over 3 to 7 days for treatment of deep venous thrombosis in heparinized patients: Results of the European thrombolysis with rt-PA in venous thrombosis (ETTT) trial. Thromb Haemost 67:306–309, 1992.
23. Comerota AJ, Aldridge SC, Cohen G, et al: A strategy of aggressive regional therapy for acute iliofemoral venous thrombosis with contemporary venous thrombectomy or catheter-directed thrombolysis. J Vasc Surg 20:244–254, 1994.
24. Semba CP, Dake MD: Iliofemoral deep venous thrombosis: Aggressive therapy with catheter-directed thrombolysis. Radiology 191:487–494, 1994.
25. Bjarnason H, Kruse JR, Asinger DA: Iliofemoral deep venous thrombosis: Safety and efficacy outcome during 5 years of

catheter-directed thrombolytic therapy. J Vasc Interv Radiol 8:405–418, 1997.

26. Verhaeghe R, Stockx L, Lacroix H, et al: Catheter-directed lysis of iliofemoral vein thrombosis with use of rt-PA. Eur Radiol 7:996–1001, 1997.

27. Heymans S, Verhaeghe R, Stockx L, et al: Feasibility study of catheter-directed thrombolysis with recombinant staphylokinase in deep vein thrombosis. Thromb Haemost 79:517–519, 1998.

28. Goldhaber SZ: Medical progress: Pulmonary embolism. N Engl J Med 339:93–104, 1998.

29. Verstraete M, Miller GAH, Bounameaux H, et al: Intravenous and intrapulmonary recombinant tissue-type plasminogen activator in the treatment of acute massive pulmonary embolism. Circulation 77:353–360, 1988.

30. Berridge DC, Niakin GS, Hopkinson BR: Local low-dose intra-arterial thrombolytic therapy, the risk of major stroke and haemorrhage. Br J Surg 76:1230–1233, 1989.

31. Dawson K, Armon A, Braithwaite B, et al: Stroke during intra-arterial thrombolysis: A survey of experience in the UK (Abstract). Br J Surg 83:568, 1996.

32. The STILE Investigators: Results of a prospective randomized trial evaluating surgery versus thrombolysis for ischemia of the lower extremity. The STILE trial. Ann Surg 220:251–268, 1994.

33. Ouriel K, Veith FJ, Sasahara AA, for the Thrombolysis or Peripheral Arterial Surgery (TOPAS) investigators: Thrombolysis or peripheral arterial surgery: Phase I results. J Vasc Surg 23:64–75, 1996.

34. Ouriel K, Veith FJ, Sasahara AA, for the Thrombolysis or Peripheral Arterial Surgery (TOPAS) Investigators: A comparison of recombinant urokinase with vascular surgery as initial treatment for acute arterial occlusion of the legs. N Engl J Med 338:1105–1111, 1998.

35. Working Party on Thrombolysis in the Management of Limb Ischemia: Thrombolysis in the management of limb peripheral arterial occlusion—a consensus document. Am J Cardiol 81:207–218, 1998.

Chapter 4 — Atherectomy

Endovascular Contributors: *Anna-Marie Belli and Tim M. Buckenham*
Surgical Contributors: *Samuel S. Ahn and Eric J. Daniels*

Percutaneous atherectomy was introduced in the 1980s as an alternative to percutaneous transluminal balloon angioplasty (PTA) in the management of peripheral vascular disease.[1] The various devices available remove plaque by cutting, shaving, or pulverizing. Atherectomy was considered theoretically more appealing than PTA, and it was hoped that the acute occlusion and restenosis rates of PTA could be lowered by the local reduction of plaque burden, thereby reducing the number of potential proliferative cells. Devices such as the Simpson Atherectomy Catheter were designed to give a larger postprocedural lumen than that provided by PTA and to avoid the fissuring and plaque disruption caused by radial balloon expansion.[2] The ideal device would remove all local plaque, leaving a smooth, nondissected lumen of physiologic size. Atherectomy seemed particularly suited to the treatment of eccentric disease, in which balloon dilatation dilates the normal wall with little or no effect on the diseased aspect. However, clinical trials show that atherectomy is at best only equal to PTA in the treatment of atherosclerosis. Because of the larger size, complexity, and cost of devices, atherectomy has not become a serious rival to PTA. Its current indications are primarily in the management of neointimal hyperplasia (NIH), eccentric atheromatous lesions, valvular obliteration of vein grafts, resection of obstructing intimal flaps,[3] and removal of lesions for which a histologic specimen is required.

MECHANISM OF ACTION

Despite the fact that percutaneous atherectomy (PA) has a different mechanism of restoring the lumen in treatment of patients with atherosclerotic arterial disease compared with that of PTA, the artery's response to injury is the same, and both are dependent on the injury to the medial smooth muscle cells and the depth of the medial injury. The precise mechanism of the medial injury is largely irrelevant.[4]

The Simpson directional atherectomy catheter (DA) has been the most extensively studied atherectomy device. Animal models have demonstrated that the large clefts formed by the cutting blade are surrounded by inflammatory cells and filled with thrombus. The thrombus is later replaced by cellular elements. The distinctive stretching and dissection effect seen with PTA is uncommon with DA despite its eccentrically positioned balloon. There has been controversy regarding the DA method of luminal gain, and some investigators have called it "facilitated angioplasty," claiming that the lumen is expanded by a Dotter effect and balloon dilatation.[5] This has been refuted by a magnetic resonance imaging (MRI) study of eccentric stenoses caused by fibrous plaque. Patients with these stenoses have been treated with DA, which indicates significant luminal gain compared with that achieved by PTA, particularly in patients who have plaques with a collagen cap. In patients with this type of plaque, PTA resulted in dilatation of the nondiseased segment. This study also confirmed evidence offered by other investigators that luminal gain is not caused by dilatation of the eccentric balloon.[6]

DEVICE TYPES

Percutaneous atherectomy devices can be divided into two broad groups according to their mode of action. These are the extirpative and ablative types.[2]

Extirpative Devices

This group of devices shaves or cuts plaque and collects fragments in a chamber that can be extracted and emptied. These devices may have a circumferential or eccentric cutting blade (Table 4–1).

SIMPSON DIRECTIONAL ATHERECTOMY CATHETER

This percutaneous device uses a rapidly rotating cup-shaped blade that is forced against the plaque by an

Table 4–1. Extirpative Atherectomy Devices

Device	Indications	Advantages
Simpson DA	Eccentric stenoses NIH Intimal flaps	Cuts lumen larger than size of catheter
Arrow-Fischell PAC	Eccentric/concentric atheroma NIH Intimal flaps	Flexible catheter Concentric cutting
Omnicath	Eccentric stenoses Intimal flaps NIH	Cuts lumen larger than size of catheter
Redha-cut	Eccentric or concentric atheroma NIH Intimal flaps	Motorless Cuts lumen larger than size of catheter Concentric cutting

DA = directional atherectomy; NIH = neointimal hyperplasia; PAC = pullback atherectomy catheter.

eccentric balloon[7, 8] (Fig. 4–1). The device can be oriented by use of fluoroscopy in conjunction with a proximal wheel that rotates the device. The battery-powered blade is advanced with a lever action that pushes the shavings into the collection chamber of the nose cone. The collection chamber can be unscrewed and emptied as required. The device comes in a range of sizes for peripheral vascular use. It is placed through a sheath (7–11 French [F]) and operated over a guide wire (either 0.018 in. or 0.035 in.), but it cannot be passed over the aortic bifurcation or steered around tight curves. Modifications, such as integral intravascular ultrasound (IVUS) or an extended collection chamber, are available.

ARROW-FISCHELL PULLBACK ATHERECTOMY CATHETER

This device differs from the Simpson DA catheter in that it has the capability of cutting circumferentially,

although a shielded device is also available for extrinsic lesions. It relies on extrinsic compression of the artery by a sphygmomanometer cuff that opposes the plaque to the cutting edge of the rapidly rotating circular blade[9, 10] (Fig. 4–2). Unlike the Simpson device, the Arrow-Fischell Pullback Atherectomy Catheter (PAC) blade is withdrawn toward the operator, and the cuttings are collected in the distal chamber (Fig. 4–3). The device is placed through a sheath and over a guide wire (0.018 in.) and is available in three sizes (2.5, 3.0, and 3.5 mm). The smallest device is used in the crural circulation. Contrast medium and saline solution can be injected through a central lumen or via the access sheath. The long, tapered nose cone of the latter device allows better transition across the diseased segment. The blade is motor driven and rotates at 2000 revolutions per minute (rpm). This circumferential cutting technique has the potential advantage of cutting in a single pass a lumen equal in diameter to that of the cutting blade while retaining coaxial alignment. The device's main limitations are that it cannot be used in the suprainguinal circulation or in incompressible vessels.

REDHA-CUT

Unlike other extirpative devices, the Redha-cut catheter is not motor driven but has 6 to 8 cutting blades that can be opened and closed like an umbrella by a mechanical back-and-forth movement of a hollow, blunt-tipped cylinder (Fig. 4–4). The cutting edges are designed to avoid vessel perforation by bending slightly inward. The device is introduced through a sheath (up to 9 F) and may be advanced without a wire or over a 0.010-inch guide wire. The cutting blades are opened beyond the diseased segment, and the catheter is then withdrawn a distance equal to the

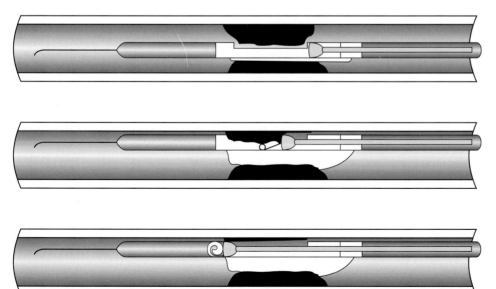

Figure 4–1. Method of action of Simpson directional atherectomy catheter.

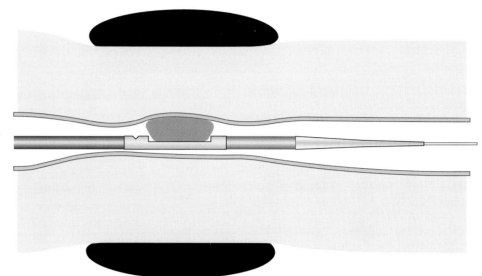

Figure 4–2. Extrinsic compression of artery by sphygmomanometer cuff.

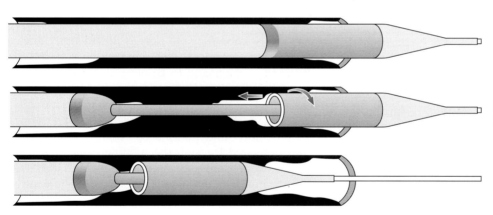

Figure 4–3. Method of action of pullback atherectomy catheter.

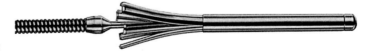

Figure 4–4. The Redha-cut device, open and closed. (Reproduced with permission of Sherine Med AG.)

length of the blades, which cut through the occluding material. This material is trapped when the cylinder is closed and removed with the device. The device can be reinserted, and further resection may be performed until the diseased segment is completely debulked. The device is available in four sizes (open diameter of 4 to 8 mm).

OMNICATH

This atherectomy catheter is similar to the Simpson device in that it uses a motor-driven 11,000 rpm eccentric cutting window that is pressed against the atheromatous material.[11] However, instead of a balloon, an extendable deflector wire provides the lateralizing force that regulates the depth of the cut, so that a single device can be applied to a variety of vessel sizes (Fig. 4–5). Constant aspiration is required because, unlike the PAC or Simpson devices, the Omnicath has no collection chamber. The disadvantage of this is that hemodilution caused by excess aspiration is possible. In addition, the device only passes over a .014-inch wire.

Ablative Devices

These devices fragment plaque and either aspirate or liberate it into the circulation as microemboli, which

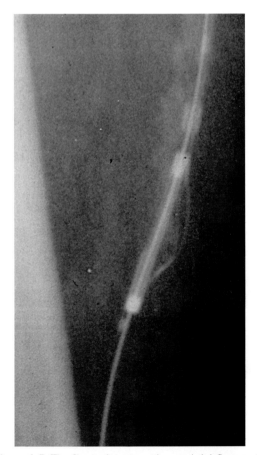

Figure 4–5. The Omnicath in situ with extended deflector wire.

are ultimately removed by the reticuloendothelial system. Many such catheters have been developed, but the main types are described herein.

AUTH ROTABLATOR

This device is characterized by its very high speed rotation of 100,000 to 200,000 rpm and its oval-shaped burr, which is coated with diamond chips that function as multiple microblades. The burrs vary in size from 1.25 to 6 mm. The burr is passed down the artery and through the occluded segment, with sequentially larger tips used until an adequate lumen is restored. The particulate matter produced is of small size (smaller than an erythrocyte) and is removed by the reticuloendothelial system. The device is placed over a guide wire and can be used for eccentric or concentric plaque. Enthusiasm for this device has been limited by its high complication rate, particularly with incidence of spasm, early rethrombosis, or recurrent stenosis. Asymptomatic gross hemagloburia is a common finding, and clinical embolic events have been reported. Most rotablator cases require adjunctive PTA.

TRAC-WRIGHT

Previously known as the Kensey atherectomy device, this system comprises a rotating cam with an internal drive cable connected to an electric motor capable of up to 100,000 rpm. It was developed to help recanalize long femoropopliteal occlusions and remove obstructing material by a combination of mechanical fragmentation and pharmacologic thrombolysis. The fluid delivered through the rotating catheter consists of physiologic saline, contrast medium, and urokinase as indicated by Kensey and associates.[12] The contrast in the fluid enables the operator to assess the point at which the catheter re-enters the patent artery. This device is available in 5-, 8-, and 10-F sizes but is unable to produce a lumen larger than the size of the device, and subsequent PTA is nearly always required.

TRANSLUMINAL EXTRACTION CATHETER

This device consists of a hollow catheter with a distal cutting blade in the shape of a cone (Fig. 4–6). The device is placed over a 0.014-inch wire and rotated at 700 rpm by a hand-held motor. As the catheter is passed through the lesion, the excised tissue is withdrawn as a result of negative pressure created by connection of the proximal end of the catheter to a vacuum bottle. The main limitation of this device is that adjunctive PTA is also required.

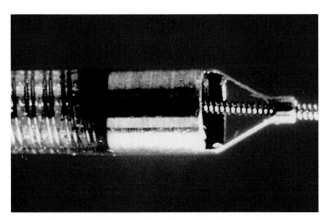

Figure 4–6. The tip of transluminal extraction catheter.

COMPLICATIONS OF ATHERECTOMY

The complications encountered with atherectomy devices are related to their size and mechanism of action.

Complications related to the size of the catheter occur at the puncture site and are more likely with larger catheters. Some devices require a 12-F sheath. The large hematoma produced by this size catheter may need surgical evacuation or it may form a pseudoaneurysm. Kim and associates[13] reported a 4% rate (3 of 77 cases) of pseudoaneurysm formation with use of the Simpson device. The incidence of hematoma formation varies from 1 to 14% and is similar for all devices.[13–15]

Complications also occur at the site of atherectomy, and these may be caused by dissection, spasm, thrombosis, or perforation. The rate of thrombosis at the atherectomy site for most devices ranges from 1 to 3%,[7, 16, 17] but patients who develop this complication are responsive to treatment with thrombolysis. In 1989, Wholey and associates[18] reported an 8% thrombosis rate with use of the Trac-Wright catheter. However, the highest reported rates of thrombosis (8 to 25%) have occurred with use of the Auth Rotablator[2, 19] and are related to a number of factors, such as creation of obstructing intimal flaps, dissection, and vasospasm. Dissection (2 to 6% rate) and spasm (11 to 23% rate) have been particular problems related to use of the Auth Rotablator, and they are attributed to the use of a large burr, long rotation sequences, and rotation speed.

Perforation at the puncture site has been reported most frequently with the Trac-Wright catheter, with rates varying from 7 to 24%.[20, 21] In these cases, perforations induced by the rotating catheter occurred mostly in heavily calcified lesions and probably were related to the catheter's tendency to take the path of least resistance.

Other potential complications at the puncture site can occur in patients who are being treated for reste-

nosis within stents. Extirpative atherectomy may cut through and resect small segments of the stent (Fig. 4–7), although no adverse effects from this have been reported. Stent entanglement can occur with the Redha-cut, and if care is not taken, the stent may become dislodged (Fig. 4–8).

Because the mechanism of action of these catheters is either to resect or pulverize obstructing material, it is possible for embolic occlusion to occur downstream from the treatment site. The purpose of extirpative devices is to remove this material by collecting it in a chamber. However, this may fail, and a distal embolization rate between 2 and 4% has been reported with use of extirpative devices.[7, 13]

Ablative devices, on the other hand, aim to reduce the debris to particulate matter smaller than the size of erythrocytes. This goal is obviously not always reached, because embolization rates of 7 to 20%[22–25] have been reported with use of both the Trac-Wright catheter and the Auth Rotablator. Gross hemoglobinuria without clinical sequelae has been reported with use of the Auth Rotablator in 63% of cases.

RESULTS

Atherosclerotic Disease

The Simpson directional atherectomy catheter has been extensively evaluated in the treatment of peripheral vascular disease, and most comparative studies have used this device. Unfortunately, many patients treated with primary atherectomy have had subsequent balloon angioplasty, which makes analysis of the data difficult (Table 4–2). One of the largest series was reported by Kim and associates in 1992.[13] In this series, 77 patients were treated. Their lesions consisted of supra- and infrainguinal atheroma and bypass grafts, and 68 patients were treated with DA

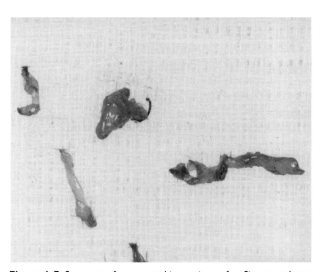

Figure 4–7. Segments of stent noted in specimen after Simpson atherectomy of stent restenosis.

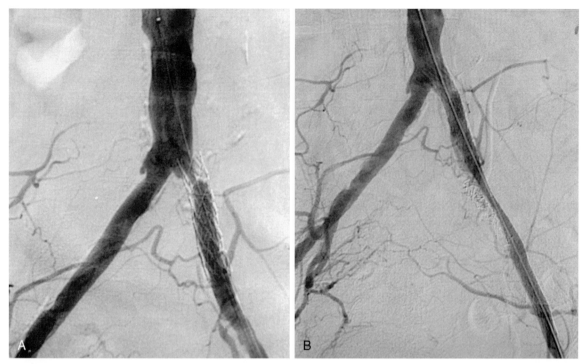

Figure 4–8. *A,* Restenosis in proximal iliac stent. *B,* Blades of Redha-cut became entangled with stent, causing stent dislodgement. Placement of new stent was required.

alone. The technical success was high (92%), but the long-term results are difficult to analyze because the majority of patients had only ankle brachial indices and clinical follow-up. No differences in patency were reported on the bases of lesion location, eccentricity, calcification, and ulceration.

Vroegindeweij and associates in 1995[26] reported a 2-year patency rate of 42%, which is similar, if not inferior, to that of PTA. They conducted a randomized prospective trial comparing PTA with Simpson (DA) catheter in the treatment of patients with femoro-popliteal lesions. After 2 years, primary angiographic patency was 67% in the PTA group and 44% in the DA group, respectively. The clinical success rate was 79% in the PTA group and 56% in the DA group. These results support the view that DA confers no advantage over PTA when it is performed below the inguinal ligament. A multicenter safety and efficacy

trial using the Arrow-Fischell PAC was published by White and coworkers.[9] Infrainguinal atherectomy was performed in 190 patients (246 lesions). Again, these data are difficult to assess because 51% of the patients underwent adjunctive PTA. The technical success rate was 99%, and there was a mean reduction of the stenosis rate from 84 to 25% ($\pm$ 17%). No follow-up data are available. Results from our own institution indicated a 97.4% technical success rate in the treatment of patients with infrainguinal lesions. However, 69.2% of patients required balloon dilatation to achieve an adequate arterial lumen[10] (Fig. 4–9).

The Omnicath has no published human data, but animal work suggests that it is technically capable of treating patients who have atherosclerotic lesions.[27] These results again emphasize that at best, extirpative atherectomy is equal in efficacy to PTA in the treatment of atherosclerotic lesions, but, in many cases, PTA is not obviated by primary atherectomy.

Ablative atherectomy has an inferior track record compared with that of extirpative atherectomy. The extensively evaluated Trac-Wright catheter has a reported technical success rate of 88 to 100% and patencies of 25 to 45% after 1 year[18, 20–23]; again, patients uniformly required adjunctive PTA. This is a particular problem with use of ablative devices, because they produce a lumen equivalent only to the size of the device. The Collaborative Rotablator Atherectomy Group (CRAG)[28] reported a disappointing patency rate of 18.6% after 2 years. Ahn and associates[25] found

Table 4–2. Simpson Atherectomy: Results

Author	Patients	Lesion	Technical Success (%)	Patency 1 Year (%)
Kim et al (1992)[13]	77	85	92	92*
Vroegindeweij et al (1995)[26]	38	38	92	42
Tielbeek et al (1997)[38]	73	73	96	—

*Calculated probable, not actual, patency.

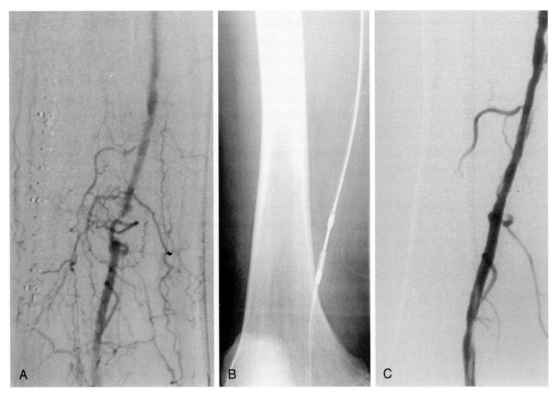

Figure 4–9. *A,* A short (SFA) occlusion before use of pullback atherectomy catheter (PAC). *B,* The pullback atherectomy catheter (PAC) is advanced over a wire through the occlusion and opened. *C,* Lumen following atherectomy and percutaneous transluminal balloon angioplasty (PTA).

a similar patency rate of 12% at 2 years and reported that the length and type of lesion did not affect the patency rate.

A report of results of use of the Redha-cut in 70 patients who had symptomatic femoropopliteal lesions showed 1-year patency rates of 81% in primary lesions, but all patients required adjunctive balloon dilatation.[29]

Restenosis, Stents, and Bypass Grafts

The primary cause of failure with use of infrainguinal vein or prosthetic bypass grafts is that patients develop anastomotic stenoses, usually located in the distal graft. These stenoses are usually within the graft and even occur in prosthetic grafts with a venous interposition cuff. Treatment of these patients with PTA has a high technical success rate but little durability. Most authors agree that surgery, such as vein patch angioplasty or graft revision, is superior to PTA.[30] DA is an alternative treatment modality that enables the operator to extract NIH. The theoretical advantage of atherectomy in treating NIH relates first to the fact that PTA does not produce the controlled tear that is seen in native vessels. Second, the conduits being treated are often prosthetic tubes that cannot dilate in the same way as a similar-sized artery. Extirpative atherectomy is the most useful tool for treating

NIH, because a lumen larger than the catheter size can be produced (Fig. 4–10). Clearly, removing NIH does not reduce the stimulus for it to form, but, theoretically, the greater the luminal size on completion, the longer the interval before significant stenosis will recur. Published results regarding atherectomy for treatment of patients with NIH are few (Table 4–3). Thirty-eight of the 70 patients with femoropopliteal lesions reported by Dai-Do and colleagues[29] had symptomatic native vessel restenoses that occurred after they underwent PTA. These patients were treated with the Redha-cut device and showed a significantly lower 1-year patency rate compared with that of patients who had primary lesions (41 vs. 81%). The Simpson device has been used in two series in the treatment of patients with anastomotic bypass grafts. Vinnacombe and colleagues[31] showed a 100% technical success rate in 7 patients, with an 86% 6-month patency rate. Dolmatch and associates[32] treated 25 patients with DA and achieved a technical success rate of 92%. They reported less than a 50% restenosis rate in 74% of the sites after 13 months. These results are encouraging, especially when compared with those of balloon angioplasty for anastomotic bypass grafts, but longer follow-up is required. Restenosis within stents has been treated with the Simpson Atherectomy Catheter[33–35] (Fig. 4–11), the Pullback Atherectomy Catheter,[10] and the Redha-cut (Fig. 4–12). Again, numbers are small and follow-up is short,

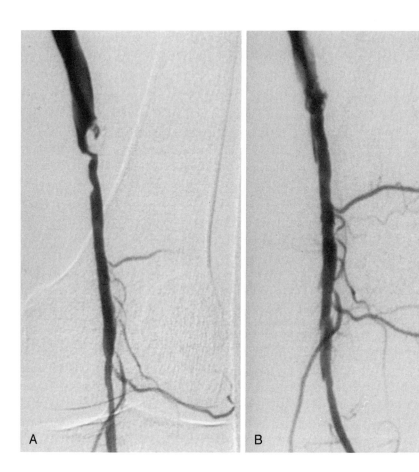

Figure 4–10. A, Neointimal hyperplasia (NIH) at distal end of polytetrafluoroethylene (PTFE) graft. B, Postatherectomy with the Simpson atherectomy catheter. No balloon dilatation was necessary.

Table 4–3. Extirpative Atherectomy: Results in the Treatment of Bypass Graft, Arterial Graft, and Stent Retenosis

Author	Conduit	Device	Lesions	Results
Dolmatch et al (1995)[32]	Bypass grafts	Simpson	n = 25	Technical success 92% <50% restenosis at 74% of sites at 13 mo
Vinnicombe et al (1995)[31]	Bypass grafts	Simpson	n = 7	Technical success 100% 6-mo patency 86%
Dai-Do et al (1998)[29]	Native arteries	Redha	n = 38	Technical success 100% 6-mo patency 62% 1-yr patency 41%
Sapoval et al (1996)[34]	Stents	Simpson	n = 2	Technical success 100% 2-yr patency 50%
Vorwerk and Guenther (1990)[33]	Stents	Simpson	n = 7	Technical success 100% 9-mo patency 71%
Ettles et al (1998)[35]	Stents	Simpson	n = 12	Technical success 95% 3 restenoses at mean 10.5 mo

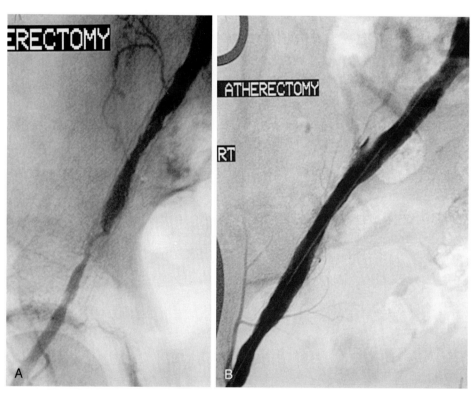

Figure 4–11. *A,* Restenosis in distal end of iliac stent. *B,* No residual stenosis following directional atherectomy (DA).

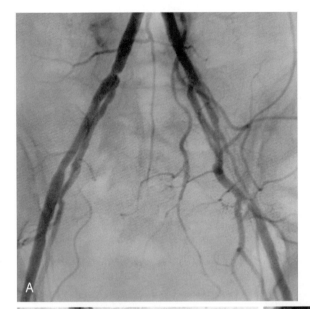

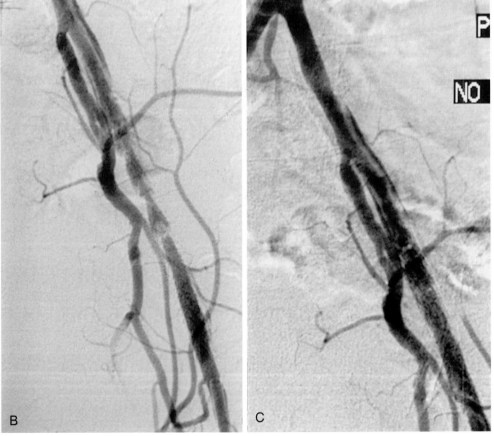

Figure 4–12. *A*, Restenosis along whole length of iliac stent. *B*, Imprint of Redha-cut device during atherectomy. *C*, End result following repeat atherectomy (no balloon dilatation).

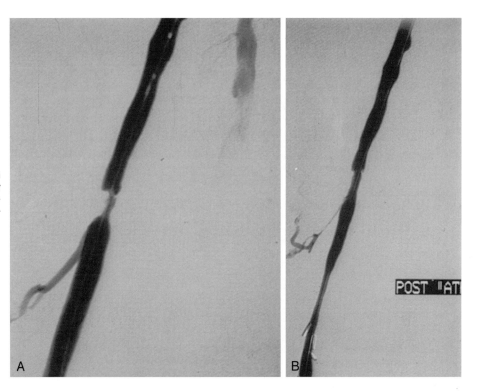

Figure 4–13. *A,* Significant stenosis in vein graft caused by valve. *B,* Postatherectomy appearance with use of the Simpson atherectomy device (no balloon dilatation performed).

but further evaluation is worthwhile in light of the disappointing results of balloon dilatation.

Obstructing Intimal Flaps and Venous Valves

Nonobstructing intimal flaps are commonly seen in patients after PTA. Occasionally, these flaps can obstruct blood flow, leading to thrombosis at the PTA site. Stenting is an acceptable method of "pinning back" such flaps, but atherectomy can be performed as an alternative. Maynar and colleagues[3] reported the use of the Simpson DA catheter to resect obstructing flaps after PTA in three femoral arteries and one common iliac artery. Grubnic and associates[10] successfully used the pullback atherectomy catheter for post-PTA obstructing intimal flaps in three femoral arteries.

Valvular obliteration in vein grafts can also be achieved by atherectomy. In situ vein grafts of venous valves are usually obliterated at the time of surgery. If only partially disrupted or missed, they are a cause of early graft failure. Various methods of postoperative disruption of these valves have been reported with use of myocardial biopsy forceps and the Wittens variable valvulotome cutter.[36] The only atherectomy catheter reported is the Simpson DA catheter[37] (Fig. 4–13), although any of the extirpative atherectomy catheters would be feasible for this purpose.

CONCLUSION

It is difficult to assess the efficacy of atherectomy because of varying reporting standards and, in particular, the confusing use of adjunctive PTA in many cases. Currently, extirpative atherectomy devices (particularly the Simpson DA catheter) have the most established role in the treatment of atheroma, and there is increasing experience in the treatment of native vessel bypass grafts or stent restenoses.

Overall, the technology is appealing, but the results are disappointing. Atherectomy has not been established as a front-line tool in the treatment of peripheral vascular disease. It may have a role in resecting NIH to maintain graft or stent patency, but, ultimately, these devices do not modify the artery's response to injury, and, therefore, occlusion and restenosis rates are high.

REFERENCES

1. Simpson JB, Johnson DE, Thapliyal HV, et al: Transluminal atherectomy: A new approach to the treatment of atherosclerotic vascular disease. Circulation 72:146, 1985.
2. Ahn SS, Concepcion B: The current status of peripheral atherectomy. Eur J Vasc Endovasc Surg 10:133, 1995.
3. Maynar M, Reyes R, Cabrera V, et al: Percutaneous atherectomy as an alternative treatment for post angioplasty obstructive intimal flaps. Radiology 170:1029, 1989.
4. Johnson DE: Directional peripheral atherectomy: Histopathologic aspects of a new interventional technique. J Vasc Intervent Radiol 1:29, 1990.
5. Safian R, Gelbfish J, Erny R, et al: Coronary Atherectomy.

Clinical, angiographic, and histological findings and observations regarding potential mechanisms. Circulation 82:69, 1990.

6. Toussaint J-F, Southern JF, Kantor HL, et al: Behaviour of atherosclerotic plaque components after in vitro angioplasty and atherectomy studied by High Field MR imaging. Magn Reson Imaging 16:175, 1998.

7. Simpson JB, Selman MR, Robertson GC, et al: Transluminal atherectomy for occlusive peripheral vascular disease. Am J Cardiol 61:96G, 1988.

8. Belli A-M, Cumberland DC: Percutaneous atherectomy—early experience in Sheffield. Clin Radiol 40:122, 1989.

9. White CJ and the PAC Investigators: Peripheral atherectomy with the pullback atherectomy catheter: Procedural safety and efficacy in a multicentre trial. J Endovasc Surg 5:9, 1995.

10. Grubnic S, Heenan SD, Buckenham TM, et al: Evaluation of the pullback atherectomy catheter in the treatment of lower limb vascular disease. Cardiovasc Intervent Radiol 19:152, 1996.

11. Mazur W, Ali NM, Rodgers GP, et al: Directional atherectomy with the OmniCath: A unique new catheter system. Cathet Cardiovasc Diagn 31:79, 1994.

12. Kensey K, Zeitler E, Rees M, et al: The Kensey catheter. In Zeitler E, Seiforth W (eds): Pros and Cons in PTA and Auxiliary Methods. Berlin, Springer-Verlag, 1989, pp 116–122.

13. Kim D, Gianturco LE, Porter DA, et al: Peripheral directional atherectomy: Four year experience. Radiology 183:773, 1992.

14. Von Polnitz A, Nerlich A, Berger H, et al: Percutaneous peripheral atherectomy. J Am Coll Cardiol 15:682, 1990.

15. Graor RA, Whitlow PL: Transluminal atherectomy for occlusive peripheral vascular disease. J Am Coll Cardiol 15:1551, 1990.

16. Wholey MH, Jarmolowski CR: New reperfusion devices: The Kensey Catheter, the atherolytic reperfusion wire device and the transluminal extraction catheter. Radiology 172:947, 1989.

17. Hinohara T, Selman MR, Robertson GC, et al: Directional atherectomy: New approaches for treatment of obstructive coronary and peripheral vascular disease. Circulation 81:79, 1990.

18. Wholey MH, Smith JAM, Godlewski P, et al: Recanalization of total arterial occlusions with the Kensey dynamic angioplasty catheter. Radiology 172:95, 1989.

19. Henry M, Amor M, Ethevenot G, et al: Percutaneous peripheral atherectomy using the Rotablator: A single center experience. J Endovasc Surg 2:51, 1995.

20. Meloni T, Carbonnato P, Mistretta L, et al: Arterial recanalization with the Kensey catheter. Radiol Med (Torino) 86:509, 1993.

21. Snyder SO, Wheeler JR, Gregory RT, et al: The Trac-Wright atherectomy device. In Ahn SS, Moore WS (eds): Endovascular Surgery. Philadephia, WB Saunders, 1992, pp 287–294.

22. Desbrosses D, Petit H, Torres E, et al: Percutaneous atherectomy with the Kensey catheter: Early and midterm results in femoropopliteal occlusions unsuitable for conventional angioplasty. Ann Vasc Surg 4:550, 1990.

23. Triller J, Do DD, Maddern G, et al: Femoropopliteal artery occlusion: Clinical experience with the Kensey catheter. Radiology 182:257, 1992.

24. Dyet JF: High speed rotational angioplasty in occluded peripheral arteries. J Intervent. Radiol 7:1, 1992.

25. Ahn SS, Yeatman LR, Deutsch LS, et al: Intraoperative peripheral rotary atherectomy: Early and late clinical results. Ann Vasc Surg 6:272, 1992.

26. Vroegindeweij D, Tielbeek AV, Buth J, et al: Direction atherectomy vs balloon angioplasty in segmental femoropopliteal artery disease: Two year follow-up with colour flow duplex scanning. J Vasc Surg 21:255, 1995.

27. Sapoval MR, Gaux JC, Bruneval P, et al: Animal evaluation of the prototype OmniCath atherectomy catheter. Cardiovasc Intervent Radiol 17:226, 1994.

28. The Collaborative Rotablator Atherectomy Group (CRAG): Peripheral atherectomy with the rotablator: A multicenter report. J Vasc Surg 19:509, 1994.

29. Dai-Do D, Triller J, Baumgartner I, et al: A new approach to plaque removal: The Redha-cut device. J Invasive Cardiol 10:578, 1998.

30. Perler BA, Osterman FA, Mitchell SE, et al: Balloon dilatation versus surgical revision of infrainguinal autogenous vein graft stenoses: Long term follow-up. J Cardiovasc Surg 31:686, 1990.

31. Vinnacombe S, Heenan S, Belli A-M, et al: Directional atherectomy in the treatment of anastomotic neointimal hyperplasia associated with prosthetic arterial grafts: Technique and preliminary results. Clin Radiol 49:773, 1994.

32. Dolmatch BL, Gray RJ, Horton KM, et al: Treatment of anastomotic bypass graft stenosis with directional atherectomy: Short term and intermediate term results. J Vasc Intervent Radiol 6:105, 1995.

33. Vorwerk D, Guenther RW: Removal of intimal hyperplasia in vascular endoprostheses by atherectomy and balloon dilatation. Am J Roentgenol 154:617, 1990.

34. Sapoval MR, Long AL, Pagny J-Y, et al: Outcome of percutaneous intervention in iliac artery stents. Radiology 198:481, 1996.

35. Ettles DF, MacDonald AW, Burgess PA, et al: Directional atherectomy in iliac stent failure: Clinical technique and histopathological correlation. Cardiovasc Intervent Radiol 21:475, 1998.

36. Cook TA, Galland RB, Torrie EPH: Percutaneous ablation of retained valve cusps following in situ femoropopliteal bypass. J Intervent Radiol 10:91, 1995.

37. Walker J, Chalmers N, Gillespie IN: A new use of the Simpson percutaneous atherectomy catheter: Resection of retained valve cusps of an in-situ vein graft. Cardiovasc Intervent Radiol 18:50, 1995.

38. Tielbeek AV, Vroegindeweij D, Gussenhoven LJ, et al: Evaluation of directional atherectomy studied by intravascular ultrasound in femoropopliteal artery stenosis. Cardiovasc Intervent Radiol 20:413, 1997.

Chapter 5 Complications of Endovascular Procedures

Endovascular Contributor: *Duncan F. Ettles*
Surgical Contributor: *Peter R. Taylor*

Although the scope and complexity of vascular interventional procedures continues to increase, many of the complications that occur are common to most endovascular techniques. Specific procedure- and site-related complications are included in subsequent chapters, whereas this section provides a more general overview of complications and possible approaches to their reduction, prevention, and management. The incidence of complications related to endovascular therapy is dependent on a number of inter-related factors. Case selection has an important influence: As interventional techniques have developed, the population referred for many procedures has become older, and patients are more likely to have serious comorbid disease as well as more severe arterial disease. For instance, elderly patients considered unfit for surgery because of cardiorespiratory illness are increasingly referred for radiologic limb salvage in the presence of extensive occlusive arterial disease, which may require multilevel treatment involving thrombolysis, conventional angioplasty, and stenting. A higher complication rate can, therefore, be anticipated in certain subgroups.

Operator experience and manual dexterity are important factors in the avoidance of complications, but even in the most experienced hands, unexpected complications inevitably occur, and realistic expectations are needed.

As technology develops, the safety and efficacy of medical devices continue to improve. The availability of hydrophilic guide wires and small-gauge angioplasty systems are good examples of this. Interventional radiologists are eager to embrace new technologies, but many published studies of new interventional devices are unsatisfactory and often lacking in objectivity. High complication rates associated with new devices are often ascribed to the "impossible lesions" tackled or the "learning curve" associated with such developments.[1] Careful prospective data collection and audit of complication rates are, therefore, important parts of any new form of therapy, because they allow valid comparison with established endovascular and surgical forms of treatment.

Complications that develop after endovascular procedures should be managed by the interventional radiologist in conjunction with the vascular surgeon. All procedures should be discussed jointly and agreement should be reached on a plan of intervention. In such a case, if complications arise, the patient is known to both interventional radiologist and surgeon and has been fully informed of the risks. It is much more difficult to deal with a patient who has never participated in this discussion and who has never met the vascular surgical team. Radiologic techniques are employed initially to deal with most complications, and surgery is required if these fail.

PUNCTURE SITE COMPLICATIONS

These remain one of the most commonly reported complications occurring in patients who undergo peripheral arterial intervention, with an incidence varying between 2 and 6%. The majority of these complications are hematomas, and differences in incidence can largely be accounted for by differences in definition of what constitutes a significant hematoma.[2, 3] Nevertheless, even small postprocedure hematomas can produce considerable discomfort, limit activity, and make future vascular access more difficult. In most cases, careful manual compression by an experienced member of staff and conservative management is sufficient, but rarely surgical evacuation and blood transfusion may be required. The occurrence of hematoma relates to several factors, including chosen puncture site, operator experience, size of device introduced, and use of anticoagulation. Patient characteristics also have a significant influence, with restless, confused, obese, or hypertensive patients being more prone to develop bleeding complications after the procedure is performed. The potentially lethal complication of retroperitoneal hematoma formation may occur as an extension of groin hematoma but is more likely in the setting of high antegrade femoral puncture, especially if the vessel is inadver-

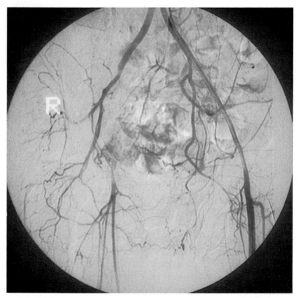

Figure 5–1. This patient underwent diagnostic coronary angiography on the previous day and manifested an acutely ischemic right leg. Surgical exploration confirmed intimal dissection at the puncture site.

tently punctured above the inguinal ligament. In the latter case, adequate manual compression is not possible, and significant blood loss may go unrecognized. If clinical observations arouse any suspicion of retroperitoneal bleeding, urgent pelvic computed tomography (CT) should be arranged after the patient has been resuscitated and blood sent for cross-matching.

Axillary puncture may be preferred as the access site for certain interventions or may be necessitated by occlusive iliac disease. This approach carries a higher risk of hematoma formation and resultant neurologic sequelae. Brachial puncture has a relatively lower risk of hematoma formation, but the added difficulties of manipulating catheters and guide wires through a much smaller vessel may be important in some interventional procedures, such as renal artery stenting.[4–6]

A variety of mechanical devices are now available to assist in hemostasis and puncture site closure. For example, an inflated plastic diaphragm can be used to compress the puncture site, with its predetermined pressure being set higher than the patient's arterial systolic pressure. Such devices work well for slim patients but are less well suited to the obese and cannot be regarded as a substitute for careful manual compression. The Angioseal device (Quinton Instrument Co., Bothell, WA) uses a small implanted collagen anchor, which is thereafter gradually resorbed, to effect hemostasis. Initial results suggest that this technique may offer important practical advantages, particularly in the aggressively anticoagulated patient, but there is a small failure rate.[7]

Intimal dissection at or close to the puncture site is uncommon and can be largely avoided by good

technique. Incomplete entry of a bevelled needle into the vessel lumen can lead to subintimal passage of the guide wire, and incorrect use of the short guide wires supplied with hemostatic sheaths may allow damage of the vessel wall by the central obturator (Fig. 5–1). Short retrograde dissections are usually of no consequence, and the typical pain often experienced by the patient should alert the operator to this immediately. Antegrade dissection is potentially more hazardous, because the direction of blood flow predisposes to persistence of the false channel. Management is most often conservative, but signs of impaired distal circulation may require a contralateral approach for endovascular treatment.

Acute vessel closure at the entry site can result from dissection, thrombosis, vessel spasm, or a combination of these factors. In the great majority of instances, successful endovascular treatment can be expected[2] (Fig. 5–2).

Arteriovenous fistula formation at the puncture site is an uncommon complication that may be predisposed by low puncture at the level where the superficial femoral artery crosses anterior to the femoral vein. Variability in the course of these vessels at the groin may lead to inadvertent transfixion of the artery and vein with subsequent fistula formation. It seems

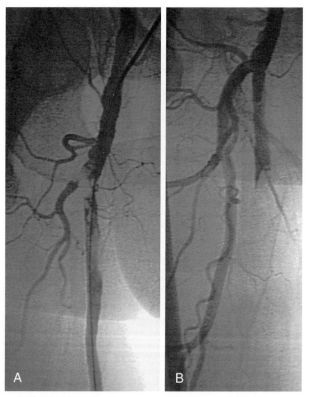

Figure 5–2. A, After performance of a technically difficult antegrade puncture in an obese patient, acute occlusion of the origin of the deep femoral artery is seen with thrombus in the proximal superior femoral artery (SFA). B, Suction embolectomy and recombinant tissue-plasminogen activator (rt-PA) were used to re-establish patency of the deep femoral artery, and overnight thrombolysis successfully cleared the SFA.

likely that the true incidence of this complication is unknown, because many patients never undergo repeat angiography (Fig. 5–3). In contrast, the occurrence of false aneurysm after arterial interventions is unlikely to be overlooked. Although it has been suggested that pseudoaneurysm formation is predisposed by low femoral puncture,[5, 8] practical experience from duplex sonography confirms that this complication can follow both low and high femoral cannulation. The use of aggressive periprocedural anticoagulation, such as occurs in coronary stenting procedures, and careless attention to hemostasis are clearly important in the pathogenesis of pseudoaneurysm (Fig. 5–4). Conservative management may be sufficient in some cases, but assessment by duplex ultrasonography and ultrasonographically guided compression are now in common use.[9] Percutaneous treatment of false aneurysms by a variety of other methods, including direct injection of thrombin, is possible,[10] and this subject is more fully discussed in Chapter 33. All arterial punctures inevitably lead to some thickening of the perivascular tissues and influence subsequent percutaneous access and surgical exposure of the vessel. Transient or permanent neural damage is a potential complication of all arterial punctures and is thought to be more common in axillary puncture in which the major divisions of the

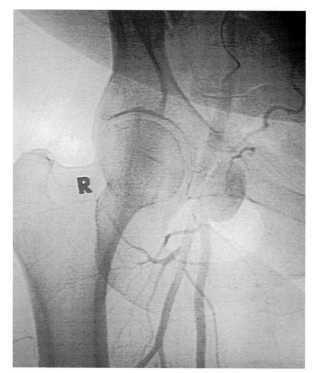

Figure 5–4. A false aneurysm is seen arising from the common femoral bifurcation. This angiogram was performed 2 days after coronary angioplasty.

brachial plexus lie in close proximity to the vessel within relatively loose connective tissue. Infection at the puncture site is very rare but has the potential to cause fatal septicemia.

TARGET SITE COMPLICATIONS

Acute closure of a stenotic vessel during attempted angioplasty or stenting can occur as a result of local dissection, vessel thrombosis, or spasm, and these may often coexist. The complexity and length of lesions influence the likelihood of acute closure as does operator experience. If recognized early, treatment by thrombolysis, antispasmodic drugs, and additional balloon inflations is usually sufficient to reopen the vessel (Fig. 5–5). Whether adjunctive treatment, such as stent insertion, is required depends on the site of the lesion and the potential effects of continued ischemia. For instance, acute closure following recanalization of a long SFA segment may require a conservative approach, accepting poor clinical outcome. On the other hand, acute iliac closure requires strenuous efforts to maintain patency, whereas carotid dissection may call for emergency surgery. The decision about treatment of dissection at the site of the lesion depends on its extent and whether it is likely to extend as a result of blood flow. Limited retrograde dissection in a vessel is unlikely to lead to hemodynamic sequelae, but antegrade dissection may extend and

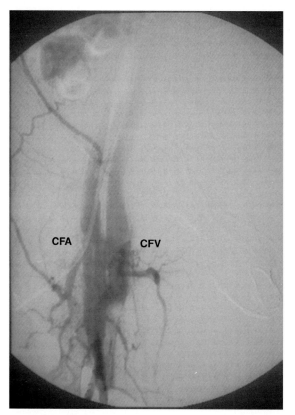

Figure 5–3. Diagnostic angiogram in a patient who had undergone previous iliac angioplasty, showing a clinically silent arteriovenous fistula. CFA = common femoral artery; CFV = common femoral vein.

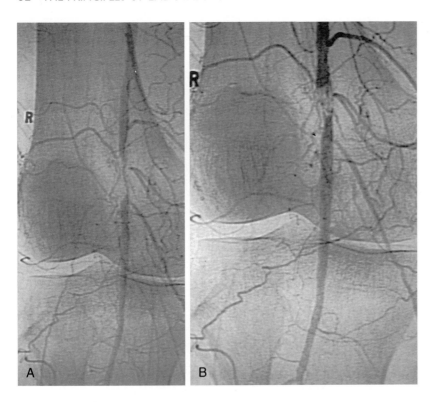

Figure 5–5. *A*, The target lesion was a short, severe popliteal stenosis. *B*, After performance of angioplasty, there was acute vessel closure. This was initially managed by endovascular means, but it later reoccluded and required surgical exploration.

limit flow as pulsatile blood flow enters the false channel and maintains its patency (Fig. 5–6). Prolonged balloon inflations (5 to 10 minutes) are often useful in successfully tamponading dissection tracts, and stents have a major role in emergency treatment

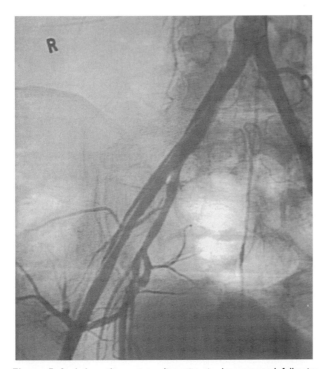

Figure 5–6. A long iliac artery dissection is demonstrated following balloon angioplasty. There was no angiographic holdup of contrast and no residual pressure gradient. Therefore, no further intervention was necessary.

when dissection and impending vessel closure are seen (Fig. 5–7).

Perforation of arteries or other structures by guide wire or catheter is uncommon and rarely of any clinical consequence. If there is significant resulting hemorrhage, balloon inflation across the damaged vessel should allow recovery (Figs. 5–8 and 5–9). Arterial rupture, which is uncommon with good technique and careful selection of balloon size, has been most often reported in the iliac vessels, where the risk may be greater in patients taking long-term steroids.[11, 12] Clinically this is recognized by severe and prolonged pain in association with a vagal response. Initial endovascular treatment is by prolonged balloon tamponade at the angioplasty site, but if this fails, placement of a covered stent should be attempted. If this is not possible or is unsuccessful, immediate surgical treatment is needed. The angioplasty balloon should be left inflated within the ruptured segment while the patient is transferred to the operating theatre.[13, 14] Aneurysm formation at the site of previous balloon angioplasty has rarely been described. Its precise prevalance in the post-treatment population is unknown, and the majority of reported cases relate to iliac artery interventions.[15]

Certain device specific complications may be encountered at the target site. In current practice, these are perhaps most often associated with the use of metallic stents where device migration and failure of deployment can occur. A variety of techniques are employed to reorientate or recover maldeployed stents but sometimes the only option is deployment

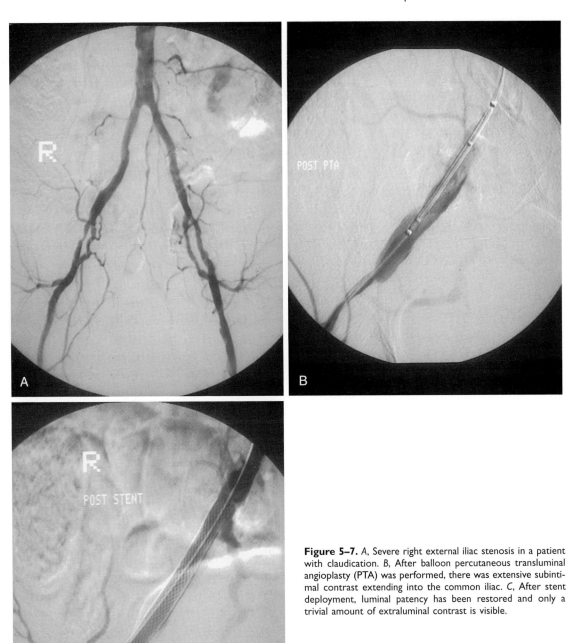

Figure 5–7. *A,* Severe right external iliac stenosis in a patient with claudication. *B,* After balloon percutaneous transluminal angioplasty (PTA) was performed, there was extensive subintimal contrast extending into the common iliac. *C,* After stent deployment, luminal patency has been restored and only a trivial amount of extraluminal contrast is visible.

at a site other than the target lesion (Fig. 5–10). Endovascular techniques that may be used to deal with such complications are discussed further in Chapter 6.

DISTAL COMPLICATIONS

The incidence of embolism distal to the target lesion is quoted as between 1.5 and 5% and is commoner during recanalization of occluded segments.[2, 16] Of course, many small thromboembolic or atheroembolic events are unlikely to have any adverse clinical sequelae and may go unnoticed, whereas larger emboli may result in acute ischemic symptoms requiring endovascular or surgical therapy. Microembolization has been shown to be a particular problem during endovascular repair of aortic aneurysms.[17]

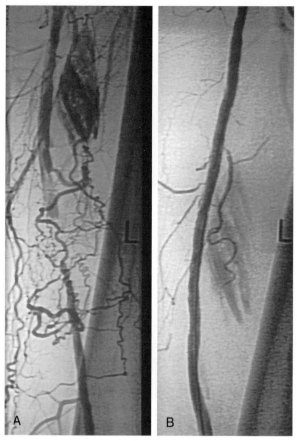

Figure 5–8. A, Inadvertent passage of the guide wire into a branch vessel of the superior femoral artery (SFA) has resulted in perforation and extravasation. B, The SFA occlusion was successfully treated and no further extravasation has occurred.

higher risk than if all three crural vessels are patent, because the effects of even small emboli may be profound. Small thromboemboli can generally be dealt with by a combination of suction embolectomy and local thrombolysis.[2] Close clinical liaison with the vascular surgeon should identify all potential limb-threatening episodes at an early stage to minimize the risks of limb loss or irreversible neuromuscular complications.

Compartment syndrome is a complication that results from revascularization of the extremity after prolonged ischemia. It is most often seen during thrombolytic therapy and relates chiefly to reperfusion coupled with increased capillary permeability. The resulting progressive increase in pressure, usually in the anterior compartment of the calf, leads to muscle necrosis and neural dysfunction. Immediate surgical fasciotomy is indicated to halt muscle necrosis and preserve limb function.

SYSTEMIC COMPLICATIONS

Cholesterol embolization, although rare, is a disastrous event in which showers of plaque cholesterol enter the visceral and peripheral arterial circulation. This is typically, although not always, a result of prolonged catheter manipulation within a heavily diseased aorta. The angiographic picture is of maintained large vessel patency accompanied by progressive renal failure, gut ischemia and cutaneous necrosis. This complication may not be evident at the end of the procedure, but the patient may later develop abdominal pain and a characteristic rash (livedo reticularis), usually from the waist down (Fig. 5–11). Treatment is essentially supportive, involving

The potential for distal occlusion must be considered in case selection and planning of the intervention. For instance, SFA angioplasty in a patient with diseased single vessel below-knee runoff carries a

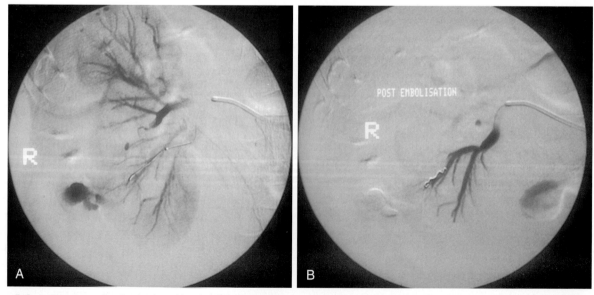

Figure 5–9. A, Capsular perforation by the guide wire after completion of renal ostial stent placement and percutaneous transluminal angioplasty (PTA) of branch vessel stenosis. B, A single, 3-mm embolization coil was sufficient to stop any further bleeding.

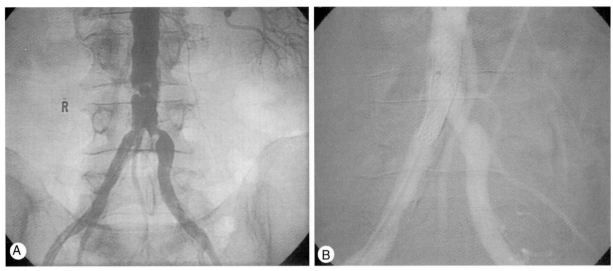

Figure 5–10. *A*, Pretreatment angiography, showing a severe complex aortic stenosis. Elective stent placement was undertaken. *B*, During deployment, the stent was placed too low and has crossed into the left iliac artery origin. The patient has been treated with warfarin and has remained asymptomatic with good femoral pulses.

fluid replacement and intravenous heparinization, but outcome is almost uniformly fatal.[18, 19]

Infective complications, including septicemia, infective arteritis, and false aneurysm formation, have been described after endovascular treatment.[20, 21] The use of antibiotic prophylaxis varies widely between operators and countries, but there is a general tendency to consider limited antibiotic prophylaxis when stent grafts as opposed to bare metallic stents are being implanted. In certain specific procedures, such as visceral embolization, there is a more cogent argument in favor of antibiotic use. Recommendations have been published for the use of antibiotic prophylaxis based on a national survey of practice by the Society for Cardiovascular and Interventional Radiology.[22]

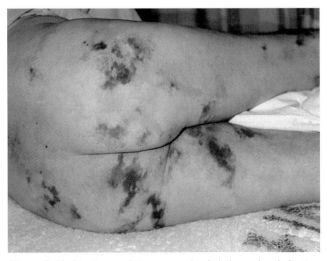

Figure 5–11. Livedo reticularis as a result of cholesterol embolization that developed after diagnostic angiography. (Courtesy of Dr. P. Birch, Consultant Radiologist, Gloucestershire Royal Hospital, England.)

DEVICE-RELATED COMPLICATIONS

Angiographic guide wires are manufactured to exacting standards, but occasional breakage and embolization have been reported. Hydrophilic wires are now in widespread use but should be used only through a catheter or a dilator. Insertion of a hydrophilic wire through arterial puncture needles may easily lead to stripping of the external coating as the wire is withdrawn (Fig. 5–12). The lack of positive "feel" that accompanies the use of such wires may predispose to arterial dissection, although this is a feature that can be exploited to advantage in subintimal recanalization of occlusions. Angioplasty balloons are able to withstand inflation pressures well beyond their quoted nominal values, and spontaneous balloon rupture is nowadays uncommon. Post dilatation of implanted stents is now a more common cause of balloon disruption if the balloon material catches on sharp edges or end wires of some types of stent. It is important to ensure compatibility between balloon catheters and hemostatic introducers before use, because subtle differences can exist between equipment even when quoted French sizes are the same (Fig. 5–13).

Mechanical devices, such as atherectomy catheters, are subject to particular types of malfunction that most often relate to improper use. Stent deployment carries its own difficulties, and the operator must be aware of the limitations of each device. For instance, some nitinol stents exhibit a tendency to move forward during deployment, whereas dislodgement from the deployment system can occur in balloon-mounted stents if they are advanced without cover by a sheath or guide catheter.

The hazards of ionizing radiation to both patient

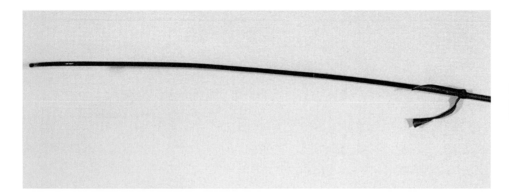

Figure 5–12. Stripping of a hydrophilic wire which has been passed through a femoral puncture needle.

and operator should always be borne in mind, and adherence should be given to the ALARA principle (as low as reasonably achievable). The great majority of endovascular interventions are completed with low screening times and total patient dose, but occasional interventions involve prolonged screening, and there have been reports of skin changes and even hair loss in patients after such exposure.

CONTRAST–MEDIA-RELATED COMPLICATIONS

The allergic, toxic, and minor contrast reactions familiar to many more senior interventional radiologists have been significantly reduced by continued developments and refinements in nonionic contrast media. Despite this, it is very difficult to be certain that the increased cost related to the introduction of newer media has resulted in any significant reduction in patient mortality. Nevertheless, the incidence of reactions interfering with or curtailing vascular interventions has been reduced and overall patient comfort has increased after the introduction of nonionic contrast media. With regard to contrast–media-related mortality, interpretation of the published data is made

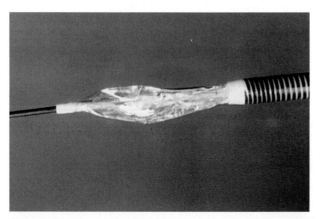

Figure 5–13. After renal stent deployment, the delivery balloon could not be retracted into a long access sheath which had been placed from the left arm. Removal of the balloon and sheath as a single unit was required.

difficult because of differing clinical practices, and the small number of mortalities even within large series. As a general guideline, the interventional radiologist is likely to encounter anaphylaxis after contrast administration in 1 of 10,000 cases and death in 1 of 40,000 cases.[23, 24] Familiarity with the management of minor and major contrast reactions is essential, and all radiologists must periodically be retrained in resuscitation techniques.

The data suggesting that any benefit is gained by the use of steroid prophylaxis in patients with a history of allergy or previous reactions are inconclusive and largely based on studies using older ionic agents. Clear guidelines on the use of steroid prophylaxis are not available and individual practice varies widely.[25, 26, 27] Many radiologists take the pragmatic approach of pretreatment with a short course of oral steroids for atopic individuals or those with a past history of reaction. Intravenous hydrocortisone is sometimes used but, to be effective, should be given hours rather than minutes before contrast is administered.

There has been a great deal of concern and publicity concerning the risks of fatal lactic acidosis in patients treated with metformin who receive iodinated contrast media.[28] Metformin is a biguanide that is excreted solely via the kidneys. It is not directly nephrotoxic but accumulates in the presence of renal impairment and predisposes the patient to develop lactic acidosis. Although the number of documented cases of lactic acidosis following contrast examinations is small, guidelines have been proposed in an attempt to minimize this complication. Essentially, these involve the cessation of metformin therapy before planned interventions, biochemical screening to detect pre-existing renal impairment, and postoperative monitoring of serum biochemistry.[29] Of course, in clinical practice it may not be possible to discontinue metformin in the emergency situation, and minimizing the contrast dose should be of primary concern.

Carbon dioxide (CO_2) digital subtraction angiography offers an important alternative in the presence of known hypersensitivity to contrast and in patients taking metformin but is still not widely available. In addition to preventing contrast reactions, CO_2 is useful in combination with conventional contrast in reducing the overall contrast dose which may be of value in patients who have pre-existing renal impairment. The technique itself carries potential risks of neurotoxicity, and, therefore, its use in the arterial circulation is restricted to the aorta and peripheral vessels.[30, 31]

REDUCING COMPLICATION RATES

Broadly speaking, there are four main components in a strategy aimed at reducing complication rates in endovascular procedures. These are the following:

1. Certified training and accreditation programs for interventional trainees
2. Local and national programs of clinical audit and quality assurance
3. Continued technologic improvements in device manufacture and safety standards
4. Careful case selection and patient management

In most countries, organized training programs are now in existence, and bodies have been appointed to introduce clinical governance in some form or another. It is the responsibility of these committees to provide clinically valid benchmarks against which individuals and institutions can compare their own morbidity and mortality data. The temptation to introduce standards beyond those that are reasonably attainable will prove to be a major test of this system.

Interventional vascular radiology is a clinical discipline, and close involvement of the radiologist is needed to ensure that patients are appropriately selected for treatment. The radiologist has a responsibility equal to that of the referring physician or surgeon to ensure that treatment of the *patient* rather than simply the *lesion* is of primary concern.

SURGICAL ASPECTS

Puncture Site Complications

The most common complication is bleeding, which may be from the anterior wall of the artery but can be from the posterior wall if the vessel has been transfixed during initial cannulation. The posterior wall of the vessel must be dissected free so that the surface can be fully inspected and any puncture wound repaired. The patient who develops a retroperitoneal hematoma after a groin puncture should undergo exploration of the access site, including the posterior wall. The hole is usually a 2- to 3-mm transverse split that requires repair with interrupted monofilament polypropylene sutures placed longitudinally

to avoid luminal narrowing. Control of the blood flow is effected by either manual compression or application of vascular clamps. Sometimes, intraluminal occlusion balloons are helpful. It is not usually necessary to give heparin before clamping owing to the short time taken for primary repair. Larger holes in smaller vessels may require a vein patch to avoid compromising the lumen. Heparin is usually given, and the vein can almost always be harvested from the same site as the incision. Synthetic material is best avoided, because infection in the hematoma can secondarily affect the prosthesis.

A variety of hemostatic devices are available to close percutaneous arterial puncture sites. Some are held in place with dissolvable sutures, which, if cut, cause the intraluminal part of the device to embolize distally. The artery should be dissected proximally and distally to the device and then clamped before the device (including the intraluminal portion) is removed. Rarely, they may be deployed wholly within the artery, causing occlusion that requires surgery.[32]

False aneurysms, which have not responded to compression with duplex ultrasonography, may need surgical repair. A separate incision to gain proximal control is useful if bleeding is uncontrolled or the aneurysm very large. However, this is usually unnecessary, and direct incision into the sac, with the aid of suction followed by manual compression, is usually all that is required to visualize the puncture site for repair. Rarely, the false aneurysm may communicate with an accompanying vein. Such arteriovenous fistulas are readily identified clinically by a machinery murmur sound that is audible on auscultation. Control of both artery and vein proximal and distal to the site of the fistula should be established after giving the patient heparin. The vessels are then repaired by either direct closure or vein patch as appropriate. The vein should berepaired first; therefore, when arterial continuity is restored, there is no venous outflow obstruction. Results of surgery are good if the referral is prompt.[33]

Complications in the Access Vessel

Hemorrhagic complications along the access vessel are usually initially hidden, as the blood enters the abdomen or thorax. Following perforation, blood flow out of the vessel is initially rapid but stops when the surrounding tissue pressure equals intraluminal pressure (Fig. 5–14). In a young patient, the only physical sign may be an unexplained tachycardia. Older patients who have compromised cardiac function and limited vascular reserve usually manifest hypotension, which may be profound. Hemorrhage is often diagnosed late, after the endovascular procedure has been completed. CT scan or ultrasonography

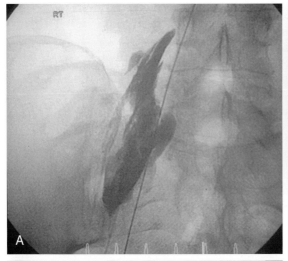
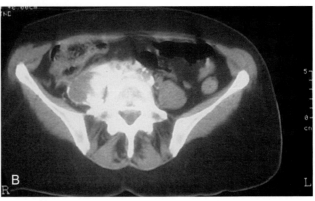
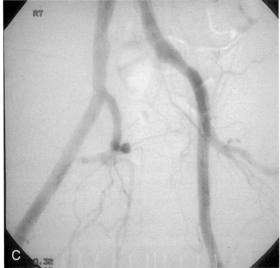

Figure 5–14. *A,* Access vessel perforation during cardiac catheterization. A guide wire is seen within the femoral vein. Contrast has been injected into the arterial sheath and there is extensive extravasation. *B,* An immediate CT examination confirms the presence of contrast within the right psoas muscle and retroperitoneal tissues. *C,* The patient was managed conservatively and follow-up angiography performed after a few hours confirms vessel patency with no active bleeding.

may be useful in confirming the hematoma but do not show the site of perforation. Angiography may demonstrate this, but a normal angiogram does not exclude bleeding from the conduit, and, in these circumstances, surgical exploration should not be delayed.

Complications at the Site of Intervention

VESSEL RUPTURE

Rupture of the vessel at the site of intervention may not always be salvageable by endoluminal techniques. Bleeding can be controlled by inflating a balloon in the vessel proximal to the tear so that the patient can be transferred to the operating theater. Tears can be repaired with patches, but severely damaged vessels may require replacement. Large vessels, such as the aorta and iliac arteries, can be repaired with synthetic polyester grafts, whereas smaller arteries require autologous vein grafts. Occasionally, com-

posite vein grafts can rupture if the balloon is incorrectly sized.[34] Rupture of a vein can result in catastrophic bleeding that is difficult to identify and control. Clamps should be avoided as they can cause further damage to these fragile vessels. Digital control or compression with swabs attached to instruments is safer. Intraluminal balloon inflation at the time of surgery may be helpful in controlling large veins. The majority of ruptured veins can be closed primarily or simply ligated or oversewn, particularly in life-threatening circumstances. If the patient's condition is stable, the vessel can be repaired with a vein patch or vein graft as appropriate. Veins that are adjacent to the site of intervention may be damaged, and arteriovenous fistulas have been reported after arterial angioplasty.[35] These require repair as described earlier, although small fistulas may not be clinically apparent and may close spontaneously.

ACUTE OCCLUSION

Peripheral pulses should be documented in all patients before the start of any endovascular procedure, preferably with Doppler pressures distal to the site of access. Any deterioration after the procedure can thus be identified immediately and measures taken to restore flow before the onset of irreversible ischemia. If there is any evidence of either motor or sensory deficit, revascularization should be performed as an emergency. Patients who have no neurologic deficit can be given therapeutic doses of heparin and managed in the light of day. If the limb is nonviable, revascularization may be dangerous. Fixed staining of the skin, which is often accompanied by muscle that feels turgid, is evidence of irreversible ischemia, for which the only surgical option is amputation.

Occlusion after catheterization in small arteries, such as the brachial artery, is usually caused by an intimal dissection. In the groin, this can follow inadvertent cannulation of the superficial femoral artery if the bifurcation is high. Systemic heparin should be given, and during surgical exploration, fresh thrombus should be removed by an embolectomy catheter. The intimal flap should be excised and the distal intima secured with interrupted polypropylene sutures to prevent further dissection. The arteriotomy is closed with a vein patch.

Two problems may arise. The first is lack of a good inflow. Careful identification of the true lumen allows an embolectomy catheter to be placed above the dissection. Inflating the balloon and withdrawing the catheter allows blood to fill the true lumen and compress the false lumen. If it is impossible to establish an adequate inflow, an anatomic or extraanatomic graft can be taken from a patent vessel. In the lower limb proximal to the inguinal ligament, a polyester or polytetrafluoroethylene graft may be used. In the upper limb and in the leg below the inguinal ligament, autologous vein is the graft of choice.

The second is lack of an adequate backflow. If this cannot be established with an embolectomy catheter, a distal vessel should be dissected and opened. Arterial reconstruction with an appropriate graft can be performed if the backflow is good. If no backflow can be established, instillation of a thrombolytic agent, such as tissue plasminogen activator, urokinase, or streptokinase can be performed.[36] On-table angiography is used to document the effects of thrombolysis and to identify any other patent distal vessel that can be used for a graft. Fasciotomy should be considered, particularly if there is muscle tenderness or if the distal part of the limb remains ischemic despite a functioning graft. These should be full length and left open for either secondary closure or skin grafting.

Revascularized limbs may have evidence of poor distal cutaneous perfusion despite a functioning graft. This may respond to infusions of vasodilators, such as iloprost or prostacyclin, and a chemical sympathectomy may be helpful. The patient should be given therapeutic doses of heparin and oral anticoagulation should be considered.

DISTAL EMBOLIZATION

Another frequent cause of arterial occlusion secondary to endovascular procedures is embolization, either from the site of intervention or from diseased vessels along the conduit. Small emboli may affect the skin, causing discrete punctate areas of necrosis. Digital arteries may be affected, causing blue digit syndrome or gangrene. Such patients are not suitable for surgical intervention; therefore, chemical sympathectomy and infusion of either prostacyclin or iloprost, together with thrombolysis, may have a role. Embolectomy catheters may be necessary to remove larger emboli that affect medium or large arteries. Failure to establish a good backflow should be treated by exploration of distal vessels and the use of thrombolysis followed by vascular reconstruction, as previously discussed. Occasionally, massive embolization of the contents of an aortic aneurysm can be fatal.[37]

Renal and Visceral Complications

Endovascular procedures can result in acute thrombosis of the renal arteries. The warm ischemia time of the kidney is approximately 60 minutes; therefore, urgent surgical referral is warranted. Rarely, the kidney may remain viable owing to collateral vessels for longer periods. Reconstruction of the renal artery may be required by thrombectomy, endarterectomy, patch angioplasty, or vascular grafting from either the aorta or the splenic artery for the left kidney, and the gastroduodenal artery for the right kidney. If reconstruction is unsuccessful, nephrectomy may be necessary for severe pain or development of uncontrolled hypertension. Removal of the kidney for cooling and extracorporeal repair may be necessary if the more distal branches of the renal artery require repair.

The small bowel may very rarely be affected by emboli showering down the superior mesenteric artery from a diseased aorta.[37] More commonly, the colon may become ischemic, particularly after endoluminal graft treatment for abdominal aortic aneurysm. This may be caused by a decrease in flow from graft occlusion of a patent inferior mesenteric artery. It may also follow therapeutic embolization of one or both internal iliac arteries, or the deliberate covering of these arteries by the stent graft to prevent backflow into the aneurysm sac. Embolization of the contents of the aneurysm into the internal iliac arteries may also affect the viability of the colon.

Mesenteric ischemia is insidious in onset, with a fever and a raised white count. The patient may subsequently develop abdominal pain and tenderness in the left iliac fossa and start passing bloody diarrhea. If the signs of peritonitis are present, laparotomy should be performed and the dead bowel removed. The ends are exteriorized and consideration given to a second-look laparotomy. This rare complication is associated with a high mortality rate.[38]

Surgical Removal of Failed Devices

Unsuccessful devices may have to be retrieved surgically. Small devices that embolize in the venous circulation impact in the lung, where they can be safely left. A large device that causes obstruction of the pulmonary artery should be removed by the cardiothoracic surgeons. Devices deployed in the arterial circulation can be retrieved at the site of access if they stay on the catheter. Small or unopened devices that move in antegrade fashion in the circulation can be snared and returned to the site of access for surgical removal. Adequate exposure of the vessel is necessary because it can be severely traumatized, requiring removal of loose intimal flaps and closure with a patch. Sometimes, attempted retrieval fails at some point along the conduit, and the device becomes impacted across the vessel wall (Fig. 5–15). This requires surgery that may involve a laparotomy. If the thoracic vessels are involved, thoracotomy or median sternotomy, with facilities for cardiopulmonary bypass, may be necessary.

Rarely, endoluminal devices, such as snares and grabbers, become entangled in the vessel wall. If the device cannot be safely withdrawn, surgical removal is the only option. The vessel is controlled proximally and distally and opened. The catheter can be cut and withdrawn from the site of access, the device can be disentangled, and the vessel can be repaired.

Late complications

OCCLUSION

Stenosis occurring after performance of endoluminal procedures can result in occlusion. If this does not respond to thrombolysis or deployment of further endovascular devices, anatomic or extra-anatomic grafts can be inserted to re-establish flow. The passage of embolectomy catheters proximally through such devices is usually unsuccessful. Great care should be taken with the vessel wall adjacent to failed endoluminal devices because it may be very friable and require operative techniques described above.

INFECTION

Infection is rare but has been reported in the literature.[39] Any foreign material, such as a stent or stent graft that has become infected, must be completely removed and the vessel reconstructed, usually with extraanatomic grafts that avoid the infected site.

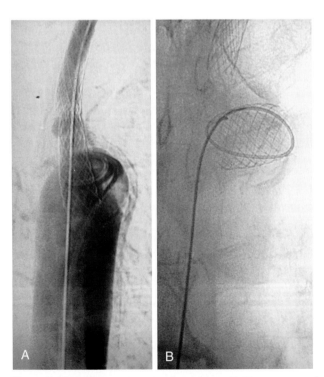

Figure 5–15. *A,* During treatment of a symptomatic false aneurysm of the proximal left subclavian artery, a second covered stent has been deployed too low and is protruding into the aortic arch. *B,* Attempts to retrieve this stent resulted in wedging the device across the aortic arch, and surgical removal was then necessary.

REFERENCES

1. Ring EJ: New interventional devices and the need for restraint. Radiology 170:945–946, 1989.
2. Belli AM, Cumberland DC, Knox AM, et al: The complication rate of percutaneous peripheral balloon angioplasty. Clin Radiol 41:380–383, 1990.
3. Gardiner GA, Meyerovitz MF, Stokes KR, et al: Complications of transluminal angioplasty. Radiology 159:201–208, 1986.
4. Heenan SD, Grubnic S, Buckenham TM, et al: Transbrachial arteriography: Indications and complications. Clin Radiol 51:205–209, 1996.
5. Hessel SJ, Adams DF, Abrams HL: Complications of angiography. Radiology 138:273–281, 1981.
6. Kaukanen ET, Manninen HI, Matsi PJ, et al: Brachial artery access for percutaneous renal artery interventions. Cardiovasc Intervent Radiol 20:353–358, 1997.
7. Beyer-Enke SA, Soldner J, Zeitler E: Immediate sealing of arterial puncture site following femoropopliteal angioplasty: A prospective randomised trial. Cardiovasc Intervent Radiol 19:406–410, 1996.
8. Rapoport S, Sniderman KW, Morse SS, et al: Pseudoaneurysm: A complication of faulty technique in femoral arterial puncture. Radiology 154:529–530, 1985.
9. Fellmeth BD, Roberts AC, Bookstein JJ, et al: Postangiographic femoral artery injuries: Nonsurgical repair with US-guided compression. Radiology 178:671–675, 1991.
10. Liau C-S, Ho F-M, Chen M-F, et al: Treatment of iatrogenic

femoral artery pseudoaneurysm with percutaneous thrombin injection. J Vasc Surg 26:18–23, 1997.

11. Johnston KW: Iliac arteries: Reanalysis of the results of balloon angioplasty. Radiology 186:207–212, 1993.

12. Lois JF, Takiff H, Schechter MS, et al: Vessel rupture by balloon catheters complicating chronic steroid therapy. Am J Roentgenol 144:276–279, 1985.

13. Joseph N, Levy E, Lipman S: Angioplasty related iliac artery rupture: Treatment by temporary balloon occlusion. Cardiovasc Intervent Radiol 10:276–279, 1987.

14. Cooper SG, Sofocleous CT: Percutaneous management of angioplasty related iliac artery rupture with preservation of luminal patency by prolonged balloon tamponade. J Vasc Intervent Radiol 9:81–83, 1998.

15. Vive J, Bolia A: Aneurysm formation at the site of percutaneous transluminal angioplasty: A report of two cases and a review of the literature. Clin Radiol 45:125–127, 1992.

16. Zeitler E: Percutaneous dilatation and recanalisation of iliac and femoral arteries. Cardiovasc Intervent Radiol 3:207–212, 1980.

17. Thompson MM, Smith J, Naylor AR, et al: Microembolisation during endovascular and conventional aneurysm repair. J Vasc Surg 25:179–186, 1997.

18. Gaines PA: Cholesterol embolisation after angiography. Lancet 19:643, 1988.

19. Henderson MJ, Manhire AR: Case report: Cholesterol embolisation following angiography. Clin Radiol 42:281–282, 1990.

20. Hoffman AI, Murphy TP: Septic arteritis causing iliac artery rupture and aneurysmal transformation of the distal aorta after iliac artery stent placement. J Vasc Intervent Radiol 8:215–219, 1997.

21. Chalmers N, Eadington DW, Gandanhamo D, et al: Case report: Infected false aneurysm at the site of an iliac stent. Br J Radiol 66:946–948, 1993.

22. Dravid VS, Gupta A, Zegel HG, et al: Investigation of antibiotic prophylaxis for vascular and nonvascular interventional procedures. J Vasc Intervent Radiol 9:401–406, 1998.

23. Ansell G, Tweedie MCK, West CR, et al: The current status of reactions to intravenous contrast media. Invest Radiol 15(suppl):S32–S39, 1980.

24. Palmer FG: The RACR survey of intravenous contrast media reactions: Final report. Australas Radiol 32:426–428, 1988.

25. Lassar EC, Berry CC, Talner LB, et al: Pretreatment with corticosteroids to alleviate reactions to intravenous contrast material. N Engl J Med 317:845–849, 1987.

26. Dawson P, Sidhu PS: Is there a role for corticosteroid prophylaxis in patients at increased risk of adverse reactions to intravascular contrast agents? Clin Radiol 48:225–226, 1993.

27. Seymour R, Halpin SF, Hardman JA, et al: Corticosteroid prophylaxis for patients with increased risk of adverse reactions to intravascular contrast agents: A survey of current practice in the UK. Clin Radiol 49:791–795, 1994.

28. Rotter A: New contraindication to intravascular iodinated contrast material (Letter). Radiology 197:545–546, 1996.

29. Nawaz S, Cleveland T, Gaines PA, et al: Clinical risk associated with contrast angiography in metformin treated patients: A clinical review. Clin Radiol 53:342–344, 1998.

30. Kerns SR, Hawkins IF: Carbon dioxide digital subtraction angiography: Expanding applications and technical evolution. Am J Roentgenol 164:735–741, 1995.

31. Seeger JM, Self S, Harward TRS, et al: Carbon dioxide gas as an arterial contrast agent. Ann Surg 217:688–698, 1993.

32. Silber S, Schon N, Seidel N, et al: Accidental occlusion of the common femoral artery after Angio-seal application. Zeitschrift fur Kardiologie 87:51–55, 1998.

33. Golledge J, Scriven MW, Fligelstone LJ, et al: Vascular trauma in civilian practice. Ann R Coll Surg Engl 77:417–420, 1995.

34. Sandison AJP, Panayiotopoulos YP, Reidy JF, et al: Inadvertent rupture of a composite vein graft by angioplasty. Cardiovasc Intervent Radiol 20:305–307, 1997.

35. Malcolm PN, King DH, Crabbe RW, et al: Arteriovenous fistula at the site of balloon dilatation complicating femoropopliteal angioplasty. Cardiovasc Intervent Radiol 20:54–56, 1997.

36. Beard JD, Nyamekye I, Earnshaw JJ, et al: Intraoperative streptokinase: A useful adjunct to balloon-catheter embolectomy. Br J Surg 80:21–24, 1993.

37. Parodi JC, Barone A, Piraino R, et al: Endovascular treatment of abdominal aortic aneurysms: Lessons learned. J Endovasc Surg 4:102–110, 1997.

38. Sandison AJP, Edmondson RA, Panayiotopoulos YP, et al: Fatal colonic ischemia after stent graft for aortic aneurysm. Eur J Vasc Endovasc Surg 13:219–220, 1997.

39. Deiparine MK, Ballard JL, Taylor FC, et al: Endovascular stent infection. J Vasc Surg 23:529–533, 1996.

Chapter 6 Intravascular Foreign Body Retrieval

George G. Hartnell

Many devices are introduced into the body for intravascular diagnosis and therapy. In spite of continued improvements in device design and materials, there is still a significant incidence of foreign bodies lost or misplaced within the vascular system. Devices that are damaged or that have deteriorated over time, such as dialysis catheters and venous cannulas, can produce fragments requiring retrieval. Unexpected design faults can also cause device fragmentation, resulting in an intravascular foreign body (e.g., after balloon rupture). In addition, devices that are meant to be deployed in the vascular system, such as embolization coils and arterial stents, can be lost within blood vessels as a result of either operator error or malfunction. More rarely, bullets and similar objects may find their way into blood vessels, where they are accessible to percutaneous removal.[1]

Although such mishaps occur relatively infrequently, there are so many intravascular procedures performed that a significant number of intravascular foreign bodies require retrieval. It is, therefore, necessary to understand the indications for foreign body removal and the various techniques that can be used to extract different types of foreign bodies from the vascular system.[1-8] Unlike the majority of interventional procedures, this subject is not suitable for study in large comparative trials. Most recommendations are, therefore, based empirically on individual experience, with a limited number of devices used in a variety of anatomic situations. No one technique or device is appropriate for removing every type of foreign body from any type of vessel. In this chapter, possible approaches are discussed for removal of foreign bodies from various anatomic locations under different sets of circumstances.

DEVICES FOR FOREIGN BODY REMOVAL

Numerous devices have been used to remove intravascular foreign bodies (Table 6–1). In the past, these were often homemade devices adapted from conventional angiographic materials[9] or devices designed for other uses, such as biopsy forceps.[8, 10] As the need to retrieve foreign bodies has increased, specially designed devices have become available. Most of these have been based on the concept of a stone-retrieval basket[6, 7] or, more commonly, a loop snare.[4, 5] Initially, the strength and self-centered design of baskets made them the preferred device for removing readily accessible intravascular foreign bodies. However, manipulation of baskets can be difficult, especially in tortuous or small-diameter vessels.

Early loop snare devices were difficult to manipulate, but current loop snares are much easier to use and their construction is much more robust than it was in the past. Loop snares can be introduced through shaped catheters, which allow easier and safer access to foreign bodies in small or tortuous vessels. They are now the device of choice for removing most intravascular foreign bodies.

A Stepwise Approach to Safe Foreign Body Removal (Table 6–2)

DOES THE FOREIGN BODY NEED TO BE REMOVED ?

The presence of an intravascular foreign body alone is not an indication for percutaneous retrieval. Removal is indicated only if the foreign body is in a position where it might cause further problems, such as thrombosis or vessel perforation. Alternatively, it might be in a safe but unstable position, so that if it were to migrate, it could cause a problem. If the foreign body is in a stable position in which it will cause no significant damage or other sequelae, it does not need to be removed.

ILLUSTRATIVE CASE 1: A coronary stent has become detached from its balloon and is impacted in a deep muscular branch of the profunda femoris artery (Fig. 6–1). The stent cannot migrate more distally and cannot cause a significant problem because thrombo-

Table 6–1. Foreign Body Retrieval Devices*

Loop Snares

Amplatz nitinol gooseneck snare
Needle's eye snare, Curry intravascular retriever; Welter retrieval loop catheter

Baskets

Dotter intravascular retriever, Schwarz biliary stone removal basket
Segura basket

Biopsy/Grasping Forceps

Endoscopic biopsy forceps
Vascular retrieval forceps, Kim stone forceps; Boren-McKinney retriever
Grasping forceps

Ancillary Devices (for placing foreign body in a more accessible position)

Pigtail catheter
Tip deflecting wires
Steerable catheter

*This table lists devices that may be of use for intravascular foreign body removal, although not all are approved for intravascular use.
Modified from Hartnell GG: Techniques for intact removal of intravascular foreign bodies. J Vasc Intervent Radiol 11:29, 1996.

Table 6–2. Steps in Planning Percutaneous Intravascular Foreign Body Retrieval

Does the foreign body need to be removed?
Can the foreign body be safely removed by percutaneous techniques?
What is the most appropriate access site and does it allow removal through a vascular sheath, or is a surgical cutdown required?
Does the foreign body need to be repositioned before deploying the retrieval device, and, if so, is this procedure safe?
What configuration of retrieval device and guiding catheter or sheath are most suited to grasp the foreign body within the vessel in question?
What can go wrong and how can possible problems be solved?

sis at this location is not clinically significant. The stent does not need to be removed.

ILLUSTRATIVE CASE 2: A Wallstent inserted for transjugular intrahepatic portosystemic shunt (TIPS) revision has become displaced and is lodged in the right ventricle (Fig. 6–2). Although it is in a stable position, there is a high risk that it will migrate and cause arrhythmias or perforate the wall of the right ventricle. Although removing the Wallstent from this

position is a challenge and not without risk, the dangers of leaving the stent in the right ventricle are very great.[11] The open surgical approach is also hazardous, and, hence, a percutaneous approach is appropriate with surgical backup. Because of the need to manipulate retrieval devices through the tricuspid valve and within the complex space of the right ventricle, the procedure was performed with transesophageal echocardiographic guidance.

CAN THE FOREIGN BODY BE SAFELY REMOVED WITH USE OF PERCUTANEOUS TECHNIQUES?

Most vessels and cardiac chambers can be reached with use of currently available devices. The ability to reach the foreign body is not enough. It is also necessary to do this without causing adjacent vessel thrombosis, dissection, or rupture. If a serious complication occurs, it is necessary to be able to treat the patient effectively and quickly. Percutaneous removal also

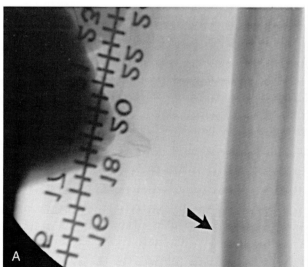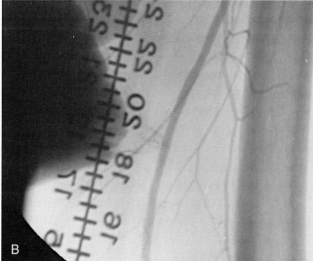

Figure 6–1. *A,* A Palmaz stent was lost during coronary stenting. Fluoroscopy over the thigh showed the stent. Notice the poor opacity of this device. *B,* A contrast arteriogram shows that the stent is aligned along a small muscular branch of the profunda femoris. In this position, it cannot move distally. Even if the vessel becomes occluded, the rich vascular network in the muscles of the thigh will provide ample circulation distal to this device.

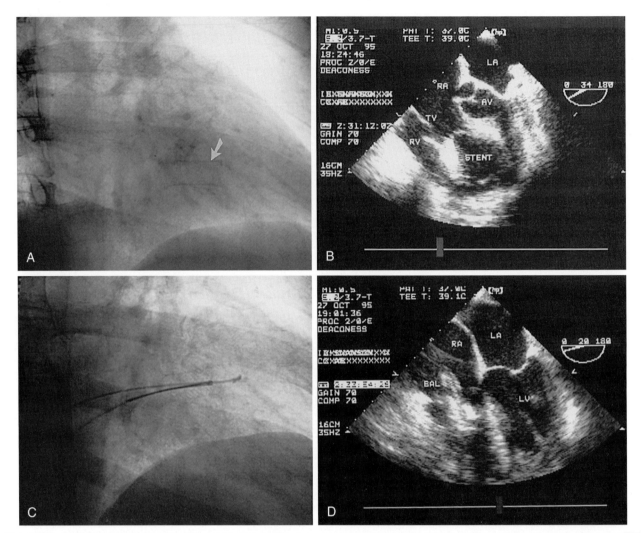

Figure 6–2. *A,* Wallstent (arrow) in the right ventricle is very difficult to see via conventional fluoroscopy. *B,* Transesophageal echocardiography (TEE) shows the stent wedged between the tricuspid valve (TV) and the apex of the right ventricle (RV). *C,* To fix the stent during withdrawal, a guide wire (arrow) was passed through the stent and snared with an Amplatz, nitinol, gooseneck snare. *D,* To smooth the passage of the open stent through the TV, a balloon (arrow) was passed through the center of the stent and inflated as shown here on TEE. The stent was removed through a 14 French femoral vein sheath.

requires the foreign body to be visible on fluoroscopy. Some catheters and stents have low radiodensity, which can make removal difficult or impossible. Digital fluoroscopy with image enhancement[12] or echocardiography[11, 13] may be used to provide adequate visualization of a low radiodensity foreign body (see Fig. 6–2).

ILLUSTRATIVE CASE 3: A patient who had received chemotherapy for malignancy was noted on chest radiograph to have a fragment of central venous catheter lodged in his right ventricle. Ultrafast computed tomography (CT) showed that this had perforated the free wall of the right ventricle at a point where the myocardium was very thin (Fig. 6–3). It was known at the time of catheter removal that the fragment must have been present for several months without causing a problem; therefore, it was unlikely to cause any problem in the future. An opinion that

open surgical removal was indicated was rejected for this reason. Although it seemed that it would be easy to snare and remove the catheter fragment, it was thought that the risk of lacerating the myocardium of the right ventricle, which would lead to hemopericardium, was too great to justify this procedure. Two years later, the fragment had not moved, and the patient had remained well.

WHAT IS THE MOST APPROPRIATE ACCESS SITE?

The access site should allow removal of the foreign object through a vascular sheath, although a surgical cutdown might be required in some cases. The best approach is one that allows easy access to the target vessel without risk of unwanted displacement of the foreign body. This is usually possible via the femoral artery or vein. Percutaneous removal of most vascular

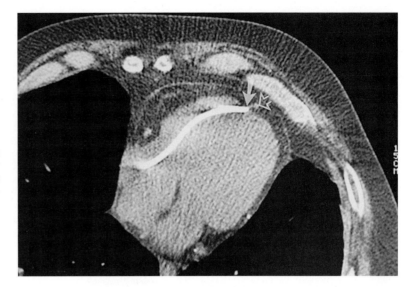

Figure 6–3. This patient was noted, as shown by routine chest radiograph, to have a fragment of central venous catheter in the right ventricle. This ultrafast computed tomographic (CT) image shows that the catheter has perforated the right ventricle without causing any problem. The tip (arrow) lies on the surface of the heart close to the left anterior descending coronary artery (open arrow). The risk of leaving a hole in the right ventricle when removing the catheter fragment was thought to be too high for intervention to be justified.

foreign bodies is usually possible through a large-bore vascular sheath, and the access site should allow the use of such a large-caliber device. If this is not possible, surgical cutdown in collaboration with a vascular surgeon is required. In particular, manipulating a foreign body in a small artery may cause significant damage close to the puncture site, requiring skilled repair.

IS THE FOREIGN BODY IN A SAFE POSITION FOR RETRIEVAL?

The foreign body may need to be repositioned before deployment of the retrieval device in such a way that it can be safely engaged (Fig. 6–4). Many snares require that one end of the foreign body lie free in the vessel. To achieve this, it may be necessary to displace the foreign body by means of a catheter or other device (Fig. 6–5). If both ends of the foreign body are embedded in branch vessels, it may be impossible to engage either end. Manipulation with a shaped catheter to engage the center of the foreign body may displace the fragment so that one end can be freed for subsequent use of a retrieval device.[14] Once this is achieved, the free end is grasped and the fragment extracted through an appropriately sized vascular sheath (see Fig. 6–5). When repositioning is attempted, consideration should be given to the possibility of migration of the foreign body into a dangerous position. This is unlikely if the flow takes the fragment into the smaller distal vessels, unless they are critical vessels, such as the carotid arteries. Migration is also unlikely if the foreign body is long and follows a curved course within the vessel (see Fig. 6–5). With venous foreign bodies, there is a risk of central migration into the heart or the pulmonary arteries. If there is such a risk, a method for fixing part of the foreign body should be used during repositioning and retrieval (see Fig. 6–2). This can be achieved by external compression of an extremity vessel, gentle inflation of an occlusion balloon against part of the foreign body, or tethering of a guide wire through the foreign body.[10, 15]

WHAT IS THE BEST COMBINATION OF RETRIEVAL DEVICE, GUIDING CATHETER, AND SHEATH?

The retrieval device should have a deployed diameter similar to that of the target vessel containing the foreign body. Biopsy forceps and similar instruments can be used, especially in smaller vessels where the foreign body is orientated across the center of the vessel lumen. Forceps may have an increased risk of vessel perforation and trauma, and in larger vessels, it is difficult to guide forceps directly onto the foreign body.

Larger vessels are less of a problem if a snare or basket is used. These should have a diameter similar to that of the vessel and should allow complete opening within the target vessel. The deployed diameter should be large enough to encircle the foreign body without excessive manipulation, because this reduces the risk of damaging the vessel wall (see Fig. 6–5). In some vessels, proprietary loop snares cannot be used because the vessel is too small or irregular to allow safe deployment. In this situation, a retrieval basket or homemade snare, made to conform to the shape and size of the target vessel, can be used.[9]

The foreign body should be grasped in such a way that it can be removed intact through a vascular sheath, eliminating the need for surgical intervention. For most soft catheter fragments, grasping the center of the fragment with a loop snare, so that it folds on itself, may be adequate, provided the sheath is of suitable size (usually 9 or 10 French for most central

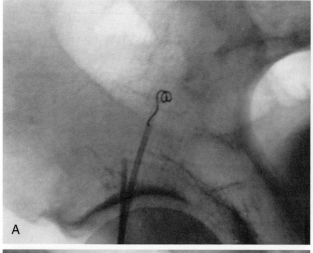

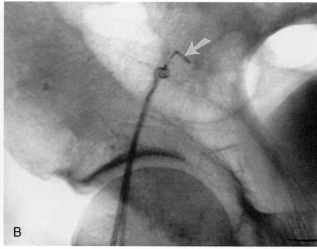

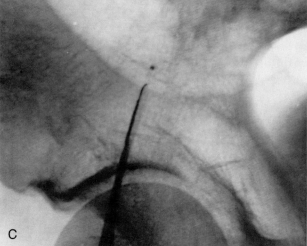

Figure 6–4. *A*, During embolization of a gastroduodenal artery, the microcatheter was displaced into the celiac artery while a coil was being deployed. More than half the length of the coil had been deployed, and it was thought that attempting to snare the coil in the celiac artery would risk dislodgment of the coil and unwanted embolization. Therefore, the coil and the microcatheter were carefully withdrawn into the iliac artery, where inadvertent embolization would be easier to control. *B*, The guiding catheter was removed and a 5-mm Amplatz nitinol gooseneck snare was introduced coaxially over the microcatheter through the arterial sheath. The loop of the snare (arrow) was opened above the coil. *C*, The loop of the snare was pulled over the coil and tightened. The coil, the snare, and the microcatheter were removed through the sheath. The embolization procedure was completed through the same sheath.

venous catheters). For larger diameter catheter fragments (e.g., dual lumen dialysis catheters), or stiffer objects (e.g., guide wires or stents), larger sheaths are required, or the object needs to be grasped at one end (Fig. 6–6). This is especially important for metal devices (e.g., stents). If these become folded over during withdrawal, they may scrape against the vessel wall and cause severe damage. If a stent becomes displaced during deployment, it usually remains around the guide wire used during introduction. To remove the misplaced stent intact and to allow completion of the stenting procedure, the stent should be grasped as closely as possible to its peripheral end, usually with a loop snare; this allows coaxial entry into the vascular sheath.[15] To allow precise snaring, it may be necessary to pass a snare from another access site around the guide wire central to the stent (Fig. 6–7).

In small-caliber vessels, or where there is extensive atheromatous disease, a retrieval basket may cause less vessel damage. The open basket is smoother than a deployed loop snare and may keep the grasped fragment orientated along the long axis of the vessel during withdrawal.

WHAT COULD GO WRONG, AND HOW MIGHT PROBLEMS BE SOLVED?

During retrieval, it is important to restrict the intravascular foreign body's potential of moving out of the range of the retrieval device. For instance, stents should be snared while still on their guide wire to prevent displacement while the snare is manipulated around them, as described earlier (see Fig. 6–7).

ILLUSTRATIVE CASE 4: A fragment of central venous catheter became lodged in a left lower lobe pulmonary artery (see Fig. 6–6). This patient was immunosuppressed, and the risk of pulmonary infarction, infection, or both, was considered to be significant, justifying percutaneous retrieval. Although retrieval required manipulation of the catheter through the heart, this was no more hazardous than performing selective pulmonary angiography. Because of its position in a medium-sized branch, more distal movement of the fragment was unlikely. Loss of the fragment on retrieval through the venous system was unlikely to have severe consequences, although retrieval from another vessel might be required should this occur. Retrieval with a 5-mm

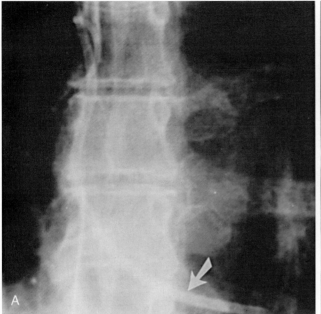
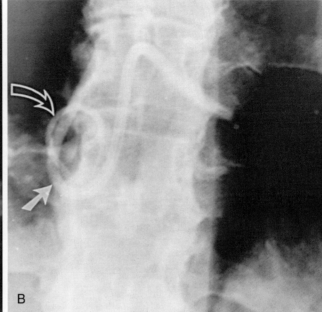
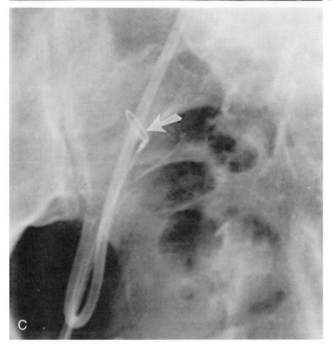

Figure 6–5. A, A long segment of venous catheter (arrow) became lodged between the lower superior vena cava and the apex of the right ventricle. The ends of the fragment could not be engaged at either end with use of a conventional snare. B, A tennis–racquet-shaped catheter (open arrow) was rotated adjacent to the center of the catheter fragment (arrow) in the right atrium. After the fragment was wound around the shaft of the pigtail catheter, both were pulled into the right external iliac vein. A loop on the lower end of the fragment prevented central migration. C, The catheter fragment was snared by a 10-mm Amplatz, nitinol gooseneck snare (arrow). This snare size was chosen because its diameter was similar to that of the external iliac vein, ensuring that when the snare was withdrawn, it would encircle the upper end of the catheter fragment.

Amplatz nitinol snare, which matched the size of the pulmonary artery, was achieved by grasping the fragment at one end. This allowed easy withdrawal through a 7 French sheath. If the catheter fragment had been grasped around its middle, a larger diameter sheath might have been required.

If the foreign body becomes displaced, use of a smaller retrieval device may be necessary to follow the foreign body into smaller branch vessels. Displacement into a larger vessel, with risk of further migration out of reach or into a hazardous position, may require a rapid snatch at any part of the foreign body to prevent further migration. Subsequent retrieval may require deployment of another retrieval

device through a second access site. Failure to withdraw the foreign body through a vascular sheath, or presence of a foreign body that is too large or irregular to pass safely though the vessels at the access site, requires that the procedure be halted. The retrieval equipment is then fixed in position and the vessel opened surgically. This also allows evacuation of any complicating thrombus and repair of any damage at the access site.

CONCLUSION

Retrieval of intravascular foreign bodies is a relatively uncommon procedure. With good understanding of

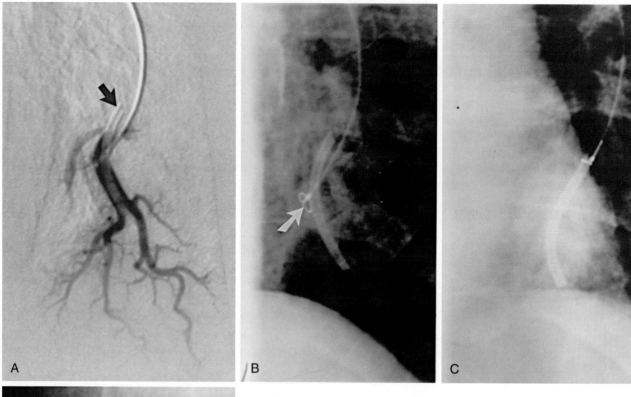

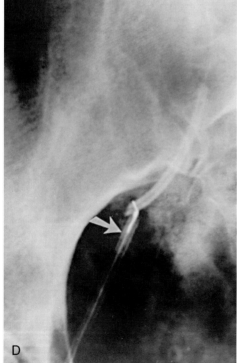

Figure 6–6. *A,* Digital subtraction pulmonary arteriogram shows a fragment of central venous catheter (arrow) in a left lower lobe pulmonary artery. *B,* A 5-mm Amplatz nitinol snare (arrow) was deployed, which had a diameter similar to that of the pulmonary artery. *C,* The snare was positioned to encircle the end of the fragment and then tightened. The fragment was pulled into the right external iliac vein. *D,* With firm traction on the snare, the catheter fragment was pulled into the end of the 7 French sheath (arrow). With the fragment grasped at one end, removal was easy.

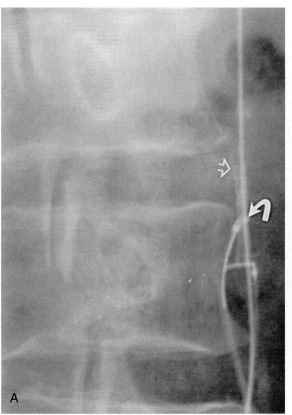

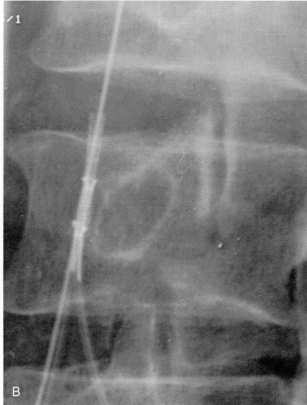

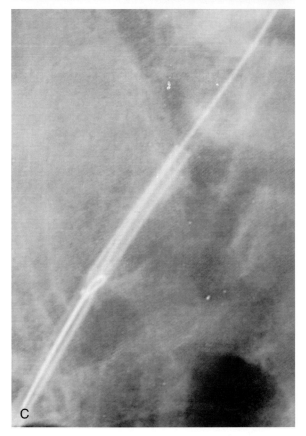

Figure 6–7. *A,* A Palmaz stent (open arrow) became partly displaced from its deployment balloon during renal angioplasty and stenting. Because of flaring of the lower end of the stent, it could not be pulled down for deployment into the external iliac artery, and it was too small to be deployed into the common iliac artery. To prevent displacement of the stent cephalad, a snare (curved arrow) was inserted from the contralateral femoral artery and passed around the guide wire above the displaced stent. This prevented migration of the stent. *B,* Because the iliac artery wall was irregular, a coaxial snare could not encircle the stent; therefore, the cephalad snare was opened and passed around the center of the stent, reducing the flare and allowing the coaxial snare to grasp the lower end of the stent. *C,* By snaring the stent at its lower end, it was possible to pull it into the arterial sheath. The stent was removed and another stent was placed in the renal artery.

vascular anatomy and appropriate choice of equipment, safe retrieval is usually a quick and easy procedure. However, awareness of potential complications of displacement and manipulation is required for less typical cases. This is one of the few situations in interventional radiology in which success brings a complete and immediate cure.

REFERENCES

1. Hartzler GO: Percutaneous transvenous removal of a bullet embolus to the right ventricle. J Thorac Cardiovasc Surg 80:153, 1980
2. Bloomfield DA: The nonsurgical retrieval of intracardiac foreign bodies: An international survey. Cathet Cardiovasc Diagn 4:1, 1978.
3. Hartnell GG: Techniques for intact removal of intravascular foreign bodies. J Intervent Radiol 11:29, 1996.
4. Cekirge S, Weiss JP, et al: Percutaneous retrieval of foreign bodies: Experience with the nitinol Goose Neck snare. J Vasc Interv Radiol 4:805, 1993.
5. Furui S, Yamauchi T, Makita K, et al: Intravascular foreign bodies: Loop-snare retrieval system with a three-lumen catheter. Radiology 182:283, 1992.
6. Endrys J, Rubacek M, Podrabsky P: Percutaneous retrieval of foreign bodies from the cardiovascular system. Cor Vasa 27:36, 1985.
7. Drabinsky M: Retrieval of embolized central venous catheters by a Dormia ureteral stone dislodger with straight filiform tip. Chest 69:435, 1976.
8. Selby JB, Tegtmeyer CJ, Bittner GM: Experience with new retrieval forceps for foreign body removal in the vascular, urinary, and biliary systems. Radiology 17:535, 1990.
9. Hartnell GG: Percutaneous retrieval of foreign bodies using preformed intravascular snare. Radiology 181:903, 1991.
10. Eeckhout E, Stauffer JC, Goy JJ: Retrieval of a migrated coronary stent by means of an alligator forceps catheter. Cathet Cardiovasc Diagn 30:166, 1993.
11. Hartnell GG, Crenshaw W, Burger AJ, et al: Percutaneous removal of a fully expanded wallstent from the right ventricle. J Vasc Intervent Radiol 17:371, 1996.
12. Wilson SC, Paul EM, Channin DS, et al: Localization of an embolized catheter tip by digital image enhancement. Am J Roentgenol 163:1230, 1994.
13. Sproat IA, Bielke D, Crummy AB, et al: Transthoracic 2D echocardiographic guidance for percutaneous removal of a nonopaque intracardiac catheter fragment. Cardiovasc Intervent Radiol 16:58, 1993.
14. Auge JM, Oriol A, Serra C, et al: The use of pigtail catheters for retrieval of foreign bodies from the cardiovascular system. Cathet Cardiovasc Diagn 10:625, 1984.
15. Hartnell GG, Jordan SJ: Percutaneous removal of the misplaced Palmaz stent. J Vasc Intervent Radiol 6:799, 1995.

Medicolegal Aspects of Endovascular Procedures and the Obligations of the Clinical Investigator

Chapter 7

Michael R. E. Dean and Gerry Dorros

MEDICOLEGAL ASPECTS OF ENDOVASCULAR PROCEDURES

During the last decade, there has been a marked increase in both the number of medical negligence cases and the amount of damages awarded to successful litigants. In the United Kingdom, medical litigation cost the National Health Service $376 million in the financial year 1996–1997, a 17% increase over the previous year. The interventional radiologist who performs endovascular procedures is by no means exempt from this growing hazard. Radiologists have not traditionally been concerned with the issues surrounding consent and direct patient management, because their work is primarily diagnostic rather than therapeutic. However, the historical working pattern of radiologists has changed since they began to perform interventional procedures, and they must take their clinical responsibilities seriously. Endovascular procedures can involve significant morbidity, and rarely, mortality; however, because these procedures are regarded as minimally invasive, the patient's expectation is that they can be performed without risk. Unforeseen complications are, therefore, more likely to be regarded as evidence of negligence than would a complication following a surgical operation. Although many endovascular procedures are well documented in the literature and are accepted as conventional therapy, a significant number are still experimental and, for this reason, it is essential to have a knowledge of the framework for introducing new devices and new procedures.

New Devices

There is general recognition that regulations for introduction of new endovascular devices are considerably less strict in Europe than they are in the United States. However, the regulations for new medical devices have now been standardized across the Member States of the European Community. A European Community Medical Devices Directive came into operation on January 1, 1995, with a transitional period lasting until June 1998. This directive allows free movement of medical devices within the European Community and ensures that the devices are safe and that they perform as the manufacturer intended. New medical devices must obtain a CE mark before they can be marketed. This CE mark indicates that the device satisfies the stated essential requirements laid out in the directive and these are designed to ensure the following:

1. A device does not compromise the clinical condition or safety of the patient, the users, or, if applicable, any third party.
2. A device achieves its intended purpose as designated by the manufacturer.
3. Any risks associated with the use of the device are judged by informed clinical opinion to be acceptable when they are weighed against the benefits to the patient and when they are compatible with a high level of protection of health and safety.

Member States of the European Community each have a competent authority who is responsible for overseeing the implementation of the Medical Devices Directive. To obtain a CE mark, a manufacturer must prove that the device conforms to the essential requirements in regard to its characteristics, performance, and safety. This proof must be based on adequate clinical data in the form of a compilation of existing scientific literature or, if this is not available, from the results of a specifically designed clinical investigation of the device. This clinical investigation must be designed in such a way as to demonstrate that the device performs in the way that the manufacturer intended, and that any side effects, in the opinion of competent clinicians, are outweighed by the clinical benefit of using the device. A manufacturer who wishes to carry out a clinical investigation of a new device must give written notice of intention to the competent authority. This submission must include full details of the investigation together with a letter of approval from the local medical ethics committee of each participating hospital or clinic. New medical devices that have not received a CE mark can be used only as part of a clinical investigation that has received the approval of the competent authority. In addition, this competent authority can designate one or more notified bodies that are expected to ensure that all medical devices demonstrate compliance with the essential requirements.

New Procedures

New endovascular procedures are by their very nature experimental because there is little accumulated experience of the likely outcome and no information about longer term follow-up. These drawbacks must be emphasized to the patient when consent is obtained. Before undertaking a new procedure, the local medical ethics committee should be consulted, and it will require an account of the perceived advantages of the new method as well as details of the proposed informed consent. In the United Kingdom, an approach should be made to the SERNIP Committee (Safety and Efficacy Register for New Interventional Procedures). This committee designates the category into which the procedure has been placed. These categories are as follows:

1. Safety and efficacy established; procedure may be used.
2. Sufficiently close to a procedure of established safety and efficacy to give no reasonable grounds for questioning safety and efficacy; procedure may be used subject to continuing audit.
3. Safety and efficacy not yet established; procedure requires a fully controlled evaluation and may be used only as part of systematic research comprising an observational study in which all interventions and their outcomes are systematically recorded.
4. Safety and efficacy not yet established; procedure requires a fully controlled evaluation and may be used only as part of systematic research comprising a randomized controlled trial; the Standing Group on Health Technology must accordingly be advised.
5. Safety, efficacy, or both have been shown to be unsatisfactory; procedure should not be used.

Reporting new procedures to SERNIP is at present voluntary, but failure to take notice of the recommended category for a procedure could lead to difficulties if adverse events should occur that could lead to subsequent litigation.

Clinical Indications, Consent, and Documentation

Before undertaking any procedure, whether new or established, the interventional radiologist must be confident of the clinical indications for the procedure, and the patient must be fully informed of the radiologist's reasons for selecting this procedure and of its potential risks. This is not just a matter of protecting the radiologist from potential litigation; it is, quite simply, a matter of good clinical practice.

The decision to carry out a particular procedure must be taken in the patient's best interests. The radiologist must not be influenced by a desire to try out a new method or a new device unless he or she is certain that this is the correct course of action for the patient's condition. It is also essential to avoid undertaking a procedure under pressure from a referring clinician if the clinical symptoms do not justify the intervention or if the radiologist considers that the procedure is not appropriate in the clinical situation.

All patients who have diagnostic angiograms or endovascular procedures must give signed consent before their arrival in the radiography department. There are no absolute rules as to what information the patient should be given about the procedure or, indeed, what details of the possible rare complications can legitimately be withheld in the patient's best interest, but the doctor who obtains consent must give patients sufficient information to enable them to make a considered decision about the proposed treatment. Medical paternalism is no longer acceptable, and the patient's interests are paramount. A senior judge, in a lecture presented in 1985 to a forum on medical communication, stated that the "sovereignty" of the patient had been reinstated.[1] He continued:

> "So all this emotive phrase means is that the medical ethic must include not only advice as to what is medically appropriate for the patient in his situation but also a respect by the doctor for the rights of the patient outside the field of medicine. And one of these rights is the right, in the light of all information available to him—family and business, as well as medical—to make his own decision as to whether or not he will accept the treatment that is being proposed."

The doctor who obtains consent must give a clear and simple description of the procedure in language that is understandable to a lay person. The patient should be given an explanation of why the intended procedure is believed to be the best course of action in the circumstances and why the alternatives (i.e., surgery or conservative treatment) were not considered appropriate. The likely chances of success of the procedure and possibility of later recurrence of the condition should also be discussed. Information about possible complications is an essential part of the process of consent. Common complications must be mentioned, but the decision as to which rare or serious complications are included in the discussion must be left to the judgment of the doctor who obtains consent. It would clearly be unproductive to mention every single rare but serious complication. This could disturb patients so much that they would decline to proceed with a course of treatment that was clearly in their best interest. The level of risk must be balanced against the severity of the patient's symptoms (e.g., risks of treating mild intermittent claudication should obviously be emphasized more than risks of treating limb-threatening ischemia). In an English court of law, the decision as to whether or not a doctor should have discussed a particular risk would be decided by the Bolam test.[2] This means that it is unlikely that a doctor would be considered to have been negligent if the court accepted the fact that a substantial number of competent doctors would not have mentioned that risk in a similar situation.

The time and place for obtaining a patient's consent is important; for example, it is unacceptable to obtain consent after the patient has arrived in the radiography department and, in particular, after the patient has been premedicated. Clearly, in the case of an emergency procedure, the consent of either the patient or his or her relatives may have to be obtained in less than ideal circumstances, but for elective procedures, consent should be obtained in such a way as to give the patient time to consider the information given. Obtaining consent after the patient's admission to hospital could, in some circumstances, be construed as exerting undue pressure for acceptance, because the patient would have to take the positive step of leaving the hospital if he or she decided, in the light of the information given, not to submit to the proposed procedure. Ideally, consent for the procedure should be obtained a few days before the patient's admission to the hospital, to give the patient time to discuss the information with relatives or friends and to formulate any questions that might arise after reflection on the advice provided. The time spent in discussion with the patient is invaluable in the event a problem should arise later.

This process of consent can be delegated to a junior physician, but only to one who is capable of performing the procedure and who is thus fully conversant with the indications and possible complications. This effectively means that the interventional radiologist should undertake the task personally. Few radiologists in the United Kingdom have outpatient clinics; however, with the legal constraints surrounding delegation and timing of consent, it will probably become standard practice in the future. The time given to obtaining consent in a relaxed atmosphere can help to develop a relationship of trust between the radiologist and the patient that may be invaluable if a complication arises during the course of the procedure. After the patient has signed the consent form, it is a good practice to write a short note in the patient case notes about the discussion. These notes may be very important if there is subsequent litigation, because the consent form signifies only that the patient has agreed to performance of the procedure. They do not include anything about the likely outcome or the possibility of complications, which should have been outlined during the discussions with the patient. Some patients may not wish to discuss any details of the intended procedure and may prefer instead to trust the physician's judgment. This refusal of full consent should also be clearly stated in the patient notes.

Just as the process of obtaining consent can be delegated to a junior physician who is capable of carrying out the procedure, so the performance of the actual procedure can be delegated, but the physician to whom it is delegated must be properly trained to carry it out unsupervised. In addition, the delegating physician must be readily available to provide advice or assistance should they be needed. If these conditions are met, this would be regarded as "proper delegation," and the junior physician would have medicolegal responsibility in the event of subsequent litigation. However, if the junior physician is not fully competent to perform the task without close supervision, or if advice and assistance are not readily available, the delegating physician is medicolegally responsible, because, under such circumstances, passing on responsibility would be regarded as "improper delegation."

At the conclusion of each procedure, a detailed record should be written in the patient notes. This should be headed with the names of the operators and the type of operation undertaken. Drugs (e.g., antibiotics, sedatives) given before the start of the procedure should be listed together with the dosages and times of administration. The practical details of the procedure must be described, and this description should include details of all the devices used or implanted. A list of drugs given during the procedure, including the type and concentration of the contrast medium used, should be stated. This account of the procedure is important for medicolegal reasons; moreover, should a repeat procedure be required at a later date, the previous notes may save considerable time (e.g., in selection of appropriate catheters for a successful approach to a lesion). The description of the procedure should conclude with clear instructions to the ward personnel for the patient's aftercare.

In the event that there is a complication, the exact circumstances and the subsequent action taken to deal with it, must be clearly recorded. If it is necessary to seek help from a clinical colleague, this should also be stated. All interventional radiologists will inevitably encounter a complication at some time in their careers, and it is important to be completely honest with the patient about the circumstances. Evasion raises distrust and suspicion in the patient's mind, and, more seriously, in the mind of any solicitor who might subsequently become involved. A completely open explanation to the patient may well prevent litigation. If the complication is potentially serious, the record of the event should be photocopied and placed in safekeeping in case the original notes should be mislaid.[3] Clinical notes should never be altered. Should an addition or correction subsequently be required, it should be added to the notes with a clear statement of the date and time that it was written. It is important to remember that inadequate medical records make a successful legal defense virtually impossible.

Good communication between interventional radiologists and their clinical colleagues is essential and allows the best results to be obtained. Regular clinical conferences improve the selection of appropriate procedures and also allow the results to be audited regularly. Although a knowledge of results from published series of cases is important, the audit of local results is vital. It is these local results that should be the basis of the discussion with the patient during the process of obtaining consent. Regular meetings between surgeons and radiologists also enable arrangements to be made for dealing with unexpected complications. Although many complications can be readily dealt with by the radiologist, certain adverse events, such as acute arterial rupture or closure, may need urgent surgical intervention, and failure to have ensured that this was readily available would be indefensible in a court of law. An accusation of medical negligence is a very distressing experience. A senior judge spoke of the pain that such incidents cause both accusers and accused.[4] He said:

> "The pain is not, however, confined to the potential plaintiffs. It is experienced also by those who delivered the health care of which complaint is made. Their ambition throughout has been to help the patient, but instead they find themselves subject to hurtful allegations of negligent mistreatment —which often surface after the carer has ceased to have any real recollection of what happened."

Maintaining the best standards of practice, ensuring that the procedure is really in the patient's best interest, considerately obtaining the patient's consent, and maintaining an honest approach in the event of a complication help to prevent the interventional radiologist from being subject to attempted litigation for medical negligence. Should the radiologist have the misfortune to face such accusations, meticulous record keeping is invaluable when all recollection of the course of events may have been forgotten.

OBLIGATIONS OF THE CLINICAL INVESTIGATOR

Historical Perspective

Endovascular procedures continue to supplant many standard medical and surgical therapies, and an increasing number of new devices and drugs are being investigated to determine whether they have a place in our therapeutic armamentarium. Consequently, the responsibilities of clinical investigators participating in these protocols have become increasingly important. Inherent in a discussion of this subject are topics that may not be readily obvious. For instance, what is the origin of the societal or religious warrant that has been granted to the individual to perform the practice of medicine; how can the physician, within these constraints, use his experience and expertise to help participate in the evolution of therapies; and what are the obligations of a clinical investigator? Within the United States, physicians, as clinical investigators, have responsibilities to abide by the regulations of the Food and Drug Administration (FDA), which, if not adhered to appropriately, could result in dire consequences.

Much of the information contained within this section has been directly quoted or paraphrased from either the Code of Medical Ethics[5] published by the American Medical Association or the Guide to Good Clinical Practice.[6] Other information is contained in Appendix II and Appendix III, including the Nuremberg Code[7] and the Declaration of Helsinki.[8]

Interventional cardiologists, radiologists, and surgeons have previously focused attention upon their own fields of training and expertise. Now, however, members of each of these specialties wish to become involved in the endovascular treatment of obliterative cardiovascular disease. This new interest has not always been met with acceptance. In particular, cardiologists' recent concern with alternative revascularization techniques for peripheral vascular obliterative disease has stimulated passionate critiques, interdisciplinary tensions, and considerable commotion. What has also occurred is a new and intense interest, which had previously been notably lacking, in the study of these peripheral vascular pathologies. This latter development offers the potential for significant improvements in better tailored and more carefully worked out treatment strategies.

The physician's unimpeded use of endovascular therapies, without a sufficient scientific basis, is to be frowned on and may be devastating to the patient as well as the physician. A cavalier approach toward patient care is unacceptable, and physicians who desire to participate in the evaluation of new endovascular therapies should be aware of their responsibilities.

Physicians and drug or device manufacturers must jointly define their protocol objectives with regard to patient care and therapeutic procedures and devices. Clearly, physicians are striving to develop new therapies that can re-establish peripheral arterial blood flow, cause minimal or no procedural complications, and eliminate lesion recurrence. Uniformly, manufacturers wish to produce an economically beneficial device that can achieve these aforementioned desires simply, safely, and effectively, when used with the skill and expertise of the average interventionist. These seem to be appropriate goals that can be attained by thoughtful and perceptive investigators who conduct well-designed investigations.

The evolution of peripheral angioplasty is no different from other recent advances in biomedical technology and therapeutic procedures that have generated a moral crisis in modern medicine. To a significant degree, we now have the ability to exercise control not only over the effects of disease but even over the very process of life and death. With the unfolding of new discoveries and techniques, the scientific and intellectual communities have developed a keen awareness of the ethical issues that arise out of man's enhanced ability to control his destiny.[9] Thus, the dilemma of new therapies that supplant other therapeutic alternatives raises a myriad of specters, including those of aberrant, immoral, and unethical clinical investigations and experiments. But the issue that must be initially addressed is the physician's responsibilities as a clinical investigator. The intertwining of historical, ethical, and moral perspectives, as well as religious precepts, has determined these responsibilities and obligations. The fabric that has been woven from these strands provides the guidelines and regulations that dictate the behavior expected of a physician performing clinical research.

First of all, what societal right entitles a person to become a physician and attempt to heal the sick? Inherent in this concept is the idea that a physician makes a great effort to heal the sick and, at the same time, attempts to be protected from familial revenge if things do not go well. From a religious perspective,[9] God has given the physician the wherewithal to heal "by earthly or natural means." Nachmanides, a 15th century Spanish physician, said that "without that warrant to treat, the physician might hesitate to treat patients for fear of fatal consequences, in that there is an element of danger in every medical procedure; that which heals one may kill another." God has granted physicians license and warrant to heal the sick, because without such, one might forget that human life is of infinite value, and physicians should not consider their needs or belongings to be more valuable than the health of their patients. Without that warrant, the practice of medicine or of clinical research could become a secondary issue to a physi-cian who would be concerned about his or her personal effects.

From the first day of medical school, the aspiring physician faces a wide range of ethical problems, including restrictions on animal experimentation for medical research and ethical concerns of sexuality and procreation as they relate to abortion, contraception, and sexual preference. Major ethical problems are related to death and dying, mercy killing, withholding treatment, heroic measures, and even discontinuation of life-support systems. How does the physician address the issues of hazardous therapy and human experimentation?

What remains paramount is the physician's obligation to use his medical skills to heal the sick. As is clearly apparent, the physician is faced with the dilemma of doing what is correct. This injunction causes difficulties, especially in the performance of clinical investigations. First, physicians must do their best for their patients, and, because of this, society has traditionally esteemed physicians. Judaism has always held the physician in high regard, and ancient and medieval Jewish writings are replete with expressions of admiration and praise for the "faithful physician." However, the Talmudic statement, "the best physician is destined for Gehenna (hell)," is very peculiar and has generated commentaries that have relevance to the question posed. Why should physicians, who spend inordinate amounts of their time, life, and energy trying to heal and help the sick and dying, be destined to hell? In the 13th century, Rabbi Hanukah Zundel ben Joseph wrote, "He who thinks of himself as the most expert physician is destined to Gehenna because through his haughtiness, he relies on his imperfect knowledge and does not consult with his colleagues, [and] . . . because of conceit may not even consider the possibility of his being in error. [Thus, the physician may not]. . . delve adequately into medical books before he administers medicinal remedies." In 1418, a further commentary indicated that the physician "should always see Gehenna opened before him should he cause the death of anyone whose health had been entrusted to him. As a consequence, the physician must carefully consider the treatment and apply all his thought to it."[9]

Physicians are among the group of communal servants who have heavy public responsibilities and who are warned against the dangers of negligence and error. The Talmudic epigram, "to hell with the best of them," is directed toward physicians who are overly confident in their craft. At the extremes, this may include those guilty of commercializing their profession, those who fail to consult with colleagues or perform medical tests when appropriate, those who fail to heal the poor and thus indirectly cause their death, those who consider themselves to be the best in their field, or those who otherwise fail to conduct themselves in an ethical and professional manner.

Thus, there is a sufficient basis for physicians to be considered select members of society who have a societal warrant to treat people, and who must continually be reminded that this warrant requires them to provide the best care possible for their patients. In this context, how can physicians who desire to implement new ideas and concepts through experimentation remain within these moral and social guidelines?

In the 5th century BC, the Oath of Hippocrates was composed to protect the rights of patients by reminding the physician of his obligations and responsibilities. The Oath of Hippocrates and Maimonides' Prayer continue to be administered to medical students before they embark on their medical careers as reminders of what is considered appropriate conduct.[5] In 1803, Thomas Percival published his Code of Medical Ethics, which addressed physician conduct within "hospitals and other charities." The American Medical Association, in 1847, amplified this concept and created a code of medical ethics that has had several major revisions between 1903 and 1994. In 1957, medical ethics was separated and distinguished from physicians' etiquette. In 1980, the Principles of Medical Ethics (Appendix I) were adopted and promulgated as a short preamble followed by 10 succinctly stated sections, which have been clarified and updated with regard to language, gender references, and contemporary legal standards.[5]

Not until the atrocities of World War II became evident did the problem of human experimentation involving unknowing, involuntary subjects bring to light the significant moral and ethical issues that relate to clinical investigation. These ideas were codified into well-defined principles for all experimenters and researchers who work with human subjects. However, what also became apparent during this codification was that the concerns of the individual patient and the needs of society could at times be in conflict. The quantifications and delineations of behavior expected of physicians and clinical researchers have been critically important in preventing clinical investigators from becoming involved with projects to such an extent that perspective is abandoned with regard to patients' rights, existing civil law, and criminal codes (Appendix II: The Nuremberg Code[7]; Appendix III: The Declaration of Helsinki[8]). Nevertheless, there are numerous examples of how investigators have performed human experimentation with almost casual disregard of the rights of the patient. The injection of mentally retarded children in the United States with hepatitis virus, the use of LSD by the United States Army in conjunction with the Central Intelligence Agency (CIA), and the exposure of human beings to radiation of plutonium by the United States Atomic Energy Commission, are some examples that have occurred since the end of World War II. Quite rightly, during the last half of the 20th century, public awareness of the ethical and legal problems associated with medical research using human subjects has become more focused and more directed, whether the research involves children, fetuses, adults, or the elderly.[10]

Introduction to General Obligations

The physician has ethical and moral responsibilities that directly impact upon his or her ability to perform clinical human research. The investigation or experiment must be conducted within a competently designed protocol whose stated purpose or purposes and methodology conform to the rigorously scientific method by which data must be collected, formatted, assessed, and interpreted to derive scientifically valid conclusions. However, the physician's zeal should not override consideration for the welfare, safety, and comfort of the patient. Furthermore, clinical investigations used as therapies do not eliminate or invalidate particular legal considerations, such as the physician-patient relationship, a degree of patient confidentiality, patient entitlement to the best medical care, and, of significance, informed and voluntary consent. Informed consent must contain certain elements, including the nature of the investigational element; the fact that the drug, device, or procedure is experimental; an explanation of the procedure and its risks as well as potential therapeutic benefits; and alternative therapies available. In addition, the patient must have the right to ask and receive answers to questions about the drug or device and maintain the right to withdraw consent or participation at anytime. The physician should give an honest, forthright, and fair explanation of the therapy and should not impart to the patient unreal or unreasonable expectations as an inducement for the patient to participate.[11, 12]

The investigator must be aware of the risk-benefit relationship that exists within the protocol regarding human subjects and must communicate that to participants. Wecht[10] has stratified this risk-benefit relationship concisely into four categories:

1. There is a reasonable belief that benefit exceeds risk to the patient, and the study involves a patient who expresses consent by coming to the physician for a low-risk diagnostic or therapeutic procedure.
2. There is a reasonable belief that benefit is at least equal to risk and may possibly exceed it. The patient is a volunteer.
3. Risk exceeds benefit to the patient, but risk is balanced by possible benefit to society. In this case, the highest degree of informed consent is essential.

4. Risk exceeds benefit. The individual is either both subject and patient or only subject. Consent of the individual has either not been obtained or has been obtained through deceit, force of authority, or other improper means.

The last of these choices is of extreme importance, because everyone in positions of authority in government, medical institutions, health-care facilities, and custodial homes appreciates that no matter how altruistic the projected humanitarian aspects of medical research may be, human beings cannot be subjected to medical experimentation without having given properly informed consent.

GENERAL OBLIGATIONS

Clinical investigations in the United States must be conducted according to FDA regulations and the sponsor's study protocol. The investigator has the responsibility to conduct the protocol according to the signed investigator agreement; to protect the rights, well-being, and safety of subjects; to obtain informed consent; to maintain absolute control over drugs, biologic agents, or devices being investigated; to retain specific records and issue reports; and to ensure that an institutional review board (IRB) monitors and reviews the study data. Investigator obligations specifically involve maintaining accurate histories; recording all observations and pertinent data; reporting serious and unexpected adverse incidents, as well as all study information, to the sponsor; accounting for all drugs, biologics, or devices received, used, and disposed; and obtaining written informed consent from the subject or subjects or their legal representatives. In addition, regarding devices, the investigator must retain all records for 2 years, allow FDA representatives to inspect the records, and provide the IRB with information for initial and continuing review of the study.[6]

RECORD REQUIREMENTS FOR INVESTIGATORS

The investigator's agreement includes an explanation of the investigator's responsibility, an outline of any relevant procedures and protocols, a description of the facility in which the study will be conducted and any other facilities that may be involved, and a listing of the IRB responsible for review and approval of the study. Furthermore, the investigator must provide the sponsor with his or her curriculum vitae. The sponsor in turn must provide the investigator with a protocol and case report forms.[6]

DELEGATION OF AUTHORITY FOR DATA MANAGEMENT

The investigator assumes responsibility for collecting information about each subject and filling out forms.

Coinvestigators may be on site, and once they sign the investigator's agreement, they are likewise responsible for the conduct of the study and adherence to regulations. The investigator can delegate the collection of data to study coordinators whose work must be reviewed periodically by the investigator. The investigator must maintain consent forms for each subject. The records (case report forms) are maintained as source documents and must be made available to FDA inspectors. The source document (paper or computer disk) must exist, and any data entries must be individually signed and dated by the person entering data, especially if more than one person performs this task. Furthermore, corrections must be initialed.

DRUG STUDY RECORDS

Information specific to drug studies includes the study identification, the sponsor's name, the dates of each subject visit, the procedures and tests ordered, any concomitant medications, any adverse experiences, a statement that the study drug was dispensed, and any specific protocol-directed procedures.

DEVICE STUDY RECORDS

The study records consist of all correspondence with other investigators, the IRB, the sponsor, the monitor, and the FDA; receipt, use and disposition of a device, subject case histories, informed consent forms, the protocol for the study, and any other records that the FDA may request.

RECORDS FOR DISPENSING, HANDLING, AND SHIPPING ARTICLES

The investigator must maintain a record of the final disposition of study articles.

RECORD RETENTION TIME PERIODS

Records must be maintained for 2 years.

INVESTIGATOR'S REPORTS

The investigator is obliged to maintain adequate case histories for all drug subject patients as well as accurate, complete, and current records for all device study patients.

DRUG STUDY REPORTS

The investigator is responsible for supplying sponsors with progress reports (including ongoing results of the study, which may be required weekly or monthly), and safety reports (describing adverse effects). Additionally, annual reports must be filed with the IRB and must describe the status of the study, any modifications to the study, and any unanticipated problems.

DEVICE STUDY REPORTS

Reports are to be supplied to the IRB, the sponsors, the monitors, and the FDA (if requested) and include unanticipated adverse effects; withdrawal of IRB approval; progress reports (to the monitor, the IRB, and the sponsor), which must be submitted at least once a year; protocol deviations (made in an emergency to protect the subject), which must be sent to the sponsor and the IRB within 5 working days; use of a device without informed consent, which must be submitted within 5 working days to the sponsor and the IRB; a final report, which must be completed within 3 months of cessation of the protocol; and accurate, complete, and current information about any aspect of the investigation, which must be sent to the FDA and the IRB upon request.[6]

REPORTING ADVERSE EXPERIENCES

Investigators are obliged to report all adverse experiences with drugs, biologics, and devices that occur during the course of the investigation. An unanticipated adverse event must be reported within 10 working days of the occurrence. Adverse experiences are categorized as *serious adverse experiences* (i.e., fatal, life-threatening, permanently disabling, requiring inpatient hospitalization), and *unanticipated adverse device effects* (i.e., a life-threatening problem or death caused by, or associated with, a device), if that effect, problem, or death was not previously identified within the protocol. The adverse event is reported to the sponsor, with an investigator's assessment of whether the adverse event was related to the device or the drug. Sponsors must assess all reports and determine whether this occurrence was an isolated incident, or whether it was related to the clinical trial. The investigator's clinical responsibility is to follow the adverse event to its resolution. The necessity of reporting the adverse experience depends upon whether the study was related to a drug or to a device.

Drug-related adverse events are tracked both during and after the clinical investigation. During the clinical trial, the FDA mandates that an adverse occurrence must be promptly reported if there is a reasonable belief that the adverse event was caused by the drug. The investigator has the responsibility of determining what constitutes an adverse drug reaction. The sponsor bears the ultimate responsibility of reporting adverse drug events to the FDA. Postmarketing surveillance of drugs is more detailed than that which occurs during the clinical investigation, but it requires reporting adverse events that are defined as any untoward effect associated with the use of a drug in humans, whether it is considered to be drug related or not.

Device-related adverse events occur only during the study period, and all unanticipated device effects must be reported within 10 working days.

INSTITUTIONAL REVIEW BOARD (IRB) INTERACTIONS

The investigator is required by an FDA mandate to communicate with the IRB, whereas sponsors are not required to do so. The investigator must communicate with, and obtain necessary approval from, the IRB. The investigator must provide the IRB with the necessary study information (the investigator's brochure, informed consent, and any advertisements used to recruit patients) to enable the IRB to make an informed decision about whether to grant approval. The investigator must inform the IRB of any proposed changes in the protocol or any adverse experiences, and an annual report must be submitted. The investigator may not start the protocol until the IRB has provided written approval of the informed consent.

The Process for Disqualifying Investigators

Within the societal warrant that grants physicians the right to practice medicine is the inherent idea that physicians should use their best judgment to find the best ways to care for patients. However, the dilemma becomes apparent when those ways may be new, untried, or even radical in conceptual approach. Under such circumstances, can physicians proceed, utilizing an unproven form of alternative care? The answer is yes, both morally and ethically. But because these new therapies, investigations, or experiments based upon rational premises place patients at unknown risks, it is obligatory for physicians to make this known to their patients. If patients understand and agree, these forms of therapy can proceed. Physicians must always remember that despite their efforts, treatment results may not occur as envisioned. Thus, physicians who are willing to walk within this no-man's land, must remember that they are bound to do their best for their patients and for society. To avoid the potentially catastrophic situations that can occur, physicians should follow the rules prescribed for a clinical investigator. However, if a physician who is participating in an experimental or investigational procedure fails to adhere to rules and regulations, the FDA can become closely involved. This FDA involvement may result in the physician's disqualification from the research protocol or may even involve criminal penalties

The FDA can disqualify a clinical investigator who repeatedly or deliberately violates FDA regulations or one who wilfully submits false information to the sponsor in a required report. An investigator's obligations under FDA regulations include maintaining drug and biologic disposition records, preparing adequate and accurate case report forms, permitting the FDA to conduct inspections, personally performing or supervising the investigation, reporting findings promptly to the sponsor, and obtaining informed consent from each subject. The majority of problems and deficiencies occur in maintaining adequate and accurate records.

The protocol sponsor is responsible for any such investigator violations and and this person may either discontinue the investigator or notify the FDA. However, once the FDA has been notified, the process of disqualification is initiated and cannot be easily stopped. The sequence of events that follows FDA notification should make a physician think seriously about avoiding involvement in such a situation.

i. An investigator inspection is initiated. This is usually conducted by the FDA district investigator, who is a member of the FDA Division of Scientific Investigations. Subsequently, the clinical investigator receives a letter (warning or standard) that describes the noncompliant event and invites a response. The FDA informs everyone of importance of the action that has been taken. This communication is usually publicly disclosed. If the FDA is not satisfied with the clinical investigator's written response, a consent agreement can place general or specific limits upon the investigator's research. If the investigator signs the consent agreement, he or she is included on a list of investigators who have some restrictions on their use of investigational products.

ii. The clinical investigator has the option of requesting an informal conference at which the deficiencies may be explained. If the explanation satisfies the FDA, the disqualification procedures can be terminated. However, this informal conference has few procedural protections, and the transcript can be used in future criminal proceedings.

iii. If the disqualification process proceeds to an informal hearing, the investigator receives written notice detailing the FDA's allegations of wrongdoing. The investigator can choose to respond or not and can participate in the hearing. If the investigator does not respond, the FDA commissioner can make a determination of disqualification. If the investigator participates in

the informal hearing, legal counsel may be present. The officer presiding over the hearing issues a recommended decision, which is used by the commissioner to make a final written decision.

iv. FDA decisions: The FDA can issue clinical hold of a study pending the outcome of the disqualification proceedings. To avoid such action, a sponsor can remove the offending investigator and choose another investigator to continue the study. Although the majority of disqualification processes are settled by consent agreement, to enter such an agreement with the FDA means that the investigator must agree to refrain from conducting further studies within the FDA's jurisdiction or must agree to restrictions in the conduct of studies. However, the FDA can perform the following actions:
   1. Refer for criminal prosecution an investigator whose errors are egregious and who knowingly or willingly submits false information to a sponsor or who includes such information in a report required by the FDA
   2. Prosecute clinical investigators under the False Statements to the Government statute
   3. In a civil suit, a disqualified clinical investigator can be held liable to a sponsor who has had a study delayed or dismissed, or to a subject who has allegedly suffered adverse effects because of the investigator's misconduct

Any involvement in the disqualification process can have lasting effects on an investigator's professional practice; therefore, it is imperative for a clinical investigator to be familiar with and adhere to FDA regulations and guidelines in conducting clinical studies.

Innovative Therapy

The investigator must understand the difference between standard and accepted therapy, innovative therapy (i.e., therapy that is derived in the best judgment of the physician to address the patient's pathologic process), and experimentation. The National Commission for the Protection of Human Subjects of Biomedical and Behavioral Research[13] defined standard practice thus:

> Interventions that are designed solely to enhance the well-being of an individual patient or client and that have a reasonable expectation of success. The purpose of medical or behavioral practice is to provide diagnosis, preventive new treatments, or therapy to particular individuals.

The commission further described innovative therapies as procedures that were:

Designed solely to enhance the well-being of an individual patient or client" but that had not been tested sufficiently to meet the standard of having "a reasonable expectation of success." Innovative therapies have been defined as activities "ordinarily conducted. . . with either pure practice intent or with varying degrees of mixed research and practice intent" that have been sufficiently tested to meet standards for acceptance or approval.

The commission then went on the describe experimentation or research as:

An activity designed to test a hypothesis, permit conclusions to be drawn, and thereby to develop or contribute to generalized knowledge (expressed, for example, in theories, principles, and statements of relationships). Research is usually described in a formal protocol that sets forth an objective and a set of procedures designed to reach that objective.

REFERENCES

1. Scarman (Lord): Consent, communication and responsibility: J R Soc Med 79:697–700, 1986.
2. Bolam v Friern Hospital Management Committee. 1 WLR 582, 1957.
3. Allison DA, Allison H: Ethics and informed consent. *In* Watkinson A, Adam A (eds): Interventional Radiology—a practical guide. Radcliffe Medical Press Ltd, Abingdon, UK, 1996, pp 12–15.
4. Woolf (Lord): The medical profession and justice. J R Soc Med 90:364–367, 1997.
5. Council on Ethical and Judicial Affairs, Code of Medical Ethics: Current opinions with annotations, 1996–1997 ed. Chicago, American Medical Association, 1996.
6. Investigators Obligations: Tables 30 and 200. *In* Ott MB, Yingling GL: Guide to Good Clinical Practice. Thompson Publishing Group, Washington, DC, 1995, pp 7–75, 7–74.
7. Trials of War Criminals Before the Nuremberg Military Tribunals, Vol I, II: The Medical Case. Washington, DC, US Government Printing Office, 1948.
8. The Declaration of Helsinki: Ann Intern Med (Suppl)67:74–75, 1967.
9. Rosner F: Modern Medicine and Jewish Ethics. New York, Yeshiva University Press, 1986.
10. Wecht CH: Legislative and Business Aspects of Medicine. Res Exp, CPT 49:711–728, 1995.
11. Levine RJ: Ethics and Regulations of Clinical Research, 2nd ed. New Haven, CT, Yale University Press, 1986.
12. Freedman B: Equipoise and the ethics of clinical research. N Engl J Med 28:141–145, 1987.
13. Title II (US Congress), Part A. para201 (a) and para202 (a) of the National Research Service Award Act of 1972. Pub. No.93-328, 88 Stat.142. Washington, DC.

The medical profession has long subscribed to a body of ethical statements developed primarily for the benefit of the patient. As a member of this profession, a physician must recognize responsibility not only to patients but also to society, to other health professions, and to self. The following Principles adopted by the American Medical Association are not laws but standards of conduct that define the essentials of honorable behavior for the physician.

I. A physician shall be dedicated to providing competent medical service with compassion and respect for human dignity.

II. A physician shall deal honestly with patients and colleagues, and strive to expose those physicians deficient in character or competence, or who engage in fraud or deception.

III. A physician shall respect the law and also recognize a responsibility to seek changes in those requirements that are contrary to the best interests of the patient.

IV. A physician shall respect the rights of patients, of colleagues, and of other health professionals, and shall safeguard patient confidences within the constraints of the law.

V. A physician shall continue to study, apply, and advance scientific knowledge; make relevant information available to patients, colleagues, and the public; obtain consultation; and use the talents of other health professions when indicated.

VI. A physician shall, in the provision of appropriate patient care, except in emergencies, be free to choose whom to serve, with whom to associate, and the environment in which to provide medical services.

VII. A physician shall recognize a responsibility to participate in activities contributing to an improved community.

Appendix *II* The Nuremberg Code

1. The voluntary consent of the human subject is absolutely essential. This means that the person involved should have legal capacity to give consent; should be so situated so as to exercise free power of choice, without the intervention of any element of force, fraud, deceit, duress, overreaching, or other ulterior form of constraint or coercion; and should have sufficient knowledge as to enable him to make an understanding and enlightened decision. This latter element requires that before the acceptance of an affirmative decision by the experimental subject, there should be made known to him the nature, duration, and purpose of the experiment; the method and means buy which it is to be conducted; all inconveniences and hazards reasonably to be expected; and the effects upon his health or person that may possibly come from his participation in the experiment. The duty and responsibility for ascertaining the quality of the consent rests upon each individual who initiates, directs, or engages in the experiment. It is a personal duty and responsibility that may not be delegated to another with impunity.
2. The experiment should be such as to yield fruitful results for the good of society, unprocurable by other methods or means of study, and not random and unnecessary in nature.
3. The experiment should be so designed and based on the results of animal experimentation and a knowledge of the natural history of the disease or other problem under study that the anticipated results will justify the performance of the experiment.
4. The experiment should be conducted as to avoid all unnecessary physical and mental suffering and injury.
5. No experiment should be conducted where there is a priori reason to believe that death or disabling injury will occur; except, perhaps, in those experiments where the experimental physicians also serve as subjects.
6. The degree of risk to be taken should never exceed that determined by the humanitarian importance of the problem to be solved by the experiment.
7. Proper preparation should be made and adequate facilities provided to protect the experimental subject against even remote possibilities of injury, disability, or death.
8. Only scientifically qualified persons should conduct the experiment. The highest degree of skill and care should be required through all stages of the experiment of those that conduct or engage in the experiment.
9. During the course of the experiment, the human subject should be at liberty to bring the experiment to an end if he has reached the physical or mental state where continuation of the experiment seems to him to be impossible.
10. During the course of the experiment, the scientist in charge must be prepared to terminate the experiment at any stage if he has probable cause to believe, in the exercise of good faith, superior skill, and careful judgment required of him, that a continuation of the experiment is likely to result in injury, disability, or death to the experimental subject.

Appendix III The Declaration of Helsinki

It is the mission of the doctor to safeguard the health of the people. His knowledge and conscience are dedicated to the fulfillment of his mission.

The Declaration of Geneva of the World Medical Association binds the doctor with the words:" The health of my patient will be my first consideration," and the International Code of Medical Ethics, which declares that "Any act or advice that could weaken physical or mental resistance of a human being may be used only in his interest."

The World Medical Association has prepared the following recommendations as a guide to each doctor in clinical research. It must be stressed that the standards as drafted are only a guide to physicians all over the world. Doctors are not relieved from criminal, civil, and ethical responsibilities under the laws of their own countries.

In the files of clinical research, a fundamental distinction must be recognized between clinical research, in which the aim is essentially therapeutic for a patient, and the clinical research, the essential object of which is purely scientific and without therapeutic value to the person subjected to the research.

Basic Principles

1. Clinical research must conform to the moral and scientific principles that justify medical research and should be based on laboratory and animal experiments or other scientifically established facts.
2. Clinical research should be conducted only by scientifically qualified persons and under the supervision of a qualified medical person.
3. Clinical research cannot legitimately be carried out unless the importance of the objective is in proportion to the inherent risk to the subject.
4. Every clinical research project should be preceded by careful assessment of inherent risks in comparison to foreseeable benefits to the subject or the others.
5. The doctor in performing clinical research in which

the personality of the subject is liable to be altered by drugs or experimental procedures should exercise special caution.

Clinical Research Combined With Professional Care

1. In the treatment of the sick person, the doctor must be free to use a new therapeutic measure if in his or her judgment it offers hope of saving life, reestablishing health, or alleviating suffering. If at all possible, consistent with patient psychology, the doctor should obtain the patient's freely given consent after the patient has been given a full explanation. In case of legal incapacity, counsel should also be procured from the legal guardian; in case of physical incapacity, the permission of the legal guardian replaces that of the patient.
2. The doctor can combine clinical research with professional care, the objective being the acquisition of new medical knowledge only to the extent that clinical research is justified by its therapeutic value for the patient.

Nontherapeutic Clinical Research

1. In the purely scientific application of clinical research carried out on a human being, it is the duty of the doctor to remain the protector of the life and health of that person on whom clinical research is being carried out.
2. The doctor must explain the nature, the purpose, and the risk of clinical research to the subject.
3. Clinical research on a human being cannot be undertaken without his free consent after he has been informed; if he is legally incompetent, the consent of the legal guardian should be procured.
4. Consent should, as a rule, be obtained in writing. However, the responsibility for clinical research always remains with the research worker; it never falls on the subject, even after consent is obtained.

5. The investigator must respect the right of each individual to safeguard his personal integrity, especially if the subject is in a dependent relationship to the investigator. At any time during the course of clinical research, the subject or his guardian should be free to withdraw permission for research to be continued. The investigator or the investigating team should discontinue the research if in his or their judgment, it may, if continued, be harmful to the individual.

Section 2

Arterial Interventions

Chapter 8 Interventions in the Aorta and Iliac Arteries

Endovascular Contributors: Dierk Vorwerk and Karl Schürmann
Surgical Contributors: Dan L. Serna, Teresa J. Chan, and Samuel Eric Wilson

Since the inception of percutaneous interventions, the aorta and the iliac arteries have been a primary field for these procedures. Easy access to the lesion, the relatively large diameter of the target vessels, and the comparably benign outcome of even major complications contribute to the wide acceptance of percutaneous interventions in this area. Over the years, indications for these procedures have increased, and they now include treatment not only of patients who have stenotic disease but also of those who have occlusive disease and aneurysms. In particular, the introduction of vascular stents has been very helpful in overcoming major problems and offering a tool to treat patients who have major complications (see Chapter 5 and, later in this chapter, the section entitled Complications) that would otherwise require surgical repair.

AORTIC DISEASE

Clinical Aspects

Although the suprarenal abdominal aorta is very rarely a target for percutaneous intervention, the infrarenal segment may undergo balloon angioplasty or related treatment. In more than 90% of cases, the cause of infrarenal aortic obstruction is atherosclerotic disease.[1] Clinically, simple infrarenal aortic stenoses that have no relation to the aortic bifurcation are infrequently found, but stenoses of both the very distal aortic segment and the common iliac arteries are much more frequent. These may be complicated by an acute or subacute thrombosis of the aortic bifurcation known as Leriche's syndrome. Small distal aortic caliber, especially in female patients, may be a predisposing factor. Atherosclerotic stenosis above the orifice of the inferior mesenteric artery is uncommon.[1]

By comparison, embolic occlusion of the distal aorta is rare but may occur in patients who have mitral valve disease. Other rare causes of aortic obstruction are fibromuscular dysplasia, Takayasu disease, or retroperitoneal fibrosis.

Typically, patients who have aortic obstruction are between 40 and 70 years of age. In aortic occlusions, 55% are located at the level of the aortic bifurcation, 8% involve the complete infrarenal segment, and 37% involve aortic segments alone.[1]

Collateral pathways are via lumbar, epigastric, and mesenteric arteries. Clinical symptoms in aortic obstruction are bilateral claudication, with predominantly upper thigh symptoms (that may mimic spinal angina), buttock pain, and erectile dysfunction in males. In occlusions, acute bilateral ischemia is present if no pre-existing stenotic process has promoted earlier development of collateral pathways.

Aortic aneurysmal disease is increasingly becoming a field of interest for interventional radiologists, and discussion of this area may be combined with that of atherosclerotic obstructive disease. Percutaneous treatment of aneurysms, however, is dealt with in a separate chapter.

Indications for Treatment

Treatment is indicated if there are clinical symptoms that have a major impact on the lifestyle and professional requirements of an individual patient. This certainly depends on the patient's age and general circumstances. In Europe, a walking distance capacity of less than 220 yd corresponds to stage 2b disease, which, according to the traditional Fontaine classification, is generally accepted as a borderline that indicates the need for interventional treatment.

Duplex scanning, determination of ankle-arm indices, and angiography, as well as magnetic resonance (MR) or computed tomography (CT) angiography are helpful in determining extent and type of obstruction. The criteria for diagnosing significant obstruction do not differ significantly from those required for other arteries (i.e., a minimum diameter stenosis of 50%).

INDICATIONS FOR PERCUTANEOUS TREATMENT

Indications for percutaneous vs. surgical treatment depend largely on the location, extension, acuteness, and type of obstruction.

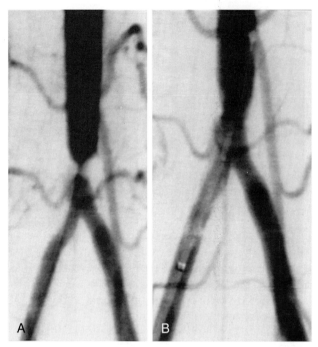

Figure 8–1. *A,* Concentric infrarenal aortic stenosis. *B,* Angioplasty alone leads to a sufficient lumen.

Accepted indications for balloon angioplasty (Fig. 8–1) are:

- Concentric segmental stenosis
- Short segment aortic bifurcational stenosis

Balloon angioplasty may be followed by stent insertion in cases of insufficient luminal gain (Fig. 8–2) after adequate balloon angioplasty has been performed. Stent placement is also appropriate if there is occurrence of significant dissection after percutaneous transluminal angioplasty (PTA).

Balloon angioplasty is contraindicated if a completely calcified ring is present at the site of obstruction, because aortic rupture has occasionally been reported under these circumstances.[2] According to LaPlace's law, the aorta is theoretically more prone to rupture than vessels of smaller diameter, such as the iliac artery. Long-segment diffuse disease of both the aorta and the iliac arteries might be considered as a contraindication, and, under these circumstances, surgical aortobifemoral bypass grafting might be a better choice.

Bifurcational aortic stenosis (Fig. 8–3) may be treated by balloon angioplasty using a simultaneous "kissing balloon" technique to dilate both distal aortic segment and both iliac orifices. Stent implantation has been increasingly used to achieve a stable postangioplasty widening by use of kissing stents in the distal aorta and both iliac arteries.

Few reports exist on the use of stents for remodeling the distal aortic segment or the aortic bifurcation of patients who have distal aortic occlusion.[3, 4] In this difficult illness, use of advanced interventional techniques is certainly of advantage over simple balloon angioplasty.

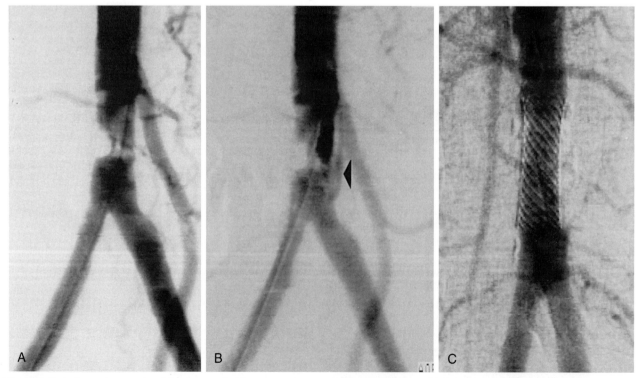

Figure 8–2. *A,* Eccentric stenosis of distal aorta. *B,* After percutaneous transluminal angioplasty (PTA), there has been no luminal gain but lateral dissection (arrow) is seen. *C,* After stent insertion (16-mm Wallstent), wide aortic lumen is restored and dissection is compressed.

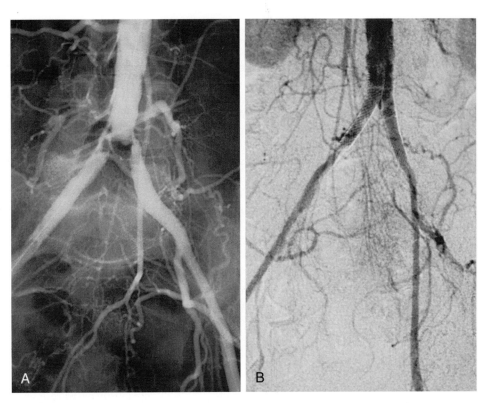

Figure 8–3. *A,* Bifurcational distal aortic stenosis with involvement of both iliac orifices. *B,* After bilateral stenting of aortic bifurcation, patency is restored.

Technical Aspects

There are no major differences between the techniques used in the aortic and iliac segments for negotiating stenoses or crossing occlusions. This is also true for balloon dilatation, which does not differ significantly from performance of angioplasty elsewhere in the body. The large diameter of the aortic lumen, however, is a particular problem.

KISSING BALLOON TECHNIQUE

Until recently, the major difficulty with this procedure was the lack of suitable balloons with sufficiently large diameters of 16 to 20 mm. Thus, a double or triple balloon technique has been recommended to open the aortic stenosis to a sufficiently large diameter. If two or three kissing balloons are inserted by a bifemoral approach respectively, an additional transbrachial approach and are inflated simultaneously, the aortic lumen can be widened to its original diameter.

A kissing technique is still recommendable for dilatation of bilateral stenosis of the aortic bifurcation and the very distal aortic segment close to the bifurcation, because this technique allows remodeling of the aortic bifurcation.

SINGLE BALLOON TECHNIQUE

More recently, large-diameter balloons (between 16 and 25 mm) have become available, and these allow use of a single-balloon technique by a unifemoral approach. To avoid overdilatation and rupture of the proximal iliac segment, it is important to locate these balloons within the aortic lumen without overriding the bifurcation.

Stent insertion into the infrarenal aortic segment follows the same rules as elsewhere. Use of a stent of appropriate size (at least 14 to 16 mm) is necessary to avoid undersizing. The largest stent diameter can be achieved by use of the balloon-expandable Palmaz XXL stent, which can be mounted on a large balloon and inflated up to 25 mm in diameter.

SINGLE-STENT TECHNIQUE

If lesions do not involve the aortic bifurcation, a single stent can be implanted with no specific technical requirements. The type of stent to be used depends on the experience of the interventionist. This is particularly true if the lesions are located a considerable distance from the bifurcation. Depending on the length of the stent or the location of the lesion, overstenting of the inferior mesenteric artery may be unavoidable.

However, if the lesion ends very close to the bifurcation, placement of a single stent, especially a balloon-expandable stent, may become difficult without overdilatation of an iliac orifice. Under these circumstances, use of a self-expanding stent may be advantageous, and the aortic bifurcation is protected by a crossover catheter inserted from a contralateral approach.

KISSING STENT TECHNIQUE

An alternative technique in the case of a very distal aortic or bifurcational lesion is the use of kissing stents. Analogous to the kissing balloon method, stents of preferably identical diameter and length are placed in kissing fashion within the distal aorta, with their distal end extending into the common iliac artery. Very frequently, the stents tend to meet the opposite aortic wall. Thus, instead of being shaped in a kissing fashion, they cross each other, forming a mirror-sided artificial iliac orifice.

There are not very many reports of this technique, and some questions remain unresolved. It is not yet known whether there are potential sequelae from using two open stents that remain partially nonendothelialized in their aortic portion. They may cause embolic disease or increase the patient's tendency for thrombosis. It is still under discussion whether covered stents would be advantageous in these cases. Use of noncovered stents is less problematic in distal aortic occlusive disease.

If a kissing stent technique is applied, it is mandatory that the proximal ends of both stents are exactly level to avoid one stent's compromising the inflow into the other. For that reason, use of noncompressible stents, such as the Palmaz stent or the new Perflex stent (which are both balloon-expandable), seems of benefit.

Results

As reported in literature, PTA of the aorta has an excellent outcome compared with those of other PTA sites.

A primary success rate of 95% and cumulative patency rates of 98% after 1 year and 80% after 5 years, respectively, have been compiled from different series.[5]

Single cases of aortic stenting of stenoses have been reported, usually with excellent outcomes. Long reported 2 cases of successful stenting in patients who had Leriche's syndrome,[6] and Dietrich reported 6 cases of chronic aortic occlusion in patients who underwent thrombolysis and stenting with Palmaz stents.[4]

Complications

Complications that may occur after aortic dilatation are not different from those in other vascular provinces; however, they may be of major clinical impact. Although severe dissection, recoil, or residual stenoses are simply treated by additional stent implantation, aortic rupture has been reported rarely but is potentially life threatening and, therefore, the patient has to undergo immediate surgery. To limit the extent of exsanguination, a large occlusion latex balloon should be positioned just below the renal arteries or placed as a covering over the site of the rupture and left inflated until the patient is prepared for surgical repair. To avoid this complication, computerized tomography is recommended before performance of the intervention to exclude complete or nearly complete circular calcification of the aortic wall, which is said to be a risk factor for rupture.

Theoretically, a covered stent graft may be placed across the site of rupture percutaneously; however, this method has as yet only been reported for iliac arterial rupture and may risk occlusion of major collateral arteries and the inferior mesenteric artery.

Embolization of atheromatous material occurs in less than 1% of cases.[5]

Subacute complications include thrombosis. This has not been reported for pure aortic dilatation or stenting but is a potential hazard in remodeling techniques of the aortic bifurcation. Thrombosis may be predisposed by adjacent aortic disease, with plaque overhanging the stent orifice and causing inflow obstruction or by adjacent outflow problems. If a poor technical result occasions placement of a stent or causes thrombosis after PTA, surgery is a reasonable option. If surgery is not elected, thrombolysis may be tried. Thanks to their large diameter, reobstruction of aortic stents occurs rarely, and they may undergo repeat balloon dilatation similar to that used for iliac stents. In kissing stents, obstruction may be caused by neointimal hyperplasia, for which the patient may undergo reballooning, atherectomy, or a second stent.

ILIAC ARTERIAL DISEASE

Clinical Aspects

Iliac disease accounts for approximately one third of lower limb occlusive arterial disease, with two thirds of cases located infrainguinally. Iliac PTA plays a major role in interventional radiologic routine because it is a well-established procedure in most institutions. A large number patients who have lesions are responsive to percutaneous treatment, and technical as well as clinical results are satisfying.

Clinically, intermittent claudication starting in the upper thigh in combination with lower limb claudication is the leading symptom. Erectile dysfunction in male patients may also be present. In isolated iliac lesions, critical ischemia is rare if it is not combined with additional subinguinal disease. Rarely, blue toe syndrome may be present if cholesterol embolization has occurred as a result of an ulcerated plaque in the iliac axis.

Weakened femoral pulses and reduced ankle-arm

index are simple clinical signs that may indicate iliac obstruction. These can be verified by direct or post-stenotic color-coded or duplex studies. For planning of a percutaneous intervention, angiography is still most helpful.

Clinical indication for treatment depends on the severity of symptoms and how they limit the daily life of an individual patient.

Indications for Percutaneous Treatment

Stent placement in patients who have stenotic lesions should be indicated from a technical point of view if angioplasty is inadequate (Fig. 8–4), as defined by visibly poor outflow or major pressure gradients. Because follow-up data are now available showing that iliac stent placement is comparatively safe, a liberal approach is justified, although primary stenting of stenosis does not seem generally justified for socio-economic reasons and potential follow-up problems.

Furthermore, primary stenting adds no benefit to successful balloon dilatation. Thus, primary stenting is only recommended if PTA fails or technical requirements compromise success of simple PTA, such as occur in patients who have iliac occlusion.

STENOSES

Although balloon angioplasty has proved to be an effective procedure, particularly in the treatment of patients who have iliac stenoses, the indication for stent placement should be restricted to lesions that are not primarily removed by PTA alone. An inadequate postangioplasty result has been suggested as a general indication for stent placement, although the term "inadequate" remains poorly defined. Examination of residual pressure gradients is certainly a useful way to assess the angioplasty result, but the borderline gradient that ultimately requires additional intervention is as yet unknown; moreover, the decision should not be made without reference to both morphologic criteria and visibly reduced flow.

Long-segment stenoses that have an irregular surface, aneurysmal formation, or markedly ulcerated plaques may be included in the group of complex lesions (Fig. 8–5). Eccentric stenoses and ostial lesions with extension to the aortic bifurcation are known not to respond well to balloon angioplasty.

A stenotic lesion may respond well to balloon inflation but may collapse after deflating the balloon.

Complications of balloon angioplasty are well treated by stent placement (see Fig. 8–5C, D). This includes intramural hematomas as well as flow-obstructing dissection that may be an acute indication for stent placement to maintain the vascular lumen and thus obviate emergency surgery.

Iliac restenosis after previous PTA does not usually require stent placement, because there is no proof that stenting prevents restenosis under such circumstances. Stenting may, however, be considered from a technical point of view in cases in which the result of balloon angioplasty remains compromised. An inadequate result after state-of-the-art balloon dilatation

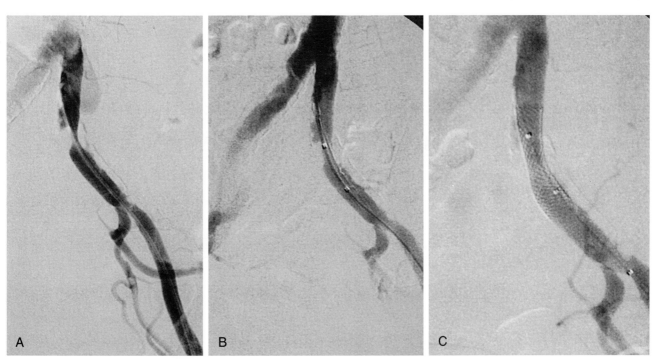

Figure 8–4. *A,* Concentric common iliac artery stenosis that appears to be ideal for percutaneous transluminal angioplasty (PTA) alone. *B,* After PTA, residual stenosis is still present. *C,* Stent placement allows full opening of lesion.

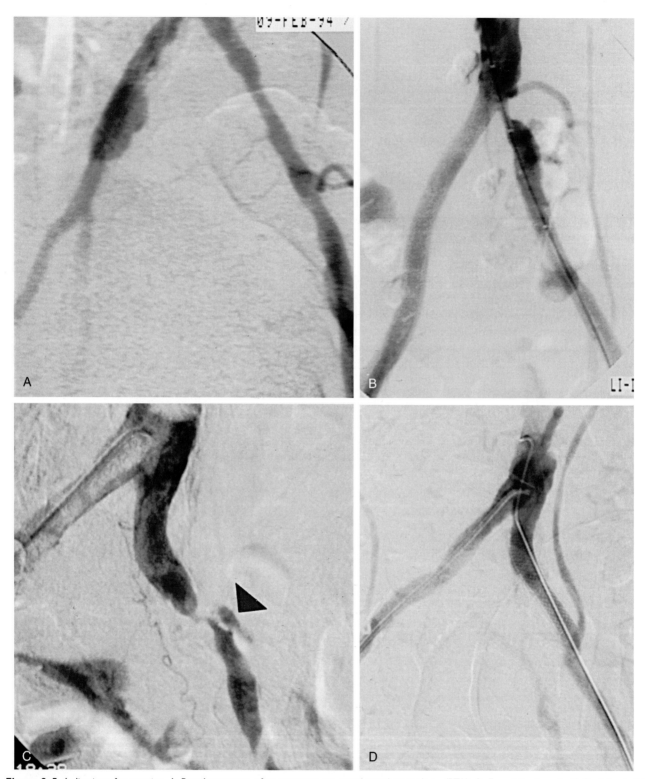

Figure 8–5. Indications for stenting. *A,* Pseudoaneurysm after percutaneous transluminal angioplasty (PTA). *B,* Eccentric stenosis. *C,* Partial arterial rupture after PTA. *D,* Partial rupture after PTA and stenting.

of the iliac stenoses is, however, a prerequisite for secondary stent placement in patients who have stenotic lesions.

OCCLUSIONS

Percutaneous treatment of patients who have iliac occlusions is technically feasible. In those who have acute thrombosis, thrombolysis as an alternative to surgical thrombectomy may precede PTA of an underlying lesion. Mechanical thrombectomy via percutaneous access is still in its infancy and cannot be recommended as a routine approach because potential risks, such as downward or crossover embolization, are possible, and no data are yet available to determine the overall complications of such an approach.

In patients who have chronic occlusions with an occlusion time exceeding 3 months, balloon angioplasty alone, thrombolysis with subsequent balloon angioplasty, elective stenting, or mechanical passage of the occlusion followed by primary stent implantation have been described as alternative techniques (Fig. 8–6).

Metallic stents, especially self-expandable endoprostheses, offer a new concept of percutaneous revascularization in patients who have chronic iliac occlusion.[7] Self-expandable stents are used to cover the occluding thrombotic material, thereby preventing peripheral dislodgment, which is a well-known complication of percutaneous recanalization of occlusions.

There should always be a technical indication for using a metallic stent in an artery. The type and morphology of the patient's lesion, the outcome of balloon angioplasty, and the complexity of the situation are important criteria, even though stenting has been tested and found to be a safe procedure.

This is particularly true for treatment of patients who have restenosis. There has been no proof up to the present that stent placement is more effective in preventing restenosis than technically successful balloon angioplasty; moreover, there is no proof that in a restenosed vessel, use of a stent would be beneficial to prevent recurrent stenosis.

Technical Aspects

BALLOON DILATATION

Balloon dilatation of iliac arteries is relatively simple to perform. A retrograde transfemoral approach is the easiest access to this type of stenotic lesion. Crossover dilatation may be performed for special indications,

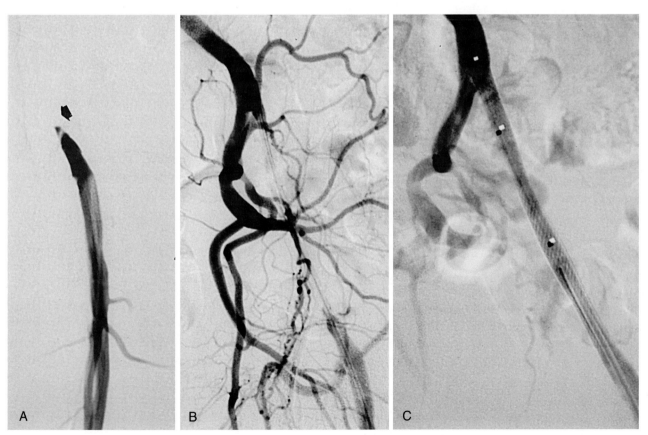

Figure 8–6. *A,* Occlusion of left external iliac artery with tapered end of occlusion (arrow). *B,* Mechanical passage of occluded segment. *C,* After stenting, patency is restored.

such as double-sided stenoses, in case both lesions should be dilated in one session, or in case an external iliac stenosis extends far down into the common femoral artery. After careful traversal of the diseased segment, a suitable balloon is placed across the lesion, and dilatation is performed either manually or by using a pressure-monitoring syringe. The size of the balloon may be decided either by film measurement or by digital subtraction angiography (DSA) images using graduated catheters that allow fairly exact measurement of the vessel size.

Imaging the postdilatation result can be accomplished by reinserting an angiographic catheter or by backflush via the sheath. Backflush angiography has been said to be a risk for retrograde dissection in cases of forceful injection. However, in our experience using DSA, this is an extremely rare event, and sequelae may be limited if the guide wire is left in place.

There is widespread agreement that both the hemodynamic relevance of a lesion as well as post-PTA success can be accurately monitored by measuring the pressure gradient across the lesion. However, there is some dispute on the appropriate level of pressure. A mean pressure gradient of 10 mm Hg or less after peripheral drug-induced vasodilation is accepted by most authors to indicate successful PTA, even if the morphologic result is not excellent. Some authors use a systolic gradient of 10 mm Hg.

There is no uniform agreement as to whether PTA of simple iliac lesions requires any additional anticoagulation afterwards. We regularly keep our patients on full heparinization (500 to 1000 IU/h) for 12 to 24 hours and recommend lifetime aspirin medication (100 mg/d).

STENT IMPLANTATION

If balloon angioplasty fails by morphologic and functional criteria, stent implantation can be considered for patients who have stenotic lesions. Techniques depend on the type of stent used. There is no preference for which type of stent should be used, because most clinical series showed similar results. The length of the lesion, its location, the experience of the investigator, and the availability of an appropriately sized device are important details that may determine preference for one type over another.

Exact placement is mandatory to avoid major complications, especially if the stent has to be placed close to the aortic bifurcation. Although self-expanding stents can be corrected to a limited extent during placement, balloon-expandable stents cannot undergo correction of their localization once inflation of the balloon has been started.

A number of different stents have been used in peripheral arterial vessels. The Wallstent, Palmaz stent, and Strecker stent have been used most exten-

sively; therefore, the longest periods of follow-up data exist for these stents. New stent devices have come into use, such as the nitinol Memotherm stent and the Cragg stent, for which only very short follow-up data are yet available.

ATHERECTOMY

Directional atherectomy does not play a major role in the treatment of patients who have iliac arterial disease. This is because the ratio of the introducer to the working diameter in most atherectomy systems is relatively low. A large introducer sheath is required to carry out atherectomy on iliac arteries between 10 and 12 mm in diameter. The Simpson atherectomy catheter system, for example, requires an 11 French (F) sheath to treat iliac lesions adequately. Atherectomy, however, plays a more important role in the removal of neointimal hyperplasia from restenosed stents.

STENT REOBSTRUCTION

For in-stent stenosis (Fig. 8–7), either directional atherectomy or balloon dilatation, or both are recommendable. If PTA is used, a balloon size according to the outer diameter of the stent in place is recom-

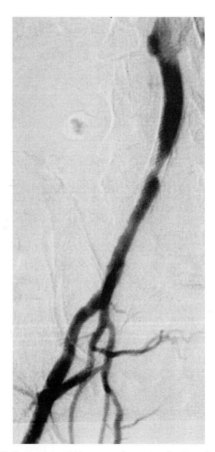

Figure 8–7. Restenosis within stent after recanalization of an iliac arterial occlusion.

mended to compress the neointima maximally, especially if compression occurs within a self-expanding stent that does not allow overexpansion. If a balloon-expandable stent is used, slight overdilatation of the stent is recommended to gain a larger diameter despite the presence of neointimal tissue. Some authors prefer atherectomy for debulking the stent. This is easily achievable in smaller stents, such as those that are used in the femoral arteries, but very large instruments (11 F) may be required in iliac stents.

In patients who have stent occlusion, treatment is more difficult. Technical problems are usually responsible for acute occlusions that occur soon after placement, and it is mandatory to overcome these problems to maintain long-term success. Recent thrombosis should be treated by thrombolysis followed by PTA, additional stent placement, or both.

Late occlusion is mainly the result of reobstruction by neointima within or adjacent to the stent. There are few data published about experience in treating patients who have complete stent occlusion at a chronic stage. Thrombolysis, atherectomy, and mechanical aspiration followed by balloon angioplasty are possible techniques. One of the easier methods is use of the stent-in-stent technique. After traversal of the occluded stent, which is generally easy to accomplish, a stent is placed within the occluded segment, bridging it at both ends. The stent is then carefully dilated, with a tendency to underdilate by 1 to 2 mm. This is considered a comparatively safe method for avoiding embolization of occluding material.

RESULTS

Balloon Dilatation

For patients who had undergone aortoiliac balloon angioplasty, Becker and coworkers compiled PTA data from the literature, including 2679 procedures that showed an average technical success rate of 92%, a 2-year patency rate of 81% (range 65 to 93%), and a 5-year-patency rate of 72% (range 50 to 87%).[8] Advanced catheter and wire technology certainly contributed to improved results with use of this technique. Gardiner and coworkers described a total complication rate of 4.5% and a major complication rate requiring surgery in 2.7% of 224 iliac procedures.[9] More recently, Tegtmeyer and coworkers reported on a single-center series of 200 patients, with a technical success rate for PTA of 88%, a total complication rate of 10.5%, and a major complication rate of 6.5%.[10] Follow-up results documented a 2-year patency rate of 90% and a 5-year patency rate of 85% in patients who were primarily successfully treated. The second-ary patency rates were 99% after 2 years and 92% after 5 years, respectively.

Improvement of these results seems difficult to achieve. The types of lesion that are treated, however, influence the technical results. Iliac lesions, for example, (including eccentric, calcified, or ulcerated plaques), dissection, or iliac occlusions have a major impact on the technical and, presumably, the follow-up results of iliac PTA. Stenting, therefore, especially in difficult cases and in patients who have complications as a result of simple balloon angioplasty, offers a solution to the problem and improves technical success.[8, 11]

Stent Implantation

WALLSTENT

In our own experience, we followed 118 patients who had iliac stenoses and stents.[11, 12] The mean length of the stenosed segment was 3 ± 2 cm; in 103 patients, the lesion was shorter than 5 cm, and in 15 patients it was longer than 5 cm. Morphologically, 85 lesions were eccentric, 73 showed major calcifications, and 52 had irregular margins.

A total of 142 stents were placed, with a mean of 1.2 ± 0.5 stents per patient. The mean stented segment was 4 ± 2 cm. The clinical stage improved in 112 patients. Eighty-nine patients improved by two or more stages, according to Fontaine. Mean ankle-arm index improved significantly to 0.92 ± 0.17.

Primary cumulative patency was 97% after 6 months, 95% after 1 year, and 88% after 2 years; the 4-year patency rate was 82%. Secondary or assisted patency was 97% after 6 months, 96 % after 1 year, and 93% after 2 years. Patency rates at 3 and 4 years were 91% each.

Chronic Iliac Occlusions

We treated 103 chronic iliac occlusions.[13] Mean length of the occluded segment was 5.1 ± 3.1 cm; in 44 patients, the occlusion was shorter than 5 cm (Society of Cardiovascular and Interventional Radiology [SCVIR class III]), and in 59 patients, it was longer than 5 cm (SCVIR class IV).[8] The lesion included the orifice of the common iliac artery in 48 patients and the orifice of the external iliac artery in 41 patients. The lesion extended into the common femoral artery in 2 patients. Mean ankle-arm index at rest was 0.48 ± 0.2 prior to treatment.

Available angiographic follow-up period was 26 ± 18 months on average, clinical follow-up period was 29 ± 17 months on average.

A total of 154 stents were placed, with a mean

placement of 1.6 ± 0.7 stents per patient. The mean stented segment was 6.1 ± 3.3 cm. Arterial flow was successfully re-established in 101 patients. In 2 patients, the stent entered the aorta subintimally and led to a compression of the stent entrance. In both of these patients, further intervention was abandoned to avoid arterial rupture, and the new channel thrombosed within 24 hours despite heparinization. Thus, the technical success rate of remodeling the vascular lumen was 98% (101 of 103 patients). The clinical stage improved in 99 patients. Mean ankle-arm index improved from 0.89 ± 0.19.

The primary patency rate was 92% after 6 months, 87% after 1 year and, 83% after 2 years. The 4-year-patency rate was 78%. The secondary or assisted patency rate was 95% after 6 months, 94% after 1 year, and 90% after 2 years. Patency rates at 3 and 4 years were 88% each.

PALMAZ AND STRECKER STENTS

For iliac stent placement, larger series with follow-up data are now available for three types of vascular endoprostheses: the Strecker stent, the Palmaz stent, and the Wallstent.[14, 15] All types of devices show different patterns of stent design, radial expansile force, and surface geometry, which may theoretically influence follow-up results in the individual type of implant.[16]

For the Palmaz stent, a multicenter study, including 486 patients, revealed a technical success rate of 99%, a complication rate of 10%, and major complications in 4.7%. The clinical follow-up patency rate was 90% after 1 year and 84% after 2 years.[15]

Strecker and coworkers reported a technical success rate of 100% with implantation of a Strecker tantalum stent in 116 patients who had iliac lesions, and a follow-up patency rate of 95% at 1 and 2 years, respectively.[14] Just recently, Long and coworkers reported on iliac implantation of Strecker stents in 64 patients.[17] Technical success rate was 98% and the complication rate was 12%, but the rate of major complications was low at 3.1%.[15] They reported restenosis in 10 patients and reocclusion in 8. Our results with the Wallstent compare well with those reported for other types of stents. These results are equal to or even better than the data reported in the literature for other types of devices. However, it remains difficult to compare the data from different series because numerous intrinsic and individual factors may also be of importance, including lesion morphology, extent of disease, outflow conditions, and others. In our series, only stenotic lesions were considered, and in comparison with patency results in iliac occlusions, those for stenoses were somewhat better.[13]

Referring to those data published on use of different types of metallic stents in iliac arteries, there are no obvious differences regarding technical success and follow-up results.

OTHER STENTS

For the time being, few clinical results are available for evaluating other stents, such as the Cragg noncovered nitinol stent and the low-profile Memotherm nitinol stent. Hausegger and coworkers reported on the first clinical results with the Cragg stent, which demonstrated a high level of technical success.[18] Starck and coworkers presented follow-up data on 203 patients who received the Memotherm stent, reporting a technical success rate of 98%. They used the stent in the iliac (44%) and femoropopliteal regions (52%) and claimed to have achieved better follow-up outcomes than those obtained with the Strecker stent.[19] These preliminary data, however, have yet to be warranted by controlled and published follow-up studies.

ATHERECTOMY

Few data are available for iliac atherectomy using Simpson directional atherectomy catheters. A technical success of 85% and a 3-year patency rate ranging from 57 to 84% were reported.[5] Maynar preferentially used the system to treat the external iliac artery, which is more accessible to atherectomy because of its smaller diameter; 18-month-patency was 87%.[20]

REOBSTRUCTION IN STENTS

In cases of reobstruction, percutaneous reintervention is feasible. We analyzed our results with reinterventions in 26 instances.[21] In 10 cases of stent stenoses, successful reintervention was possible. Stent occlusion was technically successful in 88% (14 of 16) of cases. Embolization was the major complication of reintervention (2 of 26 instances).

Patency after treatment of stent stenosis was better, with an 87% success rate after 1 year compared with patency after stent occlusion of 57% after 1 year. Recurrence of obstruction occurred in 8 of 24 successful reinterventions.

Other authors prefer atherectomy as the method of choice in stent stenosis and occlusion. Available data are limited to compare different techniques of reintervention.

Complications

Balloon angioplasty of iliac arteries is relatively safe. The overall complication rate after iliac PTA has been reported to be 8.1%, with major complications in 2.7% of cases and major complications that required surgery in 1.2%. The most frequent complications were access problems of hematomas (2.9%) and pseudoaneurysms (0.5%). Site problems, such as acute occlusion (1.9%), embolization (1.6%), and arterial rupture (0.2%), are less frequent. Mortality was very low, with an average of 0.2%.[5]

Stenting helped to improve the technical results of iliac PTA and also solved complications, such as acute occlusion. Use of stents, moreover, helped to extend the use of percutaneous techniques to cases that would otherwise be limited to surgery. Thus, potential problems in such patients seemed more likely than in those who were candidates for balloon angioplasty alone. After stenting, the rate of complications in iliac arteries was relatively small. The Wallstent was used in patients who had iliac stenoses. The total complication rate was 6.8%, with a major complication rate of 3.4%, which included subacute stent thrombosis. In iliac occlusions, complications occurred in 11.7% of cases. An additional surgical or percutaneous reintervention was necessary in 6 patients; thus, the major complication rate was 5.8%, which included arterial emboli (the most frequent type of complication in chronic arterial occlusions). Stent reobstruction occurred in our series in 7.6% of patients who had stenoses and in 17.5% of those who had occlusions. Stent stenoses occurred in 44% and stent occlusions in 56%.

SURGICAL ALTERNATIVES IN AORTOILIAC DISEASE

The lower abdominal aorta and iliac arteries are the most common areas of atherosclerotic disease and have the highest frequency of recurrence or progression requiring surgery.[22] Leriche first suggested surgical treatment of aortoiliac occlusive disease in 1940,[23] but it was in the 1950s when major advances in aortoiliac surgery occurred. In 1951, Oudot[24] described resection of an obstructed aortic segment and replacement with an arterial allograft. In 1952, Wylie[25] described aortoiliac thromboendarterectomy. Finally, in 1957, both Edwards[26] and DeBakey and coworkers[27] described the use of synthetic prostheses made of Teflon or Dacron to replace the abdominal aorta. Extra-anatomic bypass for the treatment of aortoiliac disease also evolved in the 1950s and 1960s. In 1962, Vetto[28] reported treating a series of unilateral iliac artery obstructions by means of femorofemoral bypass. Subsequently, Blaisdell and coworkers described unilateral axillofemoral bypass.[29] Simultaneous advancements were occurring in endovascular techniques. In 1983, surgical bypass between the femoral arteries was used successfully in combination with balloon dilatation.[30]

Aortoiliac Surgery

The most frequently employed operative procedure for aortoiliac occlusive disease is aortobifemoral bypass. This procedure is indicated for patients who have severe bilateral or unilateral aortoiliac disease as well as for those who have distal aortic occlusion. Out of concern for worsening disease on the contralateral side, which may eventually require intervention, most surgeons advocate placing a bifurcated aortic graft, even when unilateral iliac artery disease is present.[31] Patients who have lesions that are longer than 10 cm, multilevel occlusive disease associated with poor arterial runoff, and total occlusions involving the abdominal aorta and iliac arteries are usually treated by bypass surgery rather than endovascular techniques. In general, patients who have aortoiliac lesions less than 5 cm in length are more likely to respond to endovascular treatment than those who have lesions longer than 10 cm.[32] Aortoiliac endarterectomy may serve as an alternative to surgical bypass in selected patients who have localized lesions confined to the distal aorta, the aortic bifurcation, or the common iliac arteries. Endarterectomy offers less risk of infection than bypass and is most commonly used in young patients who have good life expectancy. Bypass surgery may be subsequently performed if endarterectomy fails. The role of endarterectomy is limited by the good success of surgical bypass, the low overall incidence of prosthetic graft complications, the technical demands of endarterectomy, the poor long-term patency of extensive endarterectomy procedures extending beyond the common iliac arteries, and the success rate of less invasive endovascular procedures in correcting localized disease. Femorofemoral bypass or axillofemoral bypass is performed in patients who have severe comorbidities and aortoiliac occlusive disease who may not tolerate a major operation. In these patients, endovascular treatment of the least diseased iliac artery may be followed by femorofemoral bypass.

Comparison of Surgical and Endovascular Results

The only multicenter, prospective, randomized clinical trial comparing PTA with bypass surgery, which was conducted in 1993, demonstrated that patients who have short (less than 10 cm), unilateral iliac artery stenosis and claudication may expect an 85% primary patency rate after surgical bypass compared with a 71% primary patency rate after treatment with PTA over a median follow-up duration of 4 years ($P = 0.055$).[33] No randomized trials of endovascular stenting vs. surgery have been performed. Other series show consistency with these findings. Long-term patency rates for aortofemoral bypass range from 85 to 90% after 5 years to 70 to 75% after 10 years to 60% after 15 years and to 55% after 20 years.[31, 34] Operative mortality for aortoiliac reconstruction ranges from 1.6% to 2.5%.[35]

Results of aortoiliac endarterectomy depend on proper patient selection and the experience of the surgeon with this technically demanding procedure. Inahara reported cumulative patency rates of 85.7% for aortoiliac endarterectomy procedures over 11 years of follow-up.[36] Duncan and coworkers found comparable patency rates between endarterectomy (93.3%) and bypass graft procedures (96.3%) in aortoiliac disease over 8 years.[37]

PTA and surgical bypass demonstrate similar patency rates for infrarenal aortic stenosis in nonrandomized studies. For 17 patients who had aortic stenosis and who received angioplasty, the success rates were 80%, 80%, and 70% at 1, 3, and 5 years, respectively.[38]

The iliac artery is a wide, high-flow vessel that is theoretically ideal for PTA and stent placements. Nevertheless, surgical revascularization of the stenosed or obstructed iliac artery, thus far, demonstrates higher and longer term patency rates than those achieved with PTA in nonrandomized studies. Although immediate success rates of greater than 95%[39] have been reported after performance of PTA for lesions located between the aortic and femoral bifurcations, 1-year limb salvage rates of 34 to 76% using PTA alone have also been reported in patients who have had severe peripheral vascular disease and prohibitive operative risk.[30] Overall, the patency rates for stenotic iliac lesions declined to 77% at 1 year, 61% at 3 years, and 54% at 5 years, with better patency observed in shorter focal lesions.[39] The 1- and 3-year patency rates for occluded iliac arteries were respectively 59 and 48% when PTA alone was used.[39]

Traditionally, extra-anatomic bypass (axillobifemoral bypass, femorofemoral bypass) has been reserved for patients who were unable to tolerate an operation involving the abdomen, such as those who had intra-abdominal infection, previous radiation therapy to the abdomen, or severe comorbidities. In such patients, extra-anatomic grafts are tunneled in subcutaneous tissue remote from the peritoneal cavity. Axillobifemoral bypass and femorofemoral bypass are two frequently used extra-anatomic techniques that may be offered in lieu of aortobifemoral bypass. Axillobifemoral bypass, however, exposes the patient to general anesthesia, is plagued by poor long-term patency, and offers only moderate hemodynamic improvement.[40]

Physicians are acquiring experience using a combination of endovascular and traditional surgical approaches for the treatment of multilevel or bilateral lesions.[41, 42] Unilateral endovascular aortofemoral bypass procedures have been used in combination with femorofemoral bypass to treat patients who have bilateral iliac artery stenosis. Such an approach is less invasive than surgical aortobifemoral bypass and may offer particular benefit to patients who have significant comorbid illness and who may not otherwise tolerate a major surgical procedure. Endovascular aortic graft replacement, in conjunction with infrainguinal arterial bypass for the treatment of patients who have multilevel aortoiliofemoral limb-threatening occlusive disease, has also been introduced. Preliminary results demonstrate that this approach is technically feasible and safe, and early evaluation gives a promise of long-term patency.[43]

CONCLUSIONS

Percutaneous interventions in the iliac arteries and the infrarenal abdominal aorta are the most widespread, effective, and durable procedures used in interventional radiology.

Although aortic angioplasty is relatively infrequent in daily routine, aortic bifurcational and iliac interventions are bread and butter procedures for most interventional radiologists. These procedures have been accepted by both surgeons and radiologists as the method of choice for treatment of patients who have atherosclerotic disease. To maintain adequate standards in performing these techniques is a prerequisite for all interventional laboratories. The role of conventional surgical bypass in patients who have aortoiliac disease is clearly diminishing. However, some clear indications for performance of surgical bypass in preference to endovascular repair remain. These include patients who have multilevel occlusive disease, total aortic occlusion, stenoses that are longer than 10 cm, and tortuous anatomy that would respond poorly to endovascular technique. For multilevel occlusive disease or bilateral iliac artery disease, endovascular techniques may also be effectively combined with conventional surgical bypass.

REFERENCES

1. Vollmar J: Rekonstruktive Chirurgie der Arterien. Stuttgart 1996, pp 207–214.
2. Berger T, Sorensen R, Konrad J: Aortic rupture. A complication of transluminal angioplasty. Am J Roentgenol 146:373, 1986.
3. Strecker E, Hogan B, Liermann D, et al: Iliac and femoropopliteal vascular occlusive disease treated with flexible tantalum stents. Cardiovasc Intervent Radiol 16:158, 1993.
4. Dietrich EB, Santiago O, Gustafson G: Preliminary observation on the use of the Palmaz stent in the distal portion of the abdominal aorta. Am Heart J 125:490, 1993.
5. Rholl, K, Van Breda A: Percutaneous intervention for aortoiliac disease. In Strandness E, Van Breda A (eds): Vascular diseases. New York, Churchill Livingstone, 1994, pp 433–466.
6. Long A, Gaux J, Raynaud A: Infrarenal aortic stents. Initial clinical experience and angiographic follow up. Cardiovasc Intervent Radiol 16:203, 1994.

7. Dietrich EB: Endovascular techniques for abdominal aortic occlusions. Int Angiol 12:270–280, 1993.
8. Becker G, Katzen B, Dake M: Noncoronary angioplasty. Radiology 170:921–940, 1989.
9. Gardiner G, Meyerovitz M, Stokes K, et al: Complications of transluminal angioplasty. Radiology 159:201, 1986.
10. Tegtmeyer CJ, Hardwell GD, Selby JB, et al: Results and complications of angioplasty in aortoiliac disease. Circulation 83:I-53, 1991.
11. Vorwerk D, Giinther RW: Mechanical revascularization of occluded iliac arteries with use of self-expandable endoprostheses. Radiology 175:411, 1990.
12. Vorwerk D, Giinther RW, Schurmann K, et al: Aortic and iliac stenoses: follow-up results of stent placement after insufficient balloon angioplasty in 118 cases. Radiology 198:45, 1996.
13. Vorwerk D, Guenther R, Schiirmann K, et al: Primary stent placement for chronic iliac artery occlusions: Follow-up results in 103 patients. Radiology 194: 745, 1995.
14. Strecker E, Hagen B, Liermann D, et al: Iliac and femoropopliteal vascular occlusive disease treated with flexible tantalum stents. Cardiovasc Intervent Radiol 16:158, 1993.
15. Palmaz JC, Labored J, Rivera F, et al: Stenting of the iliac arteries with the Palmaz stent. Experience from a multicenter trial. Cardiovasc Intervent Radiol 15: 291, 1992.
16. Schatz R: A view of vascular stents. Circulation 1989; 79:445, 1989.
17. Long A, Sapoval M, Beyssen B, et al: Strecker stent implantation in iliac arteries: Patencies and predictive factors for long-term success. Radiology 194:739, 1995.
18. Hausegger KA, Lafer M, Lammer J, et al: Iliac artery stenting—clinical experience with a nitinol prototype stent (Cragg stent) (Abstract). Cardiovasc Intervent Radiol (Suppl)16:S25, 1993.
19. Starck E, Dukiet C, Heinz C, et al: Clinical experience with a new self-expanding nitinol stent (Abstract). Cardiovasc Intervent Radiol (Suppl)18:S72, 1995.
20. Maynar M, Reyes R, Cabrera P: Percutaneous atherectomy of iliac arteries. Semin Intervent Radiol 5:253, 1988.
21. Vorwerk D, Giinther RW, Schiirmann K, et al: Percutaneous treatment of late obstruction in iliac arterial stents. Radiology 197:479, 1995
22. DeBakey ME, Lawrie GM, Gaeser DH: Patterns of atherosclerosis and their surgical significance. Ann Surg 201:115, 1985.
23. Leriche R: De la resection du carrefour aortiliaque avec double sympathectomie lombaire pour thrombose arterielle de l'aortie: Le syndrome de l'obliteration termino-aortique par arterite. Presse Med 48:601, 1940.
24. Oudot J: La greffe vasculaire dans les thromboses du carrefour aortique. Presse Med 59:234, 1951.
25. Wylie EJ: Thromboendarterectomy for arteriosclerotic thrombosis of major arteries. Surgery. 4:339, 1952.
26. Edwards WS: Plastic Arterial Grafts. Springfield, IL, Charles C. Thomas, 1957.
27. DeBakey ME, Crawford SE: Vascular prostheses. Transplant Bull 4:2, 1957.
28. Vetto RM: The treatment of unilateral iliac artery obstruction with a transabdominal subcutaneous femorofemoral graft. Surgery. 52:342, 1962.
29. Blaisdell FW, Hall AD: Axillary-femoral artery bypass for lower extremity ischemia. Surgery. 54:563, 1963.
30. Rush DS, Gewertz BL, Lu CT, et al: Limb salvage in poor-risk patients using transluminal angioplasty. Arch Surg 118:1209, 1983.
31. Piotrowski JJ, Pearch WH, Jones DN, et al: Aortobifemoral bypass: The operation of choice for unilateral iliac occlusion? J Vasc Surg 8:211, 1988.
32. Johnston KW, Rae M, Hogg-Johnston SA, et al: Five-year results of a prospective study of percutaneous transluminal angioplasty. Ann Surg 206:403, 1987.
33. Wolfe GL, Wilson SE, Cross AP, et al: Surgery or balloon angioplasty for peripheral vascular disease: A randomized clinical trial. J Vasc Intervent Radiol 4:639, 1993.
34. Nevelsteen A, Woulters L, Suy R: Aortofemoral Dacron reconstruction for aortoiliac occlusive disease: A twenty-five year survey. Eur J Vasc Surg 5:179, 1991.
35. Szilagyi DE, Hageman JH, Smith RF, et al: A thirty-year survey of the reconstructive surgical treatment of aortoiliac occlusive disease. J Vasc Surg 3:421, 1986.
36. Inahara T: Evaluation of endarterectomy for aortoiliac and aortiliofemoral occlusive disease. Arch Surg. 110:1458, 1975.
37. Duncan WC, Linton RR, Darling RC: Aortoiliofemoral atherosclerotic occlusive disease: Comparative results of endarterectomy and Dacron bypass grafts. Surgery. 70:974, 1971.
38. Johnston KW, Kalman PG, Baird RJ: Aortiliofemoral occlusive disease. *In* Veith FJ, Hobson RW, Williams RA, et al (eds): Vascular Surgery, 2nd ed. New York, McGraw-Hill, 1994, p 441.
39. Johnston KW: Iliac arteries: Reanalysis of results of balloon angioplasty. Radiology 186:207, 1993.
40. Ohki T, Marin ML, Veith FJ, et al: Endovascular aortounifemoral grafts and femorofemoral bypass for bilateral limb-threatening ischemia. J Vasc Surg 24: 984, 1996.
41. Lopez-Galarza LA, Ray LI, Rodriguez-Lopez J, et al: Combined percutaneous transluminal angioplasty, iliac stent deployment, and femorofemoral bypass for bilateral aortoiliac occlusive disease. J Am Coll Surg 184:249, 1997.
42. Walker PJ, Harris JP, May J: Combined percutaneous transluminal angioplasty and extraanatomic bypass for symptomatic unilateral iliac occlusion with contralateral iliac stenosis. Ann Vasc Surg 5:209, 1991.
43. Marin ML, Veith FJ, Sanchez LA, et al: Endovascular aortoiliac grafts in combination with standard infrainguinal arterial bypasses in the management of limb-threatening ischemia. Preliminary report. J Vasc Surg 22:316, 1995.

9 Interventions in the Femoropopliteal Arteries

Endovascular Contributor: *Luc Stockx*
Surgical Contributors: *Peter F. Lawrence, Gustavo Oderich, and Kiran Bhirangi*

The superficial femoral, profunda femoris, and the popliteal arteries are the major arterial blood vessels to the muscles of the lower extremity. Stenotic or occlusive disease of these vessels results in a decrease of blood flow and oxygen supply to the muscles of the leg and is, therefore, responsible for lower limb ischemia. Clinical symptoms are determined by the nature and location of the lesions as well as their speed of onset. Most lesions are atherosclerotic. Some obstructions are embolic, traumatic, or caused by arteritis or hypercoagulability syndromes. For the most part, the lesions involve the superficial femoral and popliteal arteries, whereas the profunda femoris artery is only occasionally involved. Moreover, the latter artery acts as a natural bypass, providing blood to the arteries of the lower limb via the collateral branches. At present, many endovascular techniques and devices are available to treat these lesions, thereby offering less invasive alternatives to surgery.

ACUTE OCCLUSIVE DISEASE

Acute extremity ischemia is caused by sudden onset of peripheral arterial occlusion and can constitute a threat to the viability of the limb. Two principal categories, thrombotic and embolic, are responsible for more than 90% of all cases of acute limb ischemia. The remaining etiologies are traumatic and iatrogenic. The most common cause of acute limb ischemia is in situ thrombosis of stenotic atherosclerotic vessels, which occurs in more than 60% of cases. Arterial emboli, the second most common cause, are of cardiac etiology in 80% of cases. Atrial fibrillation, myocardial infarction, valve vegetation, and cardiac aneurysms are the main risk factors for peripheral emboli that stem from cardiac sources. Proximal ulcerated atherosclerotic lesions and peripheral aneurysms account for 10% of arterial emboli in extremity vessels. Acute occlusion of a peripheral artery results in varying

degrees of limb ischemia, depending on the pre-existing collateral circulation. Long-standing atherosclerotic stenosis may result in only mild clinical symptoms after thrombosis if there has been development of sufficient collateral circulation over a period of years. Acute occlusion of a vessel with moderate stenosis results in more severe symptoms because of lack of collateral circulation. Differential diagnosis between embolus and thrombus is important because the therapeutic approaches for treating patients who have these problems can be different. A history of arrhythmia, myocardial infarction, or valve vegetation is indicative of acute embolic ischemia. A history of claudication or the known presence of a peripheral aneurysm suggests thrombosis as the cause of acute limb ischemia. Angiographic findings usually reveal the etiology of the lesion and are listed in Table 9–1. In our institution, percutaneous management is preferred for patients who have reversible ischemia. For patients who have embolic or thrombotic occlusions, percutaneous intra-arterial thrombolysis is our preferred treatment. If percutaneous treatment fails, a subsequent surgical procedure can be performed. The most common percutaneous treatment modalities are pharmacologic thrombolysis and percutaneous thrombectomy.

Pharmacologic Thrombolysis

This therapy requires injection of a thrombolytic drug directly into the thrombosed artery of the patient (see Chapters 3 and 12). This technique is superior to intravenous fibrinolysis of peripheral arteries. It is a useful therapy for achieving relatively rapid restoration of blood flow to an ischemic limb and for identifying underlying obstructive lesions so that patients can receive further treatment (Fig. 9–1). Two different methods of administration are described: continuous infusion and pulsed-spray. If the former method is used, the thrombolytic agent is infused at the site of

Table 9–1. Angiographic Findings: Embolus vs. Thrombosis

Embolus	Thrombosis
No associated atherosclerotic lesions	Generalized atherosclerotic disease
Sharp cut-off with reversed meniscus	Tapering vessels with irregular occlusion
Multiple locations	Mostly single location
No collateral vessels	Collateral circulation located at specific location (adductor canal)
Bifurcations	
Normal distal runoff vessels	Atherosclerosis of runoff vessels

the thrombosis; the preferred technique is to place the tip of the infusing catheter into the proximal part of the thrombus.[1] As lysis progresses, the catheter is gradually advanced. Other schemes with different drugs and infusion rates are proposed and have been described in a previous chapter. However, most experience has been obtained with urokinase and recombinant tissue plasminogen activator (rt-PA). Pulsed-spray thrombolysis is delivered by forceful injection of a spray of the thrombolytic agent into the clot via catheters with tip occlusion and multiple side holes.[2]

The injection can be done by hand with use of a tuberculin syringe, or with use of a dedicated injector. In theory, forceful intrathrombotic infusion of the thrombolytic agent accelerates thrombolysis by disrupting the thrombus and increasing the surface area available for enzymatic action. Duration of treatment should decrease, resulting in a lower complication rate and a lower cost. Reported technical success rates vary between 60 and 90%, depending on the dose, the agent, the age of the occlusion, and the endpoint. In a 3-year period, 99 patients who had acute lower limb ischemia underwent intra-arterial thrombolysis in our institution. In 60 patients, recombinant staphylokinase (STAR) was started as a 1–2 mg bolus, followed by a continuous infusion of 0.5–1 mg per hour. Alteplase (rt-PA) was infused at a rate of 3 mg per hour in the remaining 39 patients. Successful lysis was achieved in 81% of the cases (85% with STAR and 74% with alteplase). The most significant problem of thrombolysis is potential hemorrhage. The reported rate of bleeding varies from 4 to 25%. In most cases, this occurs at the puncture site, but bleeding at remote sites, including intracranial hemorrhage, has been reported. Local bleeding can generally be controlled by manual compression and termination of the infusion.

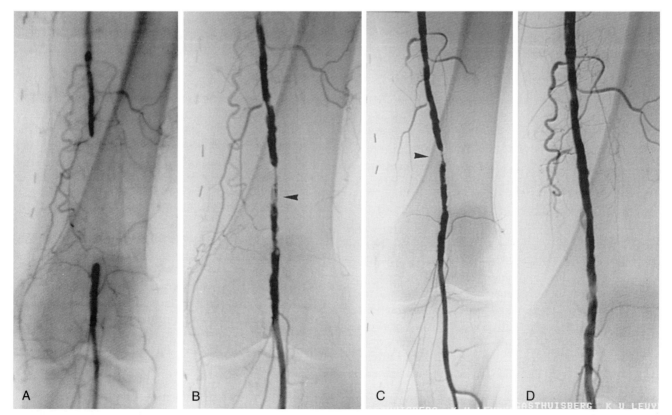

Figure 9–1. *A,* A complete occlusion of the femoropopliteal artery is demonstrated in a patient who has acute onset of ischemic rest pain in his left foot. The tip of a 4-French (F) straight diagnostic catheter is placed in the proximal part of the thrombus and intra-arterial infusion of streptokinase is initiated. *B,* Patency is partially restored after 4 hours, but residual thrombi are still present (*arrow*). The catheter is advanced, and the thrombolytic therapy is continued. *C,* After 4 additional hours, complete clearance of the thrombotic material is achieved, and an underlying stenosis is revealed (*arrow*). *D,* This lesion is successfully dilated by a percutaneous transluminal angioplasty (PTA) balloon with a diameter of 5 mm and a length of 2 cm.

Intracranial bleeding, which occurs in about 1% of cases, often has a fatal outcome. Some patients experience dramatic worsening of the ischemic symptoms during thrombolytic therapy. This is usually caused by distal embolization of thrombotic material as lysis progresses. Inadvertent catheter manipulation or overly forceful injection of contrast material or drugs can also provoke this phenomenon. It is mandatory to bridge this critical period by treating the patient with analgesic therapy, because these peripheral emboli generally resolve with continuation of the thrombolytic infusion. Sometimes, additional procedures, such as percutaneous aspiration or even surgery, may be necessary if clinical deterioration occurs.

Percutaneous Thromboembolectomy

Procedures aimed at the percutaneous mechanical removal of thromboembolic material can be divided into two techniques. The first one is dependent on operator technique and makes use of simple devices, such as catheters, sheaths, and syringes. The success of the second technique is determined by the use of sophisticated devices that have rotating, aspirating, or high-force injection capabilities.

Percutaneous Aspiration Thromboembolectomy/Percutaneous Aspiration Thromboembolectomy (PAT/PAE)

This is a relatively simple technique developed by Starck.[3] The equipment required for this procedure is basic and consists of a 6- to 8-French (F) introducer sheath with removable hemostatic valve. This removable valve is important because it prevents clot material from being trapped in the valve while it is pulled out through the sheath. For the superficial femoral and profunda femoris arteries, a 15-cm sheath can be used, whereas the popliteal artery requires longer sheaths that can measure up to 40 cm. Thin-walled aspiration (5- to 8-F) catheters with no side holes are used for aspiration because they allow a maximal diameter for aspiration and are only minimally tapered at the tip. A conventional 50-ml syringe is used to create the negative pressure for aspiration and a 0.035-inch hydrophilic guide wire is used to traverse the thrombotic or embolic occlusion and steer the aspiration catheters. Although the technique sounds very simple, there is a learning curve. An 8-F sheath is placed in an antegrade direction in the common femoral artery. The entire occlusion is recanalized with a hydrophilic guide wire. The aspiration catheter is advanced over the wire up to the proximal end of the occlusion.

For occlusions of the superficial femoral, pro-

funda femoris, or popliteal arteries, an 8-F aspiration catheter is recommended because this allows adequate aspiration. The guide wire is then removed and suction is applied with the 50-ml syringe. The tip of the catheter is slowly advanced distally. The clot material is either aspirated through the catheter into the syringe or caught at the tip of the aspiration catheter. The catheter is slowly retracted under continuous suction. The thrombus is pulled out through the sheath. To prevent entrapment of the thrombus in the hemostasis valve, the valve must be removed as soon as the thrombus enters the sheath. The catheter is extracted completely, and the contents of the syringe are expressed over a gauze-draped basin to separate the thromboemboli from the blood. The catheter is flushed, and the hemostasis valve is remounted on the sheath. If necessary, the aspiration procedure is repeated.

Angiographic assessment of the aspiration can be done via the side port of the sheath. If particles embolize further downstream, they can be aspirated by use of the same technique. Fresh thrombotic material as well as emboli can be easily removed by the aspiration technique. Detachment of wall-adherent and partially organized occlusive material can cause severe problems; in such cases, the use of a small spiral or a basket can aid removal. Intra-arterial injections of vasodilating drugs, such as nitroglycerin or papaverine, prevent spasm of the arterial wall caused by repetitive passage of large aspiration catheters. Indications for the technique include fresh thrombotic and embolic occlusions of the superficial femoral, the popliteal, and the profunda femoris arteries (Fig. 9–2). The advantage is rapid removal of the thrombus, allowing the whole interventional procedure to be accomplished in one session. If necessary, the patient can receive additional pharmacologic thrombolysis or the treatment can be completed with any other percutaneous endovascular therapy. This technique can also be used in the management of patients who have had angioplasty that is complicated by distal embolization. For patients who have thrombotic occlusions, a technical success rate of 85% can be attained, whereas cardiogenic or iatrogenic emboli can be aspirated in 90 to 100% of cases. It is best not to perform thromboaspiration from the contralateral approach, because the thrombus at the tip of the catheter may be lost and may cause embolization of the unaffected limb. Occasionally, distal embolization occurs (in approximately 30% of cases), but this can be treated easily with additional aspiration. Patients who develop vessel wall dissection, which occurs in about 3%, can be treated with prolonged balloon inflation, stenting, or atherectomy.

Mechanical Thrombectomy

A number of mechanical devices have been developed to remove thrombus. Some are rotating devices

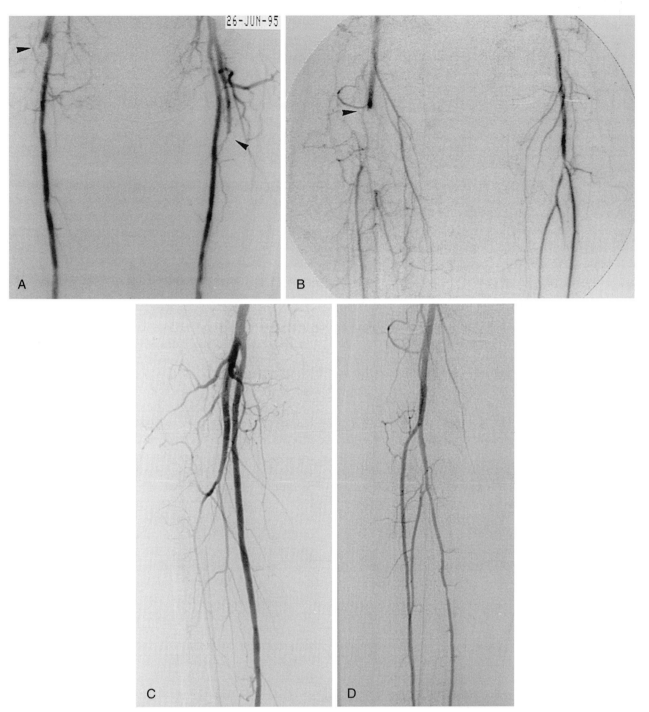

Figure 9–2. *A,* A patient with known cardiac valve vegetation presented with multiple cardiogenic emboli in the right and left profunda femoris artery and *B,* in the right popliteal artery. *C, D,* Successful percutaneous aspiration embolectomy via bilateral antegrade approach could be performed, thereby removing the embolic material and restoring the patency.

that have only a macerating effect on the thrombus, whereas others consist of hydrodynamic thrombectomy devices that not only macerate but also aspirate the thrombus. These devices are efficient only in the removal of fresh thrombus, preferably of less than 2 weeks' duration. The most common devices are described later in more detail. However, this overview is not exhaustive, and at present, several new devices are under investigation.

The Amplatz thrombectomy device consists of a 6- or 8-F polyurethane catheter with an impeller mounted on a drive shaft in 1-cm metal housing. The metal housing has two side ports that are used for recirculation. The impeller is driven by an air-powered motor at up to 150,000 rpm. The high rotational speed of the impeller enables the thrombus to be aspirated for subsequent fragmentation and recirculation of particles. At the proximal end of the catheter, the drive shaft passes through a Y-connector. Saline or contrast medium is infused through the side port of the connector to visualize the thrombus and cool the device. Because there is no end hole for the passage of a guide wire, the system has to be advanced with care to prevent dissection of the vessel wall and embolization of material. In a series of 40 patients who had acute occlusion of lower limb arteries, Rilinger and associates attained total success in completely clearing thrombi without performing an adjunctive procedure in 75% of patients. The mean thrombectomy time in these patients was 75 seconds. Partial success was achieved in 20% of patients, with incomplete clearing of the thrombi that required additional procedures, such as local thrombolysis, angioplasty, or atherectomy. No complications occurred in any of these patients.[4]

The Hydrolyzer is a straight 6- or 7-F double-lumen catheter with a 6-mm diameter oval side hole located 4 mm from the distal tip (suction nozzle). The catheter is made of nylon and has a stiff body. The distal end hole enables the system to be used over a 0.025-inch guide wire, and the catheter is introduced through a 7-F sheath. With a conventional contrast medium injector, 150 ml of normal saline solution is injected through the narrow supply channel (3 ml/s at 750 pounds per square inch [psi]). Because of resultant pressure reduction (Venturi effect), thrombus is sucked toward the side hole, fragmented, and removed as a mixture of thrombotic material and normal saline through the smaller exhaust lumen. Reekers published his initial experience with this catheter in 7 patients who had thrombotic occlusion of the superficial femoral artery. Thrombectomy was successful in all patients and the mean time required to perform the procedure was less than 20 minutes.[5]

The Angiojet consists of a 5-F double-lumen catheter that accepts a 0.018-inch guide wire. The smaller lumen of the catheter is used to supply the catheter tip with saline jets. The saline jets that emerge at the tip of the catheter are generated by an external drive unit with a positive displacement pump that generates pressures up to 10,000 psi. The saline injected into the catheter is supplied by a 1000-ml plastic bag containing normal saline solution to which 5000 IU of heparin is added. The pump creates a cyclic saline flow of 60 ml/min, and the saline jet exits at the tip of the catheter through three radially oriented holes. These jets aid in the formation of a recirculation pattern to fragment the thrombotic material. Three additional saline jets are directed retrograde into the larger exhaust lumen of the catheter. These jets create a Venturi effect that aids in the evacuation of the macerated thrombus material. The exhaust of the catheter is controlled so that the entire catheter operates in an isovolumic manner. The aspirated effluent material is collected in a bag. After the drive unit is assembled and the pump and catheter are connected, the entire unit can be activated by a foot switch. When the thrombectomy catheter is 2 cm above the lesion, the drive unit is activated, and the catheter is advanced over the guide wire through the entire thrombus. The catheter should be advanced at a constant velocity between 0.5 and 1.0 cm/sec. When the distal margin of the occlusion has been reached, the procedure can be repeated by pulling the activated catheter back over the guide wire. After the first antegrade and retrograde passage of the thrombectomy catheter, a control angiogram of the treated segment is performed, and this usually reveals creation of a small channel through the entire lesion.

To enhance the function of this device, it is possible to bend the tip of the catheter to a 30-degree curve. Curving of the catheter allows the device to be guided by the operator. After reintroduction of the catheter and advancement over the guide wire to the distal margin of the occlusion, the guide wire can be pulled back into the catheter lumen to increase efficacy of the device, because this wire obstructs the exhaust lumen partially when it is in place. The catheter is then pulled back through the occlusion in a spiral mode. Pulling the catheter in this manner allows direction of the saline jets to all parts of the arterial wall and enables evacuation of wall-adherent residual thrombi. The J-shaped catheter can also be advanced in an antegrade fashion to remove further thromboembolic material. This must be performed carefully because of the danger of dissection and subintimal passage. The amount of thromboembolic material removed can be controlled with the injection of contrast material through the side port of the sheath. The catheter can be passed through the lesion as often as necessary. However, passage is limited to a total device activation time of 15 minutes or injection of a total amount of 1000 ml of saline, because there is a possibility of increased hemolysis if the activation time is longer. Fifty patients who had acute occlusions of native lower extremity arteries (N = 39) or acute thrombosis of lower limb bypass graft (N = 11) were treated with this device in a multicenter trial.[6] The majority of thrombus material was removed, and antegrade blood flow was re-established through the formerly occluded segment in 45 (90%) of the 50 patients. In 15 (30%) patients, additional local intra-arterial thrombolysis was performed, and aspiration thrombectomy was necessary in 9 (18%) patients.[6]

CHRONIC OCCLUSIVE DISEASE

Atherosclerosis is the most common cause of chronic occlusive disease in the superficial femoral, the profunda femoris, and the popliteal arteries. Patients who have chronic occlusive disease characteristically can experience both non–limb-threatening and limb-threatening ischemia. The level and extension of the lesion, the involved artery, and the number of collateral branches determine the symptoms. Although the indication for treatment of acute limb ischemia is clear, this is not always true of chronic occlusive disease. After appropriate clinical evaluation and categorization of the patient's ischemia, angiography is performed in patients who have either failed medical management for debilitating claudication or who have critical ischemia. For patients who have significant lifestyle-limiting claudication or critical ischemia, angiographic appearance is a major determinant of whether the patient is considered a candidate for percutaneous treatment or bypass surgery.

Angioplasty

Percutaneous transluminal angioplasty (PTA) is the most commonly applied percutaneous intervention in the superficial femoral and popliteal arteries. This was first described by Dotter and Judkins in 1964[7] and further improved with the introduction of a double-lumen balloon catheter by Gruntzig and Kumpe in 1979.[8] It was originally thought that the principal mechanism of angioplasty consisted of compression and remodeling of atheromatous plaque. It is now accepted that the mechanism of PTA consists of rupture and tearing of the intima along with consequent dehiscence of this layer from the media.[9] Stretching the media and the adventitia and their subsequent reaction to the stretching are also important. The longitudinal radiolucent defects seen in angiograms made after performance of PTA, as well as the transient intramural accumulations of contrast medium originally thought to represent complicating dissections, are consequences of the rupture and dehiscence of the intima. This phenomenon is common, especially with fibrous, calcified lesions and should be interpreted as normal as long as there is no flow obstruction.

The technique and indications of peripheral PTA are well known and described in numerous journals and textbooks.[10] Either antegrade or retrograde approaches are possible for lesions of the profunda femoris or the femoropopliteal arteries. Our personal preference is use of an antegrade approach for the femoropopliteal lesion and a crossover procedure for the treatment of lesions in the profunda femoris. The most critical point of the procedure is the passage of the guide wire through the lesion. In this respect, the use of a steerable hydrophilic wire can be very helpful for crossing the stenosis. For complete occlusions, intentional creation of a new subintimal conduit can be an option (Fig. 9–3) (see Chapter 11). A control angiogram after a balloon dilatation procedure is performed with the guide wire still in place. This permits easy repeated crossing of the lesion if additional dilatations or other therapy are necessary. Major compli-

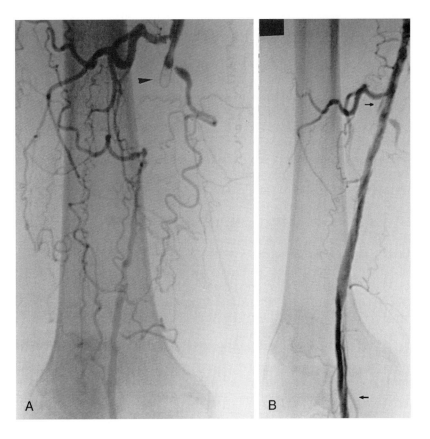

Figure 9–3. Percutaneous intentional extraluminal recanalization (PIER) of a chronic occlusion of the superficial femoral artery. *A,* Notice the loop of the tip of the guide wire (*arrow*) during performance of the extraluminal recanalization. *B,* Restoration of patency after balloon dilatation of the extraluminal space, with preservation of the major collateral arteries. Small intimal flaps (*arrows*) at the entry and re-entry sites.

A

B

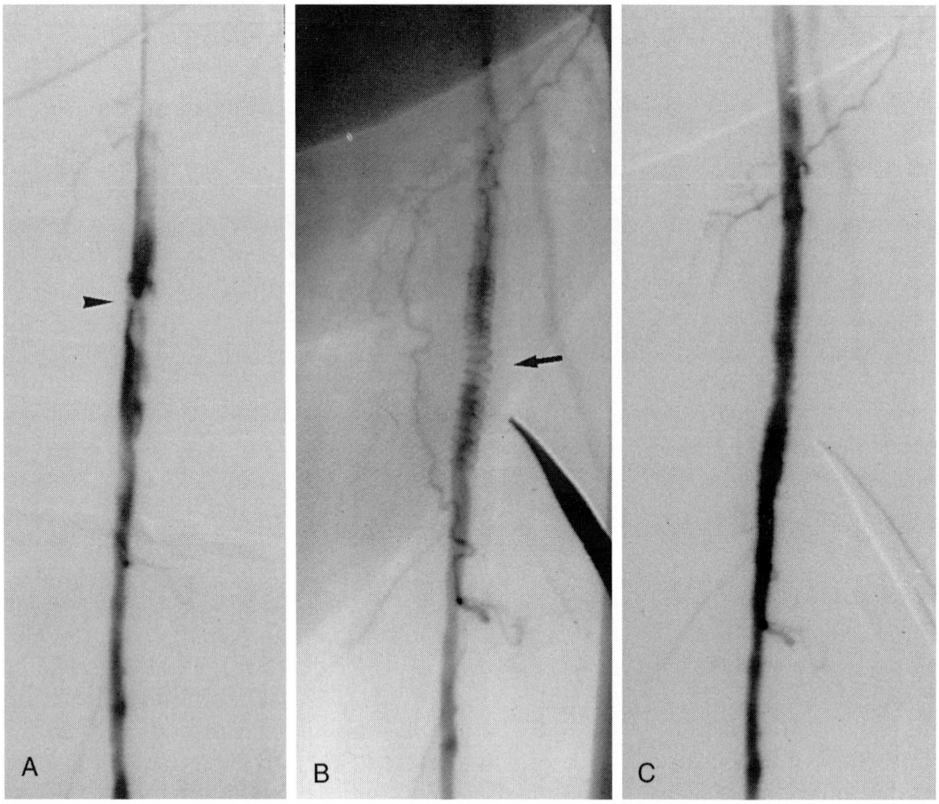

Figure 9–4. *A,* Recoil of the vessel wall is responsible for significant residual stenosis after percutaneous transluminal angioplasty (PTA). *B, C,* After insertion of a self-expandable spring coil stent, patency was restored.

cations occur in 5% of cases and can be related to the puncture site. Occasionally, these require surgical correction or at the level of the treated arterial segment. These local complications consist of perforations, flow-obstructive dissections, or distal embolization of thrombotic material. Repeated prolonged inflation (10 min) of the dilatation balloon at a low pressure is often sufficient to treat a perforation, whereas a flow obstructive dissection is one of the few remaining indications for stent placement or percutaneous atherectomy (Figs. 9–4 and 9–5). Distal emboli can be aspirated (PAT) or lysed (intra-arterial thrombolysis). The immediate technical success rate of PTA is very high. In a group of 208 femoropopliteal angioplasties, Matsi and associates obtained an overall angiographic success rate of 88%, (91% for femoropopliteal stenoses and 83% for femoropopliteal occlusions). However, the primary patency rates were disappointing. In this patient group 1-, 2-, and 3-year primary patencies were observed in 47, 41, and 43% of patients, respectively. Secondary patency was 63% at 1 year and 53% at 2 and 3 years, respectively.[11] Many factors influence short- and long-term patency after femoropopliteal PTA (Table 9–2). These may be divided into clinical and anatomic factors based on the angiogram. Of the clinical factors, the presentation mode (claudication or critical ischemia) has been proved to influence patency strongly. Patients who have claudication have a more benign overall disease process than those who have critical ischemia. Claudi-

cants are more apt to have successful early and late clinical PTA patency. Hunink and associates showed that of patients undergoing PTA for stenotic lesions, claudicants had better 5-year patency rates than those who had critical ischemia (55% vs. 29%).[12] Risk factors, such as smoking, hyperlipidemia, and hypertension have not been specifically associated with a poor femoropopliteal PTA outcome. Diabetes mellitus has been shown by some to reduce long-term patency. The patency rate is also determined by the anatomic characteristics of the lesion. A statistically significant difference was noted between patients treated for stenosis and those treated for occlusion. The stenotic group showed better long-term patency rates. Patients who have long stenotic arterial segments tend to have worse patency rates than those who have short segment involvement. Patients who have good runoff (two or three crural vessels to the ankle) and palpable

Table 9–2. Factors Associated With PTA Results

Favorable	Unfavorable
Claudication	Critical ischemia
Stenosis	Occlusion
Short lesion	Long lesion
Good runoff	Poor runoff
Concentric lesion	Eccentric lesion
No residual stenosis	Residual stenosis
Palpable pulse after PTA	No palpable pulse after PTA

PTA = percutaneous transluminal angioplasty.

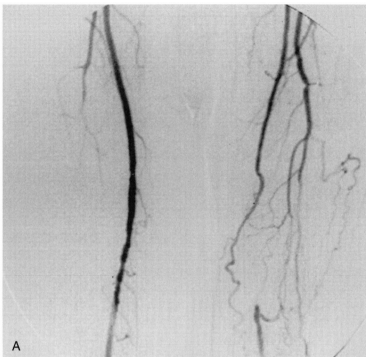

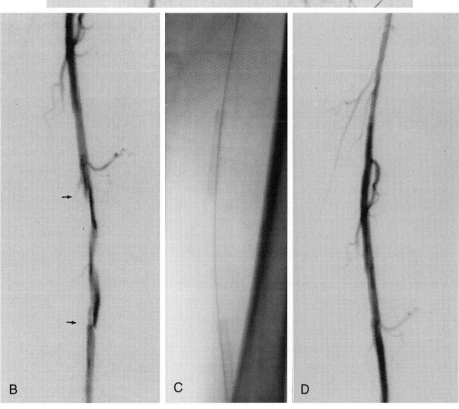

Figure 9–5. *A,* Complete occlusion of the left superficial femoral artery over a length of 15 cm in a patient suffering from claudication. After percutaneous intentional extraluminal recanalization (PIER) and percutaneous transluminal angioplasty (PTA), patency is restored, but *B,* flow-obstructive intimal flaps *(arrows)* are present at the entry and re-entry sites. *C, D,* In this situation, stent placement can be justified to avoid early rethrombosis.

peripheral pulses after the procedure is performed maintain significantly better long-term clinical patency than those who have poor runoff. Patients who have concentric lesions also show better long-term patency than those who have eccentric ones. The presence of residual stenosis after PTA is associated with poor patency rates and may be caused by vascular recoil, underdilatation, or severe intimal dissection.

Most clinical failures are seen during the first year after PTA.[13] Restenosis as a result of intimal hyperplasia occurs within months after PTA and is the most common cause of recurrence of symptoms. The most widely accepted theory for the development of intimal proliferation postulates that plaque disruption and intimal dissection from the medial layer cause deposition of platelets. The subsequent release of growth factors by platelets, leukocytes, and endothelial cells in turn causes proliferation, migration, and matrix formation of smooth muscle cell.[14] A possible solution of this problem is ablation of plaque, which improves luminal geometry and subsequently reduces residual stenosis or early reocclusion. If the plaque is removed instead of being left to disrupt and dissect, the artery regains a smooth surface, which in turn should reduce intimal hyperplasia. This was the rationale for developing new recanalization devices, such as percutaneous atherectomy systems, lasers, stents, and stent grafts.

Stents

For lesions in the superficial femoral artery (SFA) and popliteal artery, an antegrade approach is preferred, whereas for lesions in the profunda femoris, stent placement can be performed via a contralateral approach. A self-expanding stent is preferable, especially if the stent has to bridge a bending zone, such as the knee joint. Although stents have proved to be a valuable adjunct to balloon dilatation in atherosclerotic iliac artery disease, this does not seem to hold true for femoropopliteal lesions. Despite a high technical success rate, the long-term primary patency rate is no better than that achieved by conventional PTA. Intimal hyperplasia, regardless of the type of stent, is responsible for a high restenosis rate. In a comparative prospective trial Do and colleagues demonstrated that conventional femoropopliteal PTA has a 1-year primary patency rate (65%) equivalent to that of femoropopliteal Wallstents' secondary patency rate (69%).[15] In the United States, a multicenter trial of femoropopliteal Wallstents showed a 61% primary rate and an 84% secondary clinical patency rate at 1 year, with a 49% primary patency rate and a 72% secondary patency rate at 2 years. In this study, a 16.7% major complication rate was reported.[16] Similar findings were demonstrated by Sapoval, who obtained a technical success rate of 95%, and primary and secondary patency rates at 1 year of 49 and 67%, respectively.[17] Of the 21 stented arteries, 9 reoccluded: 4 in the first 30 days, and 5 in 1 to 5 months after PTA. In evaluating their series, Strecker and associates noted that the 2-year primary patency rate was significantly better for patients who had short stents (59%) than for those who had longer stents (30%), and better for patients treated for stenoses (73%) than for those treated for occlusions (33%). Multivariate analysis revealed that type and length of lesion were the most reliable predictive factors of stent failure.[18]

Approaches to the problem of intimal hyperplasia at present include prophylactic endovascular radiotherapy (brachytherapy) after stent implantation,[19] drug-coated or biodegradable stents, and covered stents. Because of the lack of demonstrable benefit in comparison with conventional PTA and the greater cost of the procedure, femoropopliteal stent placement should be reserved for patients who have suboptimal PTA results, including flow-obstructive dissection (see Fig. 9–5), thrombosis, recoil, or other situations requiring bailout.

Percutaneous Directional Atherectomy

The first atherectomy device for percutaneous use was described by Simpson (Simpson Peripheral Atherocath). This atherectomy catheter cuts and removes atheromatous material from the vessel wall, leaving behind a smooth luminal surface. The theory was that by direct removal of the plaque (debulking), the risk of peripheral embolization during conventional PTA would be reduced. Its value has not been proved, but intimal flaps that can produce abrupt arterial closure can be removed theoretically, thus reducing the lesion recurrence rate. In addition, neointima can be removed without further trauma to the arterial wall. The Simpson Atherocath device consists of a double-lumen catheter that has a cylindrical metal housing with a longitudinal window. Within this housing is a cable-driven circular cutter blade. The atherectomy catheter is positioned within the stenosis, and the window is slightly compressed to the atheroma by an eccentrically placed balloon. A battery-powered motor drive activates the cutter, which shaves the atheromatous material from the vessel wall and collects it in the distal portion of the metal housing. After this maneuver is performed, the device is withdrawn, and the atheromatous material is removed from the distal chamber and prepared for histology (an additional advantage of this procedure). The procedure must be performed via an antegrade approach. Because of the dimension of the device, which has a 7-F or larger shaft, puncture site complications are relatively common with this technique. Perforation of the vessel wall by cutting too much tissue is another possible complication. Despite an excellent technical success rate and an acceptable complication rate, angiographic follow-up results are disappointing. In a series of 183 lesions in 126 patients who were treated with the Atherocath, Dorros and associates noted a recurrence rate of stenosis of 55% after 5 months of follow-up.[20] Others have reported a clinical patency rate of 72% after 1 year.[21] Because of these data and the relatively high cost of this single-use device, this procedure should be reserved for elective cases, such as short eccentric stenoses or flow obstructive intimal flaps that are required after performance of conventional PTA (Fig. 9–6).

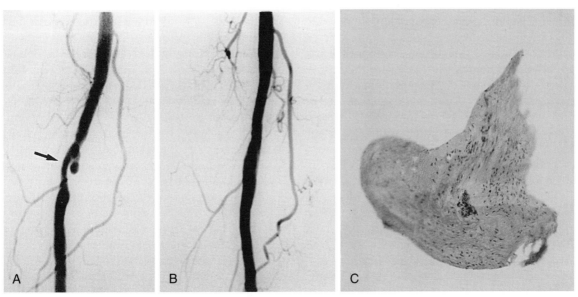

Figure 9–6. *A,* This eccentric obstructive lesion is one of the only indications for percutaneous atherectomy. *B,* This plaque can be completely removed, *B,* and thereby the smooth surface of the vessel lumen is restored. *C,* The removed material corresponds to an atheromatous plaque consisting of a strongly developed fibrous cap with proliferation of fibrous cells, smooth muscle cells, and a deposition of fibrous tissue.

Laser Angioplasty

Various lasers have been used experimentally and clinically for ablation of atherosclerotic plaque. However, the ideal laser, which would selectively ablate the obstructing material, has not yet been found. Continuous-wave laser light (Nd:YAG cw laser) is absorbed at the tissue surface. At low-power densities, coagulation, carbonization, and vaporization of plaque occur, which is the so-called photothermal effect. Pulsed lasers may have photothermal, photochemical, and photomechanical effects on tissue, depending on power density and pulse duration. The photothermal effect is caused by absorption and heat generation and is probably predominant. Because laser photon energy is higher than molecular binding energy, laser-induced dissociation results in a photochemical ablation. Absorption of Holmium-YAG photons by tissue water and of Xe-Cl excimer photons by proteins causes vaporization of tissue and bubbles, which in turn leads to mechanical tissue destruction. Lasers operate at various wavelengths: the Xe-Cl excimer laser at 308 nm, the Argon laser at 488 nm, the dye laser at 504 nm, the Nd:YAG laser at 1064 nm, and the Holmium-YAG laser at 2090 nm. Because bare fibers have a high perforation rate and cause only minimal ablation of tissue, several catheter delivery systems with different probes (hot-tip probe, sapphire probe, and spectraprobe) were developed, ensuring good contact between laser energy and tissue. The major drawback of all laser catheter systems is that they do not ablate more tissue than the area covered by the front of the catheter. In other words, a 7-F catheter can only create a channel of 2.1 to 2.5 mm in diameter. Therefore, stand-alone therapy without additional balloon angioplasty is not feasible in femoropopliteal angioplasty. Laser angioplasty creates a central core, but additional PTA is then necessary. The final procedural result and long-term patency rate thus depend on a combination of laser recanalization and mechanical balloon dilatation with all its drawbacks, such as intimal cracks, dissections, and formation of flaps. The first clinical feasibility studies using continuous wave or pulsed lasers showed initial success rates between 70 and 85% in patients who underwent recanalization of arterial occlusions. Vessel wall injuries were reported in 15 to 20% of cases and consisted of dissection and perforation.[22] Randomized trials in the early 1990s also showed no significant difference in technical success of 1-year patency rates between laser angioplasty and guide wire recanalization.[23] Laser angioplasty has, therefore, been almost completely abandoned as a treatment modality for peripheral vascular disease.

Stent Grafts

There is major interest in the use of stent grafts in treating occlusive atherosclerotic disease of the SFA.[24] Long-segment disease and complete occlusions have high restenosis rates despite initially successful PTA, whereas surgical bypass grafting with autologous vein still gives the best results. In theory, stent grafting has the potential to be as good as surgical bypass grafting. It effectively creates a relining of the vessel wall with restoration of an endoprosthetic smooth conduit. The flow dynamics should be favorable because the SFA lies in an accessible anatomic position and there are no anastomoses. Stent grafts can be divided into two major categories: unsupported and fully supported. The common prototype of the unsupported stent graft consists of a conventional segment of bypass graft with an expandable stent at one or both ends. Most of those devices are homemade and are composed of thin-walled polytetrafluoroethylene (PTFE) graft, with a 3-mm diameter, and one or two Palmaz stents. Long endoprostheses can easily be constructed by using long graft segments. The stent is generally sewn with a surgical suture at the inner side of the graft, and the whole device is then mounted on a balloon catheter. After recanalization and predilatation of the obstructed arterial segment, the stent graft is inserted through a large introducer sheath (generally 10-F) and then dilated over its entire length. Because of the characteristics of PTFE, dilatation up to 500% of the diameter of the graft can be safely performed without risk of disruption. However, after dilatation, recoil of ±25% is noticed, which makes overdilatation necessary. The distal stent has only an anchoring function and therefore acts as an endoluminal anastomosis between graft and native vessel. A variant of this self-made unsupported stent graft was developed by Boston Scientific. It consists of a constrained thin-walled PTFE graft with an anchoring nitinol stent at both ends (Fig. 9–7). The device is premounted on a balloon catheter of the same length

as the graft and can be introduced percutaneously through a 9-F introducer. Unsupported stent grafts are very flexible, with a low profile and a smooth inner surface. However, there are some major drawbacks. Because of the low radial force of the overdilated thin-walled PTFE, they are prone to external compression caused by recoil of the vessel wall. Rupture of the fabric can occur during dilatation of the part of the graft that is in close contact with sharp, calcified, atherosclerotic plaque. Flexion of hip and knee can cause kinking of the unsupported segment. Intimal hyperplasia at the level of the anchoring stent, which is the transition zone between graft and native vessel, often occurs and is responsible for restenosis.

The second group of endoprostheses are the fully supported stent grafts. These consist of a metallic skeleton covered with graft fabric. In most designs, conventional graft material, such as PTFE or polyester (Dacron), have been used to cover a nitinol or stainless steel stent or wire mesh. At present, four different devices are available in Europe. The Passager, which is a further evolution of the Cragg EndoPro System 1, consists of a nitinol self-expanding stent covered on the outside with a polyester fabric. The Hemobahn is composed of an ultra–thin-walled PTFE graft supported by a self-expanding nitinol meshwork on the external surface. The Corvita Endoluminal Graft (CEG) is made of a self-expanding braided wire mesh with highly porous, elastic coating on the inner sur-

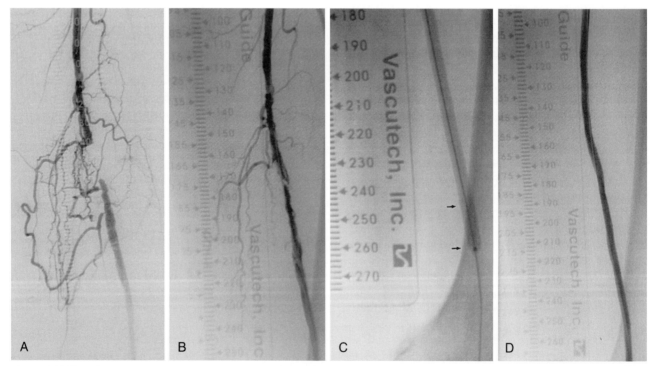

Figure 9–7. Example of an unsupported endovascular stent-graft. *A,* After percutaneous transluminal angioplasty (PTA) of a 4-cm-long occlusion, *B,* residual stenosis due to recoil of the vessel wall and an obstructive intimal flap is present in this diseased superior femoral artery (SFA). *C,* Therefore, an unsupported stent graft, which consists of a 20-cm-long polytetrafluoroethylene (PTFE) segment with an anchoring stent at both sides (*arrows indicate the stent at the distal side*) mounted on a long balloon is inserted. *D,* Patency is restored, thereby creating a smooth inner lining of the vessel wall but also risking occlusion of the major collaterals.

face, which consists of a layer of polycarbonate urethane fibers. The Jostent peripheral stent graft has ultra–thin-walled graft material placed within two balloon-expandable stainless steel stents in a sandwich construction. All these devices are intended for percutaneous use and can be inserted through an 8- to 10-F introducer sheath. Insertion of the Passager and the CEG is similar to that of the unsupported stent graft. After recanalization and predilatation of the diseased segment, the sheath is brought through the lesion and the stent graft is delivered. Postdilatation assures a good anchoring of the stent graft against the vessel wall. The Hemobahn device has a specific delivery mechanism whereby pulling back a rope results in proximal-to-distal delivery of the endoprosthesis. The Jostent peripheral stent graft is mounted on a PTA balloon and has to be deployed in the same way as a Palmaz stent. Having the metallic stent on the outer side gives a smoother lumen, which should be less thrombogenic, whereas having the stent at the inner side gives better adherence of the graft against the vessel wall. As a result of metallic support throughout the entire length of the graft, these devices have a much higher radial force and are, therefore, less prone to kinking or external compression. However, the presence of this large stent in a relatively small-caliber vessel can precipitate early thrombosis, whereas the development of intimal hyperplasia at both ends of the stent graft may be responsible for late restenosis.

Despite the enthusiastic reports of some authors, the use of stent grafts in femoral arteries is still of uncertain clinical benefit. High technical success rates can be obtained, but long-term patency has not been proved. The radial expansion force of unsupported graft material is too low to resist external compression, whereas the presence of a dense metal skeleton promotes an extensive response to injury of the vessel wall or luminal thrombosis. Finally, covering major collateral vessels with prosthetic graft material can jeopardize the viability of the limb if stent graft occlusion occurs. Refinements of these devices are, therefore, necessary if this new technique is to compete with bypass surgery. In the meantime, stent grafts should be used only under standardized investigational protocol or for specific indications.

ANEURYSMAL DISEASE

In the peripheral circulation, aneurysms of the femoropopliteal artery are the most frequently encountered disease. Men are affected 30 times more frequently than women, and more than 95% of cases are attributable to atherosclerosis. Bilateral aneurysms are seen in 30 to 60% of cases, and proximal aneurysms occur in more than 30% of patients. Although the natural

history of these aneurysms is not as well documented as that of abdominal aortic aneurysms, it is accepted that popliteal aneurysms are associated with a mean yearly complication rate of approximately 8.5%. These complications include pressure on adjacent nerves, veins, and joints, but also, and more importantly, they cause limb-threatening ischemia as a result of distal embolization or acute thrombosis. Rupture has been described but is exceptionally rare. Predisposing factors for complications are large aneurysm size, intraluminal thrombus formation, associated distortion of the popliteal artery, and pre-existing distal occlusive disease. The preferred treatment is widely agreed to be surgical and consists of local interposition or femorodistal reconstruction. Because a completely thrombosed aneurysm of the popliteal artery may mimic a simple vascular occlusion on angiography, its presence as the underlying cause is often recognized after initial thrombolysis (Fig. 9–8). The value of lysis in patients who have thrombosed popliteal aneurysms is in clearing the distal vessels to facilitate surgical reconstruction. At present, there is limited experience with use of stent grafts as treatment for patients who have femoropopliteal aneurysms. Successful treatment consists of a complete and definitive exclusion of the aneurysm (Fig. 9–9). Normal proximal and distal vessel segments are needed to achieve effective sealing of the stent graft. If possible, patients who have stent grafts should avoid crossing the knee joint, because knee flexion can result in kinking of the stent or graft. Henry and associates reported the treatment of six femoropopliteal aneurysms with placement of the Cragg EndoPro-System.[25] Exclusion of the aneurysm was possible in all of these patients. One patient died 4 days after the procedure because of a myocardial infarction; one stent graft thrombosed, necessitating surgical bypass. The use of Cragg Endopro stent grafts has been reported in 16 other patients, but 37% have occluded within 6 months despite anticoagulants, and recurrent aneurysms have been seen in 3%.

CONCLUSION

An extensive armamentarium of percutaneous endovascular procedures is available for the treatment of patients who have vascular diseases of the superficial femoral, the profunda femoris, and the popliteal arteries. For patients who have acute thrombotic occlusions, intra-arterial thrombolysis alone, or in combination with percutaneous mechanical thrombectomy procedures, is very effective, whereas patients who have embolic occlusions are preferentially treated with percutaneous aspiration embolectomy. For patients who have chronic occlusive disease, balloon angioplasty is still the best treatment, especially for short lesions. Newer techniques, such as atherectomy,

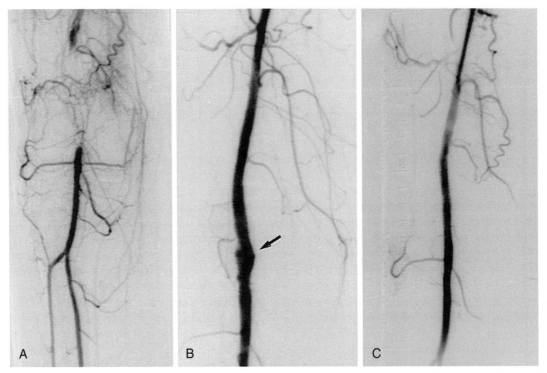

Figure 9–8. *A,* Complete thrombosis is a frequent complication of a popliteal aneurysm, which can mimic a simple vascular occlusion as demonstrated in this patient. *B,* Thrombolysis of this occlusion revealed a popliteal aneurysm with an external diameter of 1.5 cm. *C,* This could be successfully excluded with a covered stent.

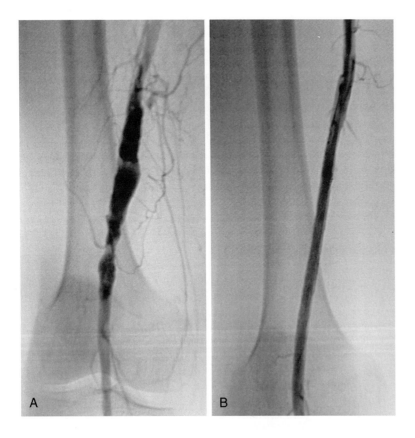

Figure 9–9. *A,* This patient presented with recurrent episodes of distal embolization from a femoropopliteal aneurysm. *B,* Exclusion of the aneurysm with restoration of the smooth inner lining of the vessel wall was performed with the insertion of the same covered stent.

laser angioplasty, and stent placement do not achieve a better long-term patency rate and, therefore, have to be reserved for specific indications. In the future, stent grafts may become of major importance.

SURGICAL ASPECTS OF FEMOROPOPLITEAL DISEASE

In the last two decades, there have been significant advances in development of endovascular procedures. Balloon angioplasty, stents, and endovascular grafts are now available to treat patients who have peripheral vascular disease.[26] Because of the high incidence of patients with atherosclerotic occlusive disease in the femoropopliteal segment and the low mortality associated with failed procedures in this location, many endovascular devices have been initially tested on infrainguinal vessels. The results of surgical treatment will be considered later, and this will allow us to propose a standard against which the results of endovascular treatment may be compared.

Occlusive Disease

Atherosclerotic occlusive disease is the most common indication for revascularization of femoropopliteal vessels. Usually the superficial femoral artery (typically at the adductor canal), the popliteal artery, or both are involved in the atherosclerotic process. The prevalence of intermittent claudication resulting from occlusive disease has been reported as 5% in men and 2.5% in women; most of these patients are smokers and are 60 years of age or older.[26] The disease is even more common and severe in the diabetic population, which represents 60% of these patients. Surgical treatment is indicated to relieve symptoms of limb-threatening ischemia, including ischemic rest pain, gangrene, and ischemic ulcers. Intermittent claudication is considered to be a relative indication for surgery, because its natural history is one of stability or slow deterioration throughout life, often without the need for surgical intervention.[26] A combination of appropriate symptoms (claudication, rest pain), physical findings (tissue loss, absent pulses, dependent rubor), and noninvasive lab tests (ankle-brachial index) is necessary to confirm significant arterial disease. The indication for revascularization in the absence of critical ischemia is based on a subjective judgment made by both patient and surgeon concerning the degree of disability imposed by claudication.

There are three surgical options for treatment of patients with femoropopliteal occlusive disease: infrainguinal bypass, profunda femoris reconstruction (profundaplasty), or both. An infrainguinal bypass is indicated when the superficial femoral artery (rarely

the common femoral artery) or the popliteal artery is occluded and angiography demonstrates luminal continuity of at least one of the three terminal branches of the popliteal artery. Generally, patients who manifest tissue loss or gangrene need an infrainguinal bypass as opposed to profundaplasty to relieve their symptoms. Immediate limb salvage is achieved in 86% of patients in whom revascularization is possible.[27] The choice of the conduit, the site of the distal anastomosis, and the number of patent runoff vessels are important factors that affect the outcome in these patients. For above-knee infrainguinal reconstructions using autologous vein, the reported 5-year primary and secondary (following revision) patency rates are 75 and 83%, respectively.[27] The limb-salvage rate varies from 84 to 90%. Despite a low mortality rate associated with the procedure (2 to 6%), only 28 to 54% of all patients who have arterial reconstruction are alive 5 years later.[26] Revascularization is often contraindicated in the presence of life-threatening sepsis, for which adequate drainage may require major amputation.

Patients who have ischemic rest pain without tissue loss theoretically have less severe disease and occasionally are treated with isolated profundaplasty. This is a controversial issue in the literature. The best results with isolated profunda femoris reconstruction are obtained when the vessel is at least 50% stenosed, the stenosis is limited to the proximal third of the artery, and the aortoiliac segment is shown by angiogram to be free of disease. A review of 17 patients subjected to profundaplasty alone demonstrated a high 30-day postoperative amputation rate of 24%.[28] The general recommendation is to use isolated profundaplasty to ensure adequate healing in patients who have an above-knee amputation in which a superficial femoral occlusion is associated with a hemodynamically significant proximal profunda femoris stenosis. The more common procedure is the association of a profundaplasty and an infrainguinal bypass, using the profunda femoris artery as the proximal anastomotic site. In a large retrospective series, there was no statistically significant difference in the 3-year patency rates for infrainguinal bypasses arising from the profunda femoris artery (96%), the common femoral artery (89%), or the superficial femoral artery (87%).[29]

An autogenous vein graft is the conduit of choice for infrainguinal bypasses. Despite considerable evidence in the literature in favor of a vein as the preferable conduit, there are some investigators who still recommend the use of prosthetic grafts for above-knee reconstructions.[28] In 1986, Veith and colleagues reported the results of a large, randomized, prospective trial comparing autogenous saphenous vein with PTFE grafts in infrainguinal bypasses[30] (Fig. 9–10). Cumulative primary patency rates remained similar

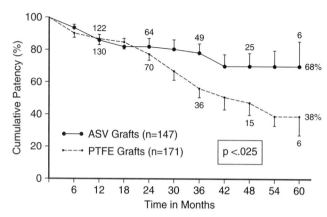

Figure 9–10. Life-table analysis for all randomized infrainguinal bypasses with autologous vein and polytetrafluoroethylene (PTFE). (Modified from Veith FJ, Gupta SK, Ascer E, et al: Six-year prospective multicenter randomized comparison of autologous saphenous vein and expanded polytetrafluoroethylene grafts in infrainguinal arterial reconstructions. J Vasc Surg 3;104, 1986.)

for the first 2 years after operation; thereafter, patency diverged, showing a significant difference after 4 years of follow-up, with a superior result in the vein group (68 vs. 38%). These differences were even more dramatic in grafts anastomosed to infrapopliteal arteries (Fig. 9–11B). A separate analysis of above-knee femoropopliteal bypasses demonstrated no statistically significant difference in patency rates. However, there was a tendency toward a higher patency rate in the vein group (see Fig. 9–11A). There was no difference in the results of saphenous vein bypass performed by either reversed or in situ techniques. The site of the distal anastomosis (above-knee, below-knee, or infrapopliteal), and the status of the runoff vessels (single, two-, or three-vessel) are the most critical factors contributing to clinical success, especially when a relatively thrombogenic prosthetic graft is elected as the conduit of choice.

Some centers use prosthetic grafts preferentially for above-knee bypasses. These recommendations are based on studies that have demonstrated equivalent patency rates for above-knee reconstructions performed with either vein or prosthetic grafts, even though there are equally compelling series showing that the results for PTFE are inferior to vein grafts.[5] The results of prosthetic grafts (PTFE) used for above-knee femoropopliteal bypasses include a 5-year primary patency rate of 22 to 59%, inferior to that reported for vein grafts. It is somewhat difficult to support the choice of a prosthetic graft on the argument that "we should save the vein for later." Most series demonstrate that only 5% of patients need vein for peripheral or coronary artery bypass.[31] The most attractive reason to use a prosthesis is to achieve lower surgical morbidity in patients who have limited life expectancy. The procedure is faster, is performed

through small incisions, and has an overall 6 to 10% rate of morbidity. This rate is superior to the higher local complication rate (20 to 40%) associated with the use of vein grafts.[26] We generally consider using prosthetic grafts in poor-risk patients who have a life expectancy of 2 to 3 years or when no autologous vein is available.

Femoropopliteal bypass is associated with a perioperative mortality of 2 to 6%, and the principal cause of death is coronary artery disease. Local complications include hemorrhage (less than 2%), wound infection (8 to 19%), and leg edema. Graft thrombosis complicates 2 to 7% of the procedures, usually in the first 24 hours, which emphasizes the importance of frequent examination of the pulses and Doppler measurements during this period.[2] Approximately 20% of vein graft bypasses require revision to maintain patency. The stenosis can frequently be identified by duplex scan and repaired with an outpatient procedure. To determine the efficacy of the competing treatment options, a combination of functional improve-

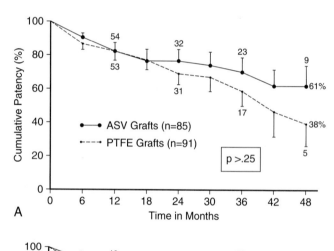

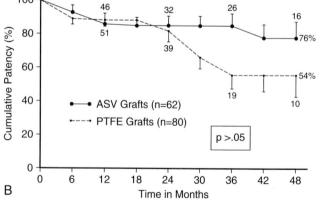

Figure 9–11. Life-table analysis for all randomized autologous vein and polytetrafluoroethylene bypasses performed to A, above-knee or B, below-knee popliteal artery. (Modified from Veith FJ, Gupta SK, Ascer E, et al: Six-year prospective multicenter randomized comparison of autologous saphenous vein and expanded polytetrafluoroethylene grafts in infrainguinal arterial reconstructions. J Vasc Surg 3:104, 1986.)

ment and improvement in noninvasive test results is required of all patients undergoing treatment.

Aneurysms

The popliteal and femoral arteries are the most common sites for peripheral artery aneurysms, accounting for nearly 90% of the aneurysms not involving the aorta.[32] Popliteal artery aneurysms are more common than femoral aneurysms, representing 70% of peripheral aneurysms. They are degenerative (atherosclerotic) in nature and occur almost exclusively in men aged 65 years or older. Bilateral aneurysms are present in 50% of patients, and another 50% have an associated aneurysm in the aorta or iliac artery. The most common clinical presentation is an asymptomatic aneurysm found on routine physical examination or during imaging studies. Occasionally, aneurysms appear as pulsatile masses and are associated with compressive symptoms in 5 to 10% of patients. Acute critical ischemia occurs in 30% of patients and results in dramatically worse clinical outcomes. For elective popliteal aneurysm repair, the 5-year patency rate with use of autogenous vein is 90%, and the 10-year patency rate is 80%.[33] The limb-salvage rate exceeds 95% at 10 years. This is in contrast to the results obtained for patients who had operations in the presence of acute symptoms; under such circumstances, the 5-year patency rate decreases to 50% and the limb-salvage rate to 80% (Fig. 9–12). Consequently, aneurysm repair is indicated in all patients who have symptoms (compression, claudication, rest pain, or gangrene). Asymptomatic patients are operated on when the aneurysm reaches 2 cm because the risk of complications increases with the size of the aneurysm. Autogenous vein is recommended as the preferable conduit based on the poor results of prosthetic grafts for distal popliteal and infrapopliteal vessels. Resection of the aneurysm is acceptable but not necessary; the surgical principle is to exclude the aneurysm from the circulation and re-establish normal distal flow through a bypass. The proximal anastomosis usually originates in the common femoral artery or superficial femoral artery proximal to the area of aneurysmal dilatation. The distal anastomosis is placed at the popliteal artery, where the vessel resumes a normal diameter. Patients who have aneurysm thrombosis represent a challenge; thrombolysis followed by aneurysm resection or bypass has yielded the best results. These patients usually have multiple emboli that occlude tibial arteries, which explains the poorer results associated with any form of therapy.

Femoral artery aneurysms are increasing in incidence and represent the second most common peripheral arterial aneurysm.[32] In contrast to popliteal aneurysms, which are mainly degenerative, femoral artery aneurysms have multiple etiologic mechanisms, including atherosclerotic, iatrogenic, anastomotic, infectious, and traumatic aneurysms. True aneurysms are degenerative or atherosclerotic in nature and are more frequently located in the common femoral artery. The most common femoral aneurysm is a pseudoaneurysm caused by an arterial puncture in the femoral artery. It is estimated that pseudoaneurysms occur at a rate of 1 in 500 femoral cannulations.[34] Most atherosclerotic aneurysms are asymptomatic; their natural history differs from that of popliteal aneurysms because only 3 to 5% of patients develop symptoms. Symptoms referable to femoral aneurysms (or pseudoaneurysms) may be grouped according to their cause: rupture (rare), compression to adjacent structures, and ischemia. Symptoms are caused more frequently by iatrogenic and anastomotic aneurysms than by atherosclerotic aneurysms. The current recommendation is to operate on all patients who have symptomatic aneurysms. Aneurysms that are degenerative in etiology can be followed closely because they have a more benign course. Enlarging aneurysms or those that become symptomatic should be repaired.

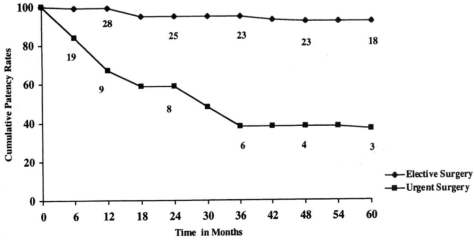

Figure 9–12. Cumulative life-table patency rates of elective vs. urgent revascularization performed in patients with popliteal aneurysms. (Modified from Ouriel K, Shortnell CK: Popliteal and femoral aneurysms. *In* Rutherford R [ed]: Vascular Surgery, 4th ed. Philadelphia, WB Saunders, 1995.)

For asymptomatic patients who have anastomotic aneurysms, the most acceptable approach is to repair the aneurysm when it reaches a diameter greater than 3 cm. Patients who have iatrogenic pseudoaneurysms related to arterial puncture have been treated with mechanical compression and injection of thrombin.[33] The surgical approach varies, depending on the cause of the aneurysm. Anastomotic aneurysms represent the greatest challenge because they result in excessive scarring and alteration of normal anatomy. They require extra surgical planning and precise technique. Arterial reconstruction is performed with a prosthetic graft of either Dacron or PTFE. In cases of associated atherosclerotic occlusion of the superficial femoral artery, a bypass from the external iliac artery to the profunda artery may be performed. The results of elective reconstruction are excellent and are translated into a 5-year primary patency rate of nearly 100%. The limb-salvage rate also approaches 100%. Aneurysms operated on in the presence of acute symptoms have an associated amputation rate of 10 to 20%.[35]

CONCLUSION

The results of angioplasty and stenting of peripheral vessels must be compared with those obtained with surgical treatment, which is considered the gold standard for patients who have femoropopliteal, occlusive, aneurysmal, or traumatic disease. At present, autogenous vein is the conduit of choice for above, below-knee, and infrapopliteal bypasses. The 5-year patency rate for patients who have these diseases is approximately 85%. The use of prosthetic grafts as conduits should be reserved for patients who do not have adequate autologous conduit. Treatment of patients before occurrence of limb-threatening ischemia and embolization is associated with the best outcome and the shortest recovery period.

REFERENCES

1. McNamara TO, Bomberger RA, Merchant RF: Intra-arterial urokinase as the initial therapy for acutely ischaemic lower limbs. Circulation 83:106, 1991.
2. Kandarpa K, Chopra PS, Aruny JE, et al: Intra-arterial thrombolysis of lower extremity occlusions: Prospective, randomized comparison of forced periodic infusion and conventional slow continuous infusion. Radiology 188:861, 1993.
3. Wagner HJ, Starck EE: Acute embolic occlusions of the infra inguinal arteries: Percutaneous aspiration embolectomy in 102 patients. Radiology 182:403, 1992.
4. Rilinger N, Görich J, Scharrer-Pamler R, et al: Short-term results with use of the Amplatz thrombectomy device in the treatment of acute lower limb occlusions. J Vasc Intervent Radiol 8:343, 1997.
5. Reekers JA, Kromhout JG, van der Waal K: Catheter for percutaneous thrombectomy: First clinical experience. Radiology 188:871, 1993.
6. Wagner HJ, Müller-Hülsbeck S, Pitton MB, et al: Rapid thrombectomy with a hydrodynamic catheter: Results from a prospective multicenter trial. Radiology 205:675, 1997
7. Dotter CT, Judkins MP: Transluminal treatment of arteriosclerotic obstructions. Circulation 30:654, 1964.
8. Gruntzig A, Kumpe DA: Technique of percutaneous transluminal angioplasty with the Gruntzig balloon catheter. AJR 132:547, 1979.
9. Zollikofer C, Ferral H, Gragg AH, et al: Percutaneous transluminal angioplasty. Part 2. In Castaneda-Zuniga WR (ed): Interventional Radiology, 3rd ed. Baltimore, Williams & Wilkins, 1997.
10. Pentecost MJ, Criqui MH, Dorros G, et al: Guidelines for peripheral percutaneous transluminal angioplasty of the abdominal aorta and lower extremity vessels. Circulation 89:511, 1994.
11. Matsi PJ, Manninen HI, Vanninen RL, et al: Femoropopliteal angioplasty in patients with claudication: Primary and secondary patency in 140 limbs with 1–3-year follow-up. Radiology 191:727, 1994.
12. Hunink MGM, Donaldson MC, Meyerovitz MF, et al: Risks and benefits of femoropopliteal percutaneous balloon angioplasty. J Vasc Surg 17:183, 1993.
13. Capek P, McLean GK, Berkowitz HD: Femoropopliteal angioplasty factors influencing long-term success. Circulation 83:I-70, 1991.
14. Roeren T, Le Veen RF, Villaneuva T, et al: Restenosis and successful angioplasty: Histologic-radiologic correlation. Radiology 172:971.
15. Do D, Triller J, Walporth BH, et al: A comparison study of self-expandable stents vs. balloon angioplasty alone in femoropopliteal artery occlusions. Cardiovasc Intervent Radiol 15:306, 1992.
16. Martin EC, Katzen BT, Benenati JF, et al: Multicenter trial of the Wallstent in the iliac and femoral arteries. J Vasc Intervent Radiol 6:843, 1995.
17. Sapoval MR, Long AL, Raynaud AC, et al: Femoropopliteal stent placement: Long-term results. Radiology: 833, 1992.
18. Strecker EP, Boos IB, Göttmann D: Femoropopliteal artery stent placement: Evaluation of long-term results. Radiology 205:375, 1997.
19. Liermann D, Bottcher HD, Kollath J: Prophylactic endovascular radiotherapy to prevent intimal hyperplasia after stent implantation in femoropopliteal arteries. Cardiovasc Intervent Radiol 17:12, 1994.
20. Dorros G, Iyer S, Lewin R, et al: Angiographic follow-up and clinical outcome of 126 patients after percutaneous directional atherectomy (Simpson Atherocat) for occlusive peripheral vascular disease. Cathet Cardiovasc Diagn 22:79, 1991.
21. Van Pölnitz A, Nerlich A, Berger H, et al: Percutaneous peripheral atherectomy: Angiographic and clinical follow-up of 60 patients. J Am Coll Cardiol 15:682, 1990.
22. Lammer J, Pilger E, Decrinis M, et al: Pulsed excimer laser versus continuous wave Nd:YAG laser versus conventional angioplasty of peripheral arterial occlusions: Prospective, controlled randomized trial. Lancet 340:1183, 1991.
23. Belli AM, Cumberland DC, Procter AE, et al: Follow-up of conventional angioplasty for femoropopliteal artery occlusions: Results of a randomized trial. J Vasc Intervent Radiol 2:485, 1991.
24. Stockx L: Stent-grafts in the superficial femoral artery. Eur J Radiol, 1998 (in press).
25. Henry M, Amor M, Cragg A, et al: Occlusive and aneurysmal peripheral arterial disease: Assessment of a stent-graft system. Radiology 201:717, 1996.
26. Weitz JI, Byrne J, Clagett P, et al: Diagnosis and treatment of chronic arterial insufficiency of the lower extremities: A critical review. Circulation 94: 3026, 1996.
27. Sanchez LA, Veith F: Femoro-popliteal-tibial occlusive disease. In Moore W (ed): Vascular Surgery—a comprehensive review, 5th ed. Philadelphia, WB Saunders, 1998, pp 497–520.
28. Harward TRS, Bergan JJ, Yao JST, et al: The demise of the profundaplasty. Am J Surg 127:126, 1988.
29. Prendiville EJ, Burke PE, Colgan MP, et al: The profunda femoris: A durable outflow vessel in aortofemoral surgery. J Vasc Surg 2:585, 1985.

30. Veith FJ, Gupta SK, Ascer E, et al: Six-year prospective multicenter randomized comparison of autologous saphenous vein and expanded polytetrafluoroethylene grafts in infrainguinal arterial reconstructions. J Vasc Surg 3:104, 1986.

31. Abbott WM: Prosthetic above-knee femoro-popliteal bypass: Indications and choice of graft. Semin Vasc Surg 10:3, 1997.

32. Dent TL, Lindenauer SM, Ernst CB, et al: Multiple arteriosclerotic arterial aneuysms. Arch Surg 105:338, 1972.

33. Dawson I, Sie RB, van Bockel JH: Atherosclerotic popliteal artery aneurysm. Br J Surg 84:293, 1997.

34. Roberts SR, Main D, Pinkerton J: Surgical therapy of femoral artery pseudoaneurysm after angiography. Am J Surg. 154:676, 1987.

35. Grahan LM, Zelenock GB, Whitehouse WM, et al: Clinical significance of arteriosclerotic femoral artery aneurysms. Arch Surg 115: 502, 1980.

10 Interventions in the Crural Arteries

Endovascular Contributor: *Jim A. Reekers*
Surgical Contributor: *Brian F. Johnson*

The primary goals for patients who are treated with infrapopliteal percutaneous transluminal angioplasty (PTA) are avoidance of major amputation and salvage of a functioning foot. These are in contrast to use of PTA in patients for whom the main goal is to achieve hemodynamic patency of the iliac or femoropopliteal arteries. Although crural PTA has been reported for severe claudication, it is still mainly a treatment for chronic critical limb ischemia.[1-3] There are, however, reports that promote use of infrapopliteal PTA in even moderately claudicated patients to increase the patency of a femoropopliteal PTA.[4]

The population treated with crural PTA is generally elderly, has extensive vascular disease, and includes more diabetic patients. Most patients who have critical limb ischemia have multilevel vascular disease.[5] Patients who have rest pain alone are reported to have a 5-year mortality rate of more than 50%.[6-7] In our own experience, however, the mortality in a group treated for critical ischemia is not greater than 20%, which suggests that for this treatment modality patient selection may play an important role. Nevertheless, less invasive therapy, such as angioplasty, can be a way to treat this very sick group of patients.

HISTORY

The Dotter technique, which has been previously discussed, demonstrated the feasibility of performing crural PTA with use of tapered catheters.[8] However, the results were poor and the complication rate was high.[9] Only after small-vessel balloons and steerable guide wires were introduced (around 1984), did the technique develop further. The use of vasodilators and the introduction of digital fluoroscopy and newer, nonionic contrast agents extended the field of PTA to the treatment of infrapopliteal arteries. Initial reports in the early 1980s were not very encouraging.[9-10] The first optimistic publication appeared in 1988 when Schwarten described the use of low-profile balloons

and steerable wires.[11] In 1991, he published an extension of his data describing use of infrapopliteal PTA in 112 patients.[3] Table 10-1 shows the most important publications regarding use of infrapopliteal PTA for treatment of patients with chronic critical ischemia. With accumulating experience, infrapopliteal PTA has become more and more accepted and successful.

INDICATIONS FOR TREATMENT

Although the use of crural angioplasty has been described in claudicant patients, most authorities agree that rest pain, ulceration, or gangrene must be present before infrapopliteal PTA is considered. Disabling claudication may be an indication if the only level of disease involves the infrapopliteal lesion (or lesions). In the author's experience, this is very rare. Ankle pressures are a good but not perfect guideline for treatment. Rest pain is associated with a resting ankle pressure of less than 40 mm Hg. We have shown that selection of patients with lesions suitable for PTA or surgery can be made with the aid of duplex ultrasonography.[12]

Before infrapopliteal PTA is considered, the patient should have all supratibial inflow lesions treated. If the patient's complaints remain 4 weeks after performance of supratibial PTA, the remaining tibial lesion(s) should receive attention. Although focal lesions have a better patency rate than that of long, diffuse lesions or occlusions, this should not be an absolute selection criterion, because even short-term local patency may be sufficient for superficial ulcers to heal.

Close cooperation between radiologist and vascular surgeon is crucial in selecting patients suitable for PTA. It is important to select the most suitable patients for this procedure rather than those who are poor surgical candidates. If PTA is the first step, and surgery is reserved for those who are poor PTA candidates or PTA failures, an equal 1-year outcome for both therapies is obtained.[13] Operator experience is

Table 10–1. Results of Infrapopliteal PTA in Patients With Chronic Critical Ischemia

Author	No. of Limbs	Critical Ischemia (%)	Initial Success (%)	Cumulative Limb Salvage at 1 Yr (%)	Cumulative Limb Salvage at 2 Yr (%)	Mean Follow-Up
Bull et al[24]	168	76	77	67	67	19 mo
Schwarten[3]	112	100	88	88	83	26 mo
Matsi et al[25]	84	100	—	56	—	12 mo
Brown et al[26]	55	84	84	60	50	26 mo
Bakal et al[23]	53	99	78	60	57	24 mo

*Only series with >50 patients and >75% critical ischemia were included.

also very important if treatment is to be successful. PTA is not a procedure that should be performed by a nonspecialist vascular radiologist.

TECHNIQUE

Crural Arteries

The technique of infrapopliteal PTA is somewhat different from that of PTA as performed on other vascular segments. Spasm can be an important problem. Most operators give spasmolytic drugs, such as nitroglycerin. In our experience, spasmolytic drugs are rarely needed if one follows a few simple rules:

1. The wire should stay in the distal runoff vessels as short a time as possible.
2. The wire should not be allowed to enter muscular side branches of the crural vessels.
3. The procedure time should be short.

There is no advantage to be gained by using expensive, low-profile infrapopliteal PTA balloons or special high-technology wires, although these are promoted by several reporters.[11]

After an antegrade puncture of the common femoral artery, a 6-French (F) sheath is introduced. Diagnostic preintervention angiography is performed through the side port of the sheath. A 0.035-inch angled hydrophilic wire and a standard 5-F PTA catheter with a 3- or 4-mm balloon is introduced. To minimize procedure time, the length of the balloon is determined by the length of the lesion We use balloons up to a length of 10 cm. The balloon is positioned in the distal popliteal artery, and a roadmap image is made. The lesion is then crossed with the wire, and the roadmap image is used as a guide. When the wire has reached the patent distal outflow vessel as seen on the roadmap image, the balloon catheter is advanced to the site of the lesion. This is done without control angiography. The lesion is dilated for 20 seconds at a pressure of 6 atmospheres (atm) (Figs. 10–1, 10–2).

Immediately after dilatation occurs, the balloon is withdrawn above the lesion with the wire still across

the lesion, and a control angiogram is performed through the side port of the sheath.

If the result is suboptimal, the procedure is repeated. When spasm is noted in the patient, a spasmolytic drug (usually nitroglycerin) is injected. When a good result is obtained, the procedure is terminated. A poor result with recoil or dissection is also terminated after three consecutive dilatations. In our experience, further dilatation does not improve the result but only jeopardizes the distal outflow. Immediately after the procedure is completed, the sheath is removed and optimal inflow is ensured.

A special and very interesting technique, not comparable to any other, is subintimal recanalization

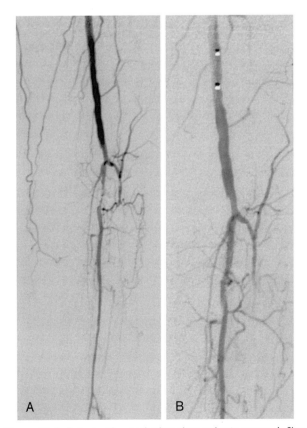

Figure 10–1. Patient with a nonhealing ulcer and pain at rest. *A,* Short stenosis at the tibioperoneal trunk, single outflow vessel. *B,* Result after percutaneous transluminal angioplasty (PTA) with a 5–French (F), 2-cm long, 3-mm balloon.

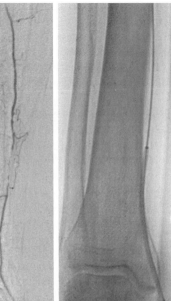
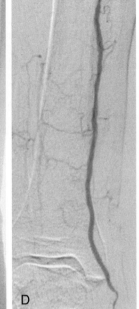
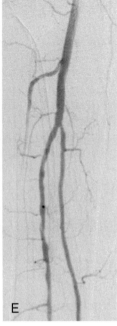

Figure 10–2. 83-year-old female with diabetes. Nonhealing ulcer at the medial malleolus of the right leg. *A,* Stenosis in the peroneal artery and poor filling of the anterior and posterior tibial arteries. *B,* Short distal occlusion in the posterior tibial artery. *C,* Dilatation of the occlusion distal in the posterior tibial artery with a 5-French (F), 10-cm long, 3-mm balloon. *D,* Good result after dilatation. *E,* Result after percutaneous transluminal angioplasty (PTA) of the stenosis in the peroneal artery. Also, improvement in flow through the posterior tibial artery, 1 month after the procedure the ulcer was healed.

of long occlusions of crural vessels, as described by Bolia and coworkers.[14] Using this technique, they are able to recanalize long crural occlusions by creating a subintimal route (dissection route) with a loop wire. After re-entry into the patent distal lumen, they dilate this subintimal route with a 3- to 4-mm balloon (Fig. 10–3).

The results are very promising and may open a new way to treat long crural occlusions[15] (see Chapter 11).

Infrapopliteal Bypass Grafts

In the first year after surgery, there is a significant risk (about 30%) that a peripheral bypass graft will develop stenosis.[16] (Fig. 10–4). Therefore, maintaining bypass surveillance is important for detecting significant lesions and treating patients before graft occlusion occurs.[17, 18] Good results with PTA for treatment of patients who have graft stenosis have been reported in several studies.[19, 20] PTA is advocated in most publications only for short, single lesions. With these, a 1-year cumulative patency of 50 to 60% can be achieved. Our own observations suggest that body-graft stenoses have better patency than stenoses at the anastomotic sites.

To obtain a good lumen diameter after PTA, long dilatation and high pressure are often necessary because the nature of these lesions is often fibrotic. The

technique, however, is not different from that used in standard infrapopliteal PTA. After a successful bypass, PTA patients should stay in the surveillance program, because a 50% rate of restenosis can be expected within the first year.

COMPLICATIONS

Complications stemming from infrapopliteal PTA are rare and are the same as those that occur when angioplasty is used with other vessels. Thrombosis, dissection, perforation, and embolization have all been described previously. A special problem is spasm, which can be managed with spasmolytic drugs. Thrombosis should be treated with local lysis, and embolization can be treated with catheter aspiration or lysis.

PHARMACOLOGIC AGENTS

Anticoagulants

It is our practice to give all patients 5000 units of heparin intra-arterially before passage of the wire and performance of PTA. All patients are treated after the procedure with intravenous heparin for a period of 24 hours, and activated clotting time (ACT) is maintained at approximately 280 seconds. Patients are also given aspirin 300 mg daily for 6 months or for the rest of their lives, if there is no contraindication.

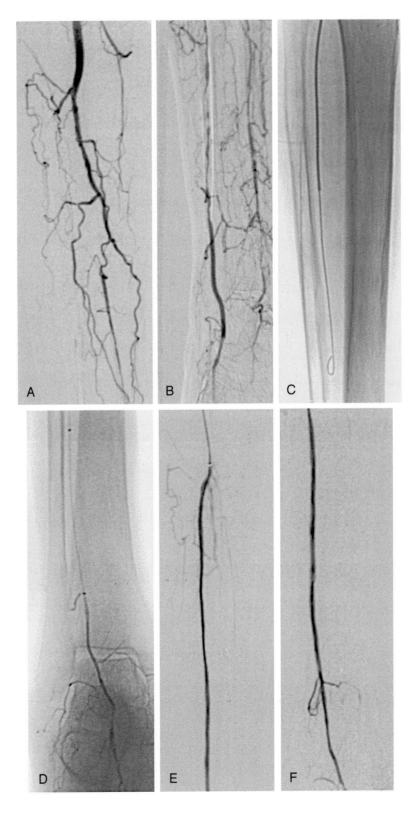

Figure 10–3. Extraluminal (subintimal) recanalization of a long occlusion of the anterior tibial artery. *A,* Occlusion of all crural vessels. 1-cm-long proximal stump of the anterior tibial artery. *B,* Refilling of the distal anterior tibial artery at the level of the ankle. *C–D,* After revascularization with the loop technique, percutaneous transluminal angioplasty (PTA) with a 10-cm, 3-mm balloon. *E–F,* End result with a good neolumen and good flow.

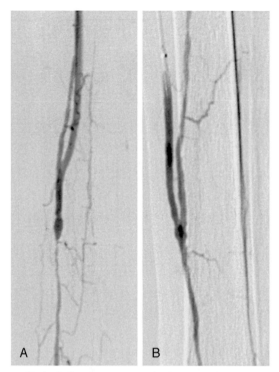

Figure 10–4. *A,* Distal stenosis in the bypass graft and also in the proximal part of the outflow artery. *B,* Result after percutaneous transluminal angioplasty (PTA) with an 8-cm-long, 3-mm balloon. Both lesions were treated at the same time to reduce procedure time.

Antispasmodics

The tibial vessels are prone to spasm, although we have found that this risk can be minimized by making the procedure as short as possible and avoiding deviation of the guide wire from the lumen of the tibial vessel into a small muscular branch. The latter occurrence has triggered spasm. We give all patients 10 mg of nifedipine orally before the procedure. If necessary, boluses of 100 to 200 μg of nitroglycerin are given locally.

Contrast

Patients may experience significant pain if contrast is used in small vessels, especially in vessels with poor runoff. This is not only uncomfortable for the patient; because of the patient's involuntary movements, there may be problems in obtaining adequate subtraction angiography and in maintaining a good roadmap. We have achieved very good results with the use of iodixanol, a dimer, as a contrast agent for these procedures. This is a nonionic, low-osmolar contrast medium. An advantage is that it causes virtually no pain in patients compared with that caused by other agents, and, therefore, produces images without motion artifacts.

RESULTS

Both patency and limb salvage rates are used to report the outcome of infrapopliteal PTA. It is known from surgical experience that patency rates for infrapopliteal PTA are 10 to 20% lower than those for limb salvage rates. If a patient is treated for critical ischemia, ulcers, or both, limb salvage is the most important endpoint. Although the initial success and primary patency of the procedure are satisfactory, there are limited data on the long-term results. This is also the main criticism of surgery.[21] However, we must emphasize the fact that appropriate patient selection is very important and that PTA and surgery are complementary procedures. We know that patients who have focal disease and good runoff can derive the greatest benefit from this procedure. Moreover, a straight-line flow to the foot, as described by Bakal and associates, improves the limb salvage rate at 2 years.[22, 23] In a series by Bull and associates, it was shown that patients who had rest pain had better clinical success than those who had tissue necrosis.[24]

In a prospective management study comparing 61 patients who underwent PTA as a first treatment option with a similar number who underwent surgery because they were not considered good PTA candidates, the 1- and 2-year limb salvage rates were equal.[25] Primary and secondary limb salvage rates for patients who underwent PTA were 81% at 1 and 2 years. For femorocrural bypass, the 1-year secondary limb salvage rate was 79%.[13]

In conclusion, limb salvage is the main objective of infrapopliteal PTA. Clinical patency achieved with use of this procedure is better than hemodynamic patency, but even a short interval of patency may be enough to improve the clinical outcome.[26] If we take into consideration that the life expectancy for patients who have critical ischemia is reduced, our aim is to optimize the risk–benefit ratio. Patient selection should always be the result of a team effort. A clinical effectiveness rate of approximately 80% at 2 years can be expected in appropriately selected patients.[22] One must always keep in mind that reocclusion of a tibial lesion after PTA does not take away the option of a surgical bypass procedure.

SURGICAL ASPECTS OF CRURAL DISEASE

Surgical bypass to the infrapopliteal arterial tree for treatment of patients with atherosclerotic occlusive vascular disease is the most challenging and technically demanding of the peripheral arterial reconstructions. Patients are often elderly, with risk factors that include coronary and cerebral artery atherosclerosis, diabetes mellitus, hypertension, renal disease, and chronic obstructive airway disease. These factors contribute to mortality figures that range from 1.2 to 6.8%.[5, 27–29] Two thirds of patients who have surgically significant crural artery disease have ulceration or gangrene, and the remaining one third have limb-threatening rest pain.[31] The principal indication for surgical bypass to tibial, peroneal, or pedal arteries is, therefore, critical leg ischemia.

The success of any bypass procedure depends on a relatively disease-free inflow vessel—a good-quality conduit—and an outflow tract that can achieve the end result of relief of ischemic rest pain and the healing of ischemic ulcers and gangrenous parts. Meticulous surgical technique and excellent perioperative care are vital in attaining a favorable outcome in crural bypass procedures. Patients who have a diagnosis of critical limb ischemia have a shortened life expectancy, and slightly fewer than half of them will be alive 5 years later.[31, 32] Protracted rehabilitation has a markedly detrimental effect on the quality of this remaining life span. Therefore, it is imperative that surgical bypass meet the ultimate objective of limb salvage.

Assessment of the Ischemic Leg

The presence of ischemic rest pain or tissue loss should prompt examination of the extremity to evaluate color, temperature, capillary refill, and peripheral pulses. If the pulses cannot be palpated, noninvasive measurement of the ankle pressure can be performed with use of a continuous-wave Doppler probe in the anterior tibial, posterior tibial, and peroneal arteries. Such a probe can also be used to obtain toe pressure, a valuable measurement in diabetic patients. Unsatisfactory ankle pressure ($\leq$50 mm Hg) or toe pressure ($\leq$30 mm Hg) is a deterrent to healing of distal ischemic lesions. However, higher pressures do not guarantee healing either, especially in a patient who has a suspected infection that must be diagnosed and treated. If a Doppler arterial signal cannot be found at the ankle when the patient is in the supine position, a dependent Doppler examination conducted while the patient is in the sitting or standing position may demonstrate a patent artery.

Intra-arterial digital subtraction angiography (IADSA) is the standard for evaluating patients preoperatively for a distal bypass. Modern imaging units demonstrate patent pedal vessels in the majority of cases. In one study, preoperative IADSA enabled planning of the distal bypass in 86% of patients' legs, but intraoperative angiography was the only means by which the outflow vessel was demonstrated in the remaining 14%.[33] No one should be turned down for crural bypass on the basis of preoperative IADSA

alone, but an artery demonstrated by dependent Doppler or by table angiography should be explored before primary amputation is considered.

Arterial Sites Used in Crural Bypass

The procedure of choice depends upon the distribution of atherosclerosis. In a study of almost 3000 patients with critical leg ischemia, significant stenosis was found both above and below the inguinal ligament in 13%, and 35% had two or more levels of significant narrowing below the inguinal ligament.[5] Unobstructed flow to the distal half of the thigh was present in a quarter of the same patients, and unobstructed flow into the upper third of the leg was present in 16%, with concomitant occlusion of all three vessels in the middle part of the leg and reconstitution of a named patent artery in the distal leg or foot.[5]

Patients who have iliac artery lesions located above distal bypass grafts are usually responsive to transluminal balloon angioplasty, and it is unusual for them to require iliocrural bypass. If surgical bypass of an iliac artery lesion is required, distal bypass may take its origin from the distal end of the proximal bypass, resulting in sequential bypass. The common femoral artery remains the usual site for proximal anastomosis of crural bypass grafts, but more distal sites of origin in the absence of inflow obstruction have included the superficial femoral and profunda femoris arteries, the popliteal artery, and even the proximal tibial artery.[5, 27–29, 32]

The outflow artery selected requires continuity to the foot to ensure healing of ulcerated or gangrenous parts. The most proximal part of the patent artery is chosen for the distal anastomosis, because shorter grafts meet with longer primary patency rates.[31] Accessible arteries include the tibioperoneal trunk in the proximal third of the leg; the anterior tibial artery throughout its course in the anterior compartment; the peroneal artery in the middle third of the leg from a lateral approach, and in the distal third of the leg from a medial approach; and the posterior tibial artery in the distal third of the leg from a medial approach. The pedal vessels available for insertion of the distal anastomosis include the dorsalis pedis artery on top of the foot and the medial and lateral plantar arteries inferior to the medial malleolus.

Conduits Used for Crural Bypass

The long saphenous vein, in situ, transposed, nonreversed, or reversed, is the bypass graft of choice.[27, 29, 30, 34–36] In the absence of usable ipsilateral long saphenous vein, either because of removal or disease, the short saphenous vein, the contralateral long saphenous vein, or an arm vein may be used. Other operators have selected prosthetic material, such as PTFE, human umbilical vein grafts, or Dacron.[28, 38–40]

Primary patency of short vein grafts was superior to that of longer vein grafts. Cumulative primary patency of vein bypass from the common femoral artery to an infrapopliteal artery in the distal third of the leg was 45%, whereas short tibiotibial bypass had a cumulative primary patency rate of 86% after 2 years.[31] Overall, 5-year primary patency rates for reversed vein grafts ranged from 29 to 69%, and the rate for in situ vein grafts was approximately 73%.[31] The choice of inflow vessel for crural bypass using autogenous saphenous vein or arm vein showed a 6-year patency rate of 65% for grafts originating from the common femoral artery, and 81% patency for grafts originating from the superficial femoral or popliteal arteries.[27] Limb salvage rates were 75 and 89%, respectively, and neither of the differences was statistically significant. The same study showed similar 6-year patency for each outflow artery: anterior tibial 78% (n = 25), posterior tibial 81% (n = 32), and peroneal 80% (n = 21). A combination of end-stage renal disease in the presence of diabetes had an adverse impact on the outcome of femorotibial and femoroperoneal bypass grafts. After 1 year, primary patency rates were 52 vs. 82%, and limb salvage rates were 63 vs. 84%.[30] In situ long saphenous vein grafts gave a 72% primary patency rate and an 82% secondary patency rate after 5 years, with a limb salvage rate of 90%.[34] Reversed vein bypass to the peroneal and pedal arteries gave a 3-year patency rate of 63% and a limb salvage rate of 75%. These rates were equivalent in statistical terms.[35] Composite veins, when spliced segments were interposed to augment insufficient vein during in situ bypasses, gave inferior but acceptable results to single-vein bypasses, with secondary patency rates after 4 years of 67 vs. 83% and limb salvage rates of 90 vs. 96%.[37]

Patency rates of prosthetic bypass are inferior to those of venous bypass. Summary reports suggest 5-year primary patency rates of 7 to 50%. Prosthetic bypass patency can be augmented by the interposition of a distal vein cuff or patch and the addition of a distal arteriovenous fistula.[28, 38–40] The patency rate was 47% after 1 year in patients who had high-risk grafts compared with 41% for those who had better risk grafts in which a fistula was not placed.[28] Another study used a distal vein patch interposition for PTFE bypass to the crural level with a cumulative graft patency rate of 91% after 6 months and 78% after 3 years with 91% limb salvage.[38] A combination of arteriovenous fistula at the distal anastomosis and chronic anticoagulation for PTFE grafts to crural vessels showed a 3-year primary graft patency rate of 70% and a limb salvage rate of 78%.[39] Without a cuff or patch, bypass to the infrapopliteal arteries gave 3-

and 5-year patency rates of 39 and 38%, respectively; secondary patency rates of 55% and 43%, respectively; and overall limb salvage rates of 71 and 67%, respectively.[40]

After bypass is performed to the tibial, peroneal, or pedal arteries, a completion study ensures quality control. Traditionally, this has been an on-table angiogram. However, physiologic studies using Doppler flow scans, conducted by experienced operators, allow angiography to be avoided when certain flow criteria are met.[41] Intraoperative duplex scanning is gaining in popularity for detecting graft imperfections and anastomoses, but data for this application are still accumulating. The use of intravascular ultrasonography (IVUS) also shows promise for the detection of graft imperfections and technical insufficiencies at anastomoses.[42]

Surveillance of Crural Bypass Grafts

Postoperative surveillance programs have been recommended on the basis that occluded bypass grafts are more difficult to rescue than grafts that are at risk but not actually thrombosed. At the point when clinical symptoms return in the situation of critical ischemia, it is often too late in the course of graft occlusion to anticipate its failure. Therefore, regular follow-up examinations, including ankle–brachial pressure index assessment and duplex assessment of graft flow, are recommended by many groups, although their value is controversial.

Bergamini and associates[43] reported an intensive program of surveillance for autogenous vein bypasses (two thirds of which were crural bypasses). They measured ankle-brachial indexes (ABI) and performed duplex scans with graft velocities at 1, 3, and 6 months after operation and every 6 months thereafter. The results were compared with those of patients who had clinical follow-up only and investigation only when clinically indicated. Findings were similar for both intensive surveillance (IS) and clinically indicated (CI) groups, with patency rates of 56 and 67%, respectively. Secondary patency and limb salvage rates at 5 years were significantly better for the IS group (80 and 94%) than for the CI group (67 and 73%).[43]

CONCLUSIONS

When performed for limb salvage, crural bypass can give good results in the medium to long term, with over 50% patency and limb salvage rates after 5 years. The best results are obtained with a single segment of vein used over the shortest distance, but acceptable results can be obtained with composite veins and prosthetic grafts, provided there is an aggressive policy in place to correct graft defects and perform secondary bypass procedures when prosthetic grafts occlude. An ideal bypass graft to the crural arteries would appear to be a short autogenous vein. The graft would be managed in an intensive postoperative surveillance program, resulting in an expectation of 80% assisted primary or secondary patency and limb salvage after 5 years. All attempts to revascularize occluded crural arteries should aspire to this high standard.

REFERENCES

1. Wagner HJ, Starck EE, McDermott JC: Infrapopliteal percutaneous transluminal revascularisation: Results of a prospective study on 148 patients. J. Intervent Radiol 8:81, 1993.
2. Bull PG, Mendel H, Hold M, et al: Distal popliteal and tibioperoneal transluminal angioplasty: Long-term follow-up. J Vasc Intervent Radiol 3:45, 1992.
3. Schwarten DE: Clinical and anatomical considerations for nonoperative therapy in tibial disease and the results of angioplasty. Circulation 83(Suppl):186, 1991.
4. Horvath W, Oertl M, Haidinger D: Percutaneous transluminal angioplasty of crural arteries. Radiology 177:565, 1990.
5. Veith FJ, Gupta SK, Wengerter KR, et al: Changing arteriosclerotic disease patterns and management strategies in lower-limb-threatening ischaemia. Ann Surg 212:402, 1990.
6. London NJM, Srinavasan R, Naylor AR, et al: Changing arteriosclerotic disease patterns and management strategies in lower-limb-threatening ischemia. Eur J Vasc Surg 8:148, 1994.
7. Cacciatore R, Inderbitzi R, Stirnemann P: Five years experience with infra inguinal arterial reconstruction: A comparison of venous with PTFE bypass. Vasa 21:171, 1992.
8. Dotter CT, Judkins MP: Transluminal treatment of arteriosclerotic obstruction: Description of a new technique and a preliminary report of its application. Circulation 30:654, 1964.
9. Sprayregen S, Sniderman KW, Sos TA: Popliteal artery branches: Percutaneous transluminal angioplasty. AJR 135:945, 1980.
10. Tamura S, Sniderman KW, Beinart C: Percutaneous transluminal angioplasty of the popliteal artery and its branches. Radiology 143:645, 1982.
11. Schwarten DE, Cutcliff WB: Arterial occlusive disease below the knee: Treatment with percutaneous transluminal angioplasty performed with low-profile catheters and steerable guide wires. Radiology 169:71, 1988.
12. Koelemay MJW, Legemate DA, de Vos H, et al: Can cruropedal colour duplex scanning and pulse generated run-off replace angiography in candidates for distal bypass surgery? Eur J Vasc Endovasc Surg 16:13, 1998.
13. Varty K, Nydahl S, Nasim A, et al: Results of surgery and angioplasty for treatment of chronic severe lower limb ischaemia. Eur J Vasc Surg 16:159, 1998.
14. Bolia A, Sayers RD, Thompson MM, et al: Subintimal and intraluminal recanalisation of occluded crural arteries by percutaneous balloon angioplasty. Eur J Vasc Surg 8:214, 1994.
15. Varty K, Bolia A, Naylor AR, et al: Infrapopliteal percutaneous transluminal angioplasty: A safe and successful procedure. Eur J Vasc Surg 9:341, 1995.
16. Grigg MJ, Nicolaides AN, Wolfe JHN: Femorodistal vein bypass graft stenoses. Br J Surg 75:737, 1988.
17. Taylor PR, Wolfe JHN, Tyrrell MR, et al: Graft stenosis: Justification for 1-year surveillance. Br J Surg 77:1125, 1990.
18. Lundell A, Lindblad B, Bergqvist D, et al: Femoropopliteal-crural graft patency is improved by an intensive surveillance program: A prospective randomized study. J Vasc Surg 21:26, 1995.
19. London NJM, Sayers RD, Thompson MM, et al: Interventional radiology in the maintenance of infrainguinal vein graft patency. Br J Surg 80:187–193, 1993.
20. Dunlop P, Varty K, Hartshorne T, et al: Percutaneous transluminal angioplasty of infrainguinal vein graft stenosis: Long-term outcome. Br J Surg 82:204, 1995.
21. Fraser SCA, Aghiad Al-Kutoubi M, Wolfe JHN: Percutaneous transluminal angioplasty of the infrapopliteal vessels: The evidence. Radiology 200:33, 1996.
22. Bakal CW, Cynamon J, Sprayregen S: Infrapopliteal percutaneous transluminal angioplasty: What we know. Radiology 200:36, 1996.
23. Bakal CW, Sprayregen S, Scheinbaum K, et al: Percutaneous transluminal angioplasty of the infrapopliteal arteries: Results in 53 patients. AJR 154:171, 1990.
24. Bull PG, Mendel H, Hold M, et al: Distal popliteal and tibioperoneal transluminal angioplasty: Long term follow-up. J Vasc Intervent Radiol 3:45, 1992.
25. Matsi PJ, Manninen HI, Suhonen MT, et al: Chronic critical lower limb ischemia: Prospective trial of angioplasty with 1–36 months follow-up. Radiology 188:381, 1993.
26. Brown KT, Moore ED, Getrajdman GI, et al: Infrapopliteal angioplasty: Long-term follow-up. J Vasc Intervent Radiol 4:139, 1993.
27. Sidawy AN, Menzoian JO, Cantelmo NL, et al: Effect of inflow and outflow sites on the results of tibioperoneal vein grafts. Am J Surg 152:211, 1986.
28. Harris PL, Campbell H: Adjuvant distal arteriovenous shunt with femorotibial bypass for critical ischaemia. Br J Surg 70:377, 1983.
29. Leather RP, Shah DM, Chang BB, et al: Resurrection of the in situ saphenous vein bypass. 1000 cases later. Ann Surg 208:435, 1988.
30. Hakaim AG, Gordon JK, Scott TE: Early outcome of in situ femorotibial reconstruction among patients with diabetes alone versus diabetes and end stage renal failure: Analysis of 83 limbs. J Vasc Surg 27:1049, 1998.
31. Ascer E, Gennaro M: Bypass operations to the infrapopliteal arteries and their terminal branches. In Strandness DE, Van Breda A (eds): Vascular Diseases: Surgical and Interventional Therapy. New York, Churchill Livingstone, 1994, pp 511–523.
32. Lyon RT, Veith FJ, Marsan BU: Eleven-year experience with tibiotibial bypass: An unusual but effective solution to distal tibial artery occlusive disease and limited autologous vein. J Vasc Surg 20:61, 1994.
33. Sayers RD, Naylor AR, London NJ, et al: The additional value of intraoperative angiography in infragenicular reconstruction. Eur J Vasc Endovasc Surg 9:211, 1995.
34. Belkin M, Knox J, Donaldson MC, et al: Infrainguinal arterial reconstruction with nonreversed greater saphenous vein. J Vasc Surg 24:957, 1996.
35. Abou-Zamzam AM, Moneta GL, Lee RW, et al: Peroneal bypass is equivalent to inframalleolar bypass for ischaemic pedal gangrene. Arch Surg 131:894, 1996.
36. Ballard JL, Killeen JD, Bunt TJ, et al: Autologous saphenous vein popliteal-tibial artery bypass for limb-threatening ischaemia: A reassessment. Am J Surg 170:251, 1995.
37. Chang BB, Darling RC III, Bock DE, et al: The use of spliced vein bypasses for infrainguinal arterial reconstruction. J Vasc Surg 21:403, 1995.
38. Neville RF, Attinger C, Sidawy AN: Prosthetic bypass with a distal vein patch for limb salvage. Am J Surg 174:173, 1977.
39. Ascer E, Gennaro M, Pollina RM: Complimentary distal arteriovenous fistula and deep vein interposition: A five-year experience with a new technique to improve infrapopliteal prosthetic bypass patency. J Vasc Surg 24:134, 1996.
40. Parsons RE, Suggs WD, Veith FJ, et al: Polytetrafluoroethylene bypasses to infrapopliteal arteries without cuffs or patches: A better option than amputation in patients without autologous vein. J Vasc Surg 23:347, 1996.
41. Bandyk DF, Cato RF, Towne JB: A low flow velocity predicts failure of femoropopliteal and femorotibial bypass grafts. Surgery 98:799, 1985.
42. van der Lugt A, Gussenhoven EJ, The SH, et al: Femorodistal venous bypass evaluated with intravascular ultrasound. Eur J Vasc and Endovasc Surg 9:394, 1995.
43. Bergamini TM, George SM Jr, Massey HT, et al: Intensive surveillance of femoropopliteal-tibial autogenous vein bypasses improves long-term graft patency and limb salvage. Ann Surg 221:507, 1995.

Chapter *11* Subintimal Angioplasty

Endovascular Contributor: *Amman Bolia*
Surgical Contributor: *Peter R. F. Bell*

Percutaneous transluminal angioplasty (PTA) as originally described by Gruntzig involves passage of a guide wire intraluminally through a stenosis or occlusion followed by subsequent balloon dilatation. The technique of subintimal angioplasty was founded in 1987 on the accidental creation of a subintimal chanel. A 15-cm popliteal occlusion was treated successfully in this manner and remained patent for 9½ years.

The technique involves the deliberate creation of a subintimal dissection plane commencing proximal to the lesion and continuing in the subintimal space before breaking back into the true lumen distal to the lesion (Fig. 11–1).

It was postulated that a false channel through a dissection probably would provide a more favorable long-term outcome compared with an intraluminal approach. Because the channel was extraluminal and therefore free of atheroma and endothelium, there would be delayed formation of neointimal hyperplasia and atheroma formation.[1] In comparison, an intraluminal approach provides a rather rough surface because of the cracked intima and atheroma following balloon angioplasty, thereby attracting platelets and thrombus formation in the short term. Also, because the atheroma is still present in the lumen, unlike in the subintimal approach, further formation of atheroma could occur. The favorable long-term results achieved with subintimal angioplasty appear to support this hypothesis.[1]

Although the technique has its main application in the femoropopliteal, tibial, and iliac arteries, anecdotally it has been used in subclavian, brachial,[2] common femoral, and profunda artery occlusions.

BASIC TECHNIQUE

The standard approach is by ipsilateral antegrade puncture of the common femoral artery, where the

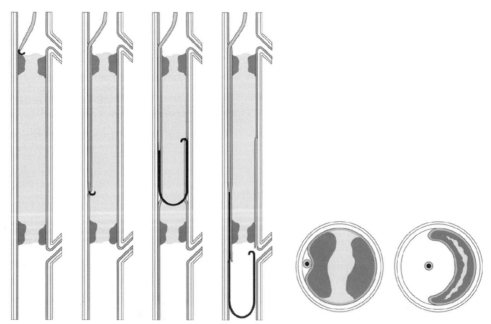

Figure 11–1. A diagrammatic representation of subintimal angioplasty. The occlusion is approached eccentrically, away from any important collaterals. Dissection is extended throughout the length of the occlusion and a large loop formed that allows re-entry into the lumen distally. Balloon dilatation of the dissected space results in a smooth, disease-free lumen.

occlusion has either a very small stump or no stump at all. When there is a reasonable length of the superficial femoral artery above the occlusion, an attempt is made to puncture this artery selectively. A 5-French Van Andel type (Cook Limited, Letchworth, UK) predilating catheter is introduced antegradely up to the origin of the occlusion. Five thousand units of heparin and 12.5 mg of tolazoline are injected before attempting to cross the lesion. Tolazoline, a vasodilator, helps to dilate the distal vessels and reduces the possibility of spasm during the procedure. A straight floppy guide wire is used to enter the occlusion. A curve is introduced on the ordinary guide wire by running the tip between the forefinger and the thumb. The tip of the curved wire is directed toward the origin of the occlusion, away from any collateral branches. A J wire (1.5 mm J, 3-cm taper, 180 cm long, 0.035-in. diameter; Meadox, Dunstable, UK) may be used instead of the straight wire. Any resistance met by the guide wire is overcome by applying pressure on the catheter to allow the force of the wire/catheter to be directed toward the path of least resistance, which is in a dissection.

Once the wire/catheter has entered the subintimal space, the position can be confirmed using a small amount of diluted contrast. At this point, an injection of contrast may cause filling of the adjacent vein. Presumably, this phenomenon of the passage of contrast from the subintimal space into the venous system occurs via the vasa vasora. The J wire once again is introduced. Looping and free movement of the guide wire will be immediately evident. The guide wire is then manipulated into a wide loop, which is usually done by allowing the tip of the wire to engage somewhere within the dissection space. Once it "catches," further advancement of the wire results in the formation of a wide loop. The diameter of the loop will appear to be much larger than the luminal diameter of the artery, once again confirming an extraluminal location of the wire. A combination of forward pressure on the wire and catheter allows the crossing of most of the length of the lesion. It is this wide loop in the guide wire that facilitates re-entry into the lumen of the artery distal to the occlusion. This occurs more favorably if the distal arterial segment is disease free. This is not surprising because the intima is likely to be much thinner in the disease-free segment. If, however, there is atheromatous disease in the artery beyond the occlusion, then the dissection may have to be extended further before re-entry can be achieved. In most cases (> 80%), successful re-entry is possible (Fig. 11–2).

Once the lesion has been crossed, a balloon catheter of appropriate size is introduced, and the entire segment undergoes angioplasty. Pressures of 10 to 12 atmospheres are used for 15-second inflations. A further aliquot of tolazoline (12.5 mg) is given at the conclusion of the procedure to facilitate vasodilation

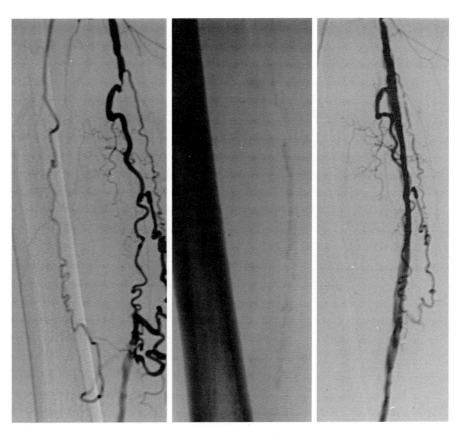

Figure 11–2. A 10-cm occlusion of the right superficial femoral artery shows large collaterals that indicate that the occlusion is of long standing. The plain film demonstrates fairly heavy calcification. A successful subintimal recanalization has been achieved.

of the distal vessels and augment flow through the segment that has undergone angioplasty.

Aspirin, if not contraindicated, is prescribed at a dose of 150 to 300 mg daily for 3 months. Oral anticoagulants are not prescribed.

INDICATIONS

Subintimal angioplasty has its widest application in the femoropopliteal segment. However, short occlusions (< 3 cm), recent occlusions (< 6 months old), and narrow vessels with extensive diffuse disease (< 4 mm in diameter) should not be attempted. However, if a dissection occurs while trying an intraluminal approach, then subintimal recanalization may be pursued.

Subintimal recanalization is generally applicable in the following situations:

1. *Chronic occlusions.* It sometimes is quite difficult to ascertain the age of an occlusion. Indicators of chronicity, however, are a demonstration of the lesion on previous arteriograms, duration of symptoms, the presence of calcification, or large collateral branches.

2. *Hard occlusions.* The hardness of an occlusion is determined by the feel imparted to the guide wire during an attempted recanalization. The harder the perceived occlusion, the longer its presence and the greater the likelihood that a dissection will occur.

3. *Long occlusions.* The longer the occlusion, the more difficult it is for the guide wire/catheter combination to be maintained intraluminally. Therefore dissection is likely to result.

4. *Diffuse disease.* When the underlying vessel has extensive disease, the guide wire likely cannot be negotiated through the occlusion while maintaining an intraluminal position. Dissection is, once again, likely to ensue.

5. *Previously failed intraluminal approach.* When an intraluminal approach has failed previously, a reattempt is unlikely to succeed intraluminally but may do well by the extraluminal approach.

6. *Presence of a large proximal collateral.* The patient may have a large collateral branch at the origin of an occlusion, and the resultant anatomy may lack the necessary "stump" to allow engagement of a guide wire. Failure of an engagement of the guide wire means that the procedure cannot be done by the intraluminal approach. Without a stump, the guide wire persistently enters the collateral. In such situations, using the subintimal approach, dissection is initiated in the main vessel, well above and opposite to the origin of the collateral. The dissection generally follows the route of the main vessel, thereby avoiding entry into the collateral branch.[1]

7. *Flush occlusion of the superficial femoral artery (SFA).* When there is no "stump" of the SFA, it is very difficult to engage a guide wire into the true lumen of the artery. It is also more difficult to maintain the guide wire in an intraluminal position in a long occlusion, which these usually are. The subintimal approach allows this situation to be tackled in most cases (Fig. 11–3).

8. *Successful recanalization after a perforation.* If a perforation of the SFA occurs during an attempted intraluminal approach, subsequent attempts at crossing the lesion usually result in the guide wire following the same path, leading into the perforation. However, using the extraluminal approach, the site of the perforation can be avoided by choosing a different route within a dissection.[3]

9. *Calcified vessels.* The presence of moderate to heavy calcification generally is regarded as unfavorable for angioplasty because of the hardness of the occlusion. Attempts at intraluminal recanalization of such a hard lesion often results in the wire taking the path of least resistance, into the subintimal space. Using subintimal angioplasty, many such lesions can have a favorable outcome.

10. *Trifurcation disease.* Subintimal angioplasty is ap-

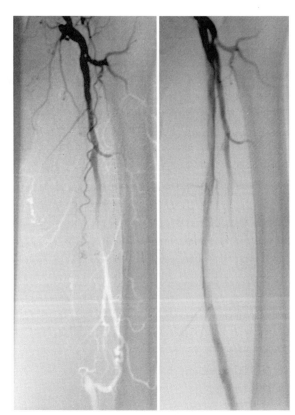

Figure 11–3. A full-length occlusion of the superficial femoral artery is present, and no stump is available. Successful subintimal recanalization has been achieved.

plicable in popliteal occlusions that extend into one or more of the runoff vessels. If the occlusion affects all three runoff vessels but there is distal patency, then the technique may allow all vessels to be recanalized.[4]

11. *Long stenoses.* When there is a reasonably disease-free segment in the proximal SFA and the distal SFA but a long segment of diffuse stenosis, subintimal angioplasty allows exclusion of this diseased segment from the neolumen, thus allowing possibly improved long-term outcome.

12. *Long tibial occlusions.* Full-length occlusions of the tibial vessels can be treated by subintimal angioplasty, which otherwise would be impossible using the intraluminal approach. The treatment is highly effective in patients with critical ischemia.

13. *SFA occlusions in the presence of an occluded graft.* Subintimal angioplasty can be effective in patients who have a femoropopliteal occlusion for which they previously have had a bypass graft, which subsequently has occluded.[5]

MATERIALS

Table 11–1 lists the essential items required to perform subintimal angioplasty in its various locations. As with any technique, the availability of the correct materials is essential if all eventualities are to be anticipated and all types of lesion tackled.

TECHNICAL VARIATIONS

Tibial Occlusions

Access to crural arteries is achieved via an ipsilateral antegrade puncture of the superficial femoral artery. If the occlusions are short, then an attempt at intraluminal recanalization is made, resorting to the subintimal route if this is unsuccessful or if a dissection is made inadvertently. Long occlusions are recanalized using the subintimal technique by choice.[6]

A diagnostic angiogram of the ipsilateral limb, before attempted recanalization, is performed through any simple catheter, positioned in the popliteal artery. The aim of this study is to obtain a good assessment of the proximal vasculature around the trifurcation, and more importantly, the quality of the distal vessels in the foot. In particular, the anterior and posterior tibial arteries at the ankle and its branches leading into the foot must be visualized. The better the quality of the vessel distally, the greater the chances of a successful recanalization.

In crural recanalization, a 5-French catheter system and 0.035-inch wires should be used because the smaller systems are not sufficiently robust.

After the diagnostic study, a balloon catheter of the appropriate size (usually a 3-mm diameter, 2-cm balloon, and 120-cm shaft) is introduced. An angled hydrophilic guide wire (180 cm long, 0.035-inch diameter) is used to make an initial entry into the occlusion. This then is used to cross the lesion in a dissection and make a re-entry into the distal vessel. However, because of the length of the occlusion and possible areas of calcification, this wire may not be strong enough. In such cases, a semistiff or stiff hydrophilic guide wire may be necessary.

Initial entry into the occlusion is made by using forward pressure on the tip of the angled hydrophilic guide wire. Dissection occurs easily with this maneuver. Once the tip of the wire is in the dissection, the balloon catheter is advanced over the wire into the occlusion. A small amount of diluted contrast medium may be used to confirm the position of the tip of the catheter and also to check that a perforation has not occurred. Once the tip of the catheter is confirmed within the dissection, the hydrophilic wire is manipulated to form a loop. This can be a difficult maneuver, but as the guide wire is advanced forward, it eventu-

Table 11–1. Items Required to Perform Subintimal Angioplasty

Guide Wires

Straight 3-cm floppy tip, 0.035-in. diameter, 180 cm long, Teflon coated

1.5 mm J with 3-cm floppy tip, 0.035-in. diameter, 180 cm long, Teflon coated

Hydrophilic wire with a curved tip, 0.035-in. diameter, 180 cm long

Stiff hydrophilic wire with curved tip, 0.035-in. diameter, 180 cm long

2 mm J, semistiff hydrophilic guide wire, 0.035-in. diameter, 180 cm long

Catheters

Van Andel catheter, 5 F, 80 cm long, preferably of Teflon construction

Celiac (7 F)/sidewinder (5 F) catheter

4-French dilator (20 cm long)

Balloon Catheters (All 5-F Size)

2.5 mm/2 cm long balloon on 120-cm shaft

3 mm/2 cm long balloon on 120-cm shaft

3.5 mm/2 cm long balloon on 120-cm shaft

4-mm up to 10-mm diameter, 4-cm long balloon on 80-cm shaft

Aspiration/Embolectomy System

F6 to F8 sheath with removable valve

F5 to F8 nontapered/wide-bore catheter, with noncollapsible wall construction

50-ml Luer lock syringe

Drugs

Aspirin 150 mg/d

Heparin up to 5000 U

Tolazoline 25 mg

Glyceryl trinitrate—500 μg

Glyceryl trinitrate patch—5 mg over 24 hrs

rt-PA or another lytic agent

F = French; rt-PA, alteplase (recombinant tissue-type plasminogen activator).

ally comes across sufficient resistance for the tip to arrest and the wire begin to loop. The balloon catheter may be advanced to enhance the formation of the loop.

The tibial vessels are delicate, and the tip of the hydrophilic guide wire is liable to cause perforation. To avoid this, care must be taken not to use undue force when the tip is its leading edge. However, once the loop has formed, it is quite safe to advance the wire forward with minimal risk of perforation.

Having formed a loop, it is usually easy to advance the wire forward, causing a dissection along the wall of the crural artery. Any resistance to progression of the loop can be overcome by advancing the balloon catheter over the wire up to the level of the loop. This strengthens one side of the loop, allowing it to advance because any force applied on the wire will be directed onto the loop. However, despite this maneuver, there may be reluctance on the part of the loop or the catheter to move forward. In such cases, the balloon is dilated sequentially, throughout the length of the occlusion that has been crossed. This has the advantage of eliminating any resistance up to the level where the loop lies. Having eliminated all the resistance proximally, any force directed on the loop and the balloon catheter will be concentrated at the site of attempted dissection. This force is usually sufficient to allow crossing of any difficult or calcified areas.

Occasionally, despite the aforementioned maneuvers, the resistance to the advancement of the balloon catheter and the loop may not be overcome, and in such situations, use of a stiff hydrophilic guide wire is indicated. The stiff wire allows crossing of almost all occlusions. The stiff wire should be replaced with the softer hydrophilic wire to complete the crossing and re-entry into the distal artery. The softer, nonstiff hydrophilic wire is gentle to the tibial arteries and is more favorable for achieving re-entry compared with the stiff-type guide wire.

Once re-entry has been achieved, the entire length of the dissection is dilated using multiple sequential 5- to 10-second inflations at 8 to 10 atmospheres of pressure (Fig. 11–4*A*, *B*).

Technical success is defined as angiographic recanalization of the occluded segment with less than 30% residual stenosis. If flow is impaired, repeat balloon dilatations are performed throughout the segment using higher inflation pressures for longer durations.

All patients receive a final intra-arterial dose of tolazoline (12.5 mg) at the conclusion of the procedure. Tolazoline causes distal vasodilation to accommodate the improved inflow from the recanalized vessel.

In all cases of critical ischemia, an attempt is

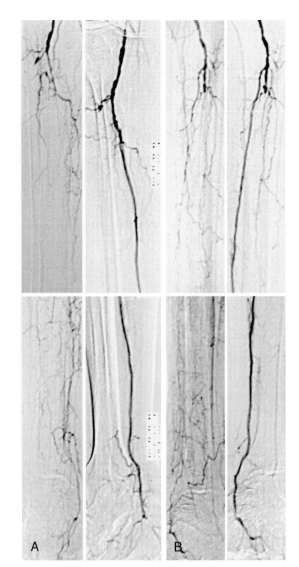

Figure 11–4. This elderly patient had critical ischemia with ulceration in both legs and no significant runoff vessels. *A*, A full-length recanalization of the left posterior tibial artery has been carried out. *B*, A full-length recanalization of the right posterior tibial artery has been carried out.

made to recanalize as many vessels as are suitable for the procedure (Fig. 11–5).

Popliteal Occlusion Extending into the Crural Vessels

Patients with critical limb ischemia may present with multilevel disease, which may include lesions in the iliac, superficial femoral, popliteal, or crural arteries. However, more commonly, the disease is distal. Arterial occlusions may occur in isolation in the crural arteries, or in the popliteal artery, extending into one or more of the crural arteries.

A popliteal artery occlusion extending into the crural arteries presents an interesting challenge.[4] During attempted recanalization, after dissecting the pop-

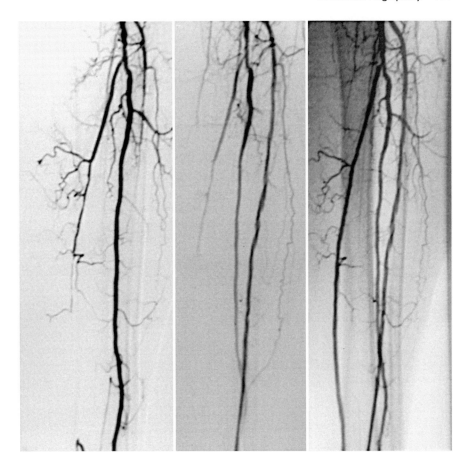

Figure 11–5. This patient had long occlusions of posterior and anterior tibial arteries. Both occlusions were successfully recanalized, the anterior tibial artery first and then the posterior tibial artery.

liteal artery, there is a choice of three vessels at the trifurcation for the guide wire to follow. The wire will enter one of the three, usually the peroneal artery, which is more or less in a straight line with the popliteal artery. Therefore, if one of the other arteries (anterior tibial or posterior tibial) is more suitable for treatment, special maneuvers must be used to guide the wire into one of these vessels. Alternatively, all three vessels may be suitable distally, and in such a situation, it would be preferable to recanalize the popliteal artery into all of these to achieve an optimum result. A different sized balloon must be used for the crural arteries (e.g., 3-mm diameter) compared with the popliteal artery (e.g., 5-mm diameter) because of disparity in diameter.

Once a diagnostic angiogram has been performed, a 5-French Van Andel predilating catheter, as previously described, is used to create a subintimal chanel in the popliteal artery down to the level of the trifurcation.

At this point, the wire is removed from the catheter and a small amount of diluted contrast confirms the extraluminal location and also the possible position of the trifurcation vessels. There may be a hint of the origin of the anterior tibial artery and the bifurcation of the tibioperoneal trunk. This helps direct the wire toward whichever vessel needs to be recanalized. A curved hydrophilic guide wire then is

introduced and directed either toward the origin of the anterior tibial artery or to the bifurcation of the tibioperoneal trunk and subsequently, the peroneal or the posterior tibial arteries (Fig. 11–6).

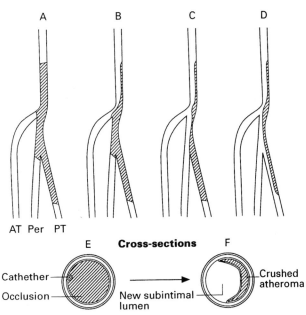

Figure 11–6. A popliteal occlusion is seen extending into all three runoff vessels. Recanalization is carried out in sequence, the anterior tibial artery first, then the peroneal artery, and, finally, the posterior tibial artery.

In some situations, the contrast may not outline the origin of the anterior tibial artery, but the tip of the curved Terumo wire usually "catches" at the site of the origin of this vessel. The wire then is persuaded to enter at the site where it "catches," and once the wire has entered a few millimeters, the Van Andel catheter is advanced over it. The recanalization then proceeds as previously described.

An appropriate balloon catheter (usually 3 mm in diameter) then is substituted for the Van Andel catheter, and dilatation is performed throughout the length of the anterior tibial artery. Subsequently, the balloon catheter is substituted for one that is more appropriate for the popliteal artery (usually 5 mm in diameter). Flow then is established through the popliteal artery into the anterior tibial artery.

If one or two of the remaining occluded crural arteries are also available for recanalization, the procedure is repeated to include these vessels also.

In this way, one or more of the crural arteries can be recanalized when the occlusion extends from the popliteal artery into the crural arteries (Fig. 11–7).

Iliac Occlusions

As previously described, a subintimal dissection is initiated in the ipsilateral iliac artery below the occlusion.[7] An attempt is made to cross the occlusion through this dissection plane via the ipsilateral approach only. However, re-entry frequently is difficult in such situations, and the tendency is for the catheter/guide wire to extend the dissection further toward the aorta. Failure of re-entry is probably a result of the thickness of the intima nearer the aorta.

Hence, with the help of a sidewinder catheter, an approach to the proximal part of the occlusion is made via crossover (see Fig. 11–8). Once again, a dissection is initiated. A hydrophilic guide wire appears to be more helpful in creating a dissection from the crossover approach. When an occlusion is hard or an aortic bifurcation steep, then the 5-French catheter may not provide sufficient strength in the system to initiate the antegrade dissection. In such cases, a 7-French celiac catheter is helpful. Once the dissection has been initiated from the proximal part of the occlusion, it is extended further distally. Because the proximal and the distal dissections are in the same plane, wire manipulations, usually with the help of the hydrophilic wire, are made such that the common channel is entered. This is achieved by converting the curved Terumo guide wire into a loop. Advancing this loop helps to re-enter the artery distally, as described previously (see recanalization of femoropopliteal occlusions). Once the guide wire has crossed the lesion, the sidewinder catheter is substituted for a balloon catheter and the false channel undergoes angioplasty, via the crossover approach (Figs. 11–8 and 11–9).

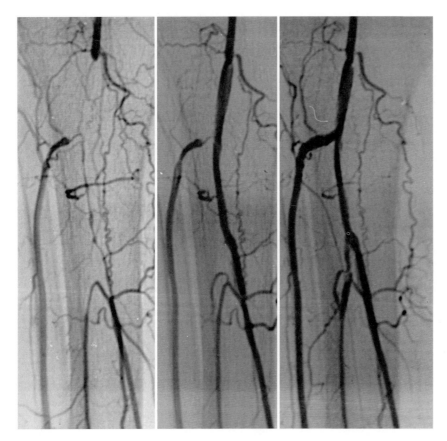

Figure 11–7. A popliteal occlusion is present that extends into all the runoff vessels. In the first instance, the posterior tibial artery was recanalized; communications were then made with peroneal and anterior tibial arteries, achieving recanalization of all three vessels.

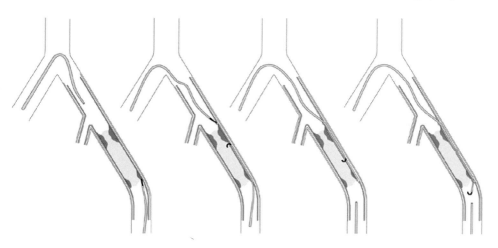

Figure 11–8. An attempt is first made to recanalize the occlusion via an ipsilateral approach, but the dissection frequently extends toward the aorta without achieving re-entry. Thus, using a sidewinder catheter, a dissection is initiated in antegrade fashion; because both dissections are in the same plane, a common channel can be found with use of wire manipulators.

EFFICACY

Large numbers of subintimal angioplasties have been performed with primary success and patency rates similar to that of conventional angioplasty.[7]

There is no significant difference in the ability to recanalize short or long occlusions. This is not surprising because the ability to cross occlusions via the subintimal route is determined by the ability to initiate a dissection then traverse and re-enter distally into the true lumen.

The literature on angioplasty of tibial lesions is limited, and the few available series have combined the treatment of stenoses and occlusions.[6–13] Comparison with subintimal recanalization is therefore difficult, but again, results appear comparable or somewhat better with primary success rates in the region of 80%.

PROCEDURE-SPECIFIC COMPLICATIONS

The common complications of subintimal angioplasty are perforation, peripheral embolism, damage to collaterals and puncture site haematoma. Of these perfo-

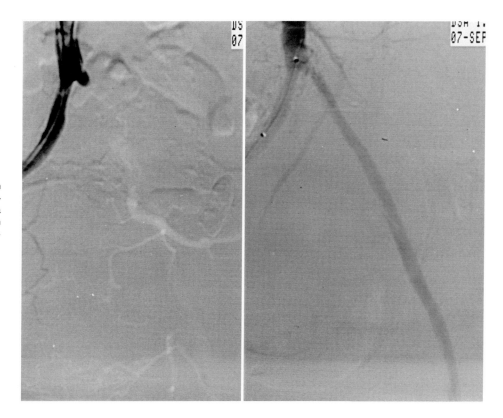

Figure 11–9. A 3-cm left common iliac occlusion was successfully repaired by angioplasty performed via a subintimal dissection. The balloon catheter was used from the contralateral approach.

rations and damage to collaterals are procedure specific.

Perforation

It is possible to treat hard and calcified occlusions with subintimal angioplasty. However, to cross a hard occlusion, a degree of force is necessary on the catheter/wire combination, and in some cases, this leads to perforation. When perforation occurs, there are three courses of action available. A successful outcome may be achieved if an alternative route to the dissection is found, thus avoiding the site of the perforation, which usually seals itself once a successful recanalization channel has been achieved. If an alternative dissection channel cannot be found, the procedure must be abandoned and a further attempt made at a later date (Fig. 11–10A,B).

If a perforation is substantial, the patient may feel

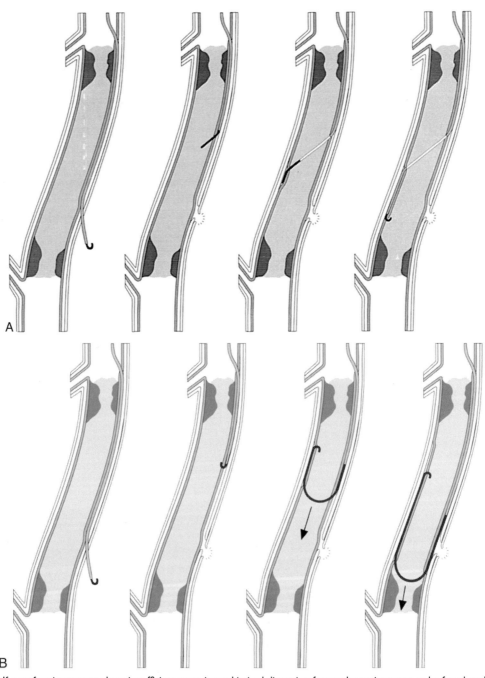

Figure 11–10. A, If a perforation occurs, there is sufficient space in a subintimal dissection for an alternative route to be found, and dissection can be continued to achieve a successful result. B, If, however, it is difficult to find an alternative dissection route with the leading edge of the wire, the wire can be converted into a loop that is too large to enter a perforation; therefore, it will usually follow the true dissection down the main vessel, and a successful result can be achieved.

a lot of discomfort because of hematoma formation around the perforation site, a result of blood loss. This is more likely in patients who are hypertensive. In such patients, the dissected segment proximal to the site of the perforation can be embolized with a coil. A further attempt at recanalization can be made after a few weeks, when the site of perforation has healed. The presence of a coil does not interfere with a subsequent attempt at recanalization.[3]

In most cases of perforation, a successful outcome can be expected (Figs. 11–11 and 11–12).

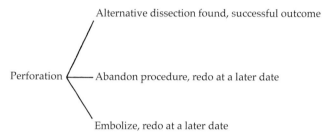

Alternative dissection found, successful outcome

Perforation — Abandon procedure, redo at a later date

Embolize, redo at a later date

Damage to Collateral Branches

This complication occurs in 1% to 1.5% of patients, in whom important collateral branches are compromised during the procedure, without achieving a successful channel. Hence, the distal circulation is compromised, and as a result, emergency bypass surgery may be necessary to restore the distal circulation.

AFTERCARE

After successful recanalization of femoropopliteal and tibial occlusions, patients do not require specialized aftercare. However, in certain situations, such as with patients who have had recanalization of a long femoropopliteal or tibial occlusion or a particularly difficult procedure, we recommend 4 doses of 5000 units of subcutaneous heparin every 6 hours to help prevent reocclusion of the segment that has undergone angioplasty. By encouraging peripheral vasodilatation in the treated leg, the resultant reduction in peripheral resistance improves flow through the treated segment, and therefore, the probability of maintaining patency during the early critical phase is increased. Hence, in most patients who have had recanalization of long femoropopliteal or tibial occlusions, a patch of glyceryl trinitrate (nitroglycerin) to the patients' treated leg—delivering 5 mg of medication over 24 hours—is beneficial.

A high puncture is required to treat flush occlusions, or occlusions with a very small stump in the

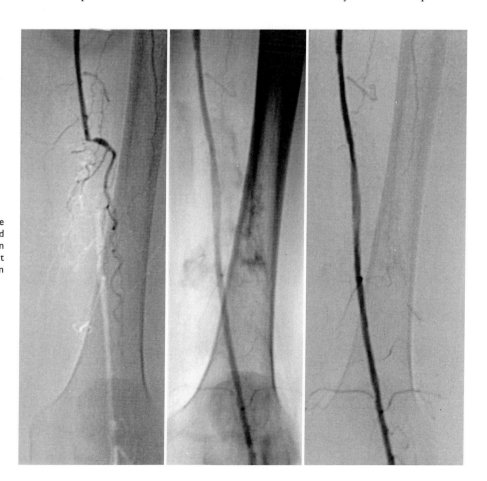

Figure 11–11. A short occlusion of the distal superficial femoral artery resulted in a perforation. An alternative dissection route was found, and a successful result was achieved. Loose contrast can be seen in the soft tissues.

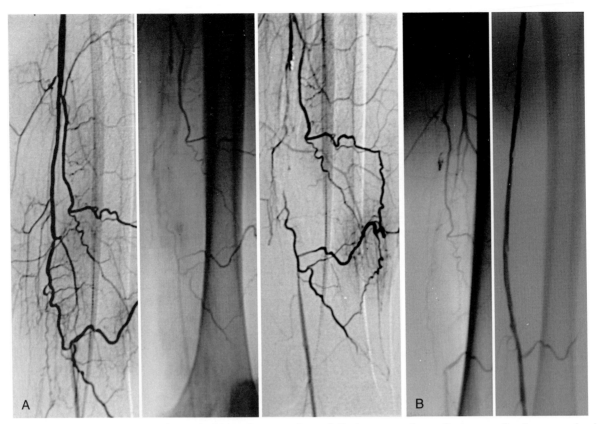

Figure 11–12. A short occlusion of the left superficial femoral artery is shown. A, During attempted recanalization, a perforation occurred and loose contrast can be seen in the soft tissues. A 3-mm coil was placed in the dissection channel and the procedure was abandoned. B, The patient was recalled 2 months later, and a successful recanalization was achieved.

superficial femoral artery. Nursing staff must be informed of the high puncture of the common femoral artery, with its increased risk of retroperitoneal hemorrhage.

SURGICAL ALTERNATIVES

Subintimal angioplasty can be applied to almost any length of occlusion in the iliac, femoropopliteal, or crural vessels. The results as set out in this chapter are excellent and provide a real alternative to existing means of treatment. However, no controlled data are available to guide us as to whether subintimal angioplasty is better or worse than conventional treatment. Also, many of the interventions performed on the femoropopliteal or iliac segments are done for patients who have moderate claudication and who would not normally be candidates for surgery. This should be kept in mind when making comparisons. Patients with critical ischemia usually have crural or multilevel disease, and the alternatives available are usually surgical.

Iliac Artery Angioplasty

The alternative to subintimal angioplasty is intraluminal angioplasty with or without stenting or surgery.

Intraluminal angioplasty has been used for some years and undoubtedly produces excellent results.[14] Recently, angioplasty alone was shown to produce good results without stenting, and there is in fact no evidence that the insertion of a stent is essential in this situation.[15] Further trials are being done to clarify this. In patients with severe claudication or resting pain, the alternative to intraluminal or subintimal angioplasty is to insert a graft between the common iliac artery, which is usually patent, and the ipsilateral femoral artery. A second possibility for unilateral disease is a crossover iliofemoral or femorofemoral graft. All these options have a low mortality and produce excellent results.[16, 17] If a patient has bilateral disease or disease involving the aorta, then an aortobifemoral graft is necessary, with an increase in mortality rate of about 5% with very good long-term patency.[18] In unfit patients, the alternative procedure is an axillobifemoral graft.[19] There have been no comparative studies between any of these techniques and angioplasty, and these must be done before angioplasty is assumed to be the answer in terms of patency and costs. For the moment, however, anecdotal data suggest that for claudication in which the lesion is usually a stenosis, angioplasty is the treatment of choice. For occlusions, if angioplasty with or without stenting or subintimal angioplasty fails, surgery using one of the aforementioned techniques is a reasonable alternative treatment.

Femoropopliteal Disease

Intraluminal angioplasty does not do well in this area unless the occlusion is less than 5 cm in length.[20] Subintimal angioplasty fares much better, but there are no surgical comparisons to make unless the claudication is severe or unless resting pain is present.[8] If that is the case, then the alternative to subintimal angioplasty is some form of bypass grafting using the patient's own long saphenous or arm veins if the lesion extends below the knee.[21] Above the knee, again long saphenous vein or some form of artificial graft, such as polytetrafluoroethylene (PTFE), will suffice. For below-the-knee lesions, the addition of a cuff of vein to the PTFE graft has been shown to produce a reasonable result.[22] This operation is straightforward, and the intermediate and long-term results are good. Vein grafts in particular are prone to stenoses in 30% of cases, and surveillance using duplex technology is essential to avoid failure from that cause.[23] Other possibilities recently explored include various endovascular options. Most of these involve the dilatation of the lesion and the insertion of a graft, usually of PTFE, through a small groin incision.[24] Other techniques involve the removal of the core of atheroma using a ring stripper and the fixer of the lower intimal flap with a stent.[25] A graft can be used to line the endarterectomized segment. These techniques are in their infancy and probably will not work because of the tendency for intimal hyperplasia to occur in the femoral artery. A third possibility is the use of surgical endarterectomy and vein patching, which has been resuscitated recently[26] and provides good results. Again, it is not possible to comment on the relative merits of subintimal angioplasty and surgery because not enough studies have been done and there is no comparative randomized trial, mainly because the patients are those who typically are not exposed to surgical treatment.

Crural Disease

In crural disease, patients typically have critical ischemia with long occlusions, and intraluminal angioplasty is not possible. In such cases, the alternative to subintimal angioplasty is a vein graft from the patent femoral or popliteal artery to one of the crural vessels distally. To do this, a reasonable vein up to 4 mm wide must be available and the vessels must run off distally into the foot. This means a femorodistal graft, which is a fairly major procedure in an older patient, but the results can be very good in specialized centers, with good limb salvage.[27] There is, however, a mortality risk because anesthesia is required, although it can be done using local anesthetic, if necessary. No comparison between this technique and subintimal angioplasty has been made yet, but the need for it exists. There is no place for stent graft combinations as low down the leg as this.

CHANGE IN SURGICAL PRACTICE BECAUSE OF SUBINTIMAL ANGIOPLASTY

There is no question that angioplasty of the iliac and femoropopliteal segments has led to a reduction in the threshold for treatment. When a patient has mild to moderate claudication and wishes to improve his or her lifestyle, the very low complication rate of subintimal angioplasty in these areas leads us to recommend this treatment earlier rather than later. By doing this, the quality of life in at least half of the patients is significantly improved. Currently, femoropopliteal grafts or endovascular procedures rarely are done because they are not usually necessary.

The situation also has changed with crural disease and critical ischemia. More than 62% of our patients currently are treated primarily by subintimal angioplasty, and the remainder receive surgical treatment.[28] Angioplasty is less traumatic, has a lower mortality than surgery, and should be recommended in this situation. Again, however, controlled studies have not been done to compare these techniques.

CONCLUSION

Subintimal angioplasty offers high success and low complication rates and good long-term patencies in patients with femoropopliteal occlusions presenting with intermittent claudication or critical ischemia. No specialized equipment or materials are necessary. It does not require extensive experience by the operator. The technique is inexpensive and therefore could potentially have widespread application as an alternative to bypass surgery.

In elderly patients presenting with critical ischemia and tibial occlusions, subintimal angioplasty is safe, effective, and cheap. It therefore offers an excellent alternative to distal reconstructive surgery for the treatment of tibial artery occlusions.

REFERENCES

1. Bolia A, Miles KA, Brennan J, et al: Percutaneous transluminal angioplasty of occlusions of the femoral and popliteal arteries by subintimal dissection. Cardiovasc Intervent Radiol 13:357–363, 1990.

2. Bolia A, Nasim A, Bell PRF: Percutaneous extraluminal (subintimal) recanalization of a brachial artery occlusion following cardiac catheterization. Cardiovasc Intervent Radiol 19:184–186, 1996.

3. Nasim A, Sayers RD, Dunlop P, et al: Intentional extraluminal recanalization of the femoropopliteal segment following perforation during percutaneous transluminal angioplasty. Eur J Vasc Endovasc Surg 12:246–249, 1996.

4. Nydal S, London NJM, Bolia A: Technical report: Recanalization of all three infrapopliteal arteries by subintimal angioplasty. Clin Radiol 51:366–367, 1996.

5. Nasim A, Sayers RD, Bell PRF, et al: Recanalization of the native artery following failure of a bypass graft. Eur J Vasc Endovasc Surg 10:125–127, 1995.

6. Bolia A, Sayers RD, Thompson MM, et al: Subintimal and intraluminal recanalization of occluded crural arteries by percutaneous balloon angioplasty. Eur J Vasc Surg 8:214–219, 1994.

7. Bolia A, Fishwick G: Recanalization of iliac artery occlusion by subintimal dissection using the ispsilateral and the contralateral approach. Clin Radiol 52:684–687, 1997.

8. London NJM, Srinivasan R, Sayers RD, et al: Subintimal angioplasty of femoropopliteal artery occlusion: The long-term results. Eur J Vasc Surg 8:148–155, 1994.

9. Bakal CW, Sprayegen S, Scheinbaum K, et al: Percutaneous transluminal angioplasty of the infrapopliteal arteries: results in 53 patients. AJR Am J Roentgenol 154:171–174, 1990.

10. Flueckiger F, Lammer J, Klein GE, et al: Percutaneous transluminal angioplasty of crural arteries. Acta Radiologica 33:152–155, 1992.

11. Scwarten DE: Clinical and anatomical considerations for nonoperative therapy in tibial disease and the results of angioplasty. Circulation 83(suppl I):86–90, 1991.

12. Schwarten DE, Cuttliff WB: Arterial occlusive disease below the knee: Treatment with percutaneous transluminal angioplasty performed with low-profile catheters and steerable guidewires. Radiology 169:71–74, 1988.

13. Buckenham TM, Loh A, Dormandy JA, et al: Infrapopliteal angioplasty for limb salvage. Eur J Vasc Surg 7:21–25, 1993.

14. Schwarten DE, Murty TS, Casteneda-Zuniga WR: Percutaneous transluminal angioplasty, part 9: Aortic iliac and peripheral arterial angioplasty. *In* Casteneda-Zuniga WR, Murty TS, Varthy S (eds): Interventional Radiology, 2nd ed. Baltimore, Williams & Wilkins, 1992, pp 378–422.

15. Tetteroo E, Van der Graf Y, Bosch JL: Randomised comparison of primary stent placement versus primary angioplasty followed by selective stent placement in patients with iliac artery occlusive disease. Lancet 351:1153–1160, 1998.

16. Kretschmer G, Niederle B, Schamper M, et al: Extra anatomic femoro-femoral cross over bypass [FF] vs unilateral orthotopic ileofemoral bypass [IF]: An attempt to compare results based on data matching. Eur J Vasc Surg 5:75–82, 1991.

17. Berce M, Sayers RD, Miller JH: Femoro-femoral cross over grafts for claudication: A safe and reliable procedure. Eur J Vasc Endovasc Surg 12:437–442, 1996.

18. Nevelsteen A, Wonters L, Suy R: Aortofemoral Dacron reconstruction for aorto iliac occlusive disease: A 25 year survey. Eur J Vasc Surg 5:179–187, 1991.

19. Passman MA, Taylor LM, Moneta GL: Comparison of axillo femoral and aorto femoral bypass for aorto iliac occlusive disease. J Vasc Surg 23:263–272, 1996.

20. Jorgensen B, Meisner S, Holstein P, et al: Early rethrombosis in femoropopliteal occlusions treated with percutaneous transluminal angioplasty. Eur J Vasc Surg 4:149–152, 1991.

21. Grass JD, Hiemer W: Results of femoropopliteal and femorotibial greater saphenous vein in situ bypass. Int Angiol 11:94–105, 1992.

22. Stonebridge PA, Howlett R, Prescott R, et al: Randomised trial comparing polytetrafluorethyline graft patients with or without a Miller collar. Br J Surg 2:555–556, 1995.

23. Murdy P, Gould DA, Harris PL: Vein graft surveillance improves patency of femoro popliteal bypass. Eur J Vasc Surg 4:117–123, 1990.

24. Spoelstra H, Casselman F, Lesceu O: Balloon expandable endobypass for femoropopliteal atherosclerotic occlusive disease: A preliminary evaluation of 55 patients. J Vasc Surg 24:4:647–654, 1996.

25. Jooston H, Ho GH, Moll FL: The Mollring Cutter—Remote endarterectomy. Crit Ischaemia 6:14–20, 1996.

26. Van der Heijden FH, Eikelboom BC, Van Reedt Dortland R, et al: Endarterectomy of the superficial femoral artery: a procedure worth randomising. Eur J Vasc Surg 6:651–658, 1992.

27. Sayers RD, Thompson MM, London NJM, et al: Selection of patients with critical limb ischaemia for femoro distal vein bypass. Eur J Vasc Surg 7:291–297, 1993.

28. Varty K, Nydhal S, Butterworth P, et al: Changes in the management of critical limb ischaemia. Br J Surg 83:953–956, 1996.

Chapter 12 Peripheral Arterial Thrombolysis

Endovascular Contributors: *Krishna Kandarpa and Melissa Graule*
Surgical Contributor: *Jonathan J. Earnshaw*

The principal objective of intra-arterial thrombolytic therapy is to restore perfusion rapidly to the ischemic limb by dissolving the occlusive thrombus. Additionally, identification of underlying lesions aids in their treatment and hence in the prevention of future thrombosis. Catheter-directed intra-arterial delivery of concentrated lytic agent directly into the thrombus is beneficial both in reducing the dose of lytic agent required and providing access for further percutaneous revascularization procedures. In patients who have thrombotic or embolic occlusion of a native artery or bypass graft, an initial trial of selective thrombolytic therapy rarely adversely compromises subsequent surgical procedures and may decrease the extent of surgery required.[1]

PATIENT SELECTION

Patients who have new-onset claudication or limb-threatening ischemia caused by either thrombotic or embolic occlusion of a native artery or bypass graft may be considered for regional thrombolytic therapy.[2-6] Before initiating therapy, a careful history and physical examination must be performed in order to minimize the risks of complications (i.e., severe internal bleeding; embolization from a remote source, such as the left ventricle; and reperfusion syndrome of a severely ischemic limb). Absolute contraindications include active internal bleeding, irreversible limb ischemia manifested by severe sensorimotor deficits and muscle rigor; recent stroke (CVA within 6–12 months or TIA within 2 months); intracranial neoplasm or craniotomy within 2 months; and the presence of a mobile, protruding, left ventricular cardiac thrombus.[2-5] In addition, there are several relative contraindications for which the benefits must clearly outweigh the risks should lytic therapy in this group of patients be considered. Careful clinical evaluation must be given to this patient group, and prophylactic measures should be employed whenever possible in order to minimize adverse events. These relative con-

traindications include a previous history of gastrointestinal bleeding; major recent surgery (within 10 days), including percutaneous biopsies, recent trauma or CPR; severe uncontrolled hypertension (diastolic pressure >125 mm Hg); history of cardiac source emboli; subacute bacterial endocarditis; coagulopathy; pregnancy, including the first 10 days of the postpartum period; severe cerebrovascular disease; and hemorrhagic diabetic retinopathy.[7]

Patients who have undergone recent vascular surgery must be given individual consideration. Traditionally, a 7- to 10-day waiting period has been employed before initiation of thrombolytic therapy to allow for wound healing. However, certain types of graft material, such as Dacron, seal by fibrin deposition within the interstices of the synthetic material as well as by the formation of a fibrin tunnel around the graft. This may take up to 3 months to accomplish, and periodically, a request for thrombolytic infusion therapy is made in the immediate postoperative period. In this situation, the extent of the problem at hand and the possible risks must be reviewed thoroughly before initiation of treatment. Additionally, clear endpoints and goals must be defined from the start. Both the surgeon and the interventional radiologist should agree on these points before commencement, and surgical backup must be available should the need arise. When the recent peripheral arterial surgical procedure has been limited to the limb in question, and when signs of bleeding from the wound site would be readily apparent on visual inspection, thrombolytic infusion may be contemplated. However, if an intra-abdominal or intrapelvic graft has been placed within the last 3 months, thrombolysis should be avoided because internal bleeding is much more difficult to detect early in these locations.

Because patients with mobile intracardiac thrombi are at greater risk of embolization during lytic therapy infusion, persons suspected of having had an embolic event should undergo echocardiography. Lytic therapy may be initiated before obtaining the echocardiogram; however, should a mobile or pro-

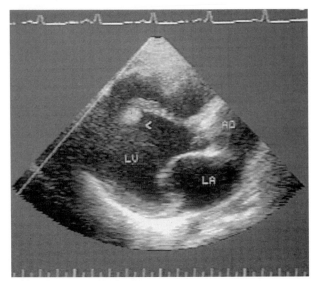

Figure 12–1. A large protruding left ventricular thrombus (*arrowed*) is demonstrated in a young patient with dilated cardiomyopathy who manifests acute pulmonary edema and distal emboli.

truding thrombus be diagnosed, prompt discontinuation of the lytic therapy must follow (Fig. 12–1). It has generally been regarded that postmyocardial infarct laminar mural thrombus may be safely dissolved by intravenous urokinase (UK) administration. There has, however, been at least one reported case of death resulting from recurrent massive embolization from the left ventricle during regional thrombolysis of a peripheral arterial occlusion.[8] Likewise, patients with

thrombosed popliteal aneurysms may be at increased risk for distal embolization during thrombolytic infusion. However, lysis may be considered in patients in whom all runoff vessels are occluded and for whom there is a need to delineate the pattern of the distal vasculature before operative bypass.[9]

Reperfusion syndrome, which may occur following rapid restoration of blood supply to an ischemic limb, occurs in less than 1% of patients undergoing thrombolytic therapy. Careful patient selection before initiation of lytic therapy is of the utmost importance, because the incidence of reperfusion syndrome is markedly increased in patients who have category III (irreversible) acute limb ischemia as defined by the Society for Vascular Surgery/International Society for Cardiovascular Surgery (SVS/ISCVS).[1] This is caused by the larger mass of ischemic muscle tissue, which results in release of metabolites from the necrotic tissue after restoration of blood flow. These metabolites, when released into the bloodstream, may cause a profound systemic acidemia and hyperkalemia that may result in cardiac dysrhythmias and death. Alternatively, patients with SVS/ISCVS category I (viable) and II (threatened) limbs have significantly lower amputation and mortality rates.[1]

TECHNIQUE

After review of the patient's history and previous radiologic studies, a physical examination should be

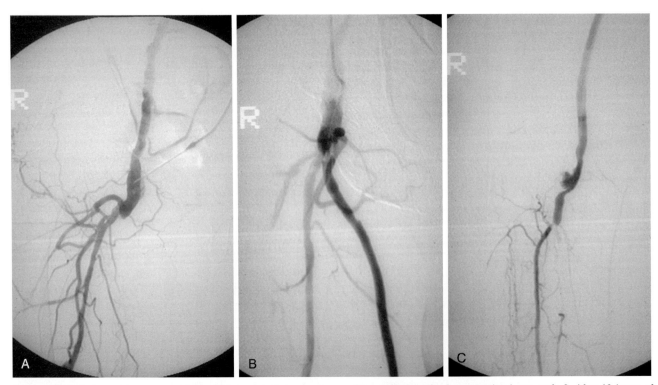

Figure 12–2. *A,* Antegrade puncture of the right common femoral artery confirms occlusion of a femoropopliteal vein graft. *B,* After 10 hours of thrombolysis, the graft is patent. *C,* A distal stenosis at the origin of the anterior tibial artery was revealed as the predisposing cause.

performed to evaluate the status of the limb in question as well as the patient's overall health. Informed consent must be obtained from the patient or guardian, including a discussion of the procedure, the possible risks and complications, and the alternatives. Laboratory values should also be reviewed to ensure that baseline hemoglobin and hematocrit levels, platelet count, electrolytes, and coagulation factors are satisfactory. Allergies should be noted, and steroids should be prescribed when applicable. Monitoring of fibrinogen levels is of limited value; however, a decrease to less than 100 mg/dl or a drop by 50% should alert the interventional radiologist to the possibility of increased risk of bleeding.

Initially, a baseline arteriogram is performed to document the site and extent of the thrombus as well as to evaluate the extent of associated vascular disease and delineate the distal runoff vessels. In selecting a puncture site, factors such as best access to the thrombus and ease of catheter manipulation must be considered. In femoral or graft thrombolysis, antegrade puncture is commonly performed (Fig. 12–2). This approach minimizes the amount of thrombogenic catheter within the patient at any given time. However, some operators prefer a contralateral retrograde puncture, especially in restless or obese patients, and this approach should also be considered when the femoral bifurcation is high lying in relation to the inguinal ligament. Inadvertently high puncture preceding thrombolysis carries a significant risk of potentially fatal retroperitoneal bleeding. The initial puncture should be made as a single-wall technique with entry into the vessel on the first attempt, if possible, to minimize potential bleeding complications during the course of therapy. The utilization of ultrasonography and a 21-gauge needle is often helpful in this regard. Use of an intra-arterial sheath is also recommended to minimize trauma at the puncture site, especially during catheter exchanges. The side-arm of the sheath may be hooked to an infusion of heparinized saline to minimize pericatheter thrombus development. In the case of a thrombosed synthetic bypass graft, careful direct puncture of the graft itself may be performed. When an upper extremity puncture is required, a high brachial puncture is favored, because the axillary region is more difficult to compress, and an axillary artery hematoma may result in injury to the brachial plexus (Fig. 12–3).

Once the occluded vessel has been selectively catheterized, an attempt should be made to cross the length of the thrombus with a straight, flexible-tipped wire. This is referred to as the guide wire traversal test. Failure to pass the wire through the thrombus is suggestive of a chronic thrombus, which may be more difficult to lyse. If the wire is unable to be passed successfully, a short trial of thrombolysis just proximal to the clot may be performed in an attempt to

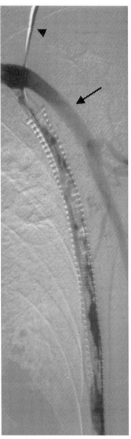

Figure 12–3. This patient had occlusion of his left axillofemoral and femorofemoral crossover grafts. Direct access was achieved by using an infraclavicular approach with ultrasonographic guidance. (Arrowhead-4F catheter, arrow-axillary artery)

soften the thrombus, thereby permitting passage of the wire and catheter. Once crossed, a J-wire may be advanced and used to gently macerate the remaining thrombus, for it is believed that this process increases the surface area of thrombus available to the lytic agent, thereby expediting lysis. This must be done with care, however, to avoid intimal damage that may result in acute rethrombosis and long-term intimal hyperplasia.

Placement of the infusion catheter across the thrombus should ensure that the entire length of the clot is maximally infused with the lytic agent. The catheter itself should be chosen to accomplish this without being occlusive to antegrade blood flow. Coaxial systems may be quite effective in accomplishing these goals.

Sullivan and associates[10] have suggested that high-dose transthrombus lacing of lytic agent significantly reduces the total time required to achieve lysis as well as the dose of lytic agent. This is accomplished by administering 100,000–250,000 units of concentrated urokinase across the length of the thrombus via a multi–side-hole catheter and pulse-spray (forced-infusion) technique. Previously, the practice of leaving a distal plug of thrombus in place was advocated; however, at our institution, we lace the entire length of the thrombus to establish prompt reperfusion distally. The occurrence of small distal emboli is rarely problematic because they usually dissolve with further infusion or may be removed by suction thrombectomy.

Once lacing has been completed, the patient is begun on a continuous slow infusion. Should a coaxial system be employed, the dose may be divided between the two catheters. Because the catheters themselves may be thrombogenic, heparin must be administered concomitantly to minimize this potential complication. This may be started as soon as the thrombus has been traversed by the guide wire. The dosage varies from patient to patient and should be adjusted to keep the prothrombin time ratio (PTT) 2.0 to 2.5 times control levels.

Before leaving the angiography suite, the sheath is sutured to the skin and the catheter secured to the sheath with sterile tape. A clear dressing is applied to facilitate visual inspection of the site. The patient is transferred to the intensive care or high-dependency unit with clear instructions provided regarding monitoring of the puncture site and the pulses of the extremity in question. The puncture site should be checked every 30 minutes for 4 hours, then every

2 hours for the duration of the infusion. Doppler evaluation of the distal pulses must also be performed at least every 4 hours. In addition to monitoring the PTT to ensure adequate anticoagulation, the hematocrit level is checked to aid in early detection of occult hemorrhage. Fluid intake and output is also closely monitored to detect acute renal failure. A Foley catheter is recommended because it minimizes patient movement and, therefore, decreases bleeding complications at the puncture site, and ensures accurate urine output recording. The fibrinogen level test may be repeated at 12 hours. Intramuscular injections should be avoided, as should shaving with a standard razor. A mechanical soft diet is recommended.

A follow-up angiogram is generally performed 8 to 12 hours after initiation of treatment to evaluate the progress of thrombolysis (Fig. 12–4). If clinically indicated, this may be performed earlier. Temporary worsening of symptoms as a result of distal embolization of clot fragments is to be expected; therefore, the patient, the ICU staff, and the referring physician should be made aware of this. Often, only clinical evaluation is required, because most small emboli resolve with continued lytic infusion. Should the follow-up angiogram indicate that a previously patent branch vessel has become occluded, suction thrombectomy or direct infusion of lytic agent, sometimes

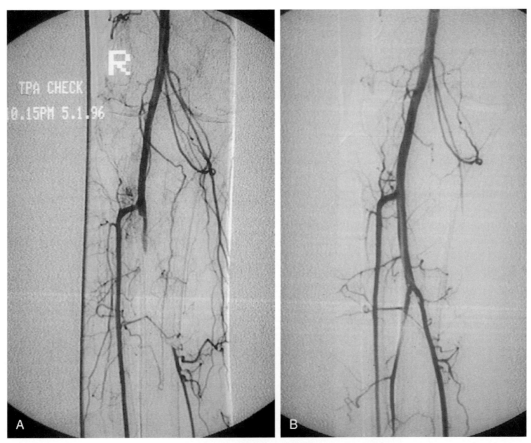

Figure 12–4. A, Embolic occlusion of the tibioperoneal trunk after femoral angioplasty. Check angiography 6 hours after shows persistent occlusion. B, After suction embolectomy and overnight lysis, patency was restored with a trivial amount of residual thrombus.

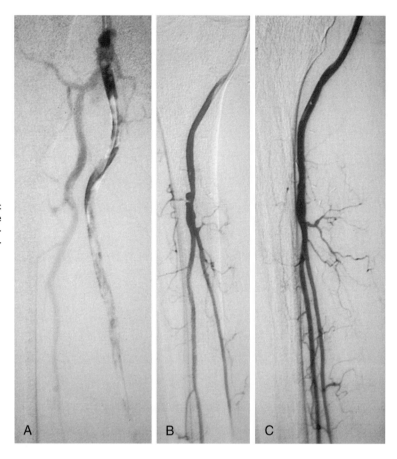

Figure 12–5. *A,* Commencement of lysis in a synthetic femoroperoneal bypass graft. *B,* After thrombolysis, a severe stenosis was demonstrated just beyond the distal anastomosis. *C,* Post percutaneous transluminal angioplasty (PTA) appearance shows an excellent angiographic result.

at an increased dose, should be administered into that area. Infusion should be terminated once successful recanalization has been documented. Infusion should also be terminated if, after a reasonable course of therapy, treatment has been deemed a failure, or if a serious complication has occurred. Minor complications, such as mild insertion-site bleeding, can often be managed by direct manual compression in combination with adjustment of the dose of heparin and lytic agent. Once it has been decided to terminate therapy, the lytic agent is discontinued. The heparin infusion may be continued based on the individual circumstances of the case. The infusion catheters are removed and the sheath is left in place with dilute heparinized saline solution infusing via the side-arm. The sheath may be removed after the patient's coagulation parameters have normalized. Underlying stenoses may be treated by percutaneous angioplasty or atherectomy (Figs. 12–5 to 12–7). More severe or diffuse disease may require surgical treatment or graft revision. Should a delay be anticipated before definitive treatment is initiated, the patient should be maintained on a therapeutic dosage of intravenous heparin. Systemic anticoagulation may be resumed approximately 6 hours after sheath removal and uncomplicated puncture site compression.

Among the thrombolytic agents currently available, urokinase and recombinant tissue plasminogen activator (rt-PA) are the most commonly used. Of these, rt-PA has been shown to have improved early lysis; however, no significant differences in clinical outcome have been demonstrated at 24 hours or 30 days.[11] Streptokinase is less frequently used in the United States because of cost issues and higher complication rates compared with those of urokinase.[12]

Given the high cost of intensive care monitoring and the fact that prolonged duration of infusion increases morbidity,[10] several infusion techniques may be employed to aid in accelerating the thrombolytic process. These include initial transthrombus lacing with the lytic agent, pulse-spray (forced infusion) technique, and use of catheters with a variety of side-hole lengths to customize the delivery of lytic agent for each particular case. Initial lacing of the thrombus with high-dose therapy has been shown to decrease the duration of therapy significantly when compared with low-dose lacing.[10] However, a recent international consensus group stated that there are no significant benefits to any one particular catheter or infusion technique.

RESULTS

It has been suggested that a positive thrombolytic outcome can be achieved in 85 to 95% of patients

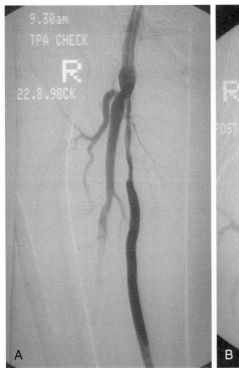 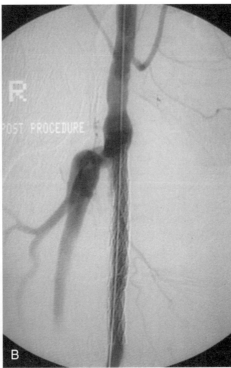

Figure 12–6. *A,* Proximal segment stenosis in an autologous vein graft after successful thrombolysis and attempted balloon angioplasty. There has been immediate recoil and threatened closure of the graft. *B,* Two balloon expandable stents have been placed with good effect. The patient was commenced on life-long oral anticoagulation.

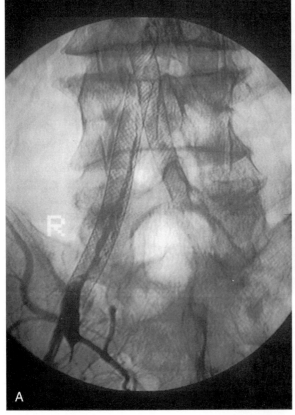 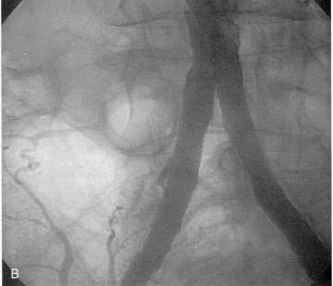

Figure 12–7. *A,* Thrombotic occlusion of a right iliac Wallstent. A catheter has been placed by a retrograde ipsilateral approach and contrast injection confirms its position. *B,* After 12 hours of thrombolysis with recombinant tissue-plasminogen activator (rt-PA), patency was restored. Atherectomy and balloon percutaneous transluminal angioplasty (PTA) were used to excise residual occlusive material and maximize the luminal diameter.

treated with urokinase.[6, 13, 14] The mean duration of infusion is approximately 24 hours, with the best prognostic indicator being presence of at least one runoff vessel below the knee.[15] Early (<2 hours) response to thrombolysis has been shown to be associated with improved initial outcome.[2] McNamara[2] has reported significantly shorter mean duration of treatment with administration of urokinase (18 hours) compared with that of streptokinase (42 hours). This may, in part, be explained by the differences in mechanism of action of the two drugs. Streptokinase, in order to catalyze plasminogen to plasmin, must first bind with another molecule of plasminogen. Additionally, streptokinase causes a more rapid and severe decrease in the circulating fibrinogen levels compared with that of urokinase or of rt-PA. This partially inhibits the body's ability to form new clots and, therefore, may result in increased bleeding complications and premature termination of thrombolysis therapy. Additionally, because streptokinase is a bacterially derived protein, patients who have previously experienced streptococcal infections may develop hypersensitivity reactions during infusion as a result of pre-existing circulating antibodies. These antibodies may also hinder lysis by decreasing the bioavailability of the drug. Similarly, patients who have previously been treated with streptokinase may make antibodies to it, requiring that repeat treatment with the drug be delayed for up to 6 months. Urokinase is also preferred to rt-PA in the treatment of peripheral arterial thrombosis because it has been reported to have a lower incidence of complications.

Another study comparing streptokinase, urokinase, and rt-PA, which was performed by Graor and associates,[14] concluded that urokinase was the safest and most efficacious of the three lytic agents. They demonstrated complete lysis and clinical improvement in 60% of streptokinase patients, 91% of rt-PA patients, and 95% of urokinase patients. The majority of complications encountered were related to streptokinase, whereas urokinase demonstrated the fewest complications. Major hemorrhage was encountered in 28% of the streptokinase patients, 12% of the rt-PA patients, and 6% of the urokinase group. The death rate was 4% for streptokinase, 2% for rt-PA, and zero for urokinase. However, it is generally acknowledged that the intracranial hemorrhage and death rates for rt-PA and urokinase are under 1%.

Long-term patency rates are better for suprainguinal grafts than for infrainguinal grafts. Obviously, timely treatment of underlying lesions is critical in aiding long-term patency. This may be accomplished either percutaneously or operatively, depending on the case in question. Each case must be evaluated individually, with the treatment plan formulated to meet the specific needs of the patient.

AVOIDANCE AND MANAGEMENT OF COMPLICATIONS

As is the case with any procedure, thrombolysis is not without risk. Thorough evaluation of the patient and his or her past medical history must be performed by the interventional radiologist before the procedure is undertaken, because careful patient selection is required to minimize the risk of complications. The probability of experiencing a major complication is increased as the duration of infusion increases. Sullivan and associates[10] have demonstrated a 4% rate of major complication after 8 hours of therapy, which is increased to 34% at 40 hours. Well-defined goals and endpoints should be considered if thrombolytic therapy is initiated to avoid unnecessarily prolonged infusion durations. The risk of intracranial hemorrhage can be minimized by excluding patients who have known recent stroke or transient ischemic attacks (TIA), or intracranial neoplasm, as previously discussed. Internal bleeding may often be an elusive clinical diagnosis early in its course. Persistent back pain or nausea should alert the physician to this possibility, and hematocrit levels should be closely monitored. Ensuring that the initial arterial puncture site is below the inguinal ligament decreases the risk of retroperitoneal hemorrhage. The close monitoring of vital signs in the intensive care unit (ICU) setting is of great benefit for the early detection of changes in the patient's hemodynamic status. Should an occult hemorrhage be suspected, both the thrombolytic agent and the heparin should be stopped, saline should be infused via the indwelling catheter to help prevent pericatheter thrombus formation, and computed tomographic (CT) examination of the abdomen and pelvis without intravenous contrast should be performed to evaluate retroperitoneal or intra-abdominal hemorrhage. Temporizing measures, such as volume replacement and transfusion, should be employed; however, if bleeding does not cease following discontinuation of lytic therapy and fresh frozen plasma (FFP) infusion, definitive treatment must take place.

Less severe bleeding, such as oozing or hematoma formation at the puncture site, can often be managed conservatively. To determine the severity of the situation, the patient should be examined by the interventional radiologist who is managing the lytic therapy. Often, the application of firm, constant manual compression at the puncture site is sufficient to provide hemostasis. Should local bleeding recur, the PTT should be checked and the heparin dose decreased accordingly. Decrease of the dose of lytic agent may also be considered. Should these measures fail, complete discontinuation of both the lytic agent and the heparin should be ordered. One must ensure that a continuous saline infusion is in place via the catheter and sheath side-arm to minimize the risk of pericatheter thrombus formation.

Should the patient experience a sudden change in mental status, both lytic agent and heparin should be stopped, and emergent, unenhanced CT of the head should be performed to evaluate the possibility of intracranial hemorrhage.

Embolization of thrombus distally is not unusual during the course of thrombolysis. This usually resolves with the continued infusion of lytic agent. Suction thrombectomy may be performed if the thromboembolus is in a critical location. Surgical embolectomy is infrequently required (Fig. 12–8).

As previously mentioned, allergic reactions are more common with use of streptokinase because of its bacterial, protein-derived nature. Patients who receive urokinase occasionally experience chills and rigors during infusion. This may be managed quite effectively with a 50-mg dose of intravenous meperidine hydrochloride (Demerol). Skin rashes, mild bronchospasm, and transient fever have been reported with all three lytic agents.

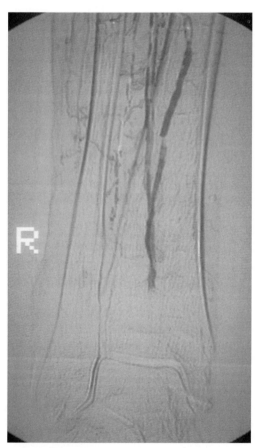

Figure 12–8. During thrombolysis, extensive embolization occurred to this patient's already diseased crural vessels. Distal surgical reconstruction was required because repeated attempts at suction embolectomy were unsuccessful.

SURGICAL ASPECTS

Choice of Surgery or Thrombolysis

Management choices for acute leg ischemia used to be much simpler in the days when the principal cause was cardiac embolism as a result of valvular heart disease. The underlying vessels were disease-free and embolectomy was a more certain procedure. Patients who have acute leg ischemia have changed in the last two decades. Pure cardiac emboli (such as atrial myxoma) are rare, and most emboli are the result of atrial fibrillation caused by ischemic heart disease (Fig. 12–9). These patients frequently have associated arterial disease, and embolectomy is more difficult. The most common cause of acute leg ischemia is thrombosis in situ. This is a disease of an elderly, frail arteriopathic patient, and embolectomy often adds further arterial damage (Fig. 12–10). Alternatively, vascular reconstruction can mean a difficult distal bypass performed as an emergency under less than ideal conditions.

With the advent of thrombolysis in the 1980s, vascular surgeons saw a solution to an increasingly complex problem. Much has been learned about the indications for and the techniques of peripheral thrombolysis, mostly from open studies. In experienced hands, about two thirds of patients with critical acute ischemia can expect successful lysis and limb salvage. The price to pay is death and a major complication rate of 10 to 20%, including a stroke rate of 2%. Some patients who have failed lysis can be salvaged by surgery, but for many it is too late. The question of whether to choose surgery or lysis as the initial treatment is one of the greatest debates in modern vascular practice.[16]

Randomized Trials of Thrombolysis vs. Surgery

Four major randomized trials have been published (Table 12–1).[17–20] The STILE study was the first and least useful because it included patients who had had symptoms for up to 6 months (i.e., chronic ischemia). In addition, experience with the techniques of thrombolysis was not widespread, so catheters could not be positioned in 28% of patients randomized to lysis. STILE was abandoned early because the composite outcome, which included failed placement and complications, was significantly better in patients randomized to initial surgery. However, the clinical outcome at 30 days was similar.[17] Subgroup analysis of patients who had had ischemia for fewer than 14 days showed that initial thrombolysis resulted in a

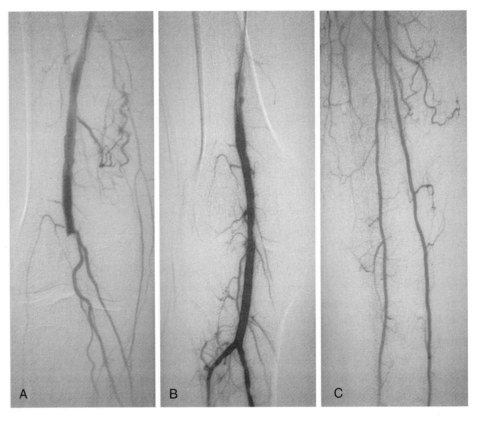

Figure 12–9. *A,* Embolic occlusion of the right popliteal artery in an elderly patient with atrial fibrillation and coronary disease. *B* and *C,* After a 16-hour thrombolysis, patency of the popliteal artery and two crural vessels has been restored. A mild popliteal stenosis is present, but angioplasty was not undertaken.

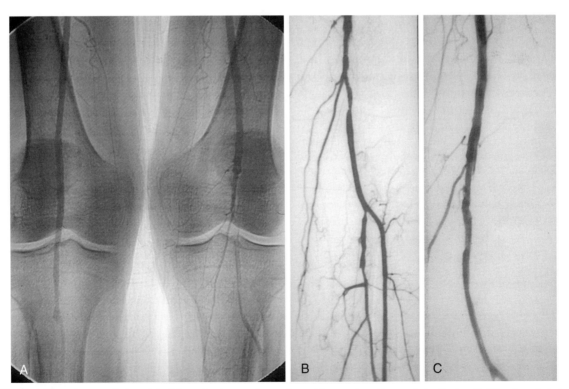

Figure 12–10. *A,* Thrombotic occlusion of the left popliteal artery in a patient with a previous history of claudication. *B,* After thrombolysis, a diffuse and distally severe popliteal stenosis was confirmed. *C,* Percutaneous transluminal angioplasty (PTA) has produced a significant improvement, although a short non–flow-limiting intimal split is noted.

Table 12–1. Thrombolysis or Surgery: The Randomized Trials. Includes All Studies of Over 100 Patients, Analyzed by "Intention to Treat"

		n	Complete Lysis	Major Hemorrhage	Stroke	One Month/Discharge		One Year amp.fs
						Death	*amp.fs*	
STILE[17]	lysis	248	75%*	6%	3	4%	91%	83%†
	surgery	144	—	1%	0	5%	89%	82%
New York[18]	lysis	57	70%	11%	1	12%	86%	84%
	surgery	57	—	—	0	18%	70%	58%
TOPAS I[19]	lysis‡	144	60–71%	2–16%	3	0–7%	83–91%	57–75%
	surgery	58	—	—	0	7%	91%	65%
TOPAS II[20]	lysis	272	68%	12.5%	4	9%	83.5%	65%
	surgery	272	—	5.5%	0	6%	89%	70%

*Excludes the 28% with failed catheter placement.
† Six month follow-up data only.
‡ Three different thrombolytic schedules used.
amp.fs = amputation-free survival.

reduced amputation rate. Later analysis of STILE patients, concentrating on native vessel occlusions only, showed that incidence of recurrent ischemia or amputation was greater at 1 year after initial thrombolysis.[21]

All the remaining trials included patients with only acute leg ischemia for fewer than 14 days. The New York study was the only one to show a significant difference in survival between surgery and lysis in favor of the latter. The reason was that patients randomized to initial surgery had a high rate of perioperative cardiorespiratory deaths.[18] The two subsequent Thrombolysis or Peripheral Arterial Surgery (TOPAS) studies were modeled on the New York trial and included larger numbers of patients, but they failed to show any differences in amputation-free survival. Initial thrombolysis, not surprisingly, reduced the need for open operation.[19, 20]

Porter has strongly criticized these results, stating that lysis has not proved advantageous and, therefore, surgeons should continue with initial surgical treatment for acute leg ischemia.[22] An alternative conclusion is that lysis has been shown to be equivalent to surgery and that it should have a role in selected patients. It is unlikely there will be further comparative trials of surgery and lysis, but it may be possible to refine the indications for lysis from other sources, such as consecutive databases. The British Thrombolysis Study Group has a collected series of over 800 cases of peripheral thrombolysis for leg ischemia. Two particular aspects have been examined: patient selection and the method of lysis used. Early analysis of the data suggests that patient selection is the most important factor affecting outcome. Elderly patients, particularly women, have a poorer outcome from thrombolysis. In addition, patients who have acute-onset claudication seem to be a high-risk group. The method of lysis used (i.e., low-dose thrombolysis or one of the various accelerated techniques) seems less important. Optimal results can be expected as a result

of cooperation between a vascular surgeon and a radiologist familiar with the full range of modern vascular surgical and thrombolytic techniques. Useful guidelines for management of acute leg ischemia based on presently available data have been constructed by an international panel of surgeons and radiologists.[23]

Surgical Techniques for Acute Leg Ischemia

The traditional management of embolectomy for all acutely ischemic legs is no longer acceptable. Preoperative diagnosis is essential and in most cases is made by angiography. Embolectomy without previous investigation is only indicated in the few patients who have severe acute ischemia (white leg or neurosensory deficit); an obvious source of emboli, such as atrial fibrillation; a short history; and normal pulses in the other leg. Preoperative angiography in the remainder may be of poor quality because collateral vessels are lacking, but supplementary angiograms may be produced intraoperatively.

Acute leg ischemia caused by in situ thrombosis is managed by use of standard surgical bypass techniques. Strategy may evolve during an operation, and the operating surgeon must be flexible and competent in all standard vascular maneuvers, such as distal bypass and intraoperative thrombolysis (see later). Management by a specialist vascular surgeon is optimal. The results of embolectomy and all bypasses should be assessed during the surgery by intraoperative angiography or another noninvasive method, such as blood-flow measurement. There is always the vexing question of when to perform a fasciotomy. This useful technique is often employed too late. If there is any doubt about the viability of leg muscle, full four-compartment fasciotomy is seldom wasted. Patients should be anticoagulated, at least in the early

Table 12–2. Method of Intra-operative Thrombolysis

1. End hole catheter situated at site of occlusion—embedding not necessary. Rubber slings passed around catheter to occlude vessel distally.
2. Inflow artery occluded with vascular clamp.
3. Lytic infusions, either:
   (a) 100,000 U streptokinase in 50 ml normal saline infused using syringe pump set to run at 99 ml/h or
   (b) three 5-mg boluses t-PA, one given every 10 min.
4. Pre- and posttreatment intraoperative angiography to assess results.
5. If there is residual trombus, repeat passage of the embolectomy catheter because thrombolysis can dislodge adherent thrombus.

postoperative phase because hypercoagulability is commonly associated with acute leg ischemia.

Intraoperative Thrombolysis

Percutaneous, catheter-directed thrombolysis was developed to deliver a high dose of lytic drug directly into the clot to maximize activity and minimize side effects. Some patients are not suitable candidates for percutaneous thrombolysis—those with failed catheter placement or ischemia too severe to wait for low-dose thrombolysis. During surgery it may not be possible to clear thrombus in small distal arteries with an embolectomy catheter. In this situation, thrombolytic drugs can be instilled into distal vessels during the operation. The techniques are described in Table 12–2 and result in minimal alteration of coagulation parameters.[24]

There are three principal situations in which intraoperative thrombolysis is helpful. Angiography, which should be done routinely after femoral embolectomy, reveals residual distal clot in about 15% of patients. Intraoperative thrombolysis can clear this in about 75% of cases. Intraoperative thrombolysis (combined with ligation and bypass) is now the accepted treatment for most patients with acute thrombosis of a popliteal aneurysm. In this situation, percutaneous thrombolysis is less helpful and can result in massive distal embolization. If used for popliteal aneurysm thrombosis, percutaneous thrombolysis should be restricted to opening distal vessels for bypass by placing the end of the infusion catheter on the distal side of the popliteal aneurysm.[25] Lastly, intraoperative thrombolysis may be helpful when distal thromboembolism occurs during arterial operation or manipulation, such as angioplasty or aortic reconstruction. The results are less certain because the rate of lysis depends on the material embolized. If atheroma is dislodged, no amount of lytic drug will help. Intraoperative lysis has been reported to clear distal embolization after aortic aneurysm repair, but hemorrhage in this situation could be disastrous.

Most of the studies of intraoperative thrombolysis are open trials with optimistic results. There is minimal systemic fibrinolysis and few complications are reported. No randomized trials exist to justify the method, and yet many vascular surgeons have found intraoperative thrombolysis occasionally useful in patients with small-vessel occlusions, and in the previously described situations.

If distal thromboembolism cannot be cleared during operation, a catheter can be left in an occlusion for postoperative thrombolytic perfusion. The risk of hemorrhage after any major operation is significant, but judicious low-dose lysis can be effective. It is helpful to insert the catheter via an arterial side branch so it can be removed after treatment without recourse to reoperation.

CONCLUSION

Intra-arterial thrombolytic therapy is now clearly established as the mainstay of treatment in many patients presenting with limb ischemia. Good radiologic technique and careful clinical audit will do much to ensure that clinical outcomes are good and that complications are reduced to a minimum. Close liaison between radiologist and vascular surgeon is essential to ensure careful patient selection and quick response to any complications which may arise. Further developments in catheter technology and thrombolytic agents will continue and may in time improve the safety of the technique.

REFERENCES

1. McNamara TO, Bomberger RA: Factors affecting initial and 6 month patency after intra-arterial thrombolysis with high dose urokinase. Am J Surg 152:709–712, 1986.
2. McNamara TO, Fischer JR: Thrombolysis in peripheral arterial and graft occlusions: Improved results using high dose urokinase. AJR 144:769–775, 1985.
3. Gardiner GA, Koltun W, Kandarpa K, et al: Thrombolysis of occluded femoropopliteal grafts. AJR 147:621–626, 1986.
4. Sullivan KL, Gardiner GA, Kandarpa K, et al: Efficacy of thrombolysis in infrainguinal bypass grafts. Circulation 83(Suppl):199–205, 1991.
5. Belkin M, Belkin B, Bucknam CA, et al: Intra-arterial fibrinolytic therapy. Efficacy of streptokinase vs urokinase. Arch Surg 121:769–773, 1986.
6. McNamara TO, Bomberger RA, Merchant RF: Intra-arterial urokinase as the initial therapy for acutely ischaemic lower limbs. Circulation 83(Suppl):1106–1119, 1991.
7. Gardiner G, Sullivan K: Complications of regional thrombolytic therapy. In Kadir S (ed): Current Practice of Interventional Radiology. Philadelphia, BC Decker, 1991, pp 87–91.
8. Paulson E, Miller F: Embolization of cardiac mural thrombus: Complication of intra-arterial thrombolysis. Radiology 169:95–96, 1988.
9. Leen VH, Shlansky-Goldberg RD, Carpenter JP, et al: Thrombolysis of thrombosed popliteal aneurysms. J Vasc Intervent Radiol 5:46, 1994.
10. Sullivan KL, Gardiner GA, Shapiro MJ, et al: Acceleration of thrombolysis with a high-dose transthrombus bolus technique. Radiology 173:805–808, 1989.
11. Meyerovitz M, Goldhaber S, Reagan K, et al: Recombinant tissue-type plasminogen activator versus urokinase in periph-

eral arterial and graft occlusions: A randomised trial. Radiology 175:75–78, 1990.

12. Janosik JE, Bettmann MA, Kaul AF, et al: Therapeutic alternatives for subacute peripheral arterial occlusion. Comparison by outcome, length of stay and hospital charges. Invest Radiol 26:921–925, 1991.

13. van Breda A, Graor RA, Katzen BT, et al: Relative cost-effectiveness of urokinase versus streptokinase in the treatment of peripheral vascular disease. J Vasc Intervent Radiol 2:77–87, 1991.

14. Graor RA, Olin JW, Bartholomew JR, et al: Efficacy and safety of intraarterial local infusion of streptokinase, urokinase to tissue plasminogen activator for peripheral arterial occlusion: A retrospective review. J Vasc Med Biol 2:769–775, 1990.

15. Clouse M, Stokes K, Perry L, et al: Percutaneous intra-arterial thrombolysis: Analysis of factors affecting outcome. J Vasc Intervent Radiol 5:93–100, 1994.

16. Earnshaw JJ: Peripheral thrombolysis: State of the art. *In* Earnshaw JJ, Gregson RHS (eds): Peripheral arterial thrombolysis. Oxford, Butterworth-Heinemann, 1994, pp 184–197.

17. The STILE Investigators: Results of a prospective randomized trial evaluating surgery versus thrombolysis for ischemia of the lower extremity. The STILE Trial. Ann Surg 220:251–268, 1994.

18. Ouriel K, Shortell CK, DeWeese JA, et al: A comparison of thrombolytic therapy with operative revascularization in the initial treatment of acute peripheral arterial ischemia. J Vasc Surg 19:1021–1030, 1994.

19. Ouriel K, Veith FJ, Sasahara A, for the TOPAS investigators: Thrombolysis or peripheral arterial surgery: Phase I results. J Vasc Surg 23:64–75, 1996.

20. Ouriel K, Veith FJ, Sasahara A: A comparison of recombinant urokinase with vascular surgery as initial treatment for acute arterial occlusion of the legs. N Engl J Med 338:1105–1111, 1998.

21. Weaver FA, Comerota AJ, Youngblood M, et al: Surgical revascularization versus thrombolysis for nonembolic lower extremity native artery occlusions: Results of a prospective randomized trial. J Vasc Surg 24:513–523, 1996.

22. Porter JM: Thrombolysis for acute arterial occlusion of the legs. N Engl J Med 338:1148–1151, 1998.

23. Working party on thrombolysis in the management of limb ischemia: Thrombolysis in the management of lower limb peripheral arterial occlusion—a consensus document. Am J Cardiol 81:207–218, 1998.

24. Earnshaw JJ, Beard JD: Intraoperative use of thrombolytic agents. BMJ 307: 638–9, 1993.

25. Thompson JF, Beard J, Scott DJA, et al: Intraoperative thrombolysis in the management of thrombosed popliteal aneurysm. Br J Surg 80:858–859, 1993.

Chapter 13 — Renal and Visceral Artery Intervention

Endovascular Contributor: Jon G. Moss
Surgical Contributor: George Hamilton

RENAL ARTERY INTERVENTION

Renal artery stenosis (RAS) is an anatomic description of renal arterial narrowing caused by a variety of pathologic processes and having a variety of clinical consequences. The most frequent etiology in the West is undoubtedly atherosclerosis, with less frequent causes such as fibromuscular dysplasia (FMD), Takayasu's arteritis, and middle aortic syndrome predominating in the younger population and children. Atherosclerotic renal artery stenosis (ARAS) is a common condition affecting up to 53% of unselected patients at autopsy.[1] A number of retrospective and recent prospective studies have confirmed the progressive nature of ARAS. Zierler and colleagues, using Doppler ultrasound in a prospective study, have shown the cumulative incidence of progression from less than 60% stenosis to more than 60% to be 48% at 3 years and from more than 60% stenosis to occlusion in 7% at 3 years.[2] The same group demonstrated the risk of losing more than 1 cm in renal length to be 19% at 1 year in kidneys with greater than 60% stenosis.[3] Atherosclerosis does not affect the renal arteries in a selective manner, and many of these patients often have evidence of more generalized arteriopathy, including coronary artery disease, peripheral vascular disease, and cerebrovascular disease. This has major implications for the treatment of ARAS.

Autoregulatory mechanisms involving the renal juxtaglomerular apparatus and the renin–angiotensin pathway enable the kidney to protect its ability to maintain filtration by inducing renal efferent arteriolar constriction in response to significant renal artery stenosis. This autoregulatory system is the basis of renovascular hypertension, and if the RAS is corrected, this rare cause of "secondary hypertension" can be cured. However, because the pharmacologic control of hypertension has improved over the years, many patients with renovascular hypertension are never recognized. Recent recommendations from the Joint National Committee of the National High Blood Pressure Education Program argue for minimal laboratory investigation of patients whose blood pressure is well controlled and whose renal function is stable.[4] This, together with an acceptance that renal revascularization rarely cures hypertension in atherosclerotic patients, has resulted in less need for renal revascularization in the purely hypertensive patient.

More recently, ARAS has been recognized as an increasingly important cause of renal insufficiency. Although the precise pathophysiology is poorly understood, clinical interest has increased with the recognition that it is a potentially reversible process with appropriate renal revascularization. The exact incidence of ARAS causing renal failure is unknown, but in the elderly (> 50 years of age), it may account for up to 14% of patients in renal replacement programs. Mailloux and associates have reported that the mortality of patients who have ARAS and who are treated with dialysis is higher than that of any other group, even including patients with diabetes mellitus.[5] The 2-year survival rate is 56%, with most patients succumbing to either comorbid vascular disease or withdrawal death.[5] These data have focused attention on preserving renal function in ARAS with the ultimate aim of preventing progression to end-stage renal replacement treatment. Hemodialysis is expensive treatment, costing approximately $32,000 per year in the United Kingdom; thus, the potential cost benefits of effective renal revascularization are obvious.

"Flash" pulmonary edema is an ill-understood condition in which the kidney's ability to excrete water is impaired because of either bilateral RAS or unilateral RAS in the uninephric patient. First described in 1988, flash pulmonary edema appears to be independent of the severity of the underlying renal impairment and hypertension but is strongly associated with coronary artery disease and bilateral RAS (or unilateral RAS in a uninephric patient). If a hypertensive patient presents with acute pulmonary edema, particularly in association with renal failure and clinical evidence of atherosclerosis, bilateral RAS should be excluded. This is particularly the case if cardiac ultrasound results demonstrate normal left ventricular function.

Renovascular hypertension, renal insufficiency, and pulmonary edema need not occur in isolation, but in combination, and in the elderly atherosclerotic patient, it is common to encounter two or even all three conditions in the same patient.

The major difficulty in renal revascularization relates to patient selection. It is well known that the discovery of RAS in a hypertensive patient or a patient with renal failure does not necessarily imply a causal relationship. Indeed, both renal arteries may become occluded without any clinical sequelae. An accurate test to predict response to revascularization remains elusive, and the only proof of renovascular hypertension is cure after treatment, which clearly is not a practical screening approach. This "suck it and see" approach can cause difficulties in patient management and undoubtedly partly explains suboptimal results of renal revascularization.

Although surgical reconstruction of renal arteries still is practiced, the rapidly aging atherosclerotic population with a multitude of adverse risk factors (because of other comorbid vascular disease) lends itself to a minimally invasive percutaneous approach. Percutaneous transluminal renal angioplasty (PTRA) and stenting both offer the advantage of a minimally invasive approach, avoiding general anesthesia, with a shorter hospital stay and lower cost. In addition, the procedure can be repeated if restenosis occurs.

Renovascular disease is not limited simply to the main renal arteries but can occur at any level in the renal bed. In conditions such as FMD, in which first-order branches can be involved, there is still the potential to revascularize these vessels. However, most patients with atherosclerotic small vessel disease usually have major parenchymal damage and as a result (Fig. 13–1) are not amenable to treatment. Similarly, revascularizing a coincidentally stenosed main renal artery in such patients is unlikely to produce clinical benefit.

Small vessel disease can progress despite satisfactory revascularization and may account for a proportion of the "deteriorated" group found in all PTRA and stent series.

Indications for Investigation and Treatment

It is not uncommon for ARAS to cause more than one clinical problem in an individual patient. The various manifestations of ARAS have been detailed previously, and in addition, it may be necessary to treat RAS in asymptomatic patients who require angiotensin-converting enzyme (ACE) inhibitors. Occasionally, patients with normal renal function are found to have

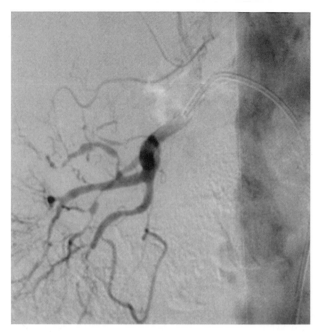

Figure 13–1. Selective renal angiogram showing extensive small vessel disease.

a single kidney with critical stenosis, and in such cases, treatment is prophylactic.

The clinical features suggestive of ARAS are asymmetrical renal size on ultrasound, unexplained renal insufficiency without significant proteinuria, deterioration of renal function with ACE inhibition, and the presence of other vascular disease, especially peripheral vascular disease.

HYPERTENSION

Any young patient with significant hypertension should be tested to exclude the causes of secondary hypertension. Although these are rare, they offer the opportunity to cure hypertension and prevent secondary end-organ damage and relieve patients of the burden of lifelong antihypertensive treatment. FMD is one of these rare causes (Fig. 13–2 *A, B*) and is usually very amenable to PTRA, with good clinical and long-term patency results.

Although FMD has been reported to progress in up to 33% of patients, this seldom progresses to occlusion nor is it associated with significant loss of renal function. FMD discovered as a coincidental finding in a normotensive patient probably should be left alone.

Older patients with ARAS and hypertension are much more difficult to assess and treat. Undoubtedly, most have essential hypertension, a small cohort of whom also have a "secondary" renovascular component. This may reveal itself in a sudden or more insidious deterioration in blood pressure control. Clearly, these patients will not be cured of hypertension, but easier pharmacologic control may be

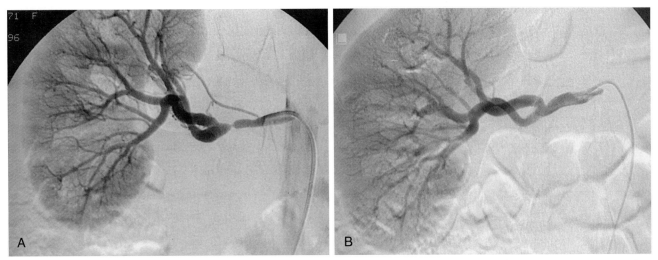

Figure 13–2. *A,* Renal angiogram in a 20-year-old hypertensive woman. A tight focal concentric stenosis is seen in the main renal artery, which is typical of fibromuscular disease. *B,* Follow-up angiogram at 6 months shows a patent vessel and a normotensive patient.

achieved. However, the benefit is limited and the risks of revascularization should be balanced carefully against the alternative of aggressive pharmacologic control. Some patients may be intolerant of their medications or have additional manifestations of renal artery stenosis dictating revascularization.

RENAL INSUFFICIENCY

Renal insufficiency is the most common indication for renal revascularization in the authors' unit. Other causes of renal insufficiency should be excluded, and the presence of significant proteinuria should suggest other nonvascular etiologies. Renal biopsy may be required to exclude other pathologies. Some workers have found renal biopsy to be useful in helping to decide whether to revascularize, and it also may predict outcome. Features such as widespread glomerular hyalinization and extensive atheroembolic disease indicate irreversible renal damage.

However, it can be difficult to decide when to investigate and intervene. Patients who present with renal deterioration after ACE inhibition therapy are an increasingly common group and perhaps the more straightforward. If possible, the ACE inhibitor should be stopped, and the renal function usually returns to normal. However, many patients stand to benefit from this class of drugs, and successful revascularization allows reintroduction. However, caution must be taken because of the risk of restenosis, and close follow-up is mandatory with this approach.

Impaired renal function itself is not necessarily an indication for revascularization. More important is the overall trend over, for example, a 6-month period. Although little is known about the natural history of untreated ischemic nephropathy, in the face of deteriorating renal function together with our knowledge from the natural history studies,[2, 3] it is difficult to

withhold revascularization, especially in bilateral disease or the uninephric patient. The exact timing of revascularization is debatable. On the one hand, it may be difficult to justify intervention with only a minor elevation of the serum creatinine (150–200 μmol/L), yet conversely, we know that the results are poor once the serum creatinine is greater than 350 μmol/L.[6] Most patients who are already receiving renal replacement therapy have irreversible ischemic damage; however, there are certain circumstances in which an attempt at revascularization may be worthwhile in this group. If there is evidence of one good-sized kidney (> 9 cm), with collateral supply on angiography together with a relatively acute presentation, then occasionally a patient can be rescued from renal dialysis. Thus, the window of opportunity for effective renal revascularization is narrow.

PULMONARY EDEMA

As stated in the previous section, this ill-understood condition commonly known as "flash" pulmonary edema responds well to renal revascularization. It appears to be independent of the severity of the underlying renal impairment and hypertension but is associated strongly with coronary artery disease and bilateral RAS (or unilateral RAS in a uninephric patient).

Angioplasty or Stenting?

The decision to stent after PTRA depends largely on the pathology and anatomy of the lesion concerned. FMD, unlike ARAS, rarely if ever affects the renal artery ostium. It responds well to PTRA, which is the treatment of choice. Occasionally, a stent may be required for an FMD-related spontaneous dissection.

The controversy regarding angioplasty and stenting revolves around atherosclerotic disease and particularly ostial ARAS. Cicuto and colleagues in 1981[7] first recognized the heterogeneous anatomy of ARAS, describing purely aortic lesions, true renal artery lesions, and a mixture of both. A variety of arbitrary measurements ranging from 2 to 5 mm taken from the contrast-laden aortic wall to the stenosis have been labeled as ostial. Spiral computerized tomography (SCT) studies recently have questioned this definition and have shown that lesions within 10 mm of the aortic wall on angiography are in fact ostial on spiral computed axial tomography (CT) (Fig. 13–3B).[8] This appears to be caused by an outpouching or infundibulum formation at the site of the renal artery origin associated with the deposition of atheroma. The implication from this study is that most atherosclerotic renal artery lesions are ostial.

Seventy-six percent of patients in Cicuto's original study with aortic or mixed lesions had poor or no clinical response to PTRA.[7] Others generally have supported this poor response in ostial RAS, although there are exceptions in the literature.[9] Aortic plaques encroaching the renal artery ostium would not be expected to respond well to PTRA simply because of elastic recoil; technical success rates have been reported as low as 25%. Until the development of stents, surgery was the treatment of choice for ostial ARAS; PTRA was reserved for nonostial disease and FMD.

Renal stents first were used in the early 1990s, and their application in the renal artery has evolved rapidly as a natural extension of their use in the iliac and coronary vessels. By virtue of their simple mechanical advantage over PTRA, renal stents have the potential to address most of the deficiencies of PTRA in ostial ARAS. Although a published randomized trial is awaited, there is a firm body of opinion developing that supports primary stenting for ostial ARAS. Restenosis after previous PTRA is a reasonable indication for stenting, especially if the original lesion was ostial. In nonostial disease, there is no evidence that stents are superior to a repeat PTRA.

A Dutch randomized trial[10] comparing stents with PTRA in ostial ARAS has shown a significantly higher procedural success rate and significant reduction in restenosis rates at 6 months with stents compared with PTRA. This study, however, has not been subjected to peer review through the publication process.

Technique

Implicit in any interventional procedure is fully informed consent. Patients should be told that although PTRA and stenting are generally safe, there is a small but real risk of damage to a kidney. There is at least a 1% chance of losing a kidney, with obvious implications for the uninephric patient. It also seems reasonable to warn atherosclerotic patients that the chances of curing hypertension are low and that improved control is the realistic aim. Similarly, patients with renal insufficiency should be warned of the possibility of worsening renal function.

RENAL ANGIOPLASTY

Initially, the patient is accessed through the femoral artery and a 6-French sheath is placed. A variety of preshaped catheters are available to select renal arteries. The authors prefer a reverse curve type, such as the Sos Omni, which can be reformed rapidly in the abdominal aorta without recourse to using the aortic

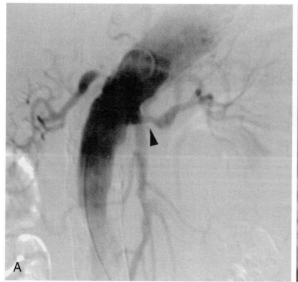
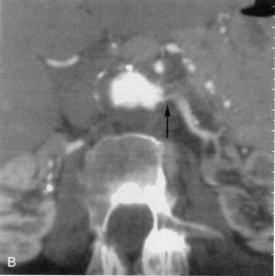

Figure 13–3. *A,* Renal angiogram showing bilateral RAS. The left-sided stenosis (arrowhead) appears nonostial. *B,* Spiral computed tomographic (CT) renal angiogram shows the left-sided stenosis (arrow) appearing as ostial, with no normal renal artery between the stenosis and the aorta.

arch. Using this catheter in combination with a soft-tipped Bentson 0.035 wire, most renal stenoses can be crossed without too much difficulty. Resist the temptation to force the catheter across the lesion without the wire leading because this risks dissecting the vessel. In circumstances in which the Bentson wire will not cross the lesion, an angled hydrophilic guide wire often will succeed. Once the catheter is across the lesion, 3000 to 5000 U of heparin and an antispasmodic (glyceryl trinitrate given in 150-μg aliquots to a maximum of 500 μg) are given through the catheter. At this stage, a tricuspid annulus diameter (TAD) 11 wire (Mallinckrodt) is placed through the catheter, and the catheter is removed. The TAD 11 wire is a tapered guide wire with a very atraumatic 0.018 platinum tip that can be placed well out in the kidney without the fear of causing spasm; the remainder of the wire rapidly thickens to 0.035 and provides good support for the angioplasty balloon catheter. A short-tipped, short-shouldered 2-cm balloon is our preference, and the balloon diameter should match that of the normal renal artery distal to the stenosis. As a guide, this is usually 6 mm in females and 7 mm in males. It is not unusual for patients to experience loin pain during balloon inflation; however, if this becomes severe, it suggests overdilatation and there is a risk of vessel rupture. Once dilatation is complete, the balloon is removed, the TAD 11 wire is left in place, and a 4-French pigtail catheter is placed alongside the TAD 11 wire through the access sheath. This allows a completion angiogram while maintaining access across the renal artery. It is not uncommon when dealing with FMD to be faced with more complex distal lesions that involve vessel bifurcation.

These are less common with atherosclerosis but do occur. It is necessary in these circumstances to use smaller balloons (typically 3 mm) and also to either protect the other branch vessel with a wire or alternatively use two balloons in a so-called "kissing" configuration (Fig. 13–4 A, B). Because these branch vessels are especially prone to spasm, it is best to use either coronary 0.018 balloon systems or one of the "balloon on wire" devices (Orion, Cordis, Johnson and Johnson), which easily slide as a pair through an 8-French guiding catheter. The guiding catheter also allows the injection of contrast and vasodilators, as required.

RENAL STENTING

The technique used to place a renal stent uses technology borrowed from conventional renal angioplasty and coronary stenting. Most of the aforementioned issues that apply to PTRA also apply to renal stents, but some are worthy of re-emphasis. A mainstream aortic injection with at least two oblique views (20° and 40° left anterior oblique [LAO]) should be obtained if not already available. This is essential to determine the most favorable projection to demonstrate the renal artery ostia in profile. It can be demonstrated by SCT that the angle of origin from the aorta varies widely. Although the right renal artery typically arises from the mid coronal plane or anterior to this, the left is less constant and can arise from anterior or posterior to the mid coronal plane. Clearly, it is not appropriate to perform renal stenting without access to a digitized "C-arm" unit. Once the decision to stent has been made, the patient should be given

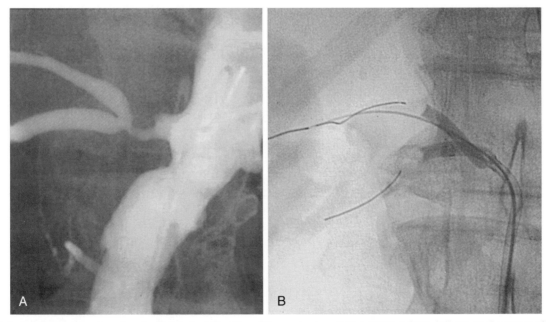

Figure 13–4. A, Atheromatous stenosis extending to the bifurcation of the renal artery. B, Two "kissing" Orion balloons on the wire in place, allowing full dilatation of the lesion and avoiding overdilatation of the branches.

intravenous heparin (5000 IU) and cefuroxime (750 mg).

Stent the entire lesion when dealing with ostial disease. The ideal aim should be to have the edge of the stent flush with the aorta. However, in most circumstances, it is unrealistic to believe one can place these stents with millimeter accuracy, and it is more usual to try to have between 1 to 3 mm protruding into the aortic lumen. This appears to have no known adverse effects, whereas if the stent is placed too distal and does not completely cover the renal ostium, then restenosis is inevitable. Therefore, the correct obliquity must be set on the "C-arm" when placing a renal stent. Some workers recommend performing an SCT study 2 weeks before stenting to determine the correct projection.

A renal curve guiding catheter is very useful because it lends added support to the system, protects the stent during passage up the aorta and across the renal lesion, and allows small repeated injections of contrast during final positioning of the stent. It is worth remembering that when using an arm approach, longer length equipment is required—that is, a 120-cm shaft-length balloon, a 90-cm guiding catheter, and a loculated (LOC) extension wire (multipurpose shape) for the TAD 11 wire.

Other techniques have been described that include a bifemoral approach, placing the stent across the renal artery unprotected. This has the disadvantage of potentially dislodging the stent while crossing the renal lesion and requires bilateral femoral punctures and increased contrast dosage because a pigtail catheter from the contralateral groin must be used. Another technique is to use a long 7-French sheath and place this across the renal lesion, the stent thereby being protected. This, however, necessitates an arm approach to avoid kinking of the sheath.

CHOICE AND TYPE OF STENT

There are at least eight different renal stents available in Europe (Table 13–1), although currently only the

Table 13–1. Renal Stents Available in European Market (1998)

Stent	Type	Material
Palmaz	Balloon expandable	SS
AVE bridge	Balloon expandable	SS
Jostent*	Balloon expandable	SS
Perflex	Balloon expandable	SS
Sinus	Self-expanding	Nitinol
Symphony	Self-expanding	Nitinol
Memotherm	Self-expanding	Nitinol
Wallstent	Self-expanding	Alloy

*Also available as a stent graft.
SS–stainless steel.

Palmaz stent has received Food and Drug Administration (FDA) approval in the United States. The ideal renal stent should have the following characteristics: good radio-opacity, no shortening; ability to negotiate acute angles; good radial strength; availability in lengths from 12 to 20 mm; and ability to attain diameters between 5 and 8 mm.

None of the current stents satisfy all these criteria, although the Palmaz, AVE renal bridge, and Jostent stents come close. The Palmaz is the stent used in most published series. The world's two largest renal stent series (the U.S. multicenter study and the European ERASMUS study, as yet unpublished) both use the Palmaz stent.

In the authors' experience, the balloon expandable stents have the advantage of more precise placement, good radio-opacity, short length, and the ability to tailor the diameter to the vessel once deployed. The length of a renal stent is important because it is only necessary to cover the lesion, which is rarely more than 10 mm long. The ideal length, therefore, should be between 10 and 20 mm. A stent that is too long may protrude unnecessarily into the aorta or alternatively interfere with any subsequent surgery if it extends too far into the kidney.

RENAL TRANSPLANTS

In many respects, renal transplants are similar to native kidneys, although there are some important differences that make PTRA and stenting technically more demanding. Cadaveric transplants invariably are anastomosed end to side to the recipient external iliac artery with a Carrel patch of donor aorta. This makes a true anastomotic stenosis very rare, and the lesion is usually several millimeters into the renal artery. Live-donor transplants usually are anastomosed end to end with the recipient internal iliac artery.

Clearly, the approach to these two situations depends on the anatomy. A live-donor transplant almost always is approached best from the contralateral groin crossing the aortic bifurcation, whereas the much more frequent cadaveric transplant often can be dealt with via an ipsilateral approach. Not uncommonly, the donor artery is longer than the vein, resulting in a tortuous and redundant vessel that can be challenging to catheterize. This tortuosity also makes a flexible stent, such as the Wallstent, more suitable for stenting transplant arteries.

TECHNICAL PROBLEMS AND HOW TO SOLVE THEM

The Wire Will Not Cross the Lesion. Switching to a hydrophilic wire, especially a curved one that can be torqued, sometimes can help in finding the channel. This often needs to be combined with a catheter with a different angle and occasionally French size must be increased for better torque control. If the problem lies in the angle that the renal artery makes with the aorta, that is, it is sharply angled inferiorly, then an arm approach may be more appropriate. This often can be assessed before the procedure. An 0.018 wire also may help but often will not support a suitable angioplasty balloon. It will, however, support the Magnum coronary balloon, which can be used to predilate the lesion up to 5 mm.

The Wire Crosses the Lesion, But the Catheter and/or Balloon Catheter Will Not Follow. The TAD 11 wire is a tapered wire that has a slightly rigid shaft and a floppy hydrophilic end. It provides excellent support. A 4-French hydrophilic ("slippy") Sidewinder or Cobra catheter may cross a lesion when others will not. The tapered end of a Van Andel catheter also can cross, but not if there is a sharp downward angle to the renal artery. A 40-cm long sheath or an 8-French guide catheter also will provide more support and help negate the effect of iliac tortuosity. Again, the "geography" of the lesion may dictate an arm approach, but the use of coronary systems to predilate lesions is probably the surest way of dealing with these lesions. They suffer the minor disadvantage of being expensive, but then so is dialysis.

AFTERCARE

There is no place for isolated renal revascularization. The decision to intervene and the aftercare should be a team approach made up of interventional radiologists, nephrologists, blood pressure physicians, and vascular surgeons. Blood pressure and urine output should be monitored closely for the first 24 hours (see Complications). Loin pain and reduced urine output should be investigated aggressively because it can indicate renal artery occlusion. Aspirin should be prescribed on a lifelong basis if tolerated. There currently is no good evidence to support the routine use of any other form of anticoagulation or antiplatelet agents.

Results

It is convenient to divide the results of percutaneous revascularization into anatomic outcome, which includes technical success, restenosis rates, and clinical outcome, the latter of which includes blood pressure, renal function, and pulmonary edema. It should not be assumed that arterial patency will be followed by a similar good clinical outcome.

TECHNICAL SUCCESS

The definition of technical success varies, but typically it means that the lesion can be crossed with a balloon and after dilatation the amount of recoil is less than 50%, and preferably less than 30%. This presents several problems. First, the "intention to treat" principle should be used when reporting technical success rates. Once the decision has been made to perform PTRA, then the patient should be included in the data. Many publications either exclude these patients or make no mention of them. Second, because of the inevitable intimal splitting after angioplasty, it can be very difficult to accurately measure the amount of vessel recoil.

To complicate matters further, most renal stent series have used stenting for either restenosis after angioplasty or vessel recoil. Hence, these patients are a select group in whom technical failure due to an inability to cross the lesion with a wire or balloon probably will be classified as angioplasty rather than stent technical failure. This may partly explain the very high technical success rates reported with stenting.

Despite the aforementioned limitations, there are some general principles and facts that can be stated. There seems little doubt that the etiology and anatomic location of a renal artery lesion are important determinants of technical success. Flechner[11] reviewed 10 series (90 patients) and found the technical success rate in FMD to be 91%. Tegtmeyer and colleagues found this excellent result to be durable, reporting an 87% 10-year predicted patency rate with FMD.[12] This excellent technical success rate is mirrored by an equally good clinical success rate, and few would argue with the recommendation that PTRA is the treatment of choice in FMD.

In contrast, the results in ARAS are less good. Work reported by Cicuto and associates[7] and then Sos and colleagues[13] in the early 1980s suggested that the technical success rate in ARAS depended on whether the lesion was ostial or nonostial. Technical failure rates for ostial ARAS were as high as 80% in contrast to 0 to 25% for nonostial lesions (Fig. 13–5 *A, B*). However, some of these early series included a significant number of occlusions and the equipment available was less refined than that currently used. More recent series have revealed somewhat better results in ostial ARAS, with Hoffman and associates reporting a 58% success rate in 50 patients (Fig. 13–6, *A* to *C*).[9] Selection bias (excluding unfavorable anatomy), improved experience, and better equipment all undoubtedly play their part in these more recent studies. However, overall the data suggest that the technical success rate for PTRA in ostial ARAS is poor and in need of improvement.

The technical success rate of renal stenting is excellent, with all studies reporting a figure in excess of 90%. Dorros and colleagues showed that not only was the residual stenosis effectively removed by stenting, but the transtenotic pressure gradient also was abol-

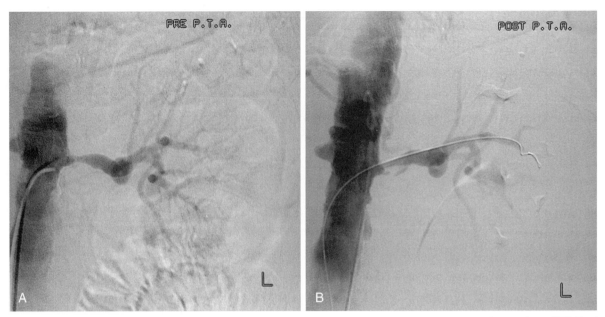

Figure 13–5. *A*, Left ostial atherosclerotic renal artery stenosis (ARAS). *B*, Following 7-mm percutaneous renal angioplasty (PTRA), showing considerable recoil.

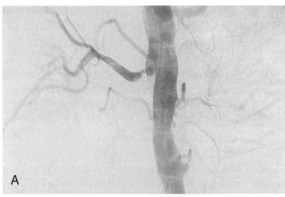

Figure 13–6. *A*, Renal angiogram showing ostial atherosclerotic renal angioplasty (ARAS) in a single right kidney. *B*, Good technical result following 6-mm percutaneous renal angioplasty (PTRA). *C*, A decision was made not to stent, and follow-up angiography at 6 months showed no evidence of restenosis.

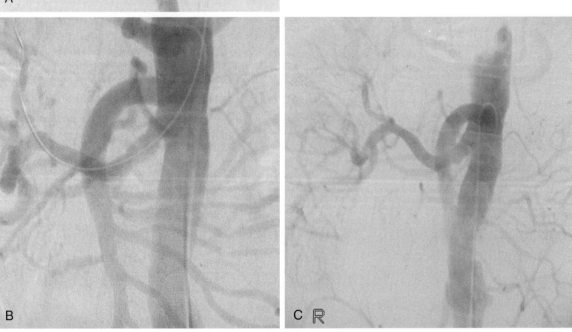

ished.[14] If primary renal stenting becomes common-place, then a slightly higher failure rate is to be expected because there will be the unavoidable small number of uncrossable stenoses hitherto classified as PTRA failures. The Dutch randomized trial[10] showed a significant difference in procedural success rates with stents (88%) vs. PTRA (57%; P < .05).

RESTENOSIS

The Achilles' heel of angioplasty is restenosis. In PTRA, there are two mechanisms that are interrelated. First is the occurrence of marked elastic recoil (usually in ostial lesions), in which the appearances immediately following PTRA look little different than before and restenosis occurs immediately (see Fig. 13–5 *A, B*); this can be addressed with a stent. Second, there is neointimal hyperplasia that can occur after any PTRA, regardless of the initial PTRA appearances, although its magnitude is related to the immediate

post-PTRA appearances (Fig. 13–7, *A to D*). Pharmacologic attempts to control this normal vascular response to trauma have been disappointing, although some encouraging work using radiation treatment is being reported.

To assess restenosis after PTRA and stenting, an angiogram is required. Herein lies the problem: because of its invasive nature, many workers have not performed routine follow-up angiography for understandable reasons. When angiography has been part of the routine patient follow-up, it often is skewed toward clinical recurrence because these patients are easier to convince of the potential benefits of an angiogram. Authors may not state the size of the total patient pool, making it impossible to calculate the angiography follow-up rate. Further problems analyzing the published data include the failure to separate patients with FMD and ARAS. The proportion of ostial lesions sometimes is not stated or can be very small compared with the nonostial lesions. To compli-

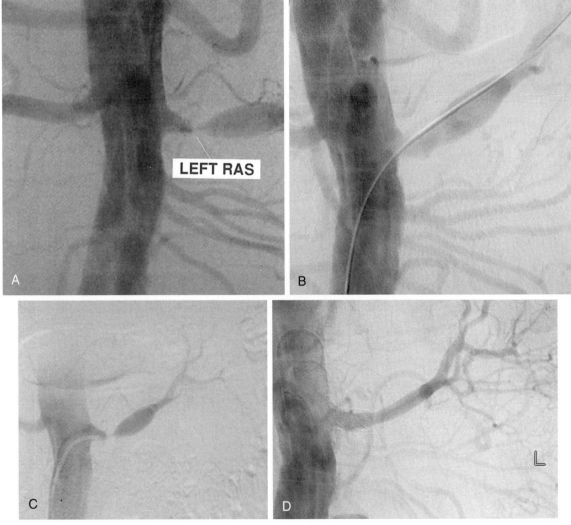

Figure 13–7. *A,* Nonostial atherosclerotic angioplasty (ARAS). *B,* After 8-mm percutaneous renal angioplasty (PTRA), a satisfactory technical result. *C,* In spite of this, the lesion restenosed at 6 months and was stented. *D,* Six months after the stent was inserted, patency was maintained.

Table 13–2. Angiographic Restenosis Data After Percutaneous Transluminal Renal Angioplasty (PTRA)

Author	Year	No. of Patients	Exclude Technical Failure	Atheroma (%)	Ostial	Angiographic Restenosis (%)
Ingrish[50]	1982	28	N/A	85	N/A	17.8–35.7
Schwarten[51]	1984	50	Yes (7%)	86	0	22.5 (ATH) 0 (FMD)
Tegtmeyer[52]	1984	109	Yes (6%)	50	?	14
Kuhlmann[53]	1985	33	Yes	58	N/A	35 (ATH) 15 (FMD)
Wilms[54]	1989	89	No	81	7.3%	14.8
Plouin[55]	1993	92	Yes	64	15%	19 (ATH) 12 (FMD)
Jensen[56]	1995	137	Yes	78	N/A	24 (ATH) 22 (FMD)
Hoffman[9]	1998	50	Yes (13%)	100	100%	27

ATH, atherosclerosis; FMD, fibromuscular disease; N/A, not available.

cate matters further, there is no standard agreement on the definition of restenosis, although most use 50% diametric narrowing. For the aforementioned reasons, the data set presented in Table 13–2 should be interpreted cautiously and at best probably gives an indication of the restenosis rate in nonostial lesions. An exception is the study by Hoffman and colleagues,[9] in which they reported a 27% restenosis rate for ostial ARAS (excluding technical failures) in a series of 50 patients.

Lessons have been learned, however, and the restenosis data on renal stents are much more precise (Table 13–3). Several points are worth elaborating when studying this data set.[15–28] Four different stents have been used, although the bulk of the data relates to the Palmaz stent. Most patients have ARAS, but in individual series, the incidence of FMD increases to 29%.[19] The incidence of ostial lesions varies from 26% to 100%, and several studies fail to classify the lesions.

All these factors plus variable angiographic follow-up rates (24–100%) may explain the wide range of reported angiographic restenosis rates (1.6–39%). The restenosis rate has, however, been decreasing significantly in the more recent publications, suggesting improved selection and/or technique. The overall angiographic restenosis rate in the 14 published series is 15.7%. Although this cannot be directly compared with the data on PTRA, it is a very acceptable result and is likely to be significantly superior to PTRA. The Dutch randomized trial[10] showed a significant difference in 6-month cumulative primary patency stents (74%) vs. PTRA (29%, P < .01).

CLINICAL RESULTS

Fibromuscular Disease. The clinical results of PTRA in FMD are good. A meta-analysis by Tegtmeyer and colleagues[29] of 370 patients revealed cure

Table 13–3. Renal Stent Data

Author	Year	No. of Patients	Stent	Ostial (%)	Nonatheroma (%)	Follow-Up Angiography Rate (%)
Rabkin[15]	1991	22	Nitinol	NR	14	ND
Rees[16]	1991	28	Palmaz	100	0	64
Kuhn[17]	1991	10	Strecker	NR	0	100
Wilms[18]	1991	11	Wallstent	54.5	9	63.6
Hennequin[19]	1994	21	Wallstent	33	29	95
Raynaud[20]	1994	18	Wallstent	26	17	88
Van de Ven[21]	1995	24	Palmaz	100	0	75
Dorros[22]	1995	76	Palmaz	NR	0	73
Henry[23]	1996	59	Palmaz	53	5	92
Iannone[24]	1996	63	Palmaz	78	2.4	ND
Rundback[26]	1996	20	Palmaz	91.6	0	60
Taylor[25]	1997	29	Palmaz	72	3	86
Blum[27]	1997	68	Palmaz	100	0	93
Boisclair[28]	1997	33	Palmaz	54	0	24
Total		482		73.5	3.9	77

*n = 274
NR = not recorded; ND = not done.

rates for hypertension ranging from 25% to 85% (mean 49%) with a further 13% to 60% (mean 43%) showing "improved" control of hypertension. Clearly, PTRA is the treatment of choice in FMD (see Fig. 13–2 *A, B*); if restenosis does occur, then the lesion can be redilated easily.

Atherosclerosis (Hypertension). It is unrealistic to expect the results of PTRA and stenting in ARAS to approach those seen in FMD. These are often elderly patients with bilateral disease, ostial lesions, and long-standing essential hypertension, which may have a renovascular component.

The Cooperative Study of Renovascular Hypertension[30] classifies outcome as either cure, improved, or no change. Although "cure" is easily defined, there are multiplicities of different definitions currently used for the "improved" group.[31] This is complicated further by a spontaneous "improvement" rate of 32% reported in a group of hypertensive patients (albeit without ARAS) receiving standard medical therapy.[32] A meta-analysis published in 1990 of 10 case series quoted a cure rate of 19%, improvement in 52%, and no benefit in 30%.[31] This study concluded that, in the context of control of hypertension, the benefit gained from PTRA in ARAS was small and its "efficacy needs to be compared with medical treatment in randomised trials." Webster and colleagues in a recently published randomized trial of PTRA vs. medical treatment in ARAS reported that only systolic blood pressure showed a significant reduction in the PTRA group, with no "cured" patients.[33] A further randomized prospective trial comparing PTRA and medical treatment recently was reported by Plouin and associates.[34] Forty-nine patients with unilateral ARAS were randomized and observed for 6 months using ambulatory blood pressure (ABP) as the primary end point. This small trial showed no significant difference in ABP between the two groups at 6 months. There was, however, a reduction in the antihypertensive drug requirement in the PTRA group, but this was at the expense of a higher complication rate.

It would appear that the value of PTRA in treating hypertension in the atherosclerotic patient has been overestimated previously in the many nonrandomized published observational studies.

The results of renal stenting are shown in Table 13–3. The overall results of the 14 studies indicate a cure rate of 7.5% and a further 52.7% showing improvement. These results are no better than the results from the PTRA series. It may be argued that the patient characteristics are less favorable in the stent series, with more elderly atherosclerotic patients with a higher incidence of bilateral ostial disease. However, the Dutch randomized study[10] showed no significant difference in blood pressure outcomes despite significantly better technical success and restenosis rates with stenting.

A reassessment of realistic therapeutic potential in hypertension for both PTRA and stenting needs to be made. When considering the increasingly aging atherosclerotic population with bilateral disease that is being treated, an overall "improvement" rate of approximately 50% would be a more practical objective. Cure of hypertension in this patient group is rare.

Atherosclerosis (Renal Insufficiency). The effect of PTRA on renal function is defined as follows: improvement greater than 20% reduction in serum creatinine over baseline, stable less than 20% increase or decrease, and failure greater than 20% increase. It should be appreciated that the relationship between serum creatinine and glomerular filtration rate (GFR) is not linear. Therefore, a 20% increase when the serum creatinine is 180 µmol/L represents a much greater loss of renal function than the same 20% increase when the serum creatinine is 500 µmol/L. Also, it is somewhat simplistic to simply compare the preintervention creatinine with the latest follow-up level available. Recently, we used a different method of assessing effect on renal function, which can be applied if there are sufficient serial data (serum creatinine) available before and after intervention.[35] This involves plotting the reciprocal slopes of serum creatinine vs. time plots for each patient before and after intervention (Fig. 13–8). This gives a much better assessment of the general trend in renal function be-

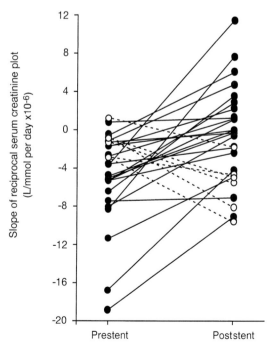

Figure 13–8. Figure showing change in renal function in 27 patients before (median 18 months) and after (median 14 months) renal stenting. Zero on the "Y" axis indicates stable renal function, a negative value deteriorating function and a positive value improving function. Patients shown in bold with solid circles have improved, whereas those shown by dotted lines with open circles have deteriorated.

fore and after revascularization. The reciprocal plot also gives a linear relationship between serum creatinine and renal function.

The authors' group showed that the rate of deterioration of renal function was significantly slowed by revascularization (stenting in this instance), the mean slope preintervention changing from 3.5 to 0.3 poststenting ($P < .03$). Although some patients continue to lose renal function after stenting, the rate of loss is less before stenting (still negative slope value, but less steep). This still may delay the need for renal replacement therapy, although it does require further long-term study.

Renal function can, however, be influenced by a variety of drugs, including antihypertensives and the ACE inhibitor group, which occasionally have been known to cause thrombosis of a high-grade renal artery stenosis.

Improvement in serum creatinine after PTRA occurs in 25% to 43% of patients with renal impairment[6] with a further third showing stabilization or no change. Ten to 35% of patients will deteriorate or continue to deteriorate. The results of renal stenting are shown in Table 13–3. The overall results of the 14 studies indicate an improvement rate of 32%, with a further 38% stabilizing. These results are not significantly better than the PTRA series. In addition, the Dutch randomized study[10] showed no significant difference in renal function outcomes despite significantly better technical success and restenosis rates with stenting.

The literature must, however, be interpreted with care. For example, in one series, 47% of patients were taking ACE inhibitors before PTRA,[36] and therefore, any improvement in renal function could be at least attributed partly to cessation of ACE inhibitor therapy rather than the PTRA. Also, the initial degree of renal impairment before revascularization is an important (if not the most important) factor influencing outcome, and our own group found that 91% of 11 patients with an initial serum creatinine greater than 500 µmol/L became dependent on dialysis within 3 months of PTRA, whereas 78% of those with an initial creatinine of 200 to 500 µmol/L improved or stabilized their renal function after PTRA or stenting.[6] However, severely impaired renal function is not always a poor prognostic indicator, and there are patients who have been rescued from hemodialysis by PTRA. This is relatively unusual, however, and most patients with severely impaired renal function have irreversible damage to the kidney.

The group of patients (10–35%) who deteriorate after PTRA or stenting are understandably a cause for concern, and some go on to require renal replacement therapy. There are a variety of possible mechanisms, including progressive small vessel disease (Fig. 13–9, A–B), cholesterol embolization, contrast nephropathy, or undiagnosed parenchymal disease. Indeed, it is one of the greatest frustrations to workers in this field to see a perfectly revascularized kidney only to be accompanied by a loss of renal function. There is much to be learned regarding patient selection and determining the optimal time for intervention.

There are no published data in the form of a randomized trial comparing renal revascularization with the best medical treatment for renal insufficiency.

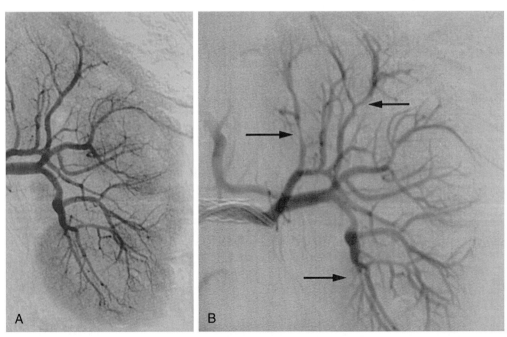

Figure 13–9. A, Selective renal angiogram at time of renal stenting, serum creatinine 286 µmol/L. B, Follow-up angiogram 2 years after stenting shows progressive small vessel changes (arrows), serum creatinine rose to 436 µmol/L.

Complications

PTRA and stenting offer the advantage of a minimally invasive approach that avoids general anesthesia, with a shorter hospital stay than surgical revascularization. However, a percutaneous approach is not a risk-free procedure. Many of the complications are by their nature common to both PTRA and stenting, although stenting carries its own additional specific complications.

Complications of PTRA reported in the literature vary in frequency from 7% to 64%. Stent series report complication rates from 0 to 66%. It is almost impossible to make comparisons because there are no agreed-on reporting standards, and many of the series are retrospective in type. It is sensible to classify complications as major, which includes serious clinical complications; minor, which includes complications of only minor significance; and radiological–technical, which indicates complications noted radiologically without clinical symptoms or signs. To make any meaningful comparison with surgical data, complications up to 30 days should be reported.

Table 13–4 shows compiled complication rates from 10 published PTRA studies (675 procedures) and 14 stent studies (512 patients). Although these are not identical series (e.g., the PTRA data are from the early 1980s and the stents from the 1990s), the minor and major complication rates are similar. There is, however, a definite trend toward slightly higher complication rates with stenting. This should not be too surprising because the delivery system is larger and there is more manipulation across the aorta and renal

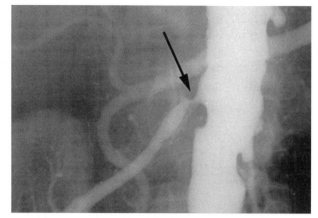

Figure 13–10. Six-month follow-up angiogram showing a restenosis of the right renal artery (arrow) caused by too distal placement of the stent.

artery with stent placement. The 6.4% radiological–technical complication rate is stent specific and results entirely from distal stent placement (Fig. 13–10).

Procedure-related deaths have been reported in the stent series, and these usually have resulted from hemorrhage from either the renal artery or access vessel damage. Perforation of a renal artery is not always catastrophic, however, and sometimes can be managed conservatively with balloon tamponade perfusing the kidney with ice cold saline (Fig. 13–11, *A* to *C*). If this fails, a stent graft can be placed. Renal artery occlusion after unsuccessful attempts to cross a tight stenosis occur occasionally (3%). In these circumstances, there is often time to rescue the kidney surgically because perfusion is maintained for several hours or more by collateral circulation. Thrombosis

Table 13–4. Complications of Renal Artery Angioplasty and Stenting (Literature Analysis)

Complication	PTRA (n = 675 procedures)		Stents (n = 512 patients)	
	Mortality		Mortality	
Major				
Permanent renal insufficiency	2 (0.3)		10 (1.9)	
Renal artery occlusion	1 (0.15)		5 (1)	
Renal artery damage	10 (1.5)		4 (0.8)	2 (+)
Segmental infarct embolization	2 (0.3)		7 (1.4)	
Retroperitoneal hematoma	5 (0.75)		7 (1.4)	
Groin complications	8 (1.2)		10 (2)	1 (+)
MI/stroke	6 (0.8)	1 (+)		
Other	3 (0.4)		2 (0.4)	
Total	47 (7)		45 (8.8)	
Minor				
Temporary renal insufficiency	25 (3.7)		16 (3.1)	
Segmental infarct	6 (0.9)			
Retroperitoneal hematoma	1 (0.15)		1 (0.2)	
Groin complications	8 (1.2)		14 (2.7)	
Other	4 (0.46)		8 (1.6)	
Total	44 (6.5)		39 (7.6)	
Radiologic	1		33 (6.4)	

MI = myocardial infarction; PTRA = percutaneous transluminal renal angioplasty.

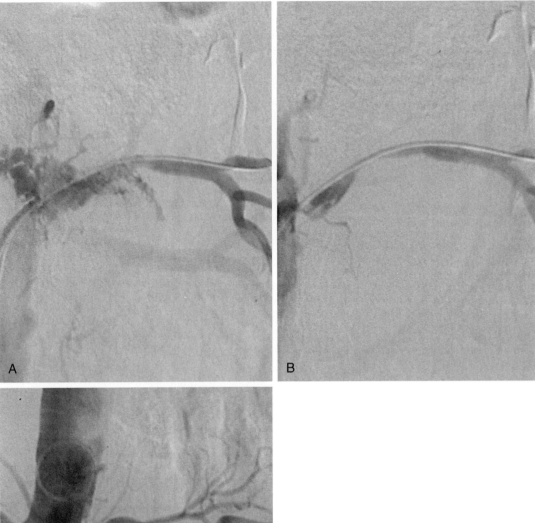

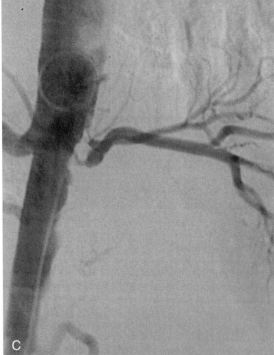

Figure 13–11. *A*, Perforation of the left renal artery following 6-mm percutaneous renal angioplasty (PTRA). *B*, Cessation of hemorrhage following 10 minutes of balloon tamponade. *C*, Six-month angiogram showing preservation of the kidney but restenosis.

of a renal stent (either acute or subacute) was a feared complication in the early series, and anticoagulation often was recommended for 3 months. This has not been supported by the published data and only occurs in 1% (most occurring with Wallstents). The use of anticoagulation in the early series may partly explain the higher hemorrhagic complication rate from stenting.

Permanent and temporary loss of renal function is the most common complication of renal PTRA and stenting, with an incidence of 4% to 6%. The etiology often is not obvious but usually is the result of either contrast toxicity and/or cholesterol embolization. Typically, contrast-associated nephropathy occurs within 12 to 24 hours of contrast administration, continues to deteriorate up to days 3 to 5, and then slowly recovers over the next 7 to 10 days. Cholesterol embolization usually reveals itself more insidiously over days to weeks. Signs suggestive of cholesterol embolization include the typical livedo reticularis rash and an elevated erythrocyte sedimentation rate (ESR) and peripheral eosinophilia. The latter usually occurs within 1 to 3 weeks of the event.

Beek and associates[37] found evidence of a definite learning curve associated with renal stenting, and it seems reasonable to suggest that PTRA and stenting should be performed only at centers at which operators have sufficient familiarity with both techniques.

Management of Early and Late Failures

Early failures most likely are caused by technical problems arising at the time of PTRA and should be addressed at that time. Problems encountered crossing the stenosis or persuading a balloon catheter to follow the guide wire usually can be solved by either gaining extra support by using a guiding catheter or changing to an arm approach, which provides considerable mechanical advantage. Other useful tricks include predilating the lesion to 3 mm with a coronary balloon or "balloon on the wire" technology; this then allows a 5-French balloon to cross. Elastic recoil, extensive dissection, and occlusion after PTRA all can be treated by stenting.

Late failures essentially are caused by restenosis. Most operators probably would elect to stent these lesions. The problem of stent restenosis is a difficult one. The choice lies between PTRA and restenting, and there are no data to support one over the other. In the future, atherectomy may become an option as more flexible devices are developed.

Surgical Aspects of Renal Artery Intervention

INVESTIGATION OF PATIENTS UNDERGOING SURGICAL RENAL REVASCULARIZATION

In addition to preoperative blood pressure and renal function measurement, measurement of renal size is important. This is achieved most easily by an experienced ultrasonographer who can reliably measure renal length and cortical thickness. A renal length of less than 8 cm is associated with poor outcome for renal revascularization. Duplex scanning to assess perfusion is useful but technically demanding and not generally available. Renal isotope scan to assess differential renal function allows selection of which kidney to revascularize in the presence of bilateral renal artery stenosis. When hypertension is difficult to control, selective renal vein renin measurements of bilateral renal artery disease may identify high renin production. This information may further help with

decisions regarding which side to revascularize and whether a small contralateral kidney producing large quantities of renin should undergo nephrectomy as part of the surgical intervention. A ratio of renal vein to inferior vena cava (IVC) renin greater than 1.5 is considered significantly abnormal.

Intra-arterial digital subtraction angiography (IADSA) is required not only to confirm the stenosis but also the presence of multiple renal arteries and segmental arterial disease. Furthermore, in the presence of an occluded renal artery, good timing in IADSA confirms distal patency of that artery as it fills from collateral vessels. The state of the visceral anterior and infrarenal aorta also must be assessed for severity and extent of atherosclerosis. The presence of a heavily diseased aorta would mitigate against procedures involving aortic clamping and indeed possibly against PTRA, in which the risks of atheroembolism are increased greatly. Routinely, biplanar views of the renal artery origins should be obtained; views of the celiac and superior mesenteric artery origins, where extra-anatomic bypass grafting is a possible option, also should be obtained. CT angiography and magnetic resonance angiography (MRA) are promising new developments. Gadolinium-enhanced renal MRA shows particular promise as a high-resolution investigation free of nephrotoxicity.

PERIOPERATIVE MANAGEMENT

Together with good patient selection, improved perioperative management has transformed the results and survival of this high-risk group of patients in comparison with earlier surgical series. Preoperative dehydration is avoided by overnight intravenous fluid administration. Similarly, a good diuresis should be maintained during the surgical procedure and in the first few days postoperatively. Hourly urine measurement is essential, with appropriate tailoring of intravenous fluid and colloid infusions to maintain this. Commonly, mannitol is given before aortic or renal clamping to maintain a diuresis. Administration of renal dosage dopamine is given traditionally, although its value is debatable. The renal warm ischemia time should be minimal, certainly no longer than 40 minutes, with most procedures comfortably undertaken within 20 minutes of renal artery clamping. Some centers advocate intrarenal perfusion of ice cold physiologic solutions, but there is no evidence that this is of any benefit. Postoperative management should be in the setting of an appropriately staffed and skilled high dependency unit or intensive care unit, with input from an anesthesiologist, a vascular surgeon, and a nephrologist.

TECHNIQUES OF SURGICAL REVASCULARIZATION

Surgery plays a pivotal role in the modern management of renal artery disease, even in the current climate of enthusiasm for endovascular stenting. Absolute indications for surgery include renal artery occlusion, renal artery aneurysm, severe renal artery stenosis, impassable guide wires or catheters, stenosis of multiple renal arteries, and the need for salvage procedures of failed endovascular revascularizations. Less absolute indications include severe stenosis in a solitary kidney, severe bilateral renal artery disease, and renal artery stenosis associated with a significant aortic occlusive or aneurysmal disease. A further indication for surgical intervention occurs when the aorta is extremely atheromatous with a high risk of atheroembolism complicating catheter procedures. There are several different approaches to renal revascularization, allowing tailoring of the surgical intervention to the underlying pathology and anatomy of the disease.

Aortorenal Bypass (Fig. 13–12). Aortorenal bypass probably has been the most commonly employed procedure, taking a bypass graft from a reasonably healthy portion of the infrarenal aorta and performing an end-to-end spatulated anastomosis onto the healthy renal artery. The procedure requires a healthy or relatively healthy portion of infrarenal aorta but also involves partial cross-clamping of the aorta, which increases left ventricular afterload. These

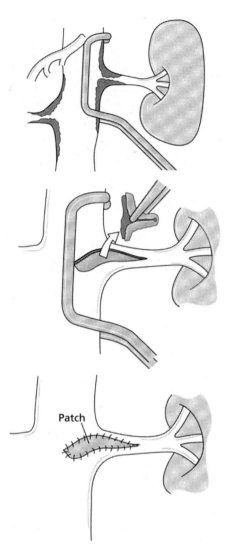

Figure 13–13. Renal endarterectomy with transverse aortorenal incision. (From Dawson K, Hamilton G: Renal and intestinal vascular disease. *In* Beard JD, Gaines PA (eds): Vascular and Endovascular Surgery. London, WB Saunders, 1998, pp 287–315.)

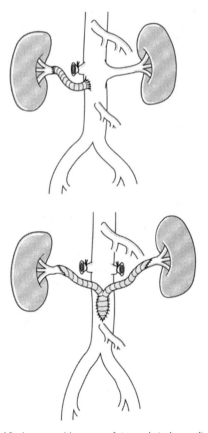

Figure 13–12. Aortorenal bypass graft in a relatively nondiseased aorta: *Top,* unilateral or *Bottom,* bilateral renal revascularization may be performed. (From Dawson K, Hamilton G: Renal and intestinal vascular disease. *In* Beard JD, Gaines PA (eds): Vascular and Endovascular Surgery. London, WB Saunders, 1998, pp 287–315.)

factors may limit significantly its applicability to the elderly patient with renal failure. With proper selection, this procedure can be performed with low morbidity and mortality. The choice of bypass graft is between saphenous vein, polytetrafluoroethylene (PTFE) or Dacron, with little difference in performance among these three. Saphenous vein in this setting tends to elongate and become aneurysmal, and therefore, its use should be avoided in the young patient in whom arterial conduits such as the internal iliac artery perform better.

Aortorenal Endarterectomy (Fig. 13–13). Aortorenal endarterectomy is a long-established procedure that also requires extensive mobilization of the juxtarenal aorta and the renal artery. Partial or complete aortic clamping also is required, with its attendant adverse effect on left ventricular function. Because most renal artery stenotic disease is really part of extensive aortic atheroma, this approach is applicable to many patients who are fit to withstand aortic clamping. Best results are obtained by direct visualization of the endarterectomy end point in the renal artery. This is achieved by a transverse aortotomy placed laterally and extending across the renal artery origin. Once endarterectomy has been completed satisfactorily, closure with a patch of Dacron or PTFE graft ensures long-term patency. An alternative method of endarterectomy is using a longitudinal aortotomy with eversion endarterectomy of the affected renal artery. However, this approach involves extensive dissection of the aorta, division of the diaphragmatic crura, and complete aortic cross-clamping. In selective patients, good long-term results for these procedures have been reported, in particular, by groups from San Francisco, California, in the United States, and Malmo, Sweden.

Combined Aortic Replacement and Renal Artery Reconstruction (Fig. 13–14). Significant occlusive or aneurysmal aortic disease with involvement of the renal arteries is the indication for a simultaneous repair. A decision to repair associated renal artery disease is based on the presence of severe hypertension and/or renal failure or a high probability of progression of renal artery disease in the near future. Less straightforward is the commonly encountered situation in which renal artery stenosis greater than 50% is found incidentally in a patient requiring an aortic procedure. There are little objective data on which to formulate decisions regarding revascularization of asymptomatic but severely stenosed renal arteries. There is little doubt from reports that simultaneous procedures in high-risk patients, particularly those with advanced renal failure, those with coronary artery disease, and those needing bilateral revascularizations, are associated with a doubling of mortality and complications.[38] For these reasons, simultaneous aortic and renal revascularization should be limited to patients with high-grade renal artery stenosis (> 80%) who are better operative risks and who have minimal renal failure. However, recently, the Seattle group reported no decrease in survival or renal function long term in a group of patients who had undergone aortic replacement but without renal revascularization of severe RAS (> 70%). The only deleterious effect noted by these authors was of an increased need for antihypertensive medication.[39]

Aortic replacement is performed using a suitably sized Dacron graft placed into the infrarenal position of the aorta without renal clamping. A sidearm graft of Dacron of PTFE, unilateral or bilateral, can be either prefashioned or anastomosed onto the aortic graft with partial clamping. End-to-end spatulated anastomosis onto one or both renal arteries then can be fashioned, keeping the warm ischemia times to 20 minutes or less.

Extra-Anatomic Bypass (Fig. 13–15). The extra-anatomic approach to renal revascularization has the considerable advantage of avoiding the aorta. This may be severely atherosclerotic, difficult to dissect and to anastomose, and prone to complications such as dissection and embolization. In the high-risk patient with significant myocardial disease, avoidance of aortic cross-clamping—and thus less ventricular stress—significantly reduces the risk of the procedure. Furthermore, the bypass can be performed using a subcostal incision similar to that used for an open cholecystectomy and can be used as part of staged unilateral or bilateral renal and aortic procedures.

The most common procedures are the hepatorenal and splenorenal bypasses. On the right side, either an interposition saphenous vein or a prosthetic graft (6–8 mm) is anastomosed end to side between the common hepatic artery at the origin of the gastroduodenal artery and end to end with the spatulated renal artery. In up to half of patients, the gastroduodenal artery is of sufficient caliber and length to allow its use as a bypass being anastomosed onto the mobilized and spatulated renal artery in front of the vena cava. Occasionally, the right renal artery with osteal disease is sufficiently long enough to allow direct end-to-side anastomosis onto the hepatic artery.

On the left side, the tortuous splenic artery is mobilized in its middle third from the superior mar-

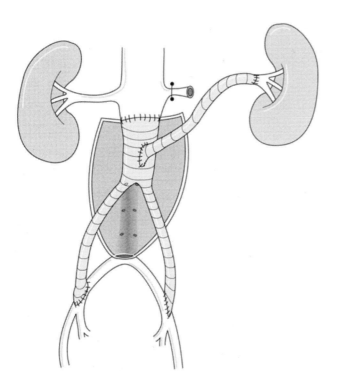

Figure 13–14. Simultaneous aortic replacement and renal revascularization. (From Dawson K, Hamilton G: Renal and intestinal vascular disease. *In* Beard JD, Gaines PA (eds): Vascular and Endovascular Surgery. London, WB Saunders, 1998, pp 287–315.)

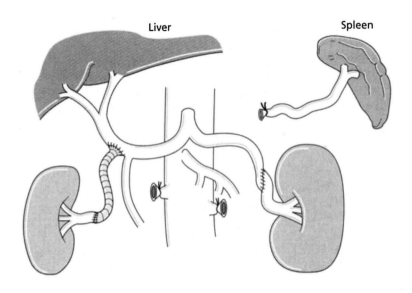

Figure 13–15. Extra-anatomic bypass: *A*, The gastroduodenal artery is of sufficient caliber to be used in up to 50% of patients to revascularize the right renal artery. *B*, Direct splenorenal anastomosis with the spleen left in situ and perfused by the short gastric and left gastroepiploic arteries. (From Dawson K, Hamilton G: Renal and intestinal vascular disease. *In* Beard JD, Gaines PA (eds): Vascular and Endovascular Surgery. London, WB Saunders, 1998, pp 287–315.)

gin of the pancreatic bed, requiring careful ligation and division of multiple small pancreatic branches. The splenic artery is divided somewhere proximal to the origin of the left gastroepiploic artery, which then together with the short gastric vessels acts as a major collateral source of blood supply to the spleen. End-to-end spatulated anastomosis between the splenic and left renal arteries then can be performed.

If it is healthy, the iliac artery supplies another easily accessible inflow for renal revascularization. Unfortunately, in the atherosclerotic patient, the iliac artery frequently is calcified and diseased, making the iliorenal bypass impossible. Mesentericorenal bypass from a healthy superior mesenteric artery has been reported as successful, but most surgeons would prefer to avoid possible compromise with this most important visceral artery.

The success of hepato- or splenorenal bypass procedures depends on a healthy celiac artery. In up to 50% of patients, the celiac artery is significantly stenosed, which should preclude these procedures. The supraceliac aorta rarely is affected severely by atherosclerosis and provides a useful inflow site for renal revascularization in this situation. A totally abdominal approach by a lateral subcostal or "rooftop" incision allows exposure of the aortic crura of the diaphragm through the lesser momentum. The fleshy crural fibers and the aortic crural tendon are divided, revealing up to 5 cm of the supraceliac aorta. With partial aortic clamping preserving distal perfusion and minimizing left ventricular stress, a Dacron graft can be anastomosed end to side onto the front of the aorta. The limb or limbs of the graft then are tunnelled gently behind the pancreas and into the relevant renal hilar beds for anastomosis. This is a well-tolerated, durable, and successful alternative to hepato- or splenorenal bypass grafting.

Extracorporal or Bench Renal Artery Surgery. Extracorporal renal artery surgery is used when there is segmental arterial disease requiring multiple anastomoses. The renal artery and vein are clamped and divided with mobilization of the kidney outside of the abdomen, usually on to the patient's flank. The ureter usually is not divided. The kidney is perfused with ice-cold Euro-Collins solution exactly as in a renal transplant harvest procedure. Complex reconstruction of segmental disease then can be undertaken at leisure, using the internal iliac artery or sections of saphenous vein from the groin. The kidney then is replaced either back into its bed by reanastomosis onto the renal artery and vein or into the iliac circulation, hence the other name for this procedure, *autotransplantation*. This is a rarely used intervention applicable mostly to FMD or segmental renal artery aneurysmal disease. Atherosclerotic segmental renal artery disease usually is too widespread to allow successful outcome from this approach.

Conclusion

There is still much to be learned in the field of renal revascularization, and many challenges lie ahead. The authors' impression is that there appears to be evidence emerging that renal stents offer significantly superior technical and patency results compared with PTRA for ARAS. However, this may not be followed necessarily with any similar gain in clinical outcome. Although renal stenting has excellent primary success, pooled data suggest that restenosis averages 15%, and this may be higher in females. Surgical rescue of stent restenosis is undoubtedly more complex, particularly in the shorter left renal artery, where bypass may not be possible except onto the segmental vessels. Therefore, the current enthusiasm for stent PTRA has the potential for causing future morbidity and mortality in addition to 30-day mortality rates similar to surgical interventions. As we enter the era of "evidence-based medicine," health-care purchasers will be looking closely at renal revascularization and asking for proof of its efficacy. The multidisciplinary team (interventional radiologist, nephrologist, blood pressure physician, and vascular surgeon) must collaborate and cooperate so that large multicenter trials can be instigated. Finally, as pharmacologic control of hypertension continues to improve, the main focus of renal revascularization will be on renal function and whether it can prevent or delay the need for long-term renal replacement therapy.

VISCERAL ARTERY INTERVENTION

Chronic mesenteric ischemia (CMI) is a rare clinical entity, which is no doubt a testimony to the three visceral arteries and their abundant collateral supply to the bowel. It generally is accepted that at least two of the three mesenteric vessels need to be significantly diseased, although as with the renal arteries, there is not a clear relationship between the angiographic findings and the clinical symptoms. There are reports of a single stenosed vessel producing symptoms, whereas occlusion of all three vessels may be completely asymptomatic. Roobottom and Dubbins, using duplex scanning, found a group of asymptomatic patients older than 65 years of age to have an 18% prevalence of significant (> 70%) disease affecting at least one mesenteric artery.[40] In patients younger than 65 years, this figure decreased to 3%. Valentine and colleagues found a prevalence of 27% in patients undergoing angiography for peripheral vascular disease.[41]

The classic symptoms of CMI are well recognized and typically include weight loss and abdominal pain, the latter of which is postprandial in nature. This may result in the patient developing a fear of eating. Other less common symptoms include diarrhea, nausea, and vomiting. The diagnosis often is made late, however (usually in excess of 1 year), and is often one of exclusion, patients having undergone a multiplicity of other gastrointestinal investigations. Other concomitant vascular disease may be present as a hallmark of the ubiquitous nature of atherosclerosis.

Although acute visceral ischemia presents as a surgical emergency and is not discussed further, it is worth noting that up to 50% of these patients are known to have presented previously with CMI.

Compression of the celiac axis by the median arcuate ligament (MAL) of the diaphragm can cause symptoms of CMI. There currently is almost universal agreement that this condition does not respond to PTRA and should be treated surgically. Features that suggest this diagnosis on angiography include a variation in the magnitude of the stenosis with respiration.

Indications for Treatment

Patients with classic symptoms of CMI with stenosis or occlusion of two vessels virtually can be guaranteed a favorable response to treatment. Angioplasty works best in stenotic disease, and there are only two reports of its use in occlusive disease of the mesenteric vessels. Patients with atypical symptoms—for example, pain that is not clearly related to eating—are featured in most published series, and as one would expect, the results are less favorable. Although there is no place for the treatment of asymptomatic disease, the situation in those about to undergo aortic surgery is less clear. A good case can be made for prophylactic PTRA of the celiac and/or superior mesenteric artery (if diseased) when the inferior mesenteric artery (IMA) is to be ligated as part of an abdominal aortic reconstruction. This may become even more pressing if the iliac vessels, particularly the internal iliac artery, also are diseased.

As mentioned in the previous section, extrinsic compression (from whatever cause) does not respond to PTRA, and the MAL syndrome should be treated surgically. It is not known whether stents will prove useful in extrinsic compression.

Angioplasty or Stenting?

There are insufficient data in the literature to answer the question of angioplasty vs. stenting. In many respects, the lesions are similar to those affecting the renal arteries, with all the limitations of angioplasty in dealing with ostial lesions. This is a controversial matter, however, and it has been suggested that ostial visceral lesions are different from ostial renal artery lesions. Several studies have reported no difference in the technical results of PTRA for visceral ostial and nonostial lesions.[42–44] The use of stents in the mesenteric circulation appears sporadic, and there are only single case reports published.[45] Therefore, the selective use of stenting in the mesenteric arteries seems reasonable. Lesions that respond poorly to PTRA with recoil and flow-limiting dissection should be stented (Fig. 13–16), and this will increase the technical success to almost 100%, as in the renal arteries.

In view of the low prevalence of CMI, it seems unlikely that a randomized trial to compare the different treatment modes ever will be done.

Technique

The reader should refer to the previous section on renal arteries because the technique of angioplasty

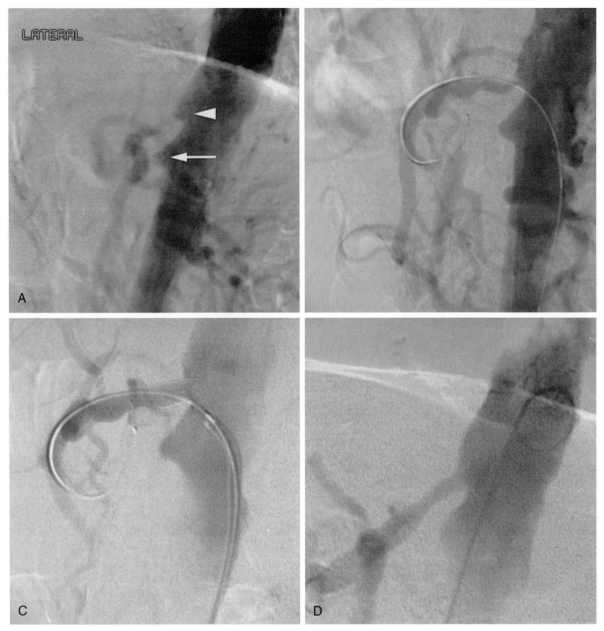

Figure 13–16. *A,* Lateral aortogram in a patient with CMI showing an occluded superior mesenteric artery (arrow) and a stenosis of the celiac trunk (arrowhead). *B,* Following 6-mm PTA there is considerable recoil. *C,* A Palmaz P154 stent was placed. *D,* Follow-up angiography at 6 months showed a 50% restenosis. However, the patient remained asymptomatic and no further treatment was undertaken.

and stenting are essentially the same in the mesenteric circulation. There is much to commend a brachial approach because of the more severe caudal angulation of the celiac and superior mesenteric arteries, which are exaggerated further in patients with a thin body habitus.

Results

There are few published data on visceral angioplasty and stenting in comparison with the renal arteries. This difference is even more apparent with visceral artery stenting, for which there is yet no published

series. The results of four published PTRA series (which include at least 10 patients) are shown in Table 13–5.[43, 44, 46, 47] Technical success is high, ranging from 79% to 95%, and this may reflect a high incidence of nonostial lesions. In some series,[43] 75% of the lesions treated were nonostial. Initial clinical success is high, with more than 80% (range 80–100%) of patients benefiting. Long-term primary clinical success is less encouraging, with only 71% (range 37.5–89%) maintaining clinical improvement. Secondary long-term success is better, although this does involve the cost and risk of a repeat intervention. True long-term results are unknown, however, and most of the PTRA series have limited follow-up of 3 to 4 years. Patency

Table 13–5. Results of Mesenteric Angioplasty*

Author, Year	No. of Patients	Technical Success†	Initial Clinical Success†	Long-Term Primary Clinical Success†	Long-Term Secondary Clinical Success†
Odurney, 1988[46]	10	8 (80)	8 (100)	3 (37.5)	3 (37)
Simonetti, 1992[47]	22	21 (95)	18 (86)	16 (89)	18 (100)
Matsumoto, 1995[44]	19	15 (79)	12 (80)	10 (83)	11 (92)
Allen, 1996[43]	19	18 (95)	15 (83)	15 (83)	17 (94)
Total	70	62 (70)	53 (85)	44 (71)	49 (79)

*Clinical results are not analyzed on an "intention to treat" principle and exclude technical failures.
†Percentages in parentheses.

data are lacking in the PTRA series, and it is likely that restenosis can occur without recurrent symptoms. McMillan and colleagues[48] found that symptomatic follow-up had a sensitivity of only 33% for surgical graft occlusion when compared with Doppler ultrasound assessment. Significantly better long-term results are available from surgical revascularization. However, in some respects, PTRA does not compete with surgery as much as offer an acceptable alternative for the high-risk patient. As the mortality rates for coronary artery disease and stroke have fallen steadily over the last 25 years, the population we treat has aged. Consequently, minimally invasive techniques such as PTRA and stenting have much to offer, albeit at the cost of inferior results compared with surgery.

Complications

There is little mention of complications in some series, and the quoted figure may well be an underestimate. Most complications are related to the access site, particularly when the arm is used. Dissection of the dilated vessel can occur and can be fatal, and stents are therefore potentially lifesaving. Clinically significant cholesterol embolization to the gut during these procedures appears to be rare.

Surgical Aspects of Visceral Artery Intervention

CHRONIC MESENTERIC ISCHEMIA

Median Arcuate Ligament Compression Syndrome. There is considerable skepticism as to whether median arcuate ligament compression syndrome truly exists. The presentation is of pain after eating, usually not as severe as in mesenteric angina but resulting in avoidance of food and weight loss. Compression of the celiac axis does occur, and in patients with this syndrome and in whom celiac angiography demonstrates a compression band, surgical interruption of the aortic crural tendon results in release of the celiac

axis. There are several reports documenting improvement of symptoms after such an operation. Possibly the syndrome can develop in those patients in whom there is a poorly developed collateral circulation between the celiac and superior mesenteric visceral beds, with pain arising in the ischemic stomach. The aortic arcuate tendon or ligament is a very strong and substantial structure. Theoretically, stent balloon angioplasty of the celiac axis could be employed but is highly unlikely to overcome the stenotic forces of this significant structure.

Chronic Intestinal Ischemia. Chronic intestinal ischemia is relatively rare, presenting with profound weight loss in a patient who typically has been investigated extensively for bowel or, more commonly, pancreatic carcinoma. All investigations for these abnormalities have been negative.

The classic history is one of pain occurring 30 to 40 minutes after eating, being very severe and relieved by vomiting or avoidance of food altogether. Therefore, patients typically have profound weight loss and food fear. These patients typically are heavy smokers, more commonly female, and examination of the abdomen reveals bruits. Careful investigation by mesenteric angiography using anterior and lateral aortic views reveal a mixture of major osteal occlusions and severe stenotic disease of the three mesenteric vessels.

Once diagnosed, the treatment is by revascularization. It is worth having a preoperative period of parenteral nutrition to treat the underlying severe state of malnourishment. In these debilitated patients, the use of endovascular means to gain revascularization is certainly attractive. However, in the absence of more objective data on the long-term efficacy of this treatment and because of the potentially catastrophic results of technical failure, angioplasty is best reserved for patients who are unfit for general anesthesia. The advent of stent angioplasty may improve these results and the reliability of the intervention, but currently there are little data on this method.

In patients who are fit for general anesthesia, excellent long-term results can be obtained by surgical revascularization (Fig. 13–17). As in renal revascularization, there are several different methods that can be

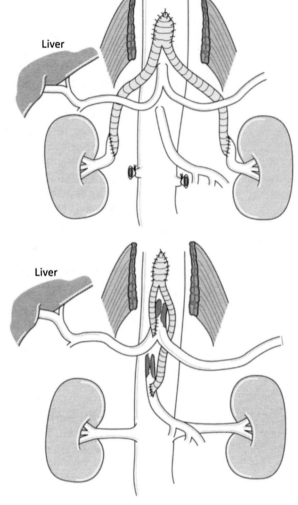

Figure 13–17. Extra-anatomical bypass using the supraceliac aorta: This approach is useful for renal, celiac, and mesenteric revascularization when the infrarenal aorta is heavily diseased. (From Dawson K, Hamilton G: Renal and intestinal vascular disease. *In* Beard JD, Gaines PA (eds): Vascular and Endovascular Surgery. London, WB Saunders, 1998, pp 287–315.)

employed. The superior mesenteric artery provides the dominant supply of blood to the gut and should be the main vessel to be treated. Surgical strategies for this include bypass grafting from the infrarenal or supraceliac aorta onto the superior mesenteric artery just distal to the osteal occlusion. The use of a bifurcated Dacron graft from the aorta is of value in revascularizing both the superior mesenteric artery and the celiac trunk. Alternatively, the superior mesenteric artery can be ligated and divided, and the healthy part reimplanted directly onto the infrarenal aorta just below its origin. Endarterectomy of the celiac and superior mesenteric artery origins is also a technically successful procedure, but this is a more major undertaking, requiring dissection and exposure of the visceral component of the aorta to allow complete aortic cross-clamping, aortotomy, and eversion endarterectomy. At the end of all of these procedures, meticu-

lous assessment of intestinal viability with resection of any frankly necrotic areas is employed, with second-look laparotomy, if indicated.

The results of surgical revascularization are good, with long-term patency rates and clinical success rates in the region of 85% to 96% and mortality rates of 5% to 10% reported.[49]

REFERENCES

1. Holley KE, Hunt JC, Brown AL, et al: Renal artery stenosis: A clinical–pathological study in normotensive and hypertensive patients. Am J Med 37:14, 1964.
2. Zierler RE, Bergelin RO, Isaacson JA, et al: Natural history of atherosclerotic renal artery stenosis: A prospective study with duplex ultrasonography. J Vasc Surg 19:250, 1994.
3. Guzman RP, Zierler RE: Renal atrophy and arterial stenosis: A prospective study with duplex ultrasound. Hypertension 23:346, 1994.
4. Joint National Committee: The sixth report of the Joint National Committee on Prevention, Detection, Evaluation and Treatment of High Blood Pressure. Arch Intern Med 157:2413, 1997.
5. Mailloux LU, Napolitano B, Bellucci B, et al: RVD causing end stage renal disease: Incidence, clinical correlates and outcomes. A 20 year experience. Am J Kidney Dis 24:622, 1994.
6. Harden PN, Sheppard D, Rodger RSC, et al: PTRA in the treatment of chronic renal failure due to renovascular disease. J Nephrol 7:186, 1994.
7. Cicuto KP, McLean GK, Oleaga JA, et al: Renal artery stenosis: Anatomical classification for percutaneous transluminal angioplasty. AJR Am J Roentgenol 137:599, 1981.
8. Kaatee R, Beek FJA, Verschuyl EJ, et al: Atherosclerotic renal artery stenosis: Ostial or truncal. Radiology 199:637, 1996.
9. Hoffman O, Carreres T, Sapoval MR, et al: Ostial renal artery stenosis angioplasty: Immediate and mid-term angiographic and clinical results. J Vasc Interv Radiol 9:65, 1998.
10. Beutler JJ, Van de Ven PJG, Beek FJA, et al: Randomised clinical trial between stent placement and balloon angioplasty in atherosclerotic renovascular hypertension (Abstract 16W). Presented at the 17th Scientific Meeting of the International Society for Hypertension, Amsterdam, June 6, 1998.
11. Flechner SM: Percutaneous transluminal dilatation: A realistic appraisal in patients with stenosing lesions of the renal artery. Urol Clin North Am 11:515, 1984.
12. Tegtmeyer CJ, Selby JB, Hartwell S, et al: Results and complications of angioplasty in fibromuscular disease. Circulation 83(suppl):I155, 1991.
13. Sos TA, Pickering TG, Sniderman K, et al: Percutaneous transluminal renal angioplasty in renovascular hypertension due to atheroma or fibromuscular dysplasia. N Engl J Med 309:274, 1983.
14. Dorros G, Prince C, Mathiak D: Stenting of a renal artery stenosis achieves better relief of the obstructive lesion than balloon angioplasty. Cathet Cardiovasc Diagn 29:191, 1993.
15. Rabkin IH, Natzvlishvili ZG, Rabkin DI, et al: Nitinol endoprosthetic reconstruction of renal arteries. J Intervent Radiol 6:87, 1991.
16. Rees CR, Palmaz JC, Becker GJ, et al: Palmaz stent in atherosclerotic stenoses involving the ostia of the renal arteries: Preliminary report of a multicenter study. Radiology 181:507, 1991.
17. Kuhn P-F, Kutkuhn B, Torsello G, et al: Renal artery stenosis: Preliminary results of treatment with the Strecker stent. Radiology 180:367, 1991.
18. Wilms GE, Peene PT, Baert AL, et al: Renal artery stent placement with use of the Wallstent endoprosthesis. Radiology 179:457, 1991.
19. Hennequin LM, Joffre FG, Rousseau HP, et al: Renal artery stent placement: Long-term results with the Wallstent endoprosthesis. Radiology 191:713, 1994.
20. Raynaud AC, Beyssen BM, Turmel-Rodrigues LE, et al: Renal

artery stent placement: Immediate and midterm technical and clinical results. J Vasc Interv Radiol 5:849, 1994.

21. Van de Ven PJG, Beutler JJ, Kaatee R, et al: Transluminal vascular stent for ostial atherosclerotic renal artery stenosis. Lancet 346:672, 1995.

22. Dorros G, Jaff M, Jain A, et al: Follow-up of primary Palmaz-Schatz stent placement for atherosclerotic renal artery stenosis. Am J Cardiol 75:1051, 1995.

23. Henry M, Amor M, Henry I, et al: Stent placement in the renal artery: Three-year experience with the Palmaz stent. J Vasc Interv Radiol 7:343, 1996.

24. Iannone LA, Underwood PL, Nath A, et al: Effect of primary balloon expandable renal artery stents on long-term patency, renal function, and blood pressure in hypertensive and renal insufficient patients with renal artery stenosis. Cathet Cardiovasc Diagn 37:243, 1996.

25. Taylor A, Sheppard D, Macleod MJ, et al: Renal artery stent placement in renal artery stenosis: Technical and early clinical results. Clin Radiol 52:451, 1997.

26. Rundback JH, Jacobs JM: Percutaneous renal artery stent placement for hypertension and azotemia: Pilot study. Am J Kidney Dis 28:214, 1996.

27. Blum U, Krumme B, Flugel P, et al: Treatment of ostial renal artery stenosis with vascular endoprosthesis after unsuccessful balloon angioplasty. N Engl J Med 336:459, 1997.

28. Boisclair C, Therasse E, Oliva VL, et al: Treatment of renal angioplasty failure by percutaneous renal artery stenting with Palmaz stents: Midterm technical and clinical results. AJR Am J Roentgenol 168:245, 1997.

29. Tegtmeyer CJ, Matsumoto AH, Angle JF: Percutaneous transluminal angioplasty in fibrous dysplasia and children. In Novick A, Scoble J, Hamilton G (eds): Renal Vascular Disease, 1st ed. London, WB Saunders, 1996, pp 363–383.

30. Maxwell MH, Bleifer KH, Franklin SS, et al: Cooperative study of renovascular hypertension: Demographic analysis of the study. JAMA 220:1195, 1972.

31. Ramsey LE, Waller PC: Blood pressure response to percutaneous transluminal angioplasty for renovascular hypertension: An overview of published series. BMJ 300:569, 1990.

32. Brawn LA, Ramsay LE: Is "improvement" real with percutaneous transluminal angioplasty in the management of renovascular hypertension? Lancet ii:1313, 1987.

33. Webster J, Marshall F, Abdalla M, et al: Randomised comparison of percutaneous angioplasty vs continued medical therapy for hypertensive patients with atheromatous renal artery stenosis. J Hum Hypertens 12:329, 1998.

34. Plouin P-F, Chatellier G, Darne B, et al: Blood pressure outcome of angioplasty in atherosclerotic renal artery stenosis: A randomised trial. Hypertension 31:823, 1998.

35. Harden PN, Macleod MJ, Rodger RSC, et al: Effect of renal artery stenting on progression of renovascular renal failure. Lancet 349:1133, 1997.

36. Donovan RM, Gutierrez OH, Izzo JL: Preservation of renal function by percutaneous renal angioplasty in high risk elderly patients: Short term outcome. Nephron 60:187, 1992.

37. Beek FJA, Kaatee R, Beutler JJ, et al: Complications during renal artery stent placement for atherosclerotic ostial stenosis. Cardiovasc Intervent Radiol 20:184, 1997.

38. Dean RH, Keyser JE III, Dupont WD, et al: Aortic and renal vascular disease: Factors affecting the value of combined procedures. Ann Surg 200:336, 1984.

39. Williamson WK, Abou-Zamzam AM, Moneta GL, et al: Prophylactic repair of renal artery stenosis is not justified in patients who require infrarenal aortic reconstruction. J Vasc Surg 28:14, 1998.

40. Roobottom CA, Dubbins PA: Significant disease of the celiac and superior mesenteric arteries in asymptomatic patients: Predictive value of Doppler sonography. AJR Am J Roentgenol 161:985, 1993.

41. Valentine JR, Martin JD, Myers SI, et al: Asymptomatic celiac and superior mesenteric artery stenoses are more prevalent with patients with unsuspected renal artery stenoses. J Vasc Surg 14:195, 1991.

42. Maleux G, Wilms G, Stockx L, et al: Percutaneous recanalization and stent placement in chronic proximal superior mesenteric artery occlusion. Eur Radiol 7:1228, 1997.

43. Allen RC, Martin GH, Rees CR, et al: Mesenteric angioplasty in the treatment of chronic intestinal ischaemia. J Vasc Surg 24:415, 1996.

44. Matsumoto AH, Tegtmeyer CJ, Fitzgerald EK, et al: Percutaneous transluminal angioplasty of visceral arterial stenoses: Results and long-term clinical follow-up. J Vasc Interv Radiol 6:165, 1995.

45. Finch IJ: Use of the Palmaz stent in ostial celiac artery stenosis. J Vasc Interv Radiol 3:633, 1992.

46. Odurney A, Sniderman KW, Colapinto RF: Intestinal angina: Percutaneous transluminal angioplasty of the celiac and superior mesenteric arteries. Radiology 167:59, 1988.

47. Simonetti G, Lupattelli L, Urigo F, et al: Interventional radiology in the treatment of acute and chronic mesenteric ischaemia. Radiol Med 84:98, 1992.

48. McMillan WD, McCarthy WJ, Bresticker MR, et al: Mesenteric artery bypass: Objective patency determination. J Vasc Surg 21:729, 1995.

49. Taylor LM, Porter JM: Treatment of chronic visceral ischaemia. In Rutherford RB (ed): Vascular Surgery, 4th ed. Philadelphia, WB Saunders, 1995, pp 1301–1311.

50. Ingrish H, Hegle T, Fry KW, et al: Angiographic control of renal artery stenosis 6 months following percutaneous transluminal angioplasty. Cardiovasc Intervent Radiol 5:249–256, 1982.

51. Schwarten DE: Percutaneous transluminal angioplasty of the renal arteries: IVDSA for follow-up. Radiology 150:369–373, 1984.

52. Tegtmeyer CJ, Kellum CD: Percutaneous transluminal angioplasty of the renal artery. Results and long-term follow-up. Radiology 153:72–84, 1984.

53. Kuhlmann U, Greminger P, Gruntzig A, et al: Long-term experience in percutaneous transluminal dilatation of renal artery stenosis. Am J Med 79:692–698, 1985.

54. Wilms G, Staessen J, Baert AL, et al: Percutaneous transluminal renal angioplasty and renal function. Radiology 29:195–200, 1989.

55. Plouin PF, Dane B, Chatellier G, et al: Restenosis after first percutaneous transluminal angioplasty. Hypertension 21:89–96, 1993.

56. Jensen G, Zachisson Bo-F, Delin K, et al: Treatment of renovascular hypertension. One year results of renal angioplasty. Kidney Int 48:1936–1945, 1995.

Chapter 14 Interventions in the Subclavian and Axillary Arteries

Endovascular Contributors: *Gerry Dorros, Lynne M. Mathiak, and Erwan Kamboj*
Surgical Contributors: *Mordechai F. Twena and Jeffrey L. Ballard*

The incidence of occlusive disease affecting the subclavian, axillary, and brachial arteries is unknown because symptoms are either minimal or disregarded and physical examination findings often are overlooked or ignored. Accumulated experience suggests that these lesions remain largely asymptomatic. However, patient symptoms or abnormal physical findings are usually the impetus for intervention.

For many years, percutaneous translaminal angioplasty (PTA) of subclavian arteries was not regarded as a viable approach to treatment because of concerns regarding possible cerebral embolic events. In 1980, however, Bachman and Kim[1] and Novelline[2] reported on their experience of angioplasty within the subclavian arteries. Despite this, the fear of cerebral thromboembolism[3] remained the main contraindication to supra-aortic intervention and was particularly feared in the presence of antegrade vertebral flow.[4] In 1984, Ringelstein and Zeumer[5] demonstrated the vertebral blood flow "delay" phenomenon. It was found that despite sufficient recanalization of the proximal subclavian lesion, the flow direction within the vertebral artery took from 20 seconds to several minutes to return to the normal antegrade direction. This phenomenon also may be coincidentally responsible for the lack of neurologic events;[6] that is, it is an inborn protective mechanism. The published incidence of complications associated with balloon angioplasty approximates 5%,[7–12] with restenosis rates of approximately 14%.[13–16] Stent revascularization techniques[17–19] have similar results. Thus, endovascular techniques employed in subclavian and innominate artery lesions appear to be safe, effective, and technically feasible (Table 14–1) in the hands of an experienced interventional radiologist.

Early in the development of these techniques, occlusion of a vessel was regarded as a contraindication to angioplasty. However, once a few reports appeared in the literature, demonstrating the feasibility of recanalizing occluded subclavian vessels,[10, 19–25] the procedure was performed more frequently. Dorros

suggested the technique of primary stent deployment used in the iliac arteries as the method of choice for the subclavian vessels.[25] It was demonstrated that primary stent deployment achieved a better physiologic result than balloon angioplasty and that stents could be deployed using low-profile percutaneous systems. In addition, potential debris that might embolize probably became entrapped within the stent struts and the arterial wall. This approach and technique in the treatment of obstructive disease for both stenotic and occluded vessels appears to be appropriate primary therapy.

The use of endovascular techniques in the subclavian and innominate arteries has met with resistance on two fronts. The first of these relates to management of complications. Rupture of a subclavian artery is difficult to deal with surgically and involves thoracotomy. The possibility of embolization of atheromatous material during such a procedure could lead to stroke and death. The second problem has been the lack of any randomized controlled data comparing the results of endovascular therapy with the traditional surgical approach. Table 14–1 lists some of the anecdotal evidence available.

Although surgical procedures have been effective, their morbidity and mortality statistics have limited their use. Transthoracic surgical approaches have a 5% mortality rate and a complication rate between 19% and 50%.[26–28] Extrathoracic surgical procedures have similar mortality and complications rates.[29–32] Thus, the use of an endovascular procedure, which can be performed relatively safely while achieving resolution of the hemodynamic abnormality, appears to have a significant therapeutic role.

INDICATIONS

Isolated exertional upper extremity ischemia or vertebrobasilar symptoms that occur in conjunction with activity of the ipsilateral extremity should prompt a

Table 14–1. Subclavian Angioplasty Published Experience

Author	Attempted PTA	Success Rate (%)	Complications (%)	Restenosis (%)	Follow-up (Mean Time [Range] in Mo)
Damuth[57]	9	100		0	13
Fields[27]	1	100			
Novelline[2]	1	100			
Bean[22]	3	100			
Ringelstein[5]	12	75			
Gordon[58]	8	63		0	20
Motarjeme[11]	15 stenosis	100	0	0	(8–60)
	6 occlusions	0			
Vitek[9]	13	100	0		
Burke[7]	30	90	7	0	
Kachel[59]	17	100			
Wilms[14]	23	91	9	14	25
Erbstein[16]	24	88	4	12	
Farina[15]	21	91	5	14	30 ± 24
Kachel[60]	44 stenosis	100	0	4	
	7 occlusions	15			
Dorros[10]	22 stenosis	100	7	5	28 (2–73)
	11 occlusions				
Hebrang[61]	43 stenosis	93	0	0	58 (8–109)
	9 occlusions	56			
Romanowski[12]	21	92	4	8	
Selby[62]	26	100		4	36 (6–48)
Millaire[13]	50	90	10	14	42 (9–101)
Bogey[63]	36	94	14		
Motarjeme[64]	67 stenosis	100	1	4	60
	13 occlusions	46			
Experiences with Stents in Subclavian and Innominate Arteries					
Queral[17]	12	92		8.3	(2–46)
Martinez[18]	17 occlusions	94	6	5.6	19 (4–56)
Kumar[19]	8 occlusions	100	7		
	23 stenoses				

PTA, percutaneous translaminal angioplasty.

thorough vascular examination. In 1961, Fisher coined the term *subclavian steal* to describe arteriographic reversal of flow in the vertebral artery as a result of an obstructing lesion in the proximal subclavian artery.[33] Symptoms associated with this syndrome may vary from drop attacks, dizziness, diplopia, and vertigo to dysarthria, bilateral motor/sensory deficits, and ataxia. Similarly, angina during ipsilateral upper extremity exertion may be the only evidence that there is a hemodynamically significant subclavian artery lesion proximal to a patent mammary-to-coronary artery bypass graft. This is referred to as "coronary steal" syndrome.[34]

Acute or chronic upper extremity ischemic symptoms may be the result of distal embolization of atherosclerotic debris from an ulcerative or stenotic plaque lesion. Thrombus within an aneurysm also can embolize distally. In this setting, the axillary and brachial arteries commonly are targeted by embolic debris. Primary or secondary aneurysmal disease of this arterial territory is rare and, when present, is more common in the subclavian artery.[35] In addition, the aneurysm may compress adjacent nerves, veins, or lymphatic vessels; rupture and infection are possi-

ble but unusual manifestations. The cause of supra-aortic arterial disease is primarily atherosclerosis, but cases of radiation-induced stenosis and aortoarteritis[36, 37] also are encountered.

Although endovascular therapy usually is aimed at the relief of symptoms, there are a few situations in which intervention may be warranted in the asymptomatic patient. This includes the planned use of the ipsilateral internal mammary artery distal to a subclavian lesion, or the requirement for axillobifemoral grafting.

TECHNIQUE

Obstructing lesions in the brachiocephalic arteries may be approached from the femoral or brachial route. The choice of access is operator dependent, but generally, simple stenoses can be readily dealt with from the femoral approach, whereas occlusions—particularly if they are flush with the aortic arch—technically may be approached more easily from the ipsilateral brachial artery. In difficult situations, a combined brachial and femoral approach, using a through-and-through wire, may be the most appropriate technique (Fig. 14–1).

Brachial Approach

The ipsilateral brachial artery is entered percutaneously with a Seldinger needle, and a 6-French sheath is inserted. Heparin (3000–5000 units) is administered. The methodology for percutaneous puncture of the brachial artery, when it cannot be palpated easily, may be a point of interest. Often, ultrasound guidance is used with either an ultrasound-guided Doppler needle or with an external ultrasound probe, which can demonstrate visually both the artery and the needle, enabling arterial puncture under direct vision. In addition, an antecubital fossa incision can be performed to allow identification and isolation of the brachial artery. In this situation, an arteriotomy or direct needle puncture can be performed, followed by the placement of the arterial sheath. A multipurpose catheter is advanced over a steerable 0.035-inch guide wire to the lesion. Brachial (distal to the lesion) arte-

rial pressure is recorded, and angiography is performed by hand injection to delineate the lesion. If the lesion is stenotic, then the guide wire is used to traverse it. When the vessel is occluded, a catheter is placed in the ascending aorta using the femoral or contralateral brachial approach. An aortic arch injection is performed, usually in the left anterior oblique position for left subclavian lesions and in the right anterior oblique for right subclavian lesions. In addition, a simultaneous contrast injection through both the brachial and femoral catheters can be performed. This helps to delineate the length of the occlusion and may provide some insight as to the direction that the guide wire and catheter have to traverse. Stenotic lesions usually are crossed with a steerable 0.035-inch Glidewire or a steerable 0.035-inch hydrophilic guide wire. If more complex maneuvers are required, then the right Judkins coronary catheter or an angled 5-French Glidecatheter is employed. Once the occlusion is crossed with the hydrophilic 0.035-inch Glidewire, the catheter then is advanced into the aorta. The unrestricted movement of the guide wire observed when the distal tip of the angled wire moves freely

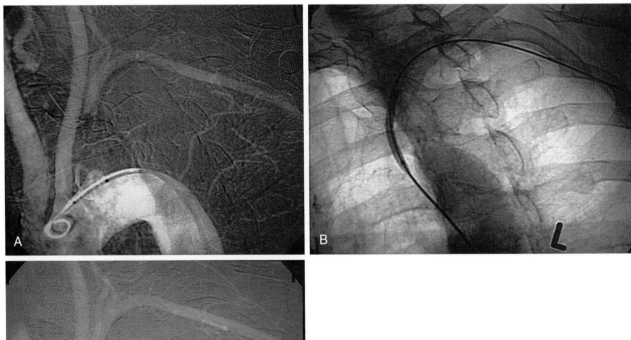

Figure 14–1. *A,* An arch aortogram in left anterior oblique projection shows occlusion of the left subclavian artery just beyond its origin. There is retrograde flow in the left vertebral artery (subclavian steal). *B,* The occlusion has been crossed from a brachial approach. A long wire has been placed in the arm and delivered through the right groin puncture site to give support through and through. The lesion is predilated with a 4-mm balloon. *C,* Completion angiography after placement of a Memotherm stent.

when rapidly rotated indicates that the guide wire has traversed the stenosis or occlusion and lies in the aortic lumen. The guide wire is removed, and the aortic pressure is recorded. When a 5-French catheter has been used through the 6-French brachial sheath, then by connecting both to transducers, simultaneous translesion pressures can be obtained. Before angioplasty, an exchange wire is placed into the aorta (preferably the descending aorta). If PTA alone is to be performed, then a 5- to 7-mm diameter, 4-cm long balloon is passed across the lesion and inflated to full dilatation for between 60 and 90 seconds. The dilatation catheter then is exchanged for an angiographic catheter. Angiography then is performed, and a pullback pressure is recorded. The angiogram determines the presence of any residual stenosis and also of any complications, such as extravasation or dissection. PTA alone is being performed less frequently. It is becoming more common to use stent-supported angioplasty using a primary deployment technique, whether the device used is a balloon expandable or a self-expanding stent. When using a balloon expandable device, once the angiographic catheter has entered the aorta, and after pressures have been recorded, an exchange wire is positioned. A long (65–90 cm) arterial sheath (6–7 French) is passed over the guide wire into the aorta. The balloon expandable stent is advanced over the guide wire and through the sheath into position. The sheath then is withdrawn, and contrast is injected through the sheath's side arm to confirm the stent's position. The balloon expandable stent (lengths vary between 12 and 30 mm) is deployed with high-pressure balloons, as previously described.[38] The sizes chosen are determined by lesion length, degree of angulation of the subclavian artery segment undergoing treatment, vessel size (6–9 mm), and the number of stents needed to be deployed to conform to vessel curvature. When self-expanding devices are used, a 7-French sheath is placed in the brachial artery. The device is passed across the lesion, and using bony landmarks or angiography to aid positioning, the device is deployed. High-pressure balloon dilatation then is undertaken to fully expand the device. After stent deployment, simultaneous gradients are recorded across the stented site (acceptable results are a systolic gradient < 10 mm mercury and a mean gradient of < 5 mm mercury). Normally, however, complete abolition of the gradient is achieved. Angiography is performed, and an acceptable result is a visual estimate of less than 10% residual diameter stenosis.

If an arteriotomy has been performed, catheter and sheath are removed and the artery is permitted to bleed until pulsatile flow is observed. If pulsatile flow is not apparent, then a Fogarty catheter is used to remove any thrombus or debris. The artery then is closed using fine suture material. After the procedure,

patients are returned to a basic ward area and usually are discharged within 24 hours. The only routine postangioplasty medication is aspirin.

Femoral Approach

The femoral artery is cannulated using a Seldinger technique and an arterial sheath is placed (6/7 French). A pigtail catheter is positioned in the ascending aorta, and arch aortography is performed. When a stenosis is present, a preformed (Simmon's sidewinder, headhunter, right Judkin's coronary or internal mammary) catheter is used to cannulate the stenotic ostium. Proximal aortic pressure has been recorded previously. After the catheter has engaged the ostium of the subclavian or innominate artery, a hydrophilic wire is used to cross the lesion. The catheter is advanced through the lesion, the guide wire is removed, and distal pressure is recorded. A 0.035-inch Amplatz extra stiff guide wire (260 cm long) then is positioned, and a long (90 cm) 6- or 7-French sheath delivery system is passed over the wire and positioned distal to the lesion without any predilatation. Once in place, either the balloon expandable or self-expanding device is deployed, as previously described. Once the device is in position, the sheath is withdrawn. Contrast can be injected to provide a clear image of the vessel's ostium and allow accurate positioning. For the femoral approach, the catheter and device lengths vary between 120 and 135 cm. Occluded vessels are crossed as has been described previously. The angiographic catheter is nudged into the ostium, and an angled hydrophilic wire is advanced into the lesion and carefully manipulated until the lesion is crossed. The catheter is advanced across the lesion, and distal pressure is recorded. The procedure is completed as described previously.

Technical Note

The aortic arch angiogram provides unique information. The left anterior oblique (or right posterior oblique) provides the best visualization for the left subclavian artery, the origin of the left vertebral artery, and the left internal mammary artery. In addition, the innominate ostium can be easily entered into and differentiated from the left common carotid and details obtained of any aberrant vessel anatomy. The major error performed during arch aortography, however, is failure to perform the right anterior oblique view. This view delineates the origins of the right subclavian and right common carotid arteries as they arise from the innominate artery. If this view is not obtained, a right subclavian origin stenosis could be missed (Fig. 14–2). If, for example, sequential innomi-

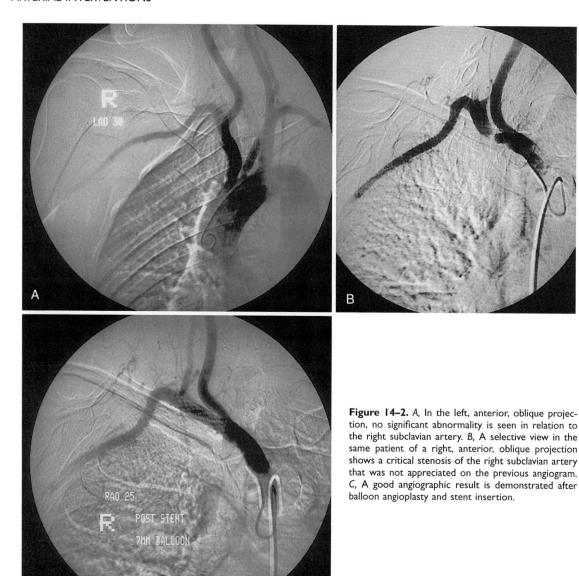

Figure 14–2. *A,* In the left, anterior, oblique projection, no significant abnormality is seen in relation to the right subclavian artery. *B,* A selective view in the same patient of a right, anterior, oblique projection shows a critical stenosis of the right subclavian artery that was not appreciated on the previous angiogram. *C,* A good angiographic result is demonstrated after balloon angioplasty and stent insertion.

nate and subclavian stenoses are present and the innominate stenosis subsequently is dilated but the subclavian stenosis is not, then the patient would have received inappropriate treatment because one of the obstructions still would be present. In addition, when stents are to be deployed at the bifurcation in the subclavian and common carotid arteries, then this view enables a clear view of the bifurcation before successful stent deployment.

RESULTS

The results from published experience of endovascular treatment of subclavian arteries is documented in Table 14–1. In our own series, the primary procedural indications (Table 14–2) were subclavian steal syndrome (35%), ipsilateral upper extremity exertional ischemia or arm fatigue (35%), and vascular access (21%).

A successful procedure (Table 14–3) was accomplished in all 11 innominate stenoses and in 111 of 117 (95%) of subclavian lesions. Of the subclavian lesions, the success rate for stenosis was 97% and for occlusions was 90%. The reason for failure was dissection in two cases and inability to cross an occlusion in four cases. The physiologic measurements

Table 14–2. Procedural Indications

Procedure	No. (%)
Subclavian steal syndrome	44 (35)
Upper extremity ischemia/fatigue	45 (35)
Vascular access to perform another intervention	27 (21)
Angina pectoris secondary to coronary steal	8 (6)
To enable use of internal mammary as coronary graft	4 (3)

Table 14–3. Procedural Success

Innominate Artery	11/11 (100%)	
Stenosis	11/11 (100%)	
Balloon PTA		4/4 (100%)
Stent		7/7 (100%)
Subclavian Artery	111/117 (95%)	
Stenosis	76/78 (97%)	
Balloon PTA		40/42 (95%)
Stent		36/36 (100%)
Occlusion	35/39 (90%)	
Balloon PTA		20/24 (83%)
Stent		15/15 (100%)

PTA, percutaneous translaminal angioplasty.

(Table 14–4) demonstrate that using postprocedural pressure gradients, stent-supported angioplasty produced a better hemodynamic result than that achieved with balloon angioplasty alone, and that the diameter stenosis after stent-supported angioplasty is significantly lower than that of balloon angioplasty. These results are statistically significant.

COMPLICATIONS

General complications related to this technique are those of angioplasty and stent insertion and include dissection, abrupt closure, thrombosis, stent malposition, and inadequate stent expansion.

The most important site-specific complication is cerebral embolization. Although this occurs in less than 1%[39] of procedures, measures to prevent it, such as carotid compression when working in the region of a carotid origin, should be undertaken. As indicated previously, vertebral embolization appears to be prevented by delay in reestablishing antegrade flow after successful subclavian recanalization.

Because the vessels are located within the thorax, emergency surgery for complications such as vessel rupture and dissection is complicated and hazardous. If possible, these complications should be dealt with either endovascularly using covered or uncovered stents (see Chapter 33) or by extrathoracic bypass, such as carotid-to-subclavian grafting for the care of

hemodynamically significant dissection without hemorrhage. Thrombosis of a brachial access artery can be avoided by adequate systemic heparinization and use of vasodilators. If thrombosis does occur, early thrombectomy (usually surgical) is mandatory to avoid hand ischemia.

SURGICAL APPROACH

DeBakey and colleagues first reported direct transthoracic reconstruction of subclavian artery stenosis in 1958.[40] Later, Crawford and others showed that transthoracic supra-aortic trunk revascularization was associated with an operative mortality rate that ranged from 6 to 19%.[41] Parrot introduced subclavian-to-carotid transposition in 1964, and this paved the way for the development of extrathoracic vascular procedures.[42] Diethrich[30] proposed carotid-to-subclavian bypass and in 1971, axilloaxillary bypass was designed for high-risk surgical patients. These procedures have excellent long-term patency and significantly lower morbidity and mortality than transthoracic reconstructions.[30, 43–51]

Clinical Presentation

Traumatic arterial injury usually presents early with objective signs such as bleeding, ischemia, nerve dysfunction, and loss of motor function.[52] History of pulsatile bleeding, stable hematoma, or other soft signs also may suggest significant vascular injury.[52]

Later, a patient may present with ischemic symptoms if a missed injury has developed into a pseudoaneurysm or arteriovenous fistula.[53] Nontraumatic causes of arterial injury are usually asymptomatic. However, a diverse group of problems may enter into the differential diagnosis. These range from atherosclerosis (more common in the subclavian artery), thoracic outlet syndrome and inflammatory arteritis, such as Takayasu's syndrome and giant cell arteritis to rheumatoid arthritis, radiation injury, fibromuscu-

Table 14–4. Procedural Measurement Results

Result	No.	Predilatation	Postdilatation
Diameter stenosis (%)	128	85 ± 16	15 ± 21
Balloon	70	85 ± 18	23 ± 24*
Stent	58	85 ± 13	6 ± 8*
Systolic gradient (mm Hg)	64	62 + 36	9 ± 19
Balloon	20	83 ± 40	20 ± 30*
Stent	44	52 ± 31	4 ± 5*
Mean gradient (mm Hg)	91	43 ± 22	6 ± 14
Balloon	47	38 ± 24	10 ± 19*
Stent	44	29 ± 20	2 + 3*

*P <.05.

lar dysplasia, and thrombosis secondary to hypercoagulable states.[43, 54] Primary or secondary aneurysmal disease of this arterial territory is rare and, when present, is more common in the subclavian artery.[35] In addition, the aneurysm may compress adjacent nerves, veins, or lymphatic vessels, whereas rupture and infection are possible but unusual manifestations.

Patient Selection

The hemodynamically unstable patient presenting with active bleeding or expanding hematoma needs prompt surgical exposure of the subclavian, axillary, or brachial artery. Extensive vascular lesions also are well suited for open surgical techniques. Endovascular intervention is best suited for focal, nonoccluding lesions, although this concept is changing with increasing application of stent technology.

Well-performed endovascular treatment options have clear advantages in the high-risk patient with multiple medical comorbidities. For instance, appropriate proximal vascular control for some clinical scenarios may require thoracotomy or median sternotomy. However, this may be avoided in the high-risk patient by obtaining proximal control with temporary balloon occlusion of the proximal subclavian or axillary artery via remote arterial cannulation. This approach combines open surgery for definitive arterial repair with endovascular methods for gaining proximal arterial control. Endovascular techniques also may be feasible for the trauma patient with a clearly defined arterial injury who is stable hemodynamically and has no signs of active bleeding. This course of action eventually may prove to be the treatment method of choice, particularly for the patient with an unstable spinal injury.

Surgical Intervention

For proximal subclavian artery lesions, the well-described transthoracic approaches provide excellent exposure and long-term patency but with associated significant morbidity and mortality.[41, 45] Exposure is based on median sternotomy with or without cervical or thoracic extension for right-sided lesions and anterolateral thoracotomy for left-sided lesions. Generally, vascular abnormalities in this territory are corrected with bypass or endarterectomy. Bypass grafts should originate from the ascending aorta and terminate well distal to the stenosis or occlusion. Side limbs may be added to reconstruct or bypass other supra-aortic trunk lesions. Bifurcated grafts in this setting are an attractive option. However, one or both limbs inevitably become compromised with sternotomy closure. Recently, the authors have used a "mini-sterno-

tomy" for great vessel reconstruction, and this has decreased significantly the morbidity associated with standard median sternotomy. In this exposure, the sternum is only opened to the third interspace and then T'd across the body of the sternum to display the ascending arch and great vessels.[55a]

Extrathoracic vascular reconstructions tend to be safer than transthoracic approaches for the patient and provide excellent long-term patency. These are essentially arterial transpositions and ipsilateral or contralateral bypass procedures. Experience with subclavian-to-carotid transposition has been quite favorable.[44] Carotid-to-subclavian or subclavian-to-subclavian bypasses usually are accomplished with synthetic material because vein grafts have proven disappointing.[44] However, the authors prefer to use vein for upper extremity bypass procedures in which the graft originates from the carotid, subclavian, or axillary artery. Axillary-to-axillary bypass is reserved for the rare patient in whom graft origin from the ipsilateral common carotid artery or contralateral subclavian or carotid artery is not possible.[45]

Acute thromboembolic lesions of the brachial or distal axillary artery are corrected readily by open thromboembolectomy via cut-down with or without patch closure of the artery. Thrombolysis is another option for the patient who still has a clearly viable hand and time considerations are unimportant. Surgical bypass with vein is preferred for extensive chronic lesions as opposed to endovascular treatment options. In extreme situations with exsanguinating hemorrhage and in some infected aneurysm cases, arterial ligation may be the safest course of action. Otherwise, if a minimal length of artery is damaged and a tension-free anastomosis is feasible, primary repair is appropriate; if not, bypass with vein is the best solution.[46–49]

Complications of Surgical Intervention

Vascular-related postoperative problems include bleeding, pseudoaneurysm, distal embolization, graft thrombosis or infection, and ischemia of the hand or brain.[44] Acute graft thrombosis generally requires re-exploration. Late failures require no intervention if they are asymptomatic. However, remedial extrathoracic reconstruction or bypass with graft origin and destination remote from the previous operative site typically are used for treatment of symptomatic late failures. Endovascular means of reconstruction are indicated when surgical re-exploration is deemed hazardous.

Nonvascular complications are predominately those of local nerve damage. These may range from brachial plexus injury or sympathetic ganglia damage with resultant Horner's syndrome to phrenic nerve

Table 14–5. Extrathoracic Vascular Reconstruction Results

	Mortality (%)	Morbidity (%)	Patency (%)	References
Bypass Procedures				
Carotid-to-subclavian	0.8–2.5	8–18	80–95	5–7
Carotid-to-axillary	0–2.2	15	82–96	9,10
Carotid-to-brachial	0	0	92–100	11,12
Axillary-to-axillary	0–2.2	0	83–88	4,10
Transposition				
Subclavian-to-carotid	1.1–1.7	17–18	99–100	5,8

injury with diaphragm dysfunction or vocal cord paralysis from recurrent laryngeal nerve injury.[45] Lymphocele or lymph fistula from injury to thoracic duct or other lymphatic channels is more common after subclavian-to-carotid transposition vs. bypass. Significant major vein injury also has been described. Cerebral steal after carotid-to-subclavian bypass or subclavian-to-carotid transposition may occur rarely if a significant proximal common carotid artery lesion is not detected preoperatively.[44, 45]

Results of Surgical Intervention

Results with different extrathoracic vascular reconstructions are displayed in Table 14–5. Overall mortality rates are less than 2.5%, and long-term graft patency rates range from 80 to 100%. Best surgical results are reported for subclavian-to-carotid transposition, and these results are least durable for axillary-to-axillary bypass. Morbidity rates range from 8 to 18%.[43–51]

Transthoracic great vessel procedures are quite durable, with patency rates that are close to 100%. However, they are associated with a mortality rate of 6 to 20%.[40, 41, 44, 45] As expected, repair of traumatic subclavian or axillary artery injuries is associated with significantly higher morbidity (25–70%) and mortality (10–20%).[55, 55a, 56] This is due in part to the presence of serious intercurrent injuries. Tufaro and colleagues[53] demonstrated that if minor intimal axillary or brachial artery injuries from penetrating trauma are observed, 95% of patients return 1 to 2 years later with distal ischemia that requires vascular intervention. Furthermore, these can prove to be troublesome operative adventures because inflammation and fibrosis obscure the usual surgical tissue planes.

CONCLUSION

Balloon angioplasty and stenting of the subclavian and innominate arteries can be accomplished simply, safely, and effectively for both stenotic and occluded vessels. The complication rates are relatively low and

clinically acceptable. Physiologic measurements and percentage diameter stenosis measurements indicate that stent-supported angioplasty achieves a better and more immediate physiologic result. The indications for endovascular treatment are broader and more encompassing than those for surgical intervention, and there are few, if any, contraindications to PTA or stent-supported PTA of the subclavian or innominate vessels.

Transthoracic vascular reconstruction of great vessel lesions and standard vascular repair of more distal lesions continue to offer patients excellent long-term benefit with relatively low risk. This is particularly true for good-risk patients with extensive pathology or multivessel disease. In contrast, poor-risk surgical patients with single-vessel disease or with prior sternotomy are better served with extrathoracic vascular approaches. Candidates for endovascular intervention include very high-risk patients, patients with "hostile necks," and patients with focal arterial lesions. The fact that multidisciplinary tools for intervention exist when dealing with this anatomically challenging area should be looked on as a blessing for both the surgeon and the patient.

REFERENCES

1. Bachman DM, Kim RM: Transluminal dilatation for subclavian steal syndrome. AJR Am J Roentgenol 135:995–996, 1980.
2. Novelline RA: Percutaneous transluminal andioplasty: Newer applications. AJR Am J Roentgenol 135:983–988, 1980.
3. Leitler E: Complications in and after PTR. *In* Leitler E, Gruntzig A, Schoop W, (eds): Percutaneous Transluminal Recanalization: Technique, Application and Clinical Results. Berlin, Springer-Verlag, 1978, pp 120–125.
4. Sharm S, Kaul V, Rajani M: Identifying high-risk patients for percutaneous transluminal angioplasty of subclavian and innominate arteries. Acta Radiol 32:381–385, 1991.
5. Ringelstein B, Zeumer H: Delayed reversal of vertebral artery blood flow following percutaneous transluminal angioplasty for subclavian steal syndrome. Neuroradiology 26:189–198, 1984.
6. Eckard DA, O'Boynick PL, Han PP: Temporary subclavian steal to reduce intraprocedural embolic risk during detachable balloon occlusion of vertebrobasilar aneurysms: Technical note with two case reports. J Endovasc Surg 3:423–428, 1996.
7. Burke DR, Gordon RL, Mishkin JD: Percutaneous transluminal angioplasty of subclavian arteries. Radiology 164:699–704, 1987.

8. Motarjeme A, Kiefer JW, Zuska AJ, Nawabi MD: Percutaneous transluminal angioplasty for treatment of subclavian steal. Radiology 155:611–613, 1985.

9. Vitek JJ: Subclavian artery percutaneous transluminal angioplasty at origin of vertebral artery. Radiology 170:407–409, 1989.

10. Dorros G, Lewin RF, Jamnadas P, Mathiak LM: Peripheral transluminal angioplasty of the subclavian and innominate arteries utilizing the brachial approach: Acute outcome and follow-up. Cathet Cardiovasc Diagn 19:71–76, 1990.

11. Motarjeme A: Percutaneous transluminal angioplasty of supraaortic vessel. J Endovasc Surg 3:171–181, 1996.

12. Romanowski CA, Fairlie NC, Proctor AE, Cumberland DC: Percutaneous transluminal angioplasty of the subclavian and axillary arteries: Initial results and long term follow-up. Clin Radiol 46:104–107, 1992.

13. Miilaire A, Trinca M, Marache P, et al: Subclavian angioplasty: Immediate and late results in 50 patients. Cathet Cardiovasc Diagn 29:8–17, 1993.

14. Wilms G, Baert A, Dewaele D, et al: Percutaneous transluminal angioplasty of the subclavian artery: Early and late results. Cardiovasc Intervent Radiol 10:123–128, 1987.

15. Farina C, Mingoli A, Schultz RD, et al: Percutaneous transluminal angioplasty versus surgery for subclavian artery occlusive disease. Am J Surg 158:511–554, 1989.

16. Erbstein RA, Wholey MH, Smoot S: Subclavian artery steal syndrome. AJR Am J Roentgenol 151:291–294, 1988.

17. Queral LA, Criado FJ: The treatment of local aortic arch branch lesions with Palmaz stents. J Vasc Surg 23:368–375, 1996.

18. Martinez R, Rodrigues-Lopez J, Torruella L, et al: Stenting for occlusion of the subclavian arteries—Technical aspects and follow-up results. Tex Heart Inst J 24:23–27, 1997.

19. Kumar K, Dorros G, Bates MC, et al: Primary stent deployment in occlusive subclavian artery disease. Cathet Cardiovasc Diagn 34:281–285, 1995.

20. Kachel R, Ritter H: Percutaneous catheter recanalization (angioplasty) of a subclavian occlusion with the subclavian steal syndrome. Rofo Fortschr Geb Rontgenstr Neuen Bildgeb Verfahr 145:107–109, 1986.

21. Burke D, Gordon R, Mishkin JD, et al: Percutaneous transluminal angioplasty of subclavian arteries. Radiology 164:699–704, 1987.

22. Bean WJ, Rodan BA, Frangui RT: Subclavian steal: Treatment with percutaneous transluminal angioplasty. South Med J 77:1044–1046, 1984.

23. Cook AM, Dyet JF: Six cases of subclavian stenosis treated by percutaneous angioplasty. Clin Radiol 40:352–354, 1989.

24. Staller B, Maleki M: Percutaneous transluminal angioplasty for innominate artery stenosis and total occlusion of subclavian artery in Takayasu's type arthritis. Cathet Cardiovasc Diagn 16:91–94, 1989.

25. Dorros G, Prince C, Mathiak L: Stenting of a renal artery stenosis achieves better relief of the obstructive lesion than balloon angioplasty. Cathet Cardiovasc Diagn 29:191–198, 1993.

26. Beebe HE, Stark C, Johnson ML, et al: Choice of operations for subclavian-vertebral arterial disease. Am J Surg 139:616–623, 1980.

27. Fields WS, Lemak NA: Joint study of extra-cranial arterial occlusion. VII Subclavian steal: A review of 168 cases. JAMA 222:1139–1143, 1972.

28. Herring M: The subclavian steal syndrome: A review. JAMA 43:220–228, 1977.

29. Crawford ES, DeBakey ME, Morris GC, Howell JF: Surgical treatment of occlusions of the innominate, common carotid and subclavian arteries: A 10 year experience. Surgery 65:17–31, 1969.

30. Diethrich EB, Garrett HE, Ameriso J, et al: Occlusive disease of the common carotid and subclavian arteries treated by carotid-subclavian bypass. Analysis of 125 cases. Am J Surg 114:800–808, 1967.

31. Edwards WH Jr, Tapper SS, Edwards WN Sr, et al: Subclavian revascularization: A quarter century experience. Ann Surg 219:673–678, 1994.

32. AbuRahma AF, Robinson PA, Khan MZ, et al: Brachiocephalic revascularization: A comparison between carotid subclavian artery bypass and axillo-axillary artery bypass. Surgery 112:84–91, 1992.

33. Editorial: A new syndrome—"The Subclavian Steal." N Engl J Med 265:912–913, 1961.

34. Ballard JL, Killeen JD: Left carotid-subclavian artery bypass for myocardial ischemia: A case report. Vasc Forum 2:70–73, 1994.

35. Gray RJ, Stone WM, Fowl RJ, et al: Management of true aneurysms distal to the axillary artery. J Vasc Surg 28:606–610, 1998.

36. Tyagi S, Gambhir DS, Kaul UA, et al: A decade of subclavian angioplasty: Aortoarteritis versus atherosclerosis. Indian Heart J 48:667–671, 1996.

37. Tyagi S, Verma PK, Gambhir DS, et al: Early and long-term results of subclavian angioplasty in aortoarteritis (Takayasu's disease): Comparison with atherosclerosis. Intervent Radiol 21:219–224, 1998.

38. Dorros G, Mathiak L: Direct deployment of the ileofemoral balloon expandable (Palmaz) stent utilizing a small (7.5 French) arterial puncture. Cathet Cardiovasc Diagn 28:80–82, 1993.

39. Becker GJ, Katzen BT, Dake MD: Noncoronary angioplasty. Radiology 170:921–940, 1989.

40. Debakey ME, Morris GC, Jordan GL, et al: Segmental thrombo-obliterative disease of branches of aortic arch. JAMA 166:988–1003, 1958.

41. Crawford ES, DeBakey ME, Morris GC, et al: Surgical treatment of occlusion of the innominate, common carotid, and subclavian arteries: A 10-year experience. Surgery 65:17–31, 1969.

42. Parrot JC: The subclavian steal syndrome. Arch Surg 88:661–665, 1964.

43. Chang JB, Stein TA, Liu JP, Dunn ME: Long-term results with axillo-axillary bypass grafts for symptomatic subclavian artery insufficiency. J Vasc Surg 25:173–178, 1997.

44. Law MM, Colburn WD, Moore WS, et al: Carotid-subclavian bypass for brachiocephalic occlusive disease: Choice of conduit and long-term follow-up. Stroke 26:1565–1571, 1995.

45. Wittwer T, Wahlers T, Dresler C, Haverich A: Carotid-subclavian bypass for subclavian artery revascularization: Long-term follow-up and effect of antiplatelet therapy. Angiology 4:279–287, 1998.

46. Vitti MJ, Thompson BW, Read RC, et al: Carotid-subclavian bypass: A twenty-two year experience. J Vasc Surg 20:411–418, 1994.

47. Edwards WH Jr, Tapper SS, Edwards WH Sr, et al: Subclavian revascularization: A quarter century experience. Ann Surg 219:673–678, 1994.

48. Criado JF, Queral LA: Carotid-axillary artery bypass: A ten-year experience. J Vasc Surg 22:717–723, 1995.

49. Owens LV, Tinsley EA Jr, Criado E, et al: Extrathoracic reconstruction of arterial occlusive disease involving the supraaortic trunks. J Vasc Surg 22:217–222, 1995.

50. Gupta A, Rubin J: Carotid brachial bypass for treating proximal upper-extremity arterial occlusive disease. Am J Surg 168:210–213, 1994.

51. Jain KM, Simoni EJ, Munn JS, Madson DL Jr: Long-term follow-up of bypasses to the brachial artery across the shoulder joint. Am J Surg 172:127–129, 1996.

52. Hyre CE, Cikrit DF, Lalka SG, et al: Aggressive management of vascular injuries of the thoracic outlet. J Vasc Surg 27:880–885, 1998.

53. Tufaro A, Arnold T, Rummel M, et al: Adverse outcome of nonoperative management of intimal injuries caused by penetrating trauma. J Vasc Surg 20:656–659, 1994.

54. Durham JR, Yao JST, Pearce WH, et al: Arterial injuries in the thoracic outlet syndrome. J Vasc Surg 21:57–70, 1995.

55. Degiannis E, Velmahoos G, Krawczykowski D, et al: Penetrating injuries of the subclavian vessels. Br J Surg 81:524–526, 1994.

55a. Sakopoulos AG, Ballard JL, Gundry SR: Minimally invasive approach for aortic arch branch vessel reconstruction. J Vasc Surg (in press).

56. Prêtre R, Hoffmeyer P, Bednarkiewicz M, et al: Blunt injury to the subclavian or axillary artery. J Am Coll Surg 179:295–298, 1994.

57. Damuth HD, Diamond AB, Rapport AS, et al: Angioplasty of subclavian artery stenosis proximal to the vertebral origin. AJNR 4:1239–1242, 1983.

58. Gordon RL, Haskell L, Hirsch M, et al: Transluminal dilatation of subclavian artery. Cardiovasc Intervent Radiol 8:14–19, 1985.
59. Kachel R, Endert E, Basche S, et al: Percutaneous transluminal angioplasty (dilatation) of carotid, vertebral and innominate artery stenosis. Cardiovasc Intervent Radiol 10:142–146, 1987.
60. Kachel R, Basche S, Heerklotz I, et al: Percutaneous transluminal angioplasty (PTA) of supra-aortic arteries, especially the internal carotid artery. Neuroradiology 33:191–194, 1991.
61. Hebrang A, Maskovic J, Tomac B: Percutaneous transluminal angioplasty of the subclavian arteries: Long term results in 52 patients. ARJ 156:1091–1094, 1991.
62. Selby JB, Matsumoto AH, Tegtmeyer CJ, et al: Balloon angioplasty above the aortic arch: Immediate and long term results. AJR 160:631–635, 1993.
63. Bogey WM, Dermasi RJ, Tripp MD, et al: Percutaneous transluminal angioplasty for subclavian artery stenosis. Am Surg 60:103–106, 1994.
64. Motarjeme A, Gordon GI: Percutaneous transluminal angioplasty of the brachiocephalic vessels: Guidelines for therapy. Int Angiol 12:260–269, 1993.

Chapter 15

Endoluminal Treatment of Carotid and Vertebral Artery Stenosis

Endovascular Contributors: Kurt Mathias and H. Jäger
Surgical Contributor: Jonathan D. Beard

CAROTID ARTERY STENOSIS

The performance of percutaneous transluminal angioplasty (PTA) of the carotid artery began in 1977 with animal experiments. Research and animal experiments continued until 1979 when a 32-year-old woman who had fibromuscular dysplasia that caused symptomatic carotid stenosis became the first human patient to be treated with balloon angioplasty.[1-3]

In more than 80% of cases, clinical symptoms of atherosclerotic carotid stenosis are caused by embolic events, and in less than 20% by hemodynamic impairment of the cerebral circulation. Therefore, the aim of invasive treatment is to remove plaque material and hence removing the source for embolus. For many years, PTA of atherosclerotic carotid stenosis was considered an unsuitable treatment because it does not remove atherosclerotic deposits. Moreover, PTA was deemed to place patients with atherosclotic carotid stenosis at risk because of their tendency to suffer cerebral artery embolism and stroke.[4]

Therefore, only patients who were poor candidates for surgery and who suffered from hemodynamic impairment of the cerebral circulation (because of smoothly delineated hourglass-like carotid stenosis in multiple vessel disease) were selected. From 1980 on, patients with atherosclerotic disease were successfully treated by PTA.[5] However, some disadvantages inherent in simple balloon angioplasty proved to be a severe obstacle for general acceptance of the method. Such factors included the heterogeneous nature of carotid stenoses, residual stenosis after PTA, risk of embolism, intimal flap formation, and dissection in the face of straightforward and effective surgical treatment.

The reluctance of vascular surgeons and neurologists in many centers to refer patients for PTA, and the absence of quantitative data on outcomes and complications of carotid PTA, slowed development of the technique. It was impossible to collect data from several centers and to establish knowledge of internal carotid artery PTA concerning feasibility, indications, and efficacy of this intervention.

In 1989, the author's group undertook the first internal carotid artery (ICA) stent placement when angiography revealed development of an intimal flap after performance of PTA, and an improvement of the PTA result was deemed necessary. The procedure was well tolerated and the patient had a good long-term result with a patent artery and no recurrent stenosis after 9 years.[6, 7]

Indications

The principal indication for stent PTA is stenosis of the internal carotid artery (ICA) exceeding 70% in a symptomatic patient (stage II) (Figs. 15–1–3). This indication has been derived from the results of surgical studies, notably the North American Study of Carotid Endarterectomy (NASCET) and the European Carotid Surgery Trial (ECST).[8-11] In asymptomatic patients (stage I), the annual stroke incidence with lesions exceeding 70% stenosis is approximately 5%. Stent PTA is performed in these patients if the degree of stenosis is greater than 80%, and if additional criteria are fulfilled, such as an occlusion of the contralateral internal carotid artery, the necessity of a major operation, or a degree of stenosis increasing more than 15% within 6 months.[12] In such cases, combined carotid and coronary angioplasty can be performed.[13]

For patients at stage IV, we recommend stent PTA if a high degree of stenosis is responsible for recurring transient ischemic attacks (TIAs) and if the infarcted area is small. These patients are in danger of developing a new stroke that may disable them more severely or that may even have a fatal outcome. Normally, the procedure is delayed for 6 to 8 weeks after the event to prevent reperfusion hemorrhage in the infarcted area.

Stenosis of the external carotid artery (ECA) is treated in only symptomatic patients with an occlusion of the ipsilateral ICA or in those with multiple-

Figure 15–1. Fifty-nine-year-old man with recurrent transient ischemic attacks (TIAs). *A,* Short stenosis (71%) of the ICA. *B,* Stent placement in the common carotid artery (CCA) and internal carotid artery (ICA) with balloon dilatation within the stent.

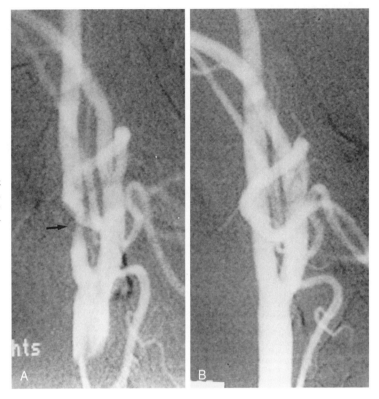

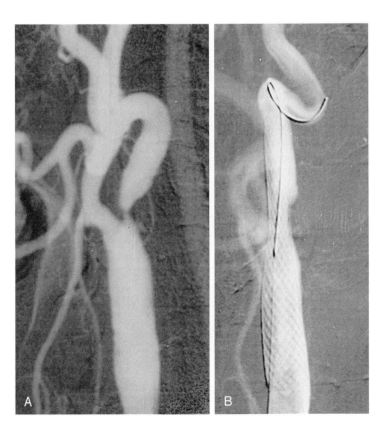

Figure 15–2. *A,* Sixty-seven-year-old man with transient ischemic attacks (TIA) and lacunar infarct of left hemisphere internal carotid artery (ICA) stenosis (82%) close to the carotid bifurcation and elongated ICA. *B,* Control angiogram over the wire with slight residual stenosis after stent percutaneous transluminal angioplasty (PTA) with the stent crossing the origin of the external carotid artery (ECA).

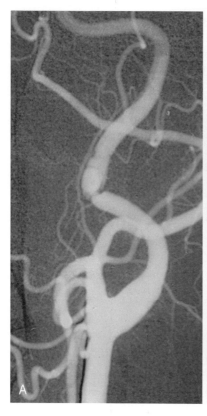
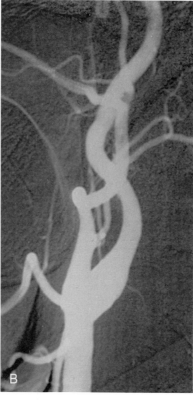

Figure 15–3. Sixty-three-year-old female with transient ischemic attacks (TIAs). Short internal carotid artery (ICA) stenosis of 78% with ulceration. *A,* the high location of the stenosis is unfavorable for carotid surgery. There is no residual stenosis after stent angioplasty with the stent distal to the bifurcation. *B,* The ICA is straightened by the stent.

vessel disease. Recurrent stenosis of the carotid artery after surgical treatment is feasible and is well suited for stent PTA.

Stent PTA can be employed more or less independently of the morphology of the underlying stenosis. Presence of irregular plaque surface, thrombus, or ulceration are not considered contraindications to the procedure, although local fibrinolysis may be necessary before dilatation and stent placement in some of these patients.[14] Major thrombus formation and thick circular or horseshoe-like calcifications are relative contraindications for stent PTA (Fig. 15–4) because overdistention of the noncalcified segment of the circumference of a calcified artery may result in false aneurysm formation or even rupture of the vessel. The degree and location of calcifications should be examined in such cases by spiral computed tomography before stent PTA is attempted (Fig. 15–5).

In patients with carotid stenosis and a so-called *hostile neck situation* after irradiation or radical neck dissection, the endovascular approach is preferred to open surgery (Fig. 15–6). Stent PTA also has a more favorable outcome in patients with severe bilateral carotid disease in whom the complication rate of vascular surgery is increased. There is no age limit for carotid stent PTA; however, technical difficulties are more frequently encountered because of elongation and tortuosity of the supra-aortic arteries and more widespread atherosclerosis in the elderly.

Choice of Stent

Several commercially produced stents are currently available; however, for carotid stent placement, some specific properties of the stent (which relate principally to the exposed position of the carotid artery and bending of the vessel with each movement of the head) are advantageous. The location of the stenotic lesion, most often at the carotid bifurcation, must also be considered, because the stent must be placed in adjoining vessels with differing diameters (Table 15–1).

The internal diameter of the ICA varies from 5 to 7 mm, and the common carotid artery (CCA) measures between 7 and 10 mm. When the stent is placed across the bifurcation, it must adapt itself to arteries with different endoluminal diameters. The stent should have close apposition with the vessel wall for neointimal overgrowth to occur. All these specifica-

Table 15–1. Properties of Stents for Carotid Placement

Self-expandable
Flexible
Noncollapsing
No interruption of blood flow during placement
Low thrombogeneity
Narrow meshwork
Tapering
Sonographically transparent

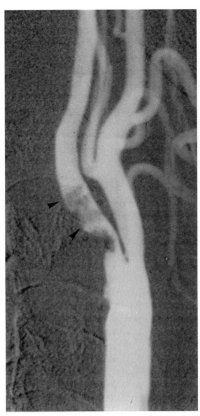

Figure 15–4. Thrombus in the internal carotid artery (ICA) *(arrowheads)* distal to an 84% stenosis; surgical treatment is the preferred modality.

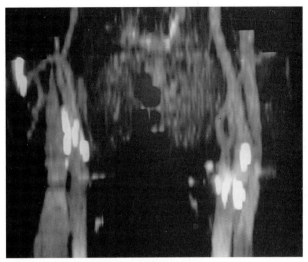

Figure 15–5. Computed tomographic (CT) angiogram reveals major streaky calcifications at both carotid bifurcations.

tions are currently best met by the Wallstent. Its narrow meshwork is also useful in preventing embolism during performance of balloon dilatation. In the authors' opinion, balloon-expandable stents should not be used at the carotid artery bifurcation because of their tendency to collapse. This happens even with the rigid Palmaz stent with a rate between 4 and 15%.[15] Accidental external pressure on the neck deforms a balloon-expandable stent, and severe stent deformity may lead to carotid occlusion and stroke. An exception to this general statement is in stent placement within the pars petrosa and the siphon of the distal ICA. These sites are protected by bony structures and, therefore, balloon-expandable stents can be used. Ostial disease of the CCA can also be treated by balloon-expandable stents, which have the advantage of more precise placement than the Wallstent.

Figure 15–6. Recurrent transient ischemic attacks (TIAs) 7 years after treatment for laryngeal carcinoma (laryngectomy, radical neck dissection, and radiation therapy). *A,* Ulcerative common carotid artery (CCA) stenosis; *B,* considerably improved by stent PTA. The stent covers the whole diseased vascular segment of the CCA.

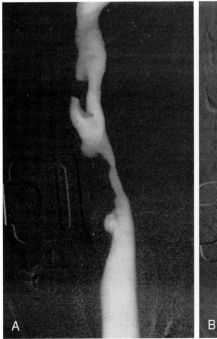
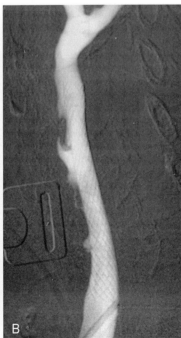

The diameter and length of the stent selected depend on the dimensions of the CCA and the extent of the stenotic lesion. They should be oversized by 1 to 2 mm compared with the vessel's diameter. The stent should be closely sized to the CCA to warrant good healing and formation of a flat neointima that will prevent thrombus apposition at that site. The diameter of the selected stent is usually between 8 and 10 mm, and a stent length of 20 to 32 mm is sufficient in most patients. In the dilated CCA, a stent with a diameter of up to 12 mm may be required, and in extensive disease involving the proximal CCA or distal ICA, a stent with a length of 45 mm may be required. If the stenosis is restricted to the ICA and situated more than 5 mm from the carotid bifurcation, a stent of suitable dimensions can be chosen to avoid crossing the origin of the ECA.

Technique of Stent Placement

ACCESS

The normal approach to the ICA is via the femoral artery. In a dilated aortic arch with deep-seated origin of the left CCA, the steep angle between the aorta and the left CCA may not provide adequate engagement of the artery and thus may not allow crossing of the stenosis and stent deployment. In these cases, a brachial or axillary approach can be used. Direct CCA puncture may rarely be used as an alternative access, but this approach has the major disadvantage that the artery recently treated by stent angioplasty must be compressed after the intervention, with an increased risk of thrombosis and stroke.[16] Therefore, the CCA approach should be reserved for special situations and is used by the authors only for the treatment of distal ICA stenosis.

Stent placement in the ICA can be performed before (primary stenting) or after (secondary stenting) balloon dilatation. For safe and easy passage of stents across the stenosis, predilatation with a 2- to 4-mm coronary balloon is recommended. Predilatation also creates enough space for deployment of the stent and reduces the amount of shortening of the Wallstent during its final dilatation with a 5- or 6-mm balloon. Otherwise, the struts of the stent tend to produce a scissors-like movement during dilatation, which may excise particles of atheroma, which may embolize after balloon deflation.

Two different techniques can be applied for carotid stenting. Our preferred technique is the *over-the-wire procedure* (85%), which is less traumatic, less expensive, and faster than the *coaxial technique* (15%), which uses a long sheath or guiding catheter. With the monocatheter technique, thinner instruments are used and less contrast medium is given. Screening

equipment with a roadmap or overlay facility is mandatory for precise placement of the stent within the stenotic lesion. Preliminary angiograms are performed with the balloon or stent catheter and sealed with a Tuhoy Borst adapter. Alternatively, the coaxial technique is necessary if the angiographic unit is not equipped with the facility for producing frozen images and if dilatation as well as stent placement must be controlled angiographically. In cases in which intravascular ultrasonography is required, use of a long, kink-resistant sheath is necessary.

OVER-THE-WIRE-TECHNIQUE

After the patient has undergone angiographic assessment, the stenosis is crossed by a steerable, floppy-tipped guide wire (0.020 inches) and a diagnostic catheter with a sidewinder or vertebral tip configuration. The guide wire should be long enough for subsequent catheter exchanges. The soft tip of the guide wire is placed in the distal ICA close to the skull base. The stenosis is predilated, most often with a 4-mm coronary balloon. The stent catheter is introduced and advanced to the stenosis via a 6-French (F) sheath inserted at the groin.

The roadmap technique is helpful in positioning the stent exactly, which might otherwise be problematic because of the variable and sometimes considerable shortening of Wallstents after deployment and balloon dilatation. During deployment, the stent is only partially uncovered, and its position is checked by a further run. It can be replaced when no more than 70% of the stent is deployed (Easy Wallstent). When the stent is deployed, its radial force reduces the degree of stenosis. The stent catheter is exchanged for a dilatation catheter, and the stenosis is dilated with the balloon in the stent up to 5 or 6 mm (see Fig. 15–1). During all of these maneuvers, the guide wire is kept in place to warrant easy access to the stenosis. To avoid any potential sawing effect on the stenotic plaque, its position should not be altered after crossing the stenosis.

COAXIAL TECHNIQUE

After cannulation of the carotid origin, a guiding catheter or a long kink-resistant sheath is introduced and advanced to the CCA. By placing the guide wire in the ECA before introduction of the sheath, accidental damage to the ICA plaque is avoided. Use of a stiff guide wire is often necessary for sheath introduction, but it may be more likely to cause vessel spasm than the over-the-wire-technique. With the sheath or guide catheter in place, the stenosis is carefully crossed by means of a steerable guide wire (0.014 to 0.018 inches), and predilatation is performed by means of a 4-mm coronary balloon dilatation catheter.

The stent is positioned and postdilated with a 5- to 6-mm balloon. Continuous flushing of the sheath or guide is needed because of this system's potential for thrombus formation.

MEDICATION

Before patients undergo stent placement and dilatation, they receive premedication with 0.5 to 1.0 mg of atropine depending on the heart rate. This prevents severe bradycardia as a result of carotid body stimulation during balloon dilatation. In the authors' experience, cardiac pacing and prophylactic placement of a pacing electrode are unnecessary. In addition, patients are given 10,000 U of heparin and 5 mg of nifedipine. For 48 hours following the intervention, heparin is given to maintain a prothrombin time of approximately 60 seconds. Long-term treatment with aspirin in a dose of 300 mg daily is commenced as well as 75 mg of clopidogrel daily for 6 weeks.

INTRAOPERATIVE MONITORING

During these procedures, the patient's blood pressure and heart rate (via electrocardiography [ECG]) are monitored continuously. Transcranial Doppler ultrasonography (TCD) and electroencephalography (EEG) are not used routinely because they do not influence treatment. It is well known that during carotid interventions, TCD detects large numbers of air emboli and thromboemboli, and this phenomenon has been published in the literature.[17, 18] It may also be useful to show the extent of flow decrease during dilatation and to give quantitative information about the efficiency of the collateral blood supply.[19] The patient's blood pressure should be carefully controlled for the first days after the intervention because approximately 20% of patients showed a decreased in blood pressure that might be explained by stent-related stimulation of the carotid body. Patients with hypertension have a risk of cerebral hyperperfusion hemorrhage.

Early Results

In the authors' unit, 538 stent PTAs and 261 simple PTAs have been performed in a total of 799 stenosed ICAs occurring in 633 patients. The mean age was 67.1 ± 5.2 years and the technical success rate was 99%. Of these patients, 564 (70.6%) were symptomatic and 235 (29.4%) were asymptomatic. 166 patients suffering from bilateral disease were treated on both sides in one or two sessions. A total of 542 Wallstents were placed, and no episode of stent migration or deformation was observed. In patients with iliac artery occlusion or unfavorable supra-aortic vessels,

Table 15–2. Protocol of Examinations Before and After Stent PTA of the Internal Carotid Artery

Before Stent PTA	Neurologic examination
	Doppler ultrasound
	MRI head
	Aortic arch and selective angiography
After Stent PTA	Neurological examination
	Doppler ultrasound, repeated every 3 months
	Control angiogram after 6 months
	MRI of head

MRI = magnetic resonance imaging; PTA = percutaneous transluminal angioplasty.

stent placement was possible by means of an axillary approach.

The data concerning 467 of these 538 patients treated by stent placement over a 9-year period were evaluated in the context of early results, complications, degree of intimal proliferation, and long-term patency, according to a study protocol. Data are incomplete in 71 cases. The follow-up protocol is detailed in Table 15–2.

In the follow-up group of 467 patients, repeat angiography at 6 months revealed normal-caliber ICA with no residual stenosis and smooth luminal contours. In all cases, cerebral angiography showed improved cerebral artery filling, and cross-flow from the contralateral side via the anterior communicating artery disappeared in all patients with a functioning A1-segment of the anterior cerebral artery.

Eleven patients with deep plaque ulcerations or false aneurysms were treated by placement of an uncovered stent. Within 6 months, 9 of the 11 false aneurysms had resolved, and in the remaining 2 patients, the size of the aneurysm had diminished. This suggests that the use of covered stents is probably indicated only in the treatment of exceptionally large aneurysms. Although distal ICA stenosis that appears in the petrous or siphon part of the ICA cannot be treated by vascular surgery, either of these locations is accessible to performance of angioplasty and stent angioplasty. In 16 of 17 patients PTA could be performed successfully.

Complications

Transient reactions and permanent deficits occurred and were caused by particle embolization (Table 15–3). During performance of carotid angioplasty, emboli are always detected by TCD, and whether the patient becomes symptomatic depends on both particle size and burden. Thirty-five of 799 carotid treatments carried out in 633 patients were accompanied by transient ischemic attacks, all of which occurred within the first 4 hours after the intervention. Thirteen patients developed minor strokes, all in the middle cere-

Table 15–3. Complications of Carotid Angioplasty and Stent Angioplasty (N = 799)

Type of Complication	N	(%)
TIA	35	4.4
Minor stroke	13	1.6
Major stroke	7	0.9
Cerebral hemorrhage	1	0.2
Amaurosis fugax	5	1
Death	2	0.4

TIA = transient ischemic attack.

bral artery territory, and 7 major strokes occurred which required intensive care management. Mortality after 30 days was low; those who died were a 66-year-old male patient with a major infarction in the middle cerebral artery territory and an 82-year-old patient with a myocardial infarction that occurred 5 days after he underwent stent angioplasty. One hypertensive patient developed a cerebral hemorrhage a few hours after he underwent carotid angioplasty; this was interpreted as a hyperperfusion injury. Cerebral hyperperfusion syndrome, which occurs in patients after they have undergone carotid endarterectomy, is a rare but well-known phenomenon. Hyperperfusion injury after angioplasty has also been observed by other authors describing two patients, one with a small putaminal hemorrhage and the other with diffuse basal subarachnoid hemorrhage. In both cases, a typical clinical hyperperfusion syndrome with headache, confusion, vomiting, and seizures occurred after angioplasty of the left carotid artery, both subclavian arteries, and the proximal vertebral arteries in one case, and carotid angioplasty in another.[20] In such cases, use of transcranial Doppler ultrasonography displays significantly elevated blood flow.

Transient neurologic complications were observed in 5.4% of patients. Permanent neurologic deficits occurred in 2.7% of patients and death in 0.4%. Minor stroke was defined according to the Rankin scale with a score of 0 to 2, and major stroke with a score of 3 to 5.

Myointimal Hyperplasia

Growth of myointimal cells, which is seen in patients after vascular surgery and stent angioplasty, represents a uniform reaction of the atherosclerotic arterial wall to the inflicted injury. After stent placement in coronary and peripheral arteries, myointimal tissue growth is of special interest, because a considerable rate of recurrent stenosis is observed. This may lead to the supposition that, as in other territories, the stented ICA will also develop myointimal prolifera-

tion and restenosis. However, this assumption has not been proved for the ICA, and the reaction of the ICA to stent placement may differ from that of other vascular territories.[21] The flow pattern of the ICA is distinct from that of other vessels, with antegrade flow in systole as well as diastole. Irrespective of a wide range of blood pressures, cerebral perfusion and flow in the carotid artery are nearly constant because of autoregulation of the cerebral circulation. This constant blood flow induces much less shear force in the vessel wall, which may be important in provoking less myointimal reaction. On the other hand, a foreign body in a pulsating artery, which is moved and bent with each movement of the head, may favor the development of myointimal proliferation.

Doppler ultrasonographic examinations performed every 3 months and selective angiography after 6 months have been used to increase our knowledge of the behavior of the vessel wall after stent placement. Doppler ultrasonography allows evaluation of the arterial lumen and the walls of the stented CCA and ICA. For quantification of myointimal hyperplasia, follow-up angiography is used as the index examination. Three different angiographic patterns can be demonstrated during follow-up, and these are included in Table 15–4. We interpreted only a concentric or eccentric narrowing of the arterial lumen as myointimal proliferation in comparison with the first control angiogram immediately after the intervention (Fig. 15–7). Stent ingrowth was defined by a normal or increased diameter of the ICA and separation of the stent from the arterial lumen by 1 or 2 mm.

Stent Ingrowth

In all patients, the stent showed a tendency to open up to its nominal diameter in the months after deployment. This phenomenon can be explained by the constant radial force generated by the stent. The stent reaches deeper layers of the vessel wall in the ICA than in the CCA. In 78 of our patients (27%), the lumen of the ICA increased during the observation period. Moreover, the Wallstent was separated from

Table 15–4. Angiographic Classification and Quantitative Distribution of Myointimal Proliferation (mip)

N = 328 arteries		
CLASSIFICATION	AMOUNT OF WALL THICKENING	NUMBER OF ARTERIES
No mip	<1 mm	179 (54.6%)*
Minor mip	1–2 mm	132 (40.2%)
Major mip	>2 mm	17 (5.2%)

*In this group of patients are included those with slight widening of the ICA (internal carotid artery).

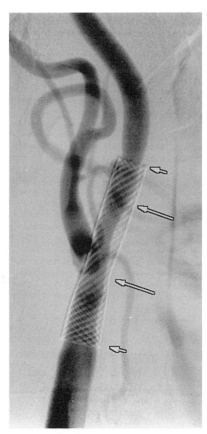

Figure 15–7. Control angiogram 6 months after intervention, with stent ingrowth and myointimal proliferation at the rear wall of the internal carotid artery (ICA) *(arrows)*, with patent external carotid artery (ECA).

the opacified inner surface of the arterial wall by 1 to 2 mm. We presume that the constant radial force of the Wallstent and its oversized dimension for the ICA (normally 8 to 10 mm) is responsible for the observed increase in arterial diameter as well as for the sinking of the stent in deeper layers of the vessel wall (Fig. 15–8). This ingrowth of the stent is comparable with the ingrowth of other devices that apply a constant pressure on the vessel wall, such as caval vein filters, in which the struts of the filter are embedded deeply in the venous wall. Over time, these struts can even penetrate the venous wall completely.

Long-Term Results

Clearly, the clinical impact of stent angioplasty of the ICA depends not only on initial results and complication rate, but also on the long-term outcome for the patient. Many patients report an improvement of higher cortical functions after stent PTA,[22] but the principal treatment objective is prevention of stroke. Do we achieve a benefit in that regard in comparison with that realized by conservative or surgical treatment?

At present, there are data available from prospec-

tive single-center studies and from the Carotid and Vertebral Artery Transluminal Angioplasty Study (CAVATAS) trial. The results of single-center studies are similar, with a complication rate of approximately 2 to 6% and a mortality rate below 1%.[23–29] In the CAVATAS study, in which 560 patients were prospectively randomized in surgical and interventional groups, the early success rate (96%) and the complication rate (10%) showed no significant difference between the two treatment modalities. The data of this trial are not yet published.

The early results of an ongoing prospective trial for the safety of percutaneous angioplasty with stenting were compared with those of retrospectively reviewed patients who were treated with carotid endarterectomy (CEA). During the same 14-month period, 273 patients underwent treatment of 310 carotid bifurcation stenoses: 107 by PTA with stenting, 166 by CEA. Indications for treatment included stroke 46 (16.8%), transient ischemic attack (TIA) 109 (39.9%), syncope 7 (2.6%), and high-grade asymptomatic stenosis 111 (40.7%). Important non-neurologic complications were evident in 6 (5.6%) stent PTA patients and 2 (1.2%) CEA patients. Six-month follow-up data were available for 193 patients (71%). Combined early stroke and death rates were 3.6% in the CEA group (7 of 166) and 3.7% in the stent angioplasty group (5 of 107).[25] If the two treatment techniques are compared it must be emphasized that the results of the interventional group included the learning curve of the team with this new technique and the limited availability of devices in the American market because of United States Food and Drug Administration (FDA) regulations.

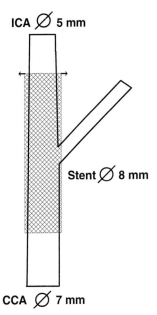

Figure 15–8. Completely expanded stent after 6 months: The part of the stent in the ICA has grown deeper into the arterial wall than that in the common carotid artery (CCA).

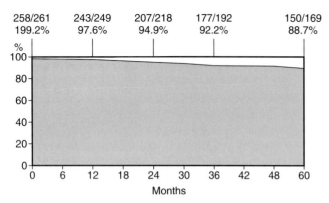

Figure 15–9. Five-year cumulative patency after balloon angioplasty (life table method; n = 261 acute coronary ischemic [ACI cases]).

Our own follow-up data give us strong evidence that stent PTA has a 5-year patency rate comparable with that of vascular surgery, with patent arteries achieved in more than 90% of treated vessels (Figs. 15–9 and 15–10). A patent artery is defined as an artery with no narrowing or a narrowing of less than 30%. Only 3 of the 288 patients with complete follow-up data developed a minor ipsilateral stroke (1%), and no death occurred as a result of ipsilateral stroke. Therefore, we have no doubts that stent PTA benefits the patient and positively influences the fate of the patient in comparison with the outcome of conservative therapy. Nevertheless, currently available data are insufficient to evaluate and compare the different aspects of treatment by surgical or endovascular techniques.

VERTEBRAL ARTERY STENOSIS

The most common site of atherosclerotic vertebral artery stenosis is at the origin of the vessel. The plaque that encircles the vertebral artery orifice is normally smooth and, therefore, well suited for PTA, but unstable plaques with embolic potential can be

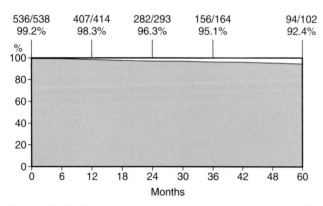

Figure 15–10. Five-year cumulative patency after stent angioplasty (life table method; n = 538 acute carotid ischemic [ACI] cases).

encountered and these must be considered when dealing with such lesions to prevent posterior fossa cerebral infarction.[30] Nonostial disease can be seen in the lower neck; this is differentiated from artery compression by the presence of bony spurs on the cervical column, where PTA is of no value. Rotational vertebrobasilar impairment of blood flow should be excluded by functional imaging.[31] The intracranial vertebral artery, after it pierces the dura, is another frequent site of occlusive disease. The left and right vertebral arteries are approximately equally affected by atherosclerosis, but there is some indication that when the two vessels are unequal in diameter, the smaller vessel is more frequently occluded. Aside from these sites of predilection, fibrous plaques and fatty streaks are distributed throughout the vertebral artery. However, ulceration in plaques occurs less frequently in the posterior circulation than in the carotid territory. The vertebral artery may be affected by non-atherosclerotic diseases, such as arteritis, dissection, and fibromuscular dysplasia. Arteritis is usually located close to the aortic arch, whereas dissection and fibromuscular dysplasia spread into the cervical part of the vertebral artery.

Indications

The indications for treatment are restricted to patients with characteristic clinical signs of vertebrobasilar insufficiency (Table 15–5).

Transient vertigo, diplopia, or headache, occurring as solitary symptoms, should not be interpreted as a vertebrobasilar TIA. Also, some patients with dizziness prove to have carotid TIA. Hence, this symptom is not a reliable indicator of the vascular

Table 15–5. Signs and Symptoms of Vertebrobasilar Insufficiency

Frequent	Rare
Ataxia	Noise or pounding in the ear or head
Dizziness	Vomiting
Diplopia (vertical or horizontal)	Hiccups
	Memory impairment
Dysarthria	Confusion
Transient vertigo	Drop attacks
Bifacial numbness	Impaired hearing
Weakness or numbness of part or all of one or both sides of the body	Deafness
	Hemiballism
	Peduncular hallucinosis
Dysphagia	Forced deviation of the eyes
Staggering	Paralysis of gaze
Veering to one side	Partial or complete blindness
Feeling of cross-eyedness	
Blurred vision	
Pupillary changes and ptosis	
Tunnel vision	

circuit that is involved. The clinical picture may vary in the vertebrobasilar system from episode to episode.

A wide range of surgical procedures is available and these can be effective. Reconstruction of the vertebral artery, bypass in the neck, and extracranial–intracranial grafts have been used to back up the flagging posterior circulation, but the indications are still uncertain and the complications are considerable. The origin of the vertebral artery is not easily accessible by surgery, and the lumen is often too small for endarterectomy. Therefore, patients are usually treated with arteriotomy and reconstruction with a venous patch. The mortality and permanent morbidity of surgical treatment exceeds 5%.

Percutaneous angioplasty of vertebral artery stenosis offers a number of advantages in comparison with those of medical and surgical treatment. Balloon angioplasty with or without stent placement removes the flow obstacle and restores normal cerebral blood supply. The intervention is more or less independent of the location of the lesion whether at the artery's origin, the cervical or intracranial part. This intervention is far less traumatic and has a lower complication rate than that of vascular surgery. The intervention should be carried out in symptomatic patients with stenosis greater than 70%. In most cases, the contralateral vertebral artery is hypoplastic, stenotic, or occluded. Stent angioplasty may also be indicated in spontaneous or traumatic dissection of the vertebral artery.[32] The clinical signs of vertebrobasilar insufficiency should be judged skeptically if only one vertebral artery is narrowed and the opposite side shows a vertebral artery of normal caliber.

Technique

The procedure is performed with coronary balloon catheters and guide wires, with a sheath in the proximal subclavian artery. Sometimes, the sheath must be stabilized by use of a double guide-wire technique in which one guide wire is placed with its tip in the brachial artery and the other wire is placed in the vertebral artery (Fig. 15–11). The guide wire in the brachial artery prevents the sheath from slipping back into the aortic arch, especially when a right-sided vertebral artery stenosis is the target lesion. Technical difficulties in cannulating the vertebral artery may arise in patients with an aberrant vessel origin at the aortic arch. The sheath should leave the origin of the vertebral artery patent to ensure a constant blood flow in the posterior cerebral circulation. Advancing the guide wire into the first segment of the vertebral artery may prove difficult if the artery is coiled and, similarly, an elongated vertebral artery loop at the C1-level may also impede easy passage of guide wire and catheter. The problem can usually be resolved by

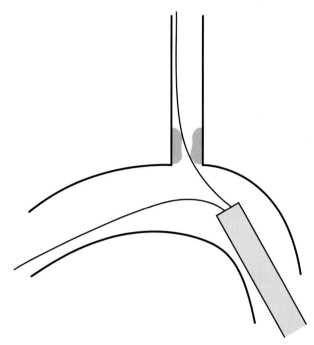

Figure 15–11. Stabilization of a sheath in the right subclavian artery for vertebral artery angioplasty with use of a double-wire technique.

using neuroradiologic microcatheters of the Tracker type to place a guide wire across the stenosis. With the guide wire in place, the microcatheter is exchanged for a dilatation catheter with a balloon diameter between 3 and 5 mm. Although balloon perfusion catheters are available, they are not normally necessary because the ischemic tolerance of the brain is higher in the posterior than in the anterior circulation. Stents are not routinely placed in all vertebral artery lesions but are reserved for patients with residual stenosis caused by plaque rupture or elastic recoil, which are more frequently seen with ostial disease. Coronary balloon-expandable stents are favored in this area. It requires experience to place the stent precisely at the origin of the vertebral artery in a way that it does not protrude into the subclavian artery or slip beyond the stenosis (Fig. 15–12).

Angioplasty of the vertebral artery can be combined with local thrombolysis in patients with vertebrobasilar thrombosis and underlying atherosclerotic stenosis.[32] Spontaneous or traumatic vertebral artery dissection should be treated by stent placement rather than angioplasty alone, because without the mechanical support of the stent the artery may occlude as we have seen in a younger male patient.[31]

Results

Vertebral artery stenosis was treated by us in 93 patients with a mean age of 66.4 ± 7.3 years. All patients had bilateral vertebral artery disease, and the

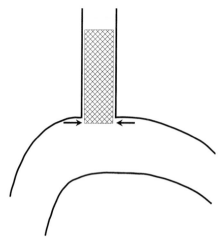

Figure 15–12. Vertebral artery ostial stent placement: Balloon-expandable stent should be deployed precisely, without protrusion into the subclavian artery.

Table 15–6. Results of Vertebral Artery Dilatation

References	Treatment Attempts	PTA Successful	Complications
Courtheux et al	24	21	1 TO
Higashida et al	42	42	3
Kachel et al	15	15	0
Kubis et al	3	3	0
Mathias et al	93	89	1 TSO; 1 TO
Motarjeme et al	35	32	0?
Qi et al	17	16	0
Storey et al	3	3	0
Vitek et al	4	4	1 TSO
Zeumer et al	9	9?	0
Total	245 (100%)	234 (95.5%)	6 (2.4%)

TO = thrombotic occlusion; TSO = transient spastic occlusion.

stenosis was successfully treated in 89 cases (96%) (Fig. 15–13). A stent was placed in 27 of the patients, nearly all of whom had ostial disease. The stenosis was located ostially in 78, cervically in 10, and intradurally in 5 patients (Fig. 15–14). In 4 cases, it was impossible to pass the stenosis with a guide wire or a balloon catheter because of tortuosity of the vertebral artery. In 1 patient with two stenotic lesions of the right vertebral artery, both stenoses could be removed. In 1 female patient with bilateral internal carotid artery occlusions, dilatation of a narrowed vertebral artery was performed uneventfully. Comparably favorable results have been reported in the literature[33–41] (Table 15–6).

Complications of vertebral artery PTA are infrequently encountered (2.4%) and have not provoked brain infarctions even in the post-PTA occlusions reported in 2 cases. Sometimes spastic reactions can be observed, which may be more common in the poststenotic segment of the artery. When a coiled or looped vessel is straightened, spasm may be induced even without damage to the vessel wall but will resolve spontaneously within 30 minutes after removal of the guide wire. Brain stem infarction is a rare complication of angioplasty.[42] Intradural dilatation of the vertebral artery has some risk of arterial rupture.

Long term-results have not been published, and randomized trials with endovascular and surgical treatment are not available. We have encountered recurrent symptomatic disease in 7 patients who required repeat angioplasty. Symptomatic improvement

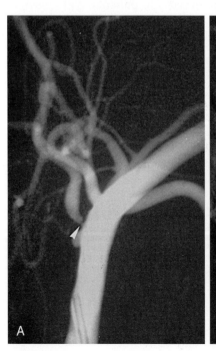
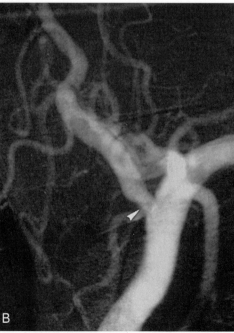

Figure 15–13. Fifty-nine-year-old patient with vertebrobasilar symptoms. Right vertebral artery hypoplastic; left vertebral artery with ostial stenosis. A, After dilatation with a 4-mm balloon normal flow and B, disappearance of symptoms.

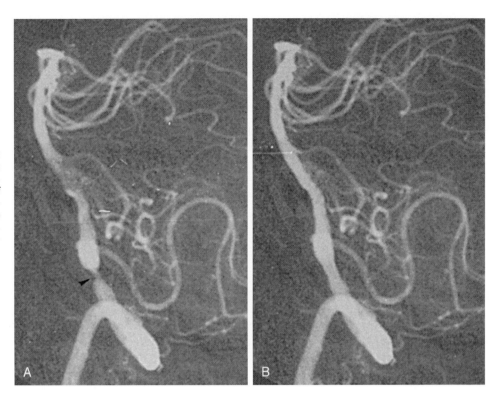

Figure 15–14. Fifty-four-year-old man with A, repeated brain stem symptoms, occlusion of the left vertebral artery distal to the origin of the posterior inferior cerebellar artery, and B, intradural stenosis of the right vertebral artery *(arrowhead)*. The stenosis was removed by dilatation with a 4-mm balloon.

is not uniform despite normalized vertebral blood flow and may relate to additional distal branch disease that is not amenable to treatment.

CONCLUSIONS AND FURTHER DEVELOPMENTS

Stent PTA has proved to be an efficient means of treatment in patients suffering from atherosclerotic stenosis of the ICA. The early results are better than those with balloon angioplasty alone in regard to residual stenosis and smoothness of the vessel wall. The complication rate of carotid stent angioplasty is low, bringing stent angioplasty into competition with vascular surgery. The European trial (CAVATAS) that is comparing thromboendarterectomy and PTA of the internal carotid artery in a prospectively randomized manner has shown no significant differences between the two methods over a period of more than 4 years. Considering the fact that the participating groups performing angioplasty have had a learning curve, whereas the vascular surgical approach is well established, these results are promising. It should not be forgotten that vascular surgery has still not proved its efficacy in comparison with the best possible medical treatment in patients older than 80 years who have contralateral carotid occlusion, tandem stenoses, severe coronary heart disease, recurrent carotid stenosis after CEA, or stenosis of nonatherosclerotic etiology.

More detailed randomized prospective trials (Carotid Randomized Endarterectomy Stent Trial—CREST; Carotid Artery Stent Arterectomy Trial—CASET; CAVATAS II) have been planned or have already been started. The endoluminal approach to atherosclerotic disease offers the advantage that additional proximal and distal carotid stenoses, contralateral carotid stenosis, or vertebral artery disease can be treated in one session, an important benefit for patients with multiple vessel disease. Nevertheless, it must be borne in mind that, because stent angioplasty is technically relatively straightforward, the danger exists that the necessary skill and experience to perform such interventions without producing complications is not appreciated, and this in turn leads to poor results or more catastrophic complications.[43]

Further development of stents will undoubtedly influence the technique in the coming years. For instance, the Wallstent has been developed to offer better visibility and less shortening. It can also be repositioned, a feature that improves accuracy of placement. We do not know if a stent with thinner struts and a narrower meshwork will be safer, because protrusion of atherosclerotic debris through the stent during performance of PTA may be better prevented and the rate of embolism reduced. Many groups are engaged in research into coated stents aimed at inhibiting thrombus formation and myointimal regrowth. The use of covered stents may have an important role in the further reduction of embolic complications in some patients, as will the further evolution of cerebral protraction systems in the distal carotid artery.

At the present time, the authors consider stent PTA as the treatment of choice in the following subgroups:

- Bilateral carotid artery stenosis
- Contralateral carotid artery occlusion
- Poor cross-flow (aplasia and hypoplasia of A1 segment of the anterior cerebral artery) and exhausted reserve capacity
- Tandem stenosis (CCA and ICA stenosis, proximal and distal ICA stenosis)
- Postoperative recurrent carotid artery stenosis
- Non atherosclerotic etiology of carotid artery stenosis (fibromuscular dysplasia, Takayasu's arteritis, after irradiation)
- Vertebral artery stenosis
- Multiple-vessel disease (carotid, vertebral, innominate, and subclavian artery obstruction)
- Increased operative risk (severe coronary heart disease)

SURGICAL ASPECTS OF CAROTID AND VERTEBRAL INTERVENTION

Percutaneous transluminal balloon angioplasty has become well established in the treatment of patients with peripheral arterial disease, but its use in the treatment of carotid artery stenosis has developed only recently. Technically, angioplasty of a short stenosis in a relatively large high-flow vessel should produce good results because the situation seems analogous to that of the iliac vessels. Large randomized controlled trials have demonstrated the clear benefit of carotid endarterectomy in symptomatic patients with severe stenosis, but asymptomatic patients may reap a small benefit as well. Neurologists now question whether endovascular intervention can produce the same benefit, based on their philosophy that "the aim of medicine is to avoid surgery." However, a world of difference may exist between the endovascular treatment of a lesion, which causes morbidity as a result of the presence of emboli, and the majority of other arterial stenoses that produce symptoms by limiting flow.

Surgery plays an important part in the management of selected patients with cerebral vascular disease. However, all patients benefit from correction of risk factors and antiplatelet therapy, which must not be forgotten. Systematic reviews of published trials indicate that reducing the systolic blood pressure by 5 mm Hg lowers the risk of stroke by 35%, and aspirin reduces the risk by 25%. Smoking must be stopped and hyperlipidemia controlled with statins if the disorder is unresponsive to diet.

Indications for and Results of Surgical Treatment

SYMPTOMATIC CAROTID ARTERY DISEASE

NASCET and ECST together comprise the largest randomized controlled trials of surgical intervention in the history of medicine.[11, 44] Patients who have suffered a recent (<120 days), nondisabling, carotid territory ischemic stroke, a transient ischemic attack (TIA), amaurosis fugax, or a retinal infarct, and ipsilateral carotid stenosis as recorded by angiography were randomized to best medical therapy (BMT) or BMT plus carotid endarterectomy (CEA). Fifty North American centers participated in the NASCET trial and 80 European centers in the ECST trial. All patients received BMT care, including antiplatelet therapy and correction of risk factors. Patients in both trials were stratified into those with high-grade stenosis (70 to 99%) and those with medium-grade stenosis (30 to 69%). The ECST trial also included a low-grade stenosis group (0 to 29%).

For the 1437 patients with severe (70 to 99%) stenosis, the conclusions of both trials were remarkably similar. Patients treated with CEA plus BMT attained six- to tenfold reduction in the long-term risk of stroke compared those who were treated with BMT alone (Fig. 15–15). This equates to an absolute risk reduction of 10 to 15% and a relative risk reduction of 44 to 54%. Men appeared to benefit more than women for the same degree of stenosis. The overall operative risk (death, all perioperative strokes, or both) was 5.8 to 7.5%, whereas the risk of death or disabling stroke, or both was 2.1 to 3.7%. The highest risk of stroke after surgery occurred in the perioperative period, and there was considerable intersurgeon

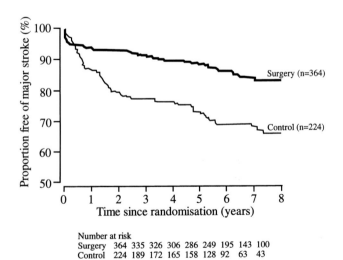

Figure 15–15. Survival curves of patients who were free of major stroke (nonstroke deaths after 30 days censored) in European Carotid Surgery Trial (ECST) surgery and control groups with symptomatic carotid artery stenosis exceeding 80% (70% North American Study of Endarterectomy [NASCET]).

variability. This implies that the maximum benefit of CEA will be realized by surgeons with a workload large enough to maintain expertise and by those who can demonstrate satisfactory results by continued audit. The same may be true for endovascular treatment.

For the 374 patients with mild stenosis (0 to 29%) in the ECST, those treated medically had little risk of ipsilateral stroke; therefore, the benefits of surgery were outweighed by the early risks. CEA conferred no additional benefit on patients with moderate stenosis (30 to 69%) who made up about half of the total number in both trials. Even if the 30 to 49% subgroup is excluded, it would still take 4 to 5 years to achieve any advantage in stroke-free life expectancy for those with a 50 to 69% stenosis. However, CEA should be offered to patients with a moderate stenosis who have continued symptoms despite optimal medical therapy. Plaque morphology may also be important because heterogeneous or ulcerated plaques appear to be associated with a higher risk of stroke.

Thus the current indications for CEA in symptomatic patients are:

- Severe stenosis (>70%) with carotid territory symptoms in the last 6 months
- Moderate stenosis (50 to 69%) with continued symptoms despite medical therapy

ASYMPTOMATIC CAROTID STENOSIS

Some patients with carotid artery disease die or sustain a disabling stroke without manifesting any previous symptoms. Although endarterectomy for treatment of patients with asymptomatic carotid stenosis (ACS) has been advocated, there is no clear evidence of benefit. Between 5 and 10% of the population who are older than 65 years of age and 20 to 30% of hospital patients with ischemic heart disease or peripheral vascular disease have a carotid artery stenosis exceeding 50%. A policy of screening and surgery to detect and treat ACS would, therefore, have major public health implications. The results of randomized trials of surgery vs. medical treatment for high-grade (>70%) ACS have been mostly inconclusive. The Mayo Clinic trial (MACE) was terminated after only 71 patients had been entered, because an excess of patients in the surgical group had myocardial infarctions. The Carotid Artery Stenosis with Asymptomatic Narrowing: Operation vs. Aspirin (CASANOVA) Trial and Veterans Administration Trial concluded that, although the risk of stroke was lower in the surgery groups, the numbers of patients required to detect a significant reduction was beyond the scope of the trials, and that meta-analysis would be required. The largest North American multicenter trial, the Asymptomatic Carotid Artery Study (ACAS)

randomized a total of 1662 patients.[8] CEA was performed by a carefully selected group of surgeons who were required to have 30-day rates of stroke, death, or both of less than 3% for their previous 50 operations. The trial demonstrated a 53% relative risk reduction from 11% in medically treated patients to 5.1% in surgical patients based on a projected life-table analysis up to 5 years. In real terms, this means that 30 CEAs would have to be performed to prevent one stroke, and the conclusion that surgery can now be justified for ACS has been criticized by the principal investigators of both NASCET and ECST trials. The ongoing Asymptomatic Carotid Surgery Trial (ACST) has recruited more than 1700 patients and may help to clarify the situation.[45] However, based on current evidence, population screening is not justified, and CEA for ACS should only be performed in the context of a randomized clinical trial.

A carotid stenosis greater than 70% is present in 2 to 4% of all patients who undergo coronary artery bypass grafting (CABG), and this increases the risk of peroperative stroke from less than 1 to 9%. A synchronous procedure avoids myocardial ischemia, which may be caused if the carotid endarterectomy is performed first, and this has been shown to reduce the stroke rate.[46] The difficulty of performing a large enough randomized trial has resulted in adopting a pragmatic approach to such patients at many centers. Common criteria for intervention include:

- Bilateral severe (>70%) stenoses
- Severe (>70%) stenosis and contralateral occlusion
- Preocclusive (>90%) stenosis

VERTEBRAL ARTERY STENOSIS

Many patients complain of dizziness, and the origin of the vertebral artery (VA) is a common site for atherosclerotic disease. Although dizziness may be associated with vertebrobasilar ischemia, it is a nonspecific symptom that can be frequently caused by cardiac and labyrinthine disorders. The diagnosis of vertebrobasilar ischemia requires the presence of two or more of the following:

- Bilateral motor and/or sensory deficit
- Ataxia of gait
- Diplopia or bilateral homonymous hemianopia
- Dysarthria or dysphagia

In the presence of such symptoms, treatment of patients with stenosis of VA origin may be justified, although evidence from randomized trials does not exist. The indications for treatment include:

- Severe (>70%) stenoses or short occlusions of both VA origins, or of only one origin if the artery is single or provides dominant supply to the basilar artery (hemodynamic indication)

- Severe (>70%) stenosis of one VA origin after recovery from a hind-brain stroke documented by CT scanning (embolic indication)

Surgical access to the VA is difficult, compared with that to the carotid artery, as it lies deep in the neck, covered by muscles and bone. This probably explains the unpopularity of surgical reconstruction. Conventional treatment of disease at the origin of the VA entails division of the artery above the stenosis or occlusion and transposition to the adjacent carotid artery.[47] Because of the difficult access, angioplasty and stenting, if required, now seem the best options for lesions of VA origin. Longer occlusions can be treated by carotid to distal VA bypass, but the indications for this procedure remain dubious.

Carotid Angioplasty vs. Surgery

CAVATAS represents the only large randomized controlled trial of endovascular therapy for carotid disease.[48] Between 1992 and 1997, 13 centers from around the world recruited 504 patients who were fit for carotid surgery. Patients with symptomatic carotid lesions exceeding 50% stenosis underwent randomization to carotid endarterectomy (N = 253) or angioplasty with stenting (N = 251), according to the uncertainty principle used in the ECST trial. The groups are matched well in terms of indication for treatment and severity of stenosis. On an intention-to-treat analysis, the 30-day death and disabling stroke rate seems no different for the two groups (6.3% for the surgical group and 6.4% for the endovascular treatment group). Some have criticized these high rates, but almost half of the events took place after randomization but before treatment. This emphasizes the need to avoid delay between randomization and treatment in future trials. The lack of a record of eligible patients who did not enter the trial, and the reasons why, represents a more serious criticism because selection bias might have occurred in some centers. Furthermore, 20 of the patients randomized to angioplasty crossed over to surgery or medical treatment because of treatment failure, and more than half of the 504 patients received treatment in just two centers.

The success of any future trial will require enrollment of a sufficient number of patients and follow-up for a minimum of 2 years to allow a comparison with adequate statistical power. To demonstrate equivalence within a margin of 2%, assuming a disabling stroke and death rate after surgery of 5%, requires 5000 patients (i.e., more than NASCET and ECST combined). Such a trial will require the establishment of teams (each composed of neurologist, vascular surgeon, and interventional radiologist) who will develop experience to avoid the problems associated with learning curves. Such experience would need careful monitoring by registries that the American Heart Association Science Advisory and Coordinating Committee[49], the Joint Working Party of the Vascular Surgical Society of Great Britain and Ireland, and the British Society of Interventional Radiologists have proposed. Longer term follow-up is required in view of high restenosis rates of up to 25% that have been reported within 12 months of angioplasty. Stents probably lower the medium-term restenosis rate. However, we have found little difference in the longer term restenosis rates between angioplasty and stenting. The majority of restenoses after CEA cause no symptoms because embolization as a result of myointimal hyperplasia is uncommon.[50] The same may not be true for restenosis after endovascular treatment.

The risk of embolization after angioplasty remains the principal concern of any surgeon who has seen the soft, "porridge-like" plaques inside carotid arteries (Fig. 15–16). Cerebral emboli can cause psychometric changes as well as strokes.[51] In Sheffield, all carotid angioplasties and endarterectomies undergo monitoring with TCD. Cerebral emboli always occur during angioplasty and in far greater numbers than those associated with endarterectomy (Fig. 15–17). This probably accounts for the 6% incidence of TIAs that we have seen during angioplasty. Plaque characterization may help identify stenoses that have a low risk of embolization, but this remains unvalidated.[52] Furthermore, there is no good evidence that balloons or stents used for cerebral protection reduce the risk of cerebral embolization.

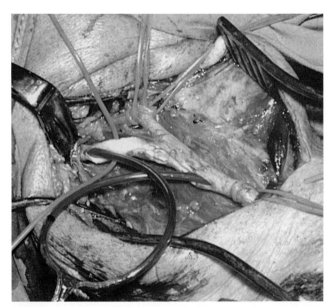

Figure 15–16. Friable atheromatous stenosis at the origin of the internal carotid artery before endarterectomy. The indwelling shunt maintains cerebral perfusion.

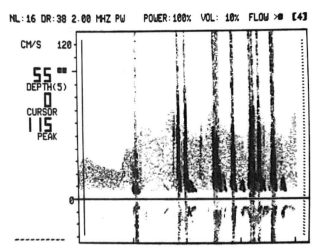

Figure 15-17. Transcranial Doppler signal from the middle cerebral artery during carotid angioplasty. The velocity increase upon deflation of the balloon is accompanied by a burst of high-intensity transients (HITS) caused by particulate emboli.

Current Indications for Endovascular Treatment

Patients naturally prefer an endovascular intervention to an operation that requires an incision. However, this patient preference depends on reassurance that the endovascular procedure has equal safety and efficacy. Patients need to know that the safety and efficacy of carotid angioplasty has not yet been fully validated. Neurologists frequently quote cranial nerve injuries as a reason for avoiding surgery. Up to 50% of patients may suffer some degree of cranial nerve injury, but most seem transitory, and patients recover within a few weeks.[53] The area of cutaneous numbness anterior to the scar also diminishes with time and does not cause long-term problems. The other quoted advantages of endovascular treatments include a shorter recovery and lower cost. This may hold true for other major vascular procedures with considerable morbidity, such as coronary bypass and aortobifemoral bypass grafting, but that is not the case with carotid endarterectomy, which represents a relatively safe and inexpensive procedure that surgeons can perform under locoregional anesthesia. Indeed, a recent comparative study has found no difference between balloon angioplasty and stenting vs. endarterectomy in terms of the length of hospitalization or total costs.[54] In the absence of a large randomized trial, CEA must remain the treatment of choice for most patients with carotid disease. However, the following situations seem appropriate for endovascular treatment:

- Primary, symptomatic carotid stenoses for which surgical access seems difficult or hazardous

- Symptomatic restenosis after conventional carotid endarterectomy

- Patients who are unfit for carotid endarterectomy

- In centers where the requisite teams and experience have already been developed, for maintenance of expertise and evaluation of new technology

The first of the aforementioned categories includes stenoses at the origin of the common carotid or brachiocephalic artery because endovascular treatment gives good results and surgical access requires a median sternotomy. Postradiotherapy stenoses of the common carotid artery and distal stenoses of the internal carotid artery represent other indications. Surgery for restenosis after carotid endarterectomy can seem technically difficult, with higher morbidity and mortality. Yadav and colleagues have reported good results after treating 25 carotid restenoses by use of stenting.[55] Conversely, symptomatic restenosis after stenting is best treated by CEA with removal of the entire atheroma–stent–hyperplasia complex (Fig. 15–18).

Almost all patients can tolerate carotid endarterectomy, especially if performed under locoregional

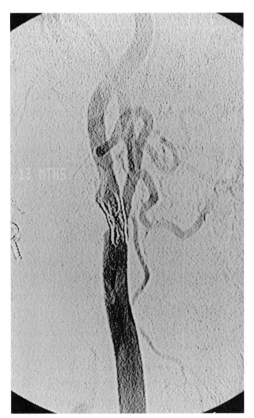

Figure 15-18. Carotid arteriogram of a patient with recurrent symptoms caused by crushing of a Strecker stent. The atheroma–stent–hyperplasia complex was successfully removed by conventional endarterectomy. (Angiogram courtesy of Mr. M. Gough, Leeds, England).

anaesthesia.[56] However, angioplasty of severe carotid stenoses before performance of coronary artery bypass grafting (CABG) might represent a reasonable alternative to a synchronous CEA in these high-risk cases. We have successfully performed 11 carotid angioplasties in patients with such stenoses before performance of CABG. Stents should only be used if the result of angioplasty is suboptimal. When required, self-expanding stents should be used, because stent deformation can occur with balloon-expandable devices (see Fig. 15–4).

SUMMARY

Two large randomized, controlled trials have shown that CEA produces a 6 to 10-fold reduction in the long-term risk of stroke in patients with severe, symptomatic carotid stenoses. Carotid angioplasty results in significantly more cerebral emboli and probably more TIAs than occur after carotid endarterectomy. Little evidence exists that cerebral protection balloons or stents reduce this risk, nor has a reliable method of selecting safe stenoses for endovascular treatment yet emerged. Endovascular treatment avoids the risk of cranial nerve damage but demonstrates few other clinical or economic advantages, especially when compared with CEA performed under locoregional anesthesia. The only randomized trial of endovascular treatment vs. surgery (CAVATAS) was too small to prove equivalence with CEA. Moreover, the long-term risk of restenosis and recurrent symptoms is not yet known. Few absolute indications for carotid angioplasty or stenting currently exist unless performed as part of a randomized, controlled trial. At the time of writing, CEA remains the treatment of choice for most patients.

REFERENCES

1. Mathias K: Ein neuartiges Katheter-System zur perkutanen transluminalen Angioplastie von Karotisstenosen. Fortschr Med 95:1007–1011, 1977.
2. Mathias K: Perkutane transluminale Katheterbehandlung supraaortaler Arterienobstruktionen. Angio 3:47–50, 1981.
3. Mathias K, Mittermayer Ch, Ensinger H, et al: Perkutane Katheterdilatation von Karotisstenosen. RöFo 133:258–261, 1980.
4. Hayward JK, Davies AH, Lamont PM: Carotid plaque morphology: A review. Eur J Vasc Endovasc Surg 9:368–374, 1995.
5. Mathias K, Bockenheimer S, von Reutern G, et al: Katheterdilatation hirnversorgender Arterien. Radiologe 23:208–214, 1983.
6. Mathias K: Percutaneous transluminal angioplasty in supraaortic artery disease. In Roubin GS, Califf RM, O'Neil WW, et al (eds): Interventional Cardiovascular Medicine, New York, Churchill Livingstone, 1994, pp 745–775.
7. Mathias K: Perkutane Rekanalisation der supraaortalen und zerebralen Arterien. In Günther RW, Thelen M (eds). Interventionelle Radiologie, Stuttgart, Thieme, pp 112–123.
8. Executive Committee for the Asymptomatic Carotid Atherosclerosis Study. Endarterectomy for asymptomatic carotid artery stenosis. JAMA 273:1421–1428, 1995.
9. Halliday AW, Thomas DJ, Mansfield AO: The asymptomatic carotid surgery trial (ACST). Int Angiol 14:18–20, 1995.
10. MRC European Carotid Surgery Trial: Interim results for symptomatic patients with severe (70–99%) or with mild (0–29%) carotid stenosis. European Carotid Surgery Trialists' Collaborative Group. Lancet 337:1235–1243, 1991.
11. North American Symptomatic Carotid Endarterectomy Trial Collaborators. Beneficial effect of carotid endarterectomy in symptomatic patients with high-grade stenosis. New Engl J Med 325:445–453, 1991.
12. Babatasi G, Massetti M, Theron J, et al: Asymptomatic carotid stenosis in patients undergoing major cardiac surgery: Can percutaneous carotid angioplasty be an alternative? Eur J Cardiothorac Surg 11:547–553, 1997.
13. Mathur A, Roubin GS, Yadav JS, et al: Combined coronary and bilateral carotid stenting: A case report. Cathet Cardiovasc Diagn 40:202–206, 1997.
14. Guterman LR, Budny JL, Gibbons KJ, et al: Thrombolysis of the cervical internal carotid artery before balloon angioplasty and stent placement: Report of two cases. Neurosurgery 38:620–630, 1996.
15. Mathur A, Dorros G, Iyer SS, et al: Palmaz stent compression in patients following carotid artery stenting. Cathet Cardiovasc Diagn 41:137–140, 1997.
16. Diethrich EB, Marx P, Wrasper R, et al: Percutaneous techniques for endoluminal carotid interventions. J Endovasc Surg 3:182–202, 1996.
17. Benichou H, Bergeron P: Carotid angioplasty and stenting: Will periprocedural transcranial Doppler monitoring be important? J Endovasc Surg 3:217–223, 1996.
18. Markus HS, Clifton A, Buckenham T, et al: Carotid angioplasty. Detection of embolic signals during and after the procedure. Stroke 25:2403–2406, 1994.
19. Eckert B, Thie A, Valdueza J, Zanella F, et al: Transcranial Doppler sonographic monitoring during percutaneous transluminal angioplasty of the internal carotid artery. Neuroradiology 39:229–234, 1997.
20. Schoser BG, Heesen C, Eckert B, et al: Cerebral hyperperfusion injury after percutaneous transluminal angioplasty of extracranial arteries. J Neurol 244:101–104, 1997.
21. Parsson H, Cwikiel W, Johansson K, et al: Deposition of platelets and neutrophils in porcine iliac arteries after angioplasty and Wallstent placement compared with angioplasty alone. Cardiovasc Intervent Radiol 17:190–196, 1994.
22. Maeshima S, Itakura T, Naka D, et al: The effect on higher cortical dysfunction of percutaneous transluminal angioplasty for internal carotid artery stenosis. No Shinkei Geka 23:971–976, 1995.
23. Bergeron P, Chambran P, Bianca S, et al: Traitement endovasculaire des artères a destinée cérébrale: Échecs et limites. J Mal Vasc 21(suppl A):123–131, 1996.
24. Diethrich EB, Ndiaye M, Reid DB: Stenting in the carotid artery: Initial experience in 110 patients. J Endovasc Surg 3:42–62, 1996.
25. Jordan WD Jr, Schroeder PT, Fisher WS, et al: A comparison of angioplasty with stenting versus endarterectomy for the treatment of carotid artery stenosis. Ann Vasc Surg 11:2–8, 1997.
26. Kachel R, Basche S: Qualitätskriterien beim Einsatz der perkutanen transluminalen Angioplastie (PTA) an supraaortalen Arterien. Zentralbl Chir 121:1076–84, 1996.
27. Roubin GS, Yadav S, Iyer SS, et al: Carotid stent-supported angioplasty: A neurovascular intervention to prevent stroke. Am J Cardiol 78:8–12, 1996.
28. Theron JG, Payelle GG, Coskun O, et al: Carotid artery stenosis: Treatment with protected balloon angioplasty and stent placement. Radiology 201:627–636, 1996.
29. Caplan LR, Amarenco P, Rosengart A, et al: Embolism from vertebral artery origin occlusive disease. Neurology 42:1505–1512, 1992.
30. Kuether TA, Nesbit GM, Clark WM, et al: Rotational vertebral artery occlusion: A mechanism of vertebro-basilar insufficiency. Neurosurgery 41:427–433, 1997.
31. Price RF, Sellar R, Leung C, et al: Traumatic vertebral arterial dissection and vertebro-basilar arterial thrombosis successfully treated with endovascular thrombolysis and stenting. AJNR 19:1677–1680, 1998.
32. Becker KJ, Crain BJ, Monsein LH, et al: Arterial changes after

thrombolysis and percutaneous transluminal angioplasty in vertebro-basilar thrombosis. AJNR 18:514–518, 1997.

33. Halbach VV, Higashida RT, Dowd CF, et al: Endovascular treatment of vertebral artery dissections and pseudoaneurysms. J Neurosurg 79:183–191, 1993.

34. Higashida RT, Tsai FY, Halbach VV, et al: Transluminal angioplasty for atherosclerotic disease of the vertebral and basilar arteries. J Neurosurg 78:192–198, 1993.

35. Kachel R, Basche S, Heerklotz I, et al: Percutaneous transluminal angioplasty (PTA) of supra-aortic arteries especially the internal carotid artery. Neuroradiology 33:191–194, 1991.

36. Kubis N, Houdart E, Merland JJ, et al: Angioplastie de sténoses athéromateuses hémodynamiques des artéres vertébrales intracraniennes. Rev Neurol Paris. 153:386–392, 1997.

37. Motarjeme A, Gordon GI: Percutaneous transluminal angioplasty of brachiocephalic vessels: Guidelines for therapy. Int Angiol 12:260–269, 1993.

38. Qi JP, Zeitler E: Katheterdilatation der arteriellen Stenosen supraaortaler Gefäße und Spätergebnisse. Röfo 155:357–362, 1991.

39. Storey GS, Marks MP, Dake M, et al: Vertebral artery stenting following percutaneous transluminal angioplasty. Technical note. J Neurosurg 84:883–887, 1996.

40. Vitek JJ: Subclavian artery angioplasty and the origin of the vertebral artery. Radiology 170:407–409, 1989.

41. Zeumer H: Vascular recanalizing techniques in interventional neuroradiology. J Neurol 231:287–291, 1985.

42. Volk EE, Prayson RA, Perl J II: Autopsy findings of fatal complication of posterior cerebral circulation angioplasty. Arch Pathol Lab Med 121:738–740, 1997.

43. Naylor AR, Bolia A, Abbott RJ, et al: Randomized study of carotid angioplasty and stenting versus carotid endarterectomy: A stopped trial. J Vasc Surg 28:326–334, 1998.

44. European Carotid Surgery Trialists' Collaborative Group. Randomised trial of endarterectomy for recently symptomatic carotid stenosis: Final results of the MRC European Carotid Surgery Trial (ECST). Lancet 351:1379–1387, 1998.

45. Halliday AW: The Asymptomatic Carotid Surgery Trial (ACST); rationale and design. Eur J Vasc Surg 8:703–710, 1994.

46. Hertzer NR, Loop FD, Beven EG, et al: Surgical staging for simultaneous coronary and carotid disease: A study including prospective randomisation. J Vasc Surg 9:455–63, 1989.

47. Berguer R, Kieffer E: Surgery of the arteries to the head. New York: Springer Verlag, 1992.

48. Brown MM, Gaines PA, Buckenham T: The carotid and vertebral artery transluminal angioplasty study (CAVATAS). Lancet (in press).

49. Bettmann MA, Katzen BT, Whisnant J, et al: Carotid stenting and angioplasty. A statement for healthcare professionals from the Councils on Cardiovascular Radiology, Stroke, Cardiothoracic and Vascular Surgery, Epidemiology and Prevention and Clinical Cardiology, American Heart Association. Circulation 97:121–123, 1998.

50. Latimer CR, Burnand KG: Recurrent carotid stenosis after carotid endarterectomy. Br J Surg 84:1206–1219, 1997.

51. Ackerstaff RGA, Janson C, Moll FL: The significance of microemboli detection by means of transcranial Doppler ultrasonography monitoring in carotid endarterectomy. Vasc Surg 21:963–970, 1995.

52. Biasi GM, Mingazzi PM: Should the type of carotid plaque determine the carotid procedure: Conventional or endovascular? *In* Greenhalgh RM (ed): Indications in Vascular and Endovascular Surgery. London, WB Saunders, 1998, pp 73–79.

53. Forsell C, Bergqvist D, Bergenz SE: Peripheral nerve injuries in carotid artery surgery. *In* Greenhalgh RM, Hollier LH (eds): Surgery for Stroke. London, WB Saunders, 1993, pp 217–234.

54. Jordan WD, Roye GD, Fisher WS, et al: A cost comparison of balloon angioplasty and stenting versus endarterectomy for the treatment of carotid artery stenosis. J Vasc Surg 27:16–22, 1998.

55. Yadav JS, Roubin GS, King P, et al: Angioplasty and stenting for restenosis after carotid endarterectomy. Stroke 27:2075–2079, 1996.

56. Tanganakul G, Counsell CE, Warlow CP: Local versus general anaesthesia in carotid endarterectomy: A systematic review of the evidence. Eur J Vasc Endovasc Surg 13:491–499, 1997.

Chapter 16 Peroperative Transluminal Angioplasty

Surgical Contributors: Brian F. Johnson and Alan R. Wilkinson

In the treatment of vascular occlusive disease, the development of percutaneous transluminal balloon angioplasty using local anesthesia for short stenoses and occlusions has proved a successful alternative to surgical bypass, which is reserved for the treatment of longer segments of arterial disease. Therefore, the treatment of arterial disease requires skills traditionally developed in the separate disciplines of vascular surgery and interventional radiology.

The combination of transluminal balloon angioplasty at the time of an open surgical approach to the arterial tree is used mainly in the treatment of occlusive peripheral vascular disease.[1-5] The combination of these two complementary techniques in a single procedure is the focus of this chapter.

INDICATIONS

The clinical indications for peroperative transluminal angioplasty are similar to those for all vascular interventions and range from severe claudication to limb-threatening ischemia.

When tandem lesions are present at two or more levels, one of which requires a surgical approach, then peroperative angioplasty may be considered. Most commonly, peroperative angioplasty is used to improve the inflow above an infrainguinal reconstruction, whether it is a femorofemoral crossover graft, a common femoral patch graft, or a femorodistal graft. In these patterns of the disease, avoiding a suprainguinal operation to increase the flow at the common femoral level reduces the surgical trauma considerably. Occasionally, transluminal balloon angioplasty of an outflow tract is used, either of the superficial femoral artery after aortobifemoral grafting or femorofemoral popliteal bypass grafting.[1-5] Although the latter is regarded as inferior to bypassing the whole segment of the diseased artery, using the patient's own vein, on occasions there is not sufficient vein either from the arm or leg to act as a conduit from the reasonably good artery to a reasonably good artery below the level of the disease. In these circumstances, using a segment of vein to overcome a more severely diseased section of the arterial tree with more distal angioplasty may be preferable to using prosthetic material. Combined disease in the aortoiliac system and in the infrainguinal arterial tree is present in 70% of patients with critical ischemia, whereas only 20% of patients with claudication have multilevel disease.[6, 7] In critical ischemia, rapid restoration of a good blood supply is necessary for pain relief and the healing of ulceration or distal amputations after the removal of necrotic material.

Another consideration for the combination of surgical bypass with peroperative angioplasty is the fitness of the patient. Almost all patients have one or more medical risk factors, including ischemic heart disease, hypertension, diabetes mellitus, chronic obstructive airway disease, obesity, and habitual tobacco smoking.[1, 3, 6] Peroperative angioplasty reduces the operating time, blood loss, and postoperative morbidity compared with surgical correction of both proximal and more distal lesions.

A further indication for peroperative angioplasty is to avoid a consecutive surgical bypass. Percutaneous angioplasty results in hematoma formation, which distorts the tissue planes and potentially increases the risk of infection in a subsequent surgical procedure. Later, after a few weeks, the scarring produced as the hematoma is organized makes surgical dissection difficult. The peroperative procedure obviates these risks.

The enthusiasm to treat every case of multilevel arterial disease by a combination of peroperative angioplasty and surgical bypass must be tempered by the knowledge that the proximal revascularization resolves the indications for a distal procedure in 66 to 90% of patients.[2, 7] However, this means that up to one third of patients will be subject to a further operative procedure with its additional risks, both surgical and anesthetic, in addition to the possibility of disease progression in an already threatened limb.

The principal advantage of peroperative angioplasty, however, lies in the ability to treat disease at more than one site. This may involve dilatation of an "inflow" stenosis of an iliac artery proximal to an infrainguinal surgical reconstruction[1-5] or the dilatation of a distal stenosis before proximal surgical reconstruction.[1, 8]

In addition to the treatment of tandem lesions, some groups have applied an "open groin" approach to arterial puncture for the treatment of single-level stenosing or occlusive disease when there was actual or anticipated difficulty with percutaneous access.[4, 5, 8] In these predominantly surgical series, one third to one half of peroperative angioplasties were performed because of difficult percutaneous access.[4, 5]

Peroperative angioplasty need not be confined only to the elective situation. When an underlying stenosis is found on completion angiography during emergency surgical thrombectomy, peroperative transluminal angioplasty may be employed to correct the lesion.

APPLICATION

Peroperative transluminal balloon angioplasty implies that a surgical incision is made to gain access to the vascular system, usually in the operating room (as opposed to the angiography suite). This approach requires that special equipment, which typically is not present, must be available in the operating room, including an x-ray lucent operating table with facility for imaging without interruption, for example, by nonlucent crossbeams, from the upper abdominal aorta to the pedal arch arteries. The availability of a modern, high-quality, portable C-arm fluoroscopy unit with digital subtraction imaging and "roadmapping" facilities is advantageous when performing this type of surgery, as is a variety of sheaths, guide wires, and angiography and balloon angioplasty catheters. Operating room sterility is usually of a higher standard than that which is available in a conventional radiology suite and must be strictly adhered to, especially when a prosthetic vascular graft is to be used.[1]

The angioplasty may be performed by a radiologist or by a surgeon trained in the technique, either by direct puncture of the femoral artery after exposure, thereby allowing pressure measurements to be taken both before and after the procedure, or by passage of a guide wire, sheath, and balloon angioplasty catheter through the arteriotomy, which later is used for anastomosis. The artery can be controlled with silastic loops, minimizing blood loss. Angioplasty or stenting then is performed under radiologic control, and completion angiogram with pressure measurements confirms a satisfactory outcome before completion of the surgical procedure.

OUTCOME

Assessment of the technical outcome of the angioplasty, in addition to that of the surgical procedure, is important. When the procedures are staged, success may be gauged by not only the final angiographic result but also by improvement in the clinical features, including pulse palpation and noninvasive assessment such as ankle-brachial pressure assessment.[2] For peroperative angioplasty, treatment of proximal lesions, in which the catheter is passed retrogradely, pull-through arterial pressure measurements allow the demonstration of a pressure decrease across the lesion, and abolition of a pressure gradient after angioplasty is extremely reassuring.[2, 3] For distal lesions in infrainguinal runoff vessels, there is a greater reliance on completion angiography for the assessment of success.

Published reports of peroperative angioplasty vary in their presentation of results. When only technically successful iliac angioplasties were considered, the 5-year primary patency rate of the distal surgical bypass was 76%, with a secondary patency rate of 88% and a limb salvage rate of 90%.[1] Graft patency rate in the series reported by van der Vliet and associates, which included vein and prosthetic femoropopliteal reconstructions and a mixture of common and external iliac angioplasties, was 100% at 1 year, 88% at 2 years, and 67% at 5 years.[3] Alimi and colleagues studied the patency of the iliac angioplasty site in 19 patients whose distal procedures included femorofemoral crossover (n = 4), ipsilateral femoropopliteal (n = 5), or tibial (n = 3) bypass or ipsilateral deep or common femoral reconstruction (n = 7); after a mean follow-up period of 20 months, a cumulative patency rate of 88% was reported.[5] In the femoropopliteal segment, duplex assessment, which is technically easier than in the iliac arteries, revealed a primary success rate (including technical failures) that was inferior to iliac angioplasty with cumulative patency rates of 78% at 1 month, 60% at 1 year, and 51% at 2 years.[8] Factors that are known to be associated with improved outcome after angioplasty include: claudication vs. limb salvage as the initial indication for treatment, dilatation of the common iliac artery vs. all other angioplasty sites, treatment of stenosis vs. an occlusion of the artery, and good runoff vs. poor runoff beyond the angioplasty site.[9] For femoropopliteal angioplasty alone, the primary patency rate was 80% in patients with stenosis less than 2 cm long, 62% for stenosis greater than 2 cm long, 42% with occlusion less than 2 cm long, and 20% for occlusions greater than 2 cm long.[8]

The initial clinical response to peroperative angioplasty and surgical reconstruction falls short of the technical success rate, with approximately 90% of patients reporting marked or moderate improvement of preoperative symptoms.[2, 3]

COMPLICATIONS

Complications of peroperative transluminal angioplasty can be of a general nature because of the surgical risk of the patient, including myocardial infarction and death, or specific to the local effects of treatment, including acute arterial thrombosis or dissection, rupture of the angioplasty balloon or rupture of the artery that has undergone angioplasty, and periarterial hematoma or false aneurysm formation.

In the series surveyed, mortality of peroperative angioplasty was 0 of 3 in Boston, 1 of 103 in Paris, 0 of 17 in Nijmegen, and 1 of 19 in Marseille, for a combined mortality of 2 of 142 (1.4%).[2, 3, 5, 8] Gross and associates did not report their specific complication rate for peroperative angioplasty, but the overall mortality for lower limb endovascular procedures was 5 of 325 (1.5%).[4] If peroperative angioplasty is to be performed in the emergency situation, the increased mortality associated with this presentation will be reflected in the outcome.

One of the perceived advantages of peroperative angioplasty is the reduction of the occurrence of some local complications associated with the percutaneous technique. Thus, false aneurysms associated with needle puncture do not occur, and arterial thrombosis, dissection, embolization, and rupture may be dealt with expeditiously, if recognized during surgery. Complications specific to the procedure may be divided into early and late categories.

Early complications are rare for peroperative iliac angioplasties. Hematomas, wound infections, lymph leaks, and arteriovenous fistulas are recorded but remain extremely uncommon. One patient with iliac thrombosis who did not respond to catheter thrombectomy required simultaneous aortofemoral and femoropopliteal bypass.[2] The risk of contrast-induced renal dysfunction should not be forgotten, but it is uncommon and usually resolves spontaneously. Peroperative infrainguinal angioplasty is associated with a higher complication rate, and 22 of 103 (21%) early failures were reported in one large series, but only 3 required immediate femoropopliteal bypass grafts.[8]

Late complications usually relate to restenosis. For proximal angioplasty, this is found most commonly after external iliac angioplasty.[9] Frequently, this is associated with graft thrombosis, although recurrent symptoms have been reported.[2] In one study distal angioplasty is associated with a relatively high frequency of late failures, with 17 (16%) having either restenosis or occlusion after a mean of 10 months.[8] The specter of graft infection occurred in one report, when sepsis of a femoral crossover graft developed 7 months after surgery, necessitating removal of the graft and performance of a contralateral axillofemoral graft.[5]

CONCLUSIONS

Peroperative angioplasty can be performed with good results, especially when there is focal disease either in the inflow or outflow vessels at the proposed site of a surgical bypass, which would preclude a simple operative approach. Not only can the treatment of multilevel arterial disease be facilitated, but some of the complications of the percutaneous approach can be avoided. We recommend a team approach for peroperative angioplasty in the belief that the cooperation of specialists with training in the disciplines of both vascular surgery and interventional radiology maximizes the chance of a beneficial outcome for the patient.

Intraoperative balloon angioplasty is an important therapeutic option with which all doctors who treat patients with arterial disease should be familiar.

REFERENCES

1. Ahn SS, Concepcion B: Endovascular surgery. *In* Moore WS (ed): Vascular Surgery: A Comprehensive Review, 5th ed. Philadelphia, WB Saunders, 1997, pp 305–329.
2. Brewster DC, Cambria RP, Darling RC, et al: Long-term results of combined iliac balloon angioplasty and distal surgical revascularisation. Ann Surg 210:324, 1989.
3. van der Vliet JA, Mulling FJ, Heijstraten FMJ, et al: Femoropopliteal arterial reconstruction with intraoperative iliac transluminal angioplasty for disabling claudication: Results of a combined approach. Eur J Vasc Surg 6:607, 1992.
4. Gross GM, Johnson RC, Roberts RM: Results of peripheral endovascular procedures in the operating room. J Vasc Surg 24:353–361, 1996.
5. Alimi Y, di Mauro P, Barthelemy P, et al: Iliac transluminal angioplasty and distal surgical revascularisation can be performed in a one-step technique. Int Angiol 16:83, 1997.
6. Parker BC, Bandyk DF, Mills JL, et al: Clinical evaluation of occlusive peripheral vascular disease. *In* Strandness DE, vanBreda A (eds): Vascular Diseases: Surgical and Interventional Therapy. New York, Churchill Livingstone, 1994, pp 423–431.
7. Horowitz JD, Durham JR: Surgical management of aortoiliac occlusive disease. *In* Strandness DE, vanBreda A (eds). Vascular Diseases: Surgical and Interventional Therapy. New York, Churchill Livingstone, 1994, pp 467–478.
8. Becquemin JP, Cavillon A, Haiduc F: Surgical transluminal femoropopliteal angioplasty: Multivariate analysis outcome. J Vasc Surg 19:495, 1994.
9. Johnston KW, Rae M, Hogg-Johnston SA, et al: Five-year results of a prospective study of percutaneous transluminal angioplasty. Ann Surg 206:403, 1987.

Section 3

Venous Interventions

Chapter 17 Lower Limb Venous Interventions

Endovascular Contributor: Charles P. Semba
Surgical Contributors: Ian Galloway and Jonathan J. Earnshaw

Endovascular therapy for lower extremity venous obstruction is emerging as a viable alternative to anticoagulation in selected patients with acute and chronic deep vein thrombosis (DVT). Although the standard of care for DVT remains centered on heparin and warfarin therapy, there is growing evidence to support early intervention with thrombolysis to preserve valve function and restore patency of the vein. This chapter provides an overview on the endovascular techniques for the treatment of acute and chronic lower extremity DVT.

DEEP VEIN THROMBOSIS: PROBLEM WITH CURRENT MANAGEMENT STRATEGIES

Deep vein thrombosis remains a common cause of morbidity in the United States, with approximately 300,000 new cases annually.[1] The standard of care remains anticoagulation, with supportive measures including leg elevation, compression stockings, and bed rest. Systemic anticoagulation traditionally involves unfractionated intravenous heparin therapy until the patient is therapeutically anticoagulated using oral warfarin and requires several days of hospitalization. The recent introduction of subcutaneously administered low molecular weight heparin (LMWH) compounds offers significant pharmacoeconomic advantages over unfractionated heparin because there is no need for hospitalization and no laboratory values to measure.[2] Despite the availability of LMWH, the overall goals toward approaching DVT have not changed—the purpose of systemic anticoagulation is to prevent thrombus propagation, reduce the risk of recurrent DVT, and decrease the risk of pulmonary emboli. Three major problems exist with current management strategies: (1) anticoagulation is ineffective in actively removing acute thrombus; (2) treatment algorithms are based solely on the presence or absence of thrombus, without consideration to the extent and length of the involved venous segment; and (3) treatment of an underlying anatomic problem within the vein is underappreciated.

Anticoagulation is ineffective in removing acute thrombus. Although anticoagulation remains the cornerstone of DVT therapy, neither unfractionated heparin, LMWH, or sodium warfarin enzymatically breaks down thrombus. Restoration of patency of the occluded vessel is dependent solely on the endogenous fibrinolytic capacity of the involved venous segment. Based on our 6-year clinical experience in treating patients with DVT, spontaneous recanalization of large diameter veins (>10 mm) seldom, if ever, occurs when anticoagulants alone are used. If the vein does recanalize spontaneously, the venous lumen often is obstructed partially by synechiae and fibrous tissue and probably contributes to the increased risk of recurrent DVT in these patients. Only 10% of patients have spontaneous lysis of their DVT within 10 days of heparin therapy, and up to 40% of patients continue to have propagation of thrombus despite treatment with heparin.[3, 4]

All types of DVT are treated the same despite differences in long-term outcome. The decision to treat DVT with anticoagulants is based primarily on sonographic detection of thrombus in the deep veins, and the workup is essentially a binary process: patients with documented DVT receive anticoagulation; patients with a negative ultrasound study are evaluated for other causes of leg pain and swelling. The problem with binary methodology is that no distinctions are made in treating patients with small thrombus volumes and relatively good clinical outcomes, for example, isolated popliteal DVT, vs. patients with extensive thrombosis (iliofemoral thrombosis) and at high risk of long-term morbidity. There are several studies demonstrating that iliofemoral DVT in particular is associated with the highest risk in the development of postphlebitic syndrome (PPS). PPS is a constellation of clinical findings, including chronic leg edema, pain, hyperpigmentation, venous claudication, and in advanced cases, venous stasis ulcers. PPS is caused by chronic ambulatory venous hypertension from either venous outflow obstruction, valvular incompetence, or both.[5] Long-term studies over 5- and 10-year periods have shown that despite adequate long-term anticoagulation, in 50% of patients with iliofemoral DVT, venous claudication and significant occupational disability developed from their venous disease, venous stasis ulcers developed in 88%, 95% lost valvular competency, and all patients had chronic leg edema.[6, 7] Although it initially may appear that the use of LMWH agents is more cost-effective in the initial treatment of DVT, the long-term socioeconomic consequences of managing the late sequelae of extensive lower extremity DVT often are neglected.

Anatomic abnormalities of the iliac vein are a frequent cause of iliofemoral thrombosis. Traditional concepts on the etiology of lower extremity DVT describe the pathogenesis of thrombus arising in the soleal sinuses and ascending into the popliteal and femoral veins. However, since the advent of catheter-directed thrombolysis, it has been our observation that iliofemoral DVT behaves differently and that most of these patients have an underlying stenosis of the iliac vein and subsequent downward propagation of thrombus.[8] The high incidence of an iliac vein stenosis previously has been unappreciated because most patients historically have received only anticoagulation and no attempts have been made to lyse the thrombus and "unmask" possible venous lesions.

SYSTEMIC THROMBOLYTIC THERAPY VS. ANTICOAGULATION IN ACUTE DEEP VEIN THROMBOSIS

There is abundant clinical evidence to demonstrate that systemic infusion of thrombolytic agents through a peripheral intravenous line in the antecubital vein has significant advantages over standard unfractionated heparin. A meta-analysis of 13 clinical trials involving more than 600 patients comparing systemic streptokinase vs. heparin demonstrated the clinical benefits of lytic therapy compared with heparin alone.[9] In lower extremity DVT, the streptokinase treatment group had a complete thrombolysis rate of 45% vs. 4% for the heparin-only group. However, in long-segment iliofemoral DVT, systemic lytic infusions tended to be ineffective, presumably because of the inability of the agent to bind directly to the surface of the thrombus in the occluded vein and dispersal of the agent through collateral pathways instead.[10]

There are four thrombolytic agents that are currently available in the United States: streptokinase, alteplase, reteplase, and urokinase. All four agents directly or indirectly convert plasminogen into plasmin. Plasmin binds to fibrin and enzymatically breaks it apart, causing the thrombus to dissolve (see Chapter 3).[11–13]

CATHETER-DIRECTED THROMBOLYSIS FOR ILIOFEMORAL DEEP VEIN THROMBOSIS

Rationale

Although systemic infusion of thrombolytic agents can improve the resolution of DVT better than standard heparin therapy, administration of the lytic agent through a peripheral arm vein is inefficient. Catheter-directed thrombolysis has been the standard approach in treating a wide variety of arterial thrombotic and embolic ischemic occlusions for the past two decades. Delivering urokinase or another lytic agent directly into the thrombus using a catheter improves the efficiency of drug delivery, decreases the total quantity of urokinase required, and provides venous access for adjunctive techniques such as angioplasty and stent placement. The goals of catheter-based therapy are to rapidly restore patency to the occluded vein, to preserve valve function, and to detect and treat underlying venous stenoses.[14, 15]

Acute Iliofemoral Deep Vein Thrombosis: Indications for Treatment

Patients enrolled into our protocol must have symptomatic acute iliofemoral DVT (≤10 days) or phlegmasia that is documented by conventional venography or color Doppler ultrasound of the lower extremities (Fig. 17–1). Patients must be eligible for thrombolytic therapy and anticoagulation; contraindications include active internal bleeding, history of a cerebrovascular accident, recent (within 12 months) intracranial or intraspinal surgery, pregnancy, and/or coagulopathy. Patients are usually otherwise healthy and active, with a normal life expectancy. Inferior vena cava filters are placed only if the patient has had recurrent pulmonary emboli despite anticoagulation or has a true "free-floating" thrombus identified in the iliac veins or inferior vena cava. If patients are therapeutically anticoagulated (international normalized ratio [INR] 2.0–3.0) using warfarin, we usually do not reverse their anticoagulation status. This allows us to discharge the patient after the completion of our procedure without the need for additional hospitalization.

Technique

After placement of a Foley urinary bladder catheter, the patient is positioned prone on the angiography table, and the popliteal fossa is prepared. Catheterization of the popliteal vein is performed with a 5 French

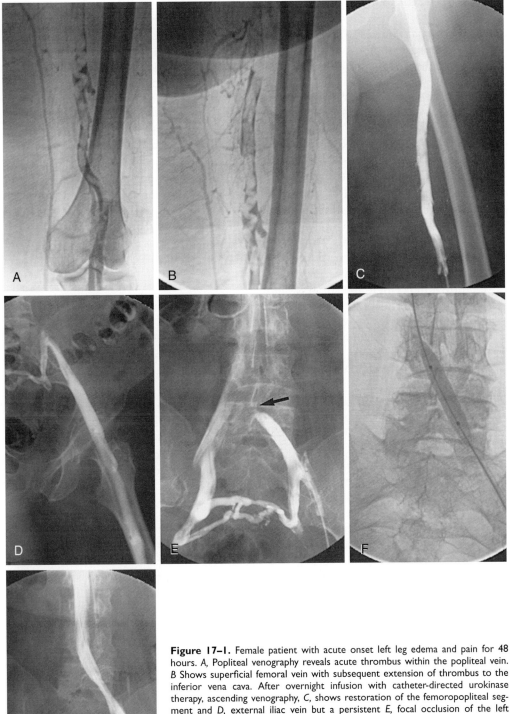

Figure 17–1. Female patient with acute onset left leg edema and pain for 48 hours. *A,* Popliteal venography reveals acute thrombus within the popliteal vein. *B* Shows superficial femoral vein with subsequent extension of thrombus to the inferior vena cava. After overnight infusion with catheter-directed urokinase therapy, ascending venography, *C,* shows restoration of the femoropopliteal segment and *D,* external iliac vein but a persistent *E,* focal occlusion of the left common iliac vein (*arrow*) caused by compression by the overriding iliac artery. The occlusion was treated using *F,* balloon angioplasty followed by stent placement to restore *G,* continuity of venous outflow. Patient remains asymptomatic at 2-year follow-up with no recurrent thrombosis or residual leg edema.

microaccess set under ultrasound guidance using a 21-gauge needle and an 0.018-inch diameter guide wire, with care taken to perform a single wall puncture and avoid the popliteal artery. If there is extensive calf vein and popliteal thrombus, the posterior tibial vein can be used instead.[16] After ascending venography through the 5-French dilator, a 6-French sidearm sheath is inserted over a 0.035-inch hydrophilic guide wire, and a 5-French hydrophilic end-hole catheter is used to negotiate the wire into the inferior vena cava. After removal of the end-hole catheter, a 5-French, 65-cm multiside-hole, valve-tipped infusion catheter is embedded in the thrombus. Urokinase is administered in split doses of 80,000 IU/hour through both the sidearm of the popliteal sheath and the multiside-hole infusion catheter (total infusion dose, 160,000 IU/hour). Patients are anticoagulated systemically with heparin after a preliminary bolus of 5000 units. Overnight monitoring occurs in a coronary step-down unit where the support staff are familiar with managing indwelling vascular lines and anticoagulation regimens. Fibrinogen and partial thromboplastin times (PTTs) are obtained at 4 and 24 hours after the start of therapy. The fibrinogen is maintained above 100 mg/dl, and the desired PTT range is 60 to 90 seconds. On the evening of the first hospital day, patients receive a 10-mg loading dose of warfarin. For patients already therapeutically anticoagulated with warfarin, we do not use additional systemic intravenous heparin.

After overnight thrombolytic infusion with urokinase, venography is performed the next day in the angiography suite. The Stanford algorithm is as follows: (1) if there is complete thrombolysis and no underlying stenosis, no further intervention is required; 2) if there is complete thrombolysis and an underlying iliac vein stenosis, angioplasty followed by endovascular stent placement is performed; 3) if there is complete thrombolysis and an underlying femoral vein stenosis, angioplasty is performed only; 4) if there is partial thrombolysis, urokinase infusion is continued for 1 additional night; and 5) if there is no thrombolysis of the iliac and femoral vein, the case is considered a technical failure and no further intervention is performed because the thrombus is too organized. All patients are placed on warfarin therapy for a minimum of 6 months (INR 2.0–3.0) after completion of the procedure.

In most cases (70%), a residual obstructive lesion within the iliac vein is identified after complete or partial thrombolysis. These lesions rarely respond to angioplasty alone, and a stent is required to reconstruct the vein. In general, we prefer to use the large diameter (10–16 mm) Wallstents because of their longitudinal flexibility and ability to accommodate the curvature of the iliac vein. After predilation using an 8- or 10-mm angioplasty balloon, the iliac vein is stented from the popliteal approach. For the common iliac vein, the Wallstent (12–16 mm) initially is deployed partially in the inferior vena cava until 50% of the device is unsheathed. Under fluoroscopic control, the Wallstent delivery catheter is gently pulled inferiorly to allow the distal end of the stent to align with the orifice of the iliocaval junction. The stent then is fully deployed and dilated using the appropriate diameter balloon. We do not advocate stent placement in the superficial femoral or popliteal veins. The overall role of mechanical thrombectomy devices is not well defined. We usually reserve the use of these devices to dissolute any remaining small thrombus fragments after a course of urokinase therapy.

Follow-up is performed using Doppler evaluation immediately postprocedure, at 3, 6, and 12 months, and annually thereafter.

ILIAC VEIN COMPRESSION SYNDROME

Iliofemoral DVT is three to five times more common in the left leg than the right because of compression of the left common iliac vein by the overlying right common iliac artery, known as "May–Thurner" or "Cockett's" or "iliac vein compression" syndrome (Fig. 17–2). Despite renewed interest in this syndrome, the anatomic phenomenon was described first by Rudolf Virchow in 1851.[17] Based on the clinical experience of lower extremity venous thrombolysis at

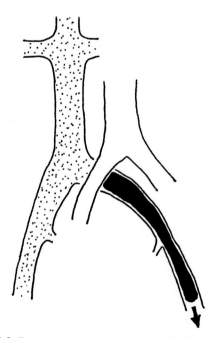

Figure 17–2. Iliac vein compression syndrome. The right common iliac artery crosses anteriorly to the left common iliac vein and can lead to venous compression, stasis, and subsequent "downward" propagation of thrombus.

Stanford, it is our contention that iliac vein compression syndrome is a common entity and a major cause of left lower extremity iliofemoral DVT and highly suited for treatment with endovascular methods. An overview of iliac vein compression syndrome is essential because it is highly likely that interventionalists will encounter this disorder in practice.

Historical Background

1851—Virchow[17] observes that pelvic vein thrombosis occurs five times more frequently on the left than the right and postulates that the artery resting on the vein leads to venous obstruction.

1908—McMurrich[18] first describes spur-like projections in the iliac vein and proposes that these were congenital anomalies.

1943—Krumbhaar and Ehrich[19] describe spur-like projections in the left iliac vein in fetuses and further advocate a congenital etiology; however, no other group was able to confirm their findings.

1957—May and Thurner[20] describe their findings in 430 cadavers, including 88 fetuses, and describe three types of "spurs" within the iliac vein: (1) lateral spur, (2) central spur, and (3) partial obliteration. The spurs were eight times more likely in the left iliac vein (vs. right) and found in 22% of cases. No evidence could be found for congenital iliac "spurs."

1965—Cockett and Thomas[21] note that iliofemoral deep vein thrombosis tends to be predisposed to the left leg and call the anatomic entity "iliac vein compression syndrome." Four variants of compression are described. Cross-saphenous bypass surgery is proposed as a solution to relieving the venous outflow obstruction.

1983—Ferris and associates[22] describe May–Thurner syndrome in the radiologic literature as a cause of chronic leg edema (due to obstructive venous hypertension).

1991—Okrent[23] describes thrombolytic therapy and angioplasty for treating an acutely thrombosed left common iliac vein.

1994—Catheter-directed thrombolysis and endovascular stents are proposed for treating iliofemoral deep venous thrombosis and iliac vein compression syndrome.[14]

Although some investigators argue that May–Thurner syndrome and Cockett's syndrome are two different entities, it is our opinion that they represent the same pathologic process—obstruction of the vein by arterial compression, which eventually leads to venous stenosis or thrombosis of the iliac vein. The "spurs" described by May and Thurner probably are the result of intimal hyperplasia caused by direct wall contact of the anterior and posterior surfaces of the vein and subsequent formation of endothelial tissue bridges. The normal histology of the intima and media of the vein is replaced largely by well-organized connective tissue covered with endothelium, which tends to support the concept that these synechiae or "spurs" result from compression with secondary irritation and tissue reaction from chronic pulsatile trauma to the vein. Surgeons have described a dense fibrotic reaction that tends to enshroud both the artery and vein at the point of contact. Cockett[21] was able to identify at least four patterns of arterial compression, and others have since described variations: type I—the most common (80%): compression of the left common iliac vein by the right common iliac artery (see Fig. 17–2); type II—compression of the distal cava by the aortic bifurcation (Fig. 17–3 *A*); type III—compression of the right external iliac vein by the right iliac artery (see Fig. 17–3 *B*); type IV—compression of the left external iliac vein by the iliac artery at the inguinal ligament (see Fig. 17–3 *C*); type V—compression of the left common iliac vein by the left internal iliac artery[24]; and type VI—compression of the left common iliac vein by a tortuous left common iliac artery.[25]

Clinical and Angiographic Findings of Iliac Vein Compression Syndrome

Review of the surgical and radiologic literature reveals that these patients tend to be young, postpartum

Figure 17–3. Variants of iliac vein compression syndrome.

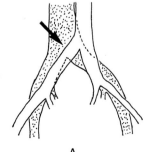
A

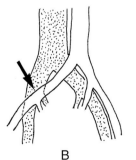
B

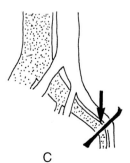
C

females who complain of persistent left leg edema due to either chronic venous outflow obstruction from compression-related iliac vein stenosis or subsequent iliofemoral DVT. Other findings include hyperpigmentation, superficial venous collaterals, cyanosis, venous ulcers, and a history of venous claudication. In a summation of several clinical reports, there were 128 patients who underwent treatment for iliac vein compression syndrome (IVCS)[26]; 69.5% of the patients were female, and the average age was 35.5 years.

The diagnosis should be suspected with a young, otherwise healthy patient who presents with chronic left-leg edema with or without a history of iliofemoral DVT or a patient who presents with an acute left-sided iliac vein thrombosis. Typically, these patients remain symptomatic despite conservative management (anticoagulation, venous stockings, leg elevation). Duplex venography or another noninvasive examination such as magnetic resonance angiography can confirm the presence of thrombus and assess iliac vein patency. We usually reserve venography with the intent to treat and do not use it solely for diagnostic purposes.

Pelvic venography usually demonstrates a focally stenotic common left iliac vein resulting from external compression with abundant left-to-right presacral venous collaterals and hypertrophied ascending paralumbar veins. In our practice, many patients present with an acute left-sided iliofemoral DVT, and the underlying stenosis is not revealed until after catheter-directed thrombolysis. The natural impression of the iliac artery on the left iliac vein can be seen in asymptomatic patients; however, in our experience, most symptomatic patients demonstrate collateral venous pathways. Cockett[27] proposed that a difference in left vs. right external iliac vein pressures greater than 2 mm Hg is a sign of clinically significant obstruction.[27] We have not found pressures measurements to be entirely helpful, and at times, they are unreliable because the patient is supine.

Surgical Approach Toward Treatment of Iliac Vein Compression Syndrome

The optimal surgical treatment for IVCS remains controversial, with mixed results. Several types of operative repairs have been described to treat IVCS. Cockett and Thomas used a cross-femoral venous bypass using the contralateral saphenous vein (Palma procedure),[21] but long-term results were poor. Others proposed dissecting the iliac artery off the vein followed by venotomy and placing the vein over the artery, whereas other surgeons created a sling around the iliac artery by using fascia to suspend the vessel and prevent it from reobstructing the vein,[28] suspending the artery over the vein using a silastic bridge,[29] or

wrapping the vein in reinforced polytetrafluoroethylene (PTPE) to prevent arterial compression.[30] Use of reinforced PTFE grafts to bypass the venous occlusion combined with small arteriovenous fistulas has been used successfully with success[31]; however, there is emerging support for simply dividing the artery and placing it underneath the iliac vein and joining the artery end to end with or without an interposition graft.[32] With acute iliofemoral thrombosis, surgical thrombectomy combined with temporary creation of an arteriovenous fistula has been proposed for patients who are not candidates for anticoagulation or thrombolytic therapy.[33]

Endovascular Approach Toward Treatment of Iliac Vein Compression Syndrome

The endovascular approach toward managing IVCS has several advantages: (1) diagnostic venography allows for direct assessment of the degree of venous obstruction and collateralization; (2) intravenous synechiae and webs can be disrupted using angioplasty; (3) large acute thrombus burdens can be cleared using catheter-directed thrombolysis; and (4) the compressed iliac vein can be stented safely without apparent long-term harm to the overriding artery and recreate a smooth lumen. There is a rapidly evolving body of clinical experience worldwide using endovascular techniques with good initial and mid-term success, but long-term studies are not available. Thus, IVCS is a common problem and should be suspected in a young female patient who presents with a spontaneous left-sided iliofemoral DVT. Although several surgical strategies exist, we propose that endovascular techniques eventually will prove to be the optimal treatment strategy in most of these patients.

CHRONIC ILIAC VEIN OCCLUSION

Isolated chronic iliac vein occlusion can be a late sequelae of iliofemoral DVT in which the femoropopliteal segment recanalizes but the iliac outflow vessels remain thrombosed. Clinically, these patients often present with a history of iliofemoral DVT months to years earlier and remain symptomatic despite long-term anticoagulation and supportive therapy. Symptoms usually consist of leg edema and pain, which tend to be exacerbated with moderate activity (venous claudication). Most of these individuals in our practice have competent venous valves but are symptomatic from a chronic venous outflow obstruction.

Indications for Treatment

Endovascular techniques can be used to reconstruct the iliac vein and relieve the outflow obstruction. Most patients already are therapeutically anticoagulated with warfarin and have documented Doppler or venographic evidence of a patent femoropopliteal system and iliac vein occlusion. Indications for treatment include patients with a history and physical findings consistent with venous hypertension and active lifestyles limited by venous claudication. For isolated iliac vein occlusions greater than 6 weeks in duration, we usually do not use antecedent thrombolytic therapy, nor do we reverse their anticoagulation status.

Technique

After placement of a Foley bladder catheter, the patient is positioned prone on the angiography table, and the popliteal fossa is prepared. After access into the popliteal vein using ultrasound guidance and a micropuncture set, ascending venography is performed to document patency of the femoropopliteal segment and to define the iliac vein occlusion and collateral pathways (Fig. 17–4). After placement of a 6-French sidearm sheath into the popliteal vein, the iliac vein occlusion is probed using a stiff hydrophilic guide wire in combination with an angle-tapered end-hole 5-French hydrophilic catheter. The wire is negotiated through the occluded vein and passed into the inferior vena cava. Dilation of the occluded iliac segment is performed using a 6- or 8-mm diameter angioplasty balloon to break apart the organized synechiae and fibrotic tissue within the lumen. Wallstents are used to reconstruct the entire venous outflow as discussed previously, starting with the common iliac segment using a 12- to 16-mm diameter device. A second Wallstent is required to cover the external iliac vein into the common femoral segment. Typically, we use a 10- to 12-mm diameter stent and provide approximately 2 to 3 mm of overlap with the initially deployed Wallstent. Stent placement at the common femoral vein usually terminates between the level of the mid-femoral head to the level of the lesser trochanter. Despite concerns about stenting across the inguinal ligament, we have not had any delayed sequelae from stent placement at the groin. The completed ascending venogram from the popliteal sheath should demonstrate direct "in-line" flow with significantly reduced opacification of large collateral veins and no stasis or puddling of contrast. Follow-up is performed using Doppler evaluation immediately postprocedure, at 3, 6, and 12 months, and annually thereafter. We recommend warfarin therapy with an INR between 2.0 and 3.0 for at least 3 to 6 months poststenting.

RESULTS

Based on the clinical experience at Stanford, the overall technical success rates are 90% in treating acute iliofemoral thrombosis and isolated chronic iliac vein occlusions. Endovascular stents for the treatment of underlying iliac lesions are required in 70% of the thrombolysis cases and all cases of chronic isolated iliac vein occlusions. Iliac vein stent patency rate at 12 months for all patients is 93% based on follow-up serial Doppler studies. The success of catheter-directed thrombolysis is correlated directly with duration of the patient's symptomatology. Patients with complete lysis tend to present within the first 7 to 10 days, those with partial lysis present within 4 weeks, and no significant lysis is generally seen in patients with symptoms of greater than 4 weeks duration. Valve competency at 12 months is preserved in 91% of patients who received lytic therapy. Almost all patients report symptomatic improvement with decreased edema and leg pain after successful restoration of flow in the deep system. Although we encourage the use of graded compression hose after endovascular therapy, patient compliance is often low because of the cosmetic appearance of the appliance and general discomfort.

COMPLICATIONS

Complications include access site hematomas, bleeding complications, and acute thrombosis of the treated segment. The overall minor complication rate is approximately 3%, and there have been no instances of cerebrovascular hemorrhage, pulmonary emboli, massive bleeding requiring operative intervention, or death. Pulmonary emboli have not occurred, and we no longer advocate routine placement of prophylactic inferior vena cava filters in patients undergoing endovascular therapy. Thrombosis of the treated segment tends to occur within the first days to weeks after intervention. All patients who were patent at 3 months follow-up also were patent at 12 months. Patients who have reoccluded acutely have had evidence of poor flow through the treated segment or areas of contrast stasis on the completion venogram. Therefore, it is imperative that a hemodynamically "perfect" result is achieved because veins are much more susceptible to thrombosis (compared with arteries) because of lower flow rates and decreased pressures.

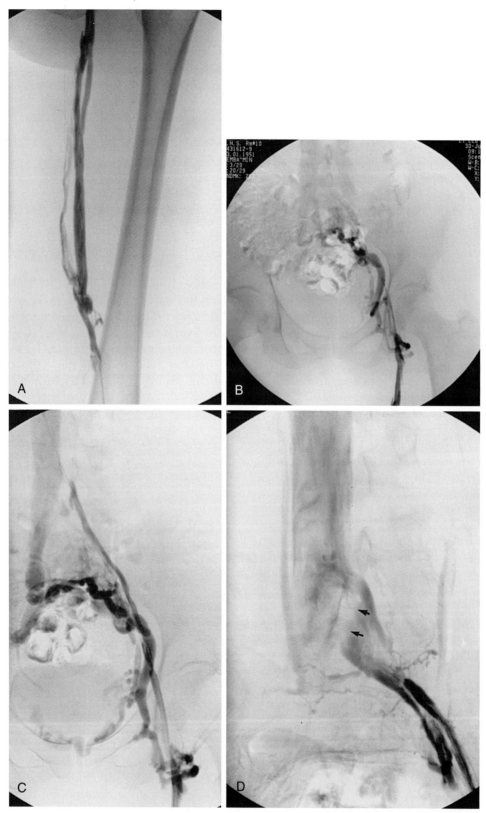

Figure 17–4. A 38-year-old woman with a history of left leg iliofemoral deep vein thrombosis (DVT) 8 months ago. Complaints of persistent left-sided leg edema and pain that are aggravated by exercise. *A,* Ascending popliteal venography reveals a recanalized and patent femoropopliteal segment. *B,* There is occlusion of the iliac vein and opacification of numerous pelvic collateral veins. *C,* The iliac vein is recanalized directly without antecedent thrombolysis using initial angioplasty alone. *D,* Closer examination demonstrates compression of the left common iliac vein by the overlying iliac artery (*arrows*).

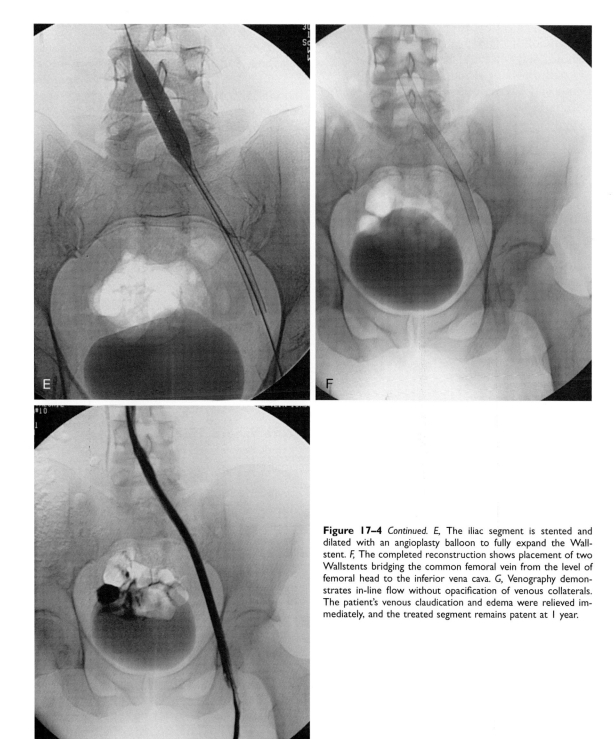

Figure 17–4 *Continued. E,* The iliac segment is stented and dilated with an angioplasty balloon to fully expand the Wallstent. *F,* The completed reconstruction shows placement of two Wallstents bridging the common femoral vein from the level of femoral head to the inferior vena cava. *G,* Venography demonstrates in-line flow without opacification of venous collaterals. The patient's venous claudication and edema were relieved immediately, and the treated segment remains patent at 1 year.

MANAGEMENT OF EARLY AND LATE FAILURES

Early failures usually involve acute thrombosis of the treated segment, as described previously. Catheter-directed thrombolysis is repeated to clear out the fresh thrombus, and careful inspection of the venous outflow is performed to define any possible nidus for re-thrombosis. Any residual intimal flap, partially occlusive thrombus, or organized material is removed either using a stent or by thrombectomy techniques. Patients receiving an iliac vein stent have been observed for up to 6 years, and we have not had any documented late thrombosis of the stents; however, we have not had the opportunity to evaluate all patients, and thus, this information remains anecdotal. In our opinion, iliac vein stents provide an intraluminal lattice for the regeneration of new endothelium. After a period of approximately 6 weeks, the stent surface is incorporated fully into the wall of the vessel, and the vein literally is reconstructed. The use of stents for the treatment of IVCS and isolated chronic iliac vein occlusion appears durable and curative.

SURGICAL ASPECTS OF VENOUS DISEASE

The past 40 years have seen major advances in the operative management of arterial disease. There has been little corresponding progress in the treatment of venous disease. Understanding of the etiology and pathogenesis of the disease has improved, and our ability to prevent acute DVT has increased. However, mortality from pulmonary embolism remains unchanged, the incidence of chronic venous insufficiency has increased, and surgery has achieved little in relief of this condition.

Knowledge of the anatomic distribution and physiologic consequences of venous disease has been revolutionized by noninvasive investigation in the vascular laboratory. Ambulatory venous pressure, formerly the gold standard[34] for assessing venous insufficiency, currently is rarely required. Venography is used infrequently in diagnosis and reserved for occasional road-mapping before surgery. Many noninvasive techniques such as photoplethysmography, strain-gauge plethysmography, and foot volumetry have been used and largely abandoned. Most situations can be assessed fully by color duplex ultrasonography, supplemented where necessary by pneumoplethysmography.[35]

The aim of treatment for venous thromboses of the leg is to prevent pulmonary embolism, to protect the limb from extension of thrombosis, and to minimize the late sequelae of thrombosis. Systemic anticoagulation with heparin fulfills most of the treatment requirements. Only rarely is a limb placed at risk from extensive venous thrombosis, and even patients with massive iliofemoral venous thrombosis and venous gangrene usually can be treated successfully by extreme elevation and anticoagulation. Occasionally, venous gangrene does not respond to conservative measures, and urgent intervention with thrombolysis or venous thrombectomy may be required. Published reports with both of these methods are sparse, but both can be effective, and there is no evidence that one is superior.

Venous gangrene is rare, although troublesome sequelae of deep vein thrombosis are common. In most patients investigated 10 years after venous thrombosis in the leg, deep venous insufficiency has developed. This postphlebitic syndrome can result in a variety of problems, ranging from leg swelling and discomfort to chronic venous ulceration. Severe sequelae are more likely to occur after extensive proximal iliofemoral thrombosis. The natural history of the postphlebitic syndrome may be modified by wearing graduated compression stockings after venous thrombosis. The cause of the postphlebitic syndrome is damage to the deep venous valves. The question remains whether thrombolytic treatment for selected severe thromboses could preserve venous valve function and reduce the risk of late complications.

Acute Venous Thrombosis

SUPERFICIAL THROMBOPHLEBITIS

The most common cause of superficial thrombophlebitis is intravenous cannulation and infusions. This usually is localized, should be exclusively in the upper limb, and, although it causes pain, is self-limiting. Hirudin creams hasten resolution, and surgery is indicated for rare suppuration. Superficial thrombophlebitis of the lower limb mainly occurs in varicose veins after trauma. It usually remains localized to a cluster of veins in the calf, where it causes marked symptoms and is slow to resolve. In the acute phase, conservative management with hirudin cream, elastic support, and mobilization suffices. When the proximal short sphenous vein is involved, there is a risk of popliteal vein occlusion, and proximal long saphenous involvement may similarly affect the femoral vein. In these circumstances, pulmonary embolism may occur.[36] Intraluminal thrombus extends many centimeters proximal to the hard, tender, inflamed superficial vein. Duplex scan confirms this and has the added benefit of excluding coexisting DVT, which is prone to develop where initial therapy for superficial thrombophlebitis has included enforced inactivity.

In phlebitis involving the proximal saphenous

vein, flush ligation after removal of any protruding thrombus and resection of several centimeters of the thrombosed vein are required. This must be coupled with phrophylactic subcutaneous LMWH.

When thrombophlebitis, initially responding to conservative measures, recurs in varicose veins, surgical treatment of the veins is indicated. In these circumstances, repeated episodes are typical.

DEEP VEIN THROMBOSIS

DVT and its sequelae of pulmonary embolism and chronic venous insufficiency continue to present major challenges. Despite increasing knowledge of prevention, implementation of these measures remains patchy.[37] There is general acceptance of the THRIFT guidelines,[38] but strategies for increasing compliance have had limited success. Improved uptake in general and orthopaedic surgery has not been matched in general medical wards, where utilization remains low despite the high prevalence of DVT in conditions such as cardiac failure.

When DVT is suspected, it should be confirmed objectively because clinical diagnosis, even by experts, is notoriously inaccurate.[39] Color duplex ultrasonography is the investigation of choice. It can determine the presence or absence of thrombosis from the calf veins to the inferior vena cava in expert hands. Management of established DVT remains conservative in most cases. Anticoagulation, initially with LMWH and then warfarin, aiming for an INR of 2.0 to 2.5 can be administered safely on an outpatient basis.[40] The optimum duration of warfarin treatment remains unclear, but recent studies suggest a minimum of 3 to 6 months. In the acute phase, measures to prevent development of chronic venous insufficiency often are ignored. Below-knee graduated compression stockings can reduce this,[41] but physician and patient compliance with these measures is poor.

In a minority of patients, anticoagulants alone are insufficient. In extensive iliofemoral DVT with phlegmasia alba or cerulea dolens or impending venous gangrene, measures to restore venous return are required.

VENOUS THROMBECTOMY

In the 1960s, there was considerable enthusiasm for venous thrombectomy and excellent results were reported—especially in DVT associated with the high estrogen contraceptive pill.[42] However, subsequent reports were less favorable, and the procedure was largely abandoned. Interest has been renewed by reports from Scandinavia, where thrombectomy with adjuvant arteriovenous fistula has been shown to reduce chronic venous insufficiency.[43] This will be required in a minority of cases and should be reserved for phlegmasia cerulea dolens not resolving with anticoagulants and steep elevation of the legs, or where there are signs of impending venous gangrene.

THROMBOLYTIC THERAPY

Systemic thrombolytic therapy for iliofemoral thrombosis has given disappointing results, and early experience of local infusion was also poor. However, delivery of the thrombolytic agent directly into the thrombus has produced encouraging results. Semba and Dake reported complete lysis in 72% of 25 limbs with acute iliofemoral DVT and partial lysis in a further 20%.[14] They demonstrated a high association with iliac vein compression and common iliac vein webs, which can be overcome by balloon angioplasty and stenting. This was a major reason for incomplete thrombectomy and re-thrombosis and opens a new avenue for successful restoration of venous integrity and reduction of venous insufficiency.

After venous thrombectomy and thrombolysis, long-term (at least 6 months) warfarin is essential and should be coupled with graduated compression stockings to minimize the risks of chronic venous insufficiency.

CHRONIC VENOUS DISEASE

Varicose Veins

Varicose veins develop in 10 to 20% of the adult population of the United Kingdom, and operations for their control remain among the most common procedures performed in the west. At least 10% of these operations are for recurrences, indicating a very high failure rate, often technical, of the primary procedure. Despite this, assessment, management, and operation on such patients is commonly left to inexperienced and untrained surgeons.

The indications for varicose vein operations frequently are poorly considered. Cosmetic operations performed for minor varicose veins in the morbidly obese or on elderly patients with advanced degenerative disease are not justified. Assessment of the need for operation by a surgeon with training, experience, and an interest in venous surgery is essential before outcomes can be improved.

Not all patients need treatment for varicose veins. Many patients seek advice because they fear DVT, venous ulceration, or increase in their veins. Reassurance is often all that is required. It is necessary to establish that the varicose veins are the cause of symptoms. The major indications for treatment are:

1. Cosmesis: This is relative and not an indication in the presence of significant comorbidities.

2. Aching: Pain is rare in uncomplicated varicose veins, but localized and more general aches are both common. Exclude other causes such as joint, arterial, or neurologic disease.

3. Recurrent Superficial Thrombophlebitis: A single episode of phlebitis does not constitute an absolute indication for operation in the absence of other symptoms.

   However, when phlebitis recurs, operation is required because further episodes can be expected. Even when the varices are quite small, determine by duplex ultrasonography the stem vein involved and deal with this.

4. Venous Insufficiency and Ulceration: It had long been held that primary varicose veins did not cause venous insufficiency and ulceration. More recent evidence suggests that they are a major factor in up to 60% of cases of venous insufficiency.[44] Treatment of the superficial vein reflux results in ulcer healing provided that the deep veins are patent, even if their valves are incompetent.

CHRONIC VENOUS INSUFFICIENCY

Chronic venous insufficiency is the result of venous hypertension in the gaiter area secondary to venous obstruction or reflux or calf pump failure. This is postthrombotic in 70% of cases, but in 30% is a consequence of primary valve dysfunction. This results in edema, pigmentation, eczema, lipodermatosclerosis, and ulceration. More rarely, venous claudication is the major symptom.

Only 80% of patients presenting with lower limb ulceration have evidence of venous insufficiency.[45, 46] Arterial insufficiency, which occurs in the other 20%, either in isolation or in association with diabetes or rheumatoid arthritis, should be excluded by Doppler pressure studies. This is especially so where other stigmata of venous insufficiency are not apparent. In elderly patients who spend long spells with their legs dependent and immobile, ulceration can result from stasis edema and intracuticular blistering with superadded infection in the absence of significant venous disease.

Knowledge of the underlying mechanisms in venous insufficiency has been increased by noninvasive investigation, especially by duplex ultrasonography. Reflux appears to be more important than outflow obstruction. Reflux in the popliteal vein is thought to be critical. Many ingenious techniques to overcome such reflux, including valve repair by internal[47] and external[48] valvuloplasty and valve transposition,[49] have been employed. Unfortunately, these techniques are applicable only in a minority of patients.[50] Long-term results are poor, often because of secondary phlebitis. Where there has been clinical benefit, it has

not been clear whether this has resulted from the reconstructive surgery or associated procedures for superficial varicose veins or incompetent perforators. More surgical literature has resulted from these procedures than clinical benefit. It seems unlikely that they will have a continuing place in the vascular surgical repertoire.

Operations for the relief of outflow obstruction, such as the Palma femorofemoral venous crossover graft, with or without arteriovenous fistula, are similarly likely to have limited indications. Even enthusiasts, such as May and colleagues, only performed 50 procedures over a 19-year period. Their best results were in the unusual circumstances of thigh claudication of venous origin.[51]

The most significant recent observation has been the high incidence of chronic venous insufficiency and ulceration due to superficial venous reflux. Duplex studies have demonstrated isolated superficial reflux in 57% of limbs with skin changes.[44] In many of these, there is long saphenous reflux without obvious superficial varicose veins. The reflux is transmitted from groin to ankle level without producing dilation of intervening tributaries.

The long saphenous vein lies in a deep plane and rarely is dilated and palpable. Full assessment of this reflux requires duplex ultrasonography, which is essential in all cases of venous ulceration. Correction of superficial reflux by varicose vein surgery improves venous insufficiency and leads to ulcer healing, even in the presence of deep venous incompetence.[52]

SUMMARY

Despite increased understanding of the etiology and pathogenesis of venous disease, our ability to influence it by surgery remains extremely limited. Conservative management has improved but frequently is implemented inadequately. The most significant surgical advances have been the realization that varicose vein surgery requires attention to detail and, when properly performed, can relieve venous insufficiency and ulceration in a large proportion of cases.

REFERENCES

1. Moser KM: Pulmonary thromboembolism. *In* Isselbacher KJ, Braunwald E, Wilson JD (eds): Harrison's Principles of Internal Medicine, 18th ed. New York, McGraw-Hill, 1994, pp. 1214–1220.
2. Hull RD, Raskob GE, Pineo GF, et al: Subcutaneous low-molecular weight heparin vs. warfarin for prophylaxis of deep venous thrombosis following hip or knee implantation: An economic perspective. Arch Intern Med 157:298–303, 1997.
3. Sherry S: Thrombolytic therapy for deep venous thrombosis. Semin Intervent Radiol 4: 331–337, 1985.
4. Krupski WC, Bass A, Dilley RB, et al: Propagation of deep

venous thrombosis identified by duplex ultrasonography. J Vasc Surg 12:467–475, 1990.

5. Johnson BF, Manzo RA, Bergelin RO, Strandness DE: Relationship between changes in the deep venous system and the development of the postthrombotic syndrome after an acute episode of lower limb deep vein thrombosis: A one to six year follow-up. J Vasc Surg 21:307–312, 1995.

6. O'Donnell TF, Browse WL, Burnand KE, Thomas ML: Socioeconomic effects of an iliofemoral deep venous thrombosis. J Surg Res 22:483–488, 1977.

7. Akesson H, Brudin L, Dahlstrom JD, et al: Venous function assessed during a five year period after acute iliofemoral venous thrombosis treated with anticoagulation. Eur J Vasc Surg 4:43–48, 1990.

8. Hill SL, Holtzman GI, Martin D, et al: The origin of lower extremity deep vein thrombi in acute venous thrombosis. Am J Surg 173:485–490, 1997.

9. Comerota AJ, Aldridge S: Thrombolytic therapy for acute deep vein thrombosis. Semin Vasc Surg 5:76–81, 1992.

10. Hill SL, Martin D, Evans P: Massive vein thrombosis of the extremities. Am J Surg 158:131–136, 1989.

11. van Breda A, Graor RA, Katzen BT, et al: The relative cost-effectiveness of urokinase versus streptokinase in the treatment of peripheral vascular disease. J Vasc Intervent Radiol 2:77–87, 1991.

12. Verhaege R, Stockx L, Lacroix H, et al: Catheter-directed lysis of iliofemoral vein thrombosis with use of rt-PA. Eur Radiol 7:996–1001, 1997.

13. Fox D, Ouriel K, Green RM, et al: Thrombolysis with prourokinase versus urokinase: an in vitro comparison. J Vasc Surg 23:657–666, 1996.

14. Semba CP, Dake MD: Iliofemoral deep venous thrombosis: Aggressive therapy using catheter-directed thrombolysis. Radiology 191:487–494, 1994.

15. Bjarnason H, Kruse JR, Asinger DA, et al: Iliofemoral deep venous thrombosis: Safety and efficacy outcome during 5 years of catheter-directed thrombolytic therapy. J Vasc Intervent Radiol 8:405–418, 1997.

16. Cragg AH: Lower extremity deep venous thrombosis: A new approach to obtaining access. J Vasc Intervent Radiol 7:283–288, 1996.

17. Virchow R: Uber die Erweiterung kleiner Gefasse. Arch Pathol Anat 3:427, 1851.

18. McMurrich JP: The occurrence of congenital adhesions in the common iliac veins and their relation to the thrombosis of the femoral and iliac veins. Am J Med Sci 135:142–147, 1908.

19. Krumbhaar EB, Ehrich WE: A frequent obstructive anomaly of the mouth of the left common iliac vein. Am Heart J 26:737–739, 1943.

20. May R, Thurner J: The cause of the predominately sinistral occurrence of thrombosis of the pelvic veins. Angiology 8:419–427, 1957.

21. Cockett FB, Thomas ML: The iliac vein compression syndrome. Br J Surg 52:816–821, 1965.

22. Ferris EJ, Lim WN, Smith PL, Casali R: May-Thurner syndrome. Radiology 147:29–31, 1983.

23. Okrent D, Messersmith R, Buckman J: Transcatheter fibrinolytic therapy and angioplasty for left iliofemoral venous thrombosis. J Vasc Intervent Radiol 2:195–197, 1991.

24. Steinberg JB, Jacocks MA: May-Thurner syndrome: A previously unreported variant. Ann Vasc Surg 7:577–581, 1993.

25. Hassell DR, Reifstock JE, Harshfield DL, Ferris EJ: Unilateral left leg edema: A variation of the May-Thurner syndrome. Cardiovasc Intervent Radiol 10:89–91, 1987.

26. Taheri SA, Taheri PA, Schultz R, et al: Ileocaval compression syndrome. Contemp Surg 40:9–14, 1992.

27. Cockett FB, Thomas ML, Negus D: Iliac vein compression: Its relation to iliofemoral thrombosis and the post-thrombotic syndrome. Br Med J 2:14–19, 1967.

28. Rigas A, Vomvoyannis A, Tsardakas E: Iliac vein compression syndrome: Report of ten cases. J Cardiovasc Surg 11:389–392, 1970.

29. Trimble C, Bernstein EF, Pomerantz M, et al: A prosthetic bridging device to relieve iliac venous compression. Surg Forum 23:249–251, 1972.

30. Calvignac JL, Giraud C, Bastide G: Syndrome de Cockett, Traitment par enveloppement veineux dans une prosthese armee. Presse Med 13:97–98, 1984.

31. Alimi YS, DiMauro P, Fabre D, Juhan C: Iliac vein reconstructions to treat acute and chronic venous occlusive disease. J Vasc Surg 25:673–681, 1997.

32. Jasczak P, Mathieson FR: The iliac compression syndrome. Acta Chir Scand 144:133–136, 1978.

33. Comerota AJ, Aldridge SC, Cohen G, et al: A strategy of aggressive regional therapy for acute iliofemoral venous thrombosis with contemporary thrombectomy or catheter-directed thrombolysis. J Vasc Surg 20:244–254, 1994.

34. Criado E: Laboratory evaluation of the patient with chronic venous insufficiency. In Rutherford RB (ed): Vascular Surgery, 4th ed. Philadelphia, WB Saunders, 1995.

35. Christopoulos DG, Nicolaides AN, Cook A, et al: Pathogenesis of venous ulceration in relation to calf muscle pump function. Surgery 106:829, 1989.

36. Galloway JMD, Karmody AM, Mavor GE: Thrombophlebitis of the long saphenous vein complicated by pulmonary embolism. Br J Surg 56:360–361, 1969.

37. Morris GK, Mitchell JRA: Prevention and diagnosis of venous thrombosis in patients with hip fractures. Lancet ii:867–869, 1976.

38. Thromboembolic Risk Factors (THRIFT) Group: Risk of and prophylaxis for venous thromboembolism in hospital patients. Br Med J 305:567–574, 1992.

39. Hull R, Hirsh J, Sackett D, et al: Clinical validity of a negative venogram in patients with clinically suspected venous thrombosis. Circulation 64:622–625, 1981.

40. Levine M, Gent M, Hirsch J, et al: A comparison of low-molecular-weight heparin administered primarily at home with unfractionated heparin administered in hospital for proximal deep-vein thrombosis. N Engl J Med 334:677–681, 1996.

41. Milne AA, Ruckley CV: The clinical course of patients following extensive deep venous thrombosis. Eur J Vasc Surg 8:56–59, 1994.

42. Mavor GE, Galloway JMD: Iliofemoral venous thrombosis. Br J Surg 56:45–59, 1969.

43. Plate G, Akesson H, Einarsson E, et al: Long-term results of venous thrombectomy combined with a temporary arteriovenous fistula. Eur J Vasc Surg 4:483, 1990.

44. Lees TA, Lambert D: Patterns of venous reflux in limbs with skin changes associated with chronic venous insufficiency. Br J Surg 80:725–728, 1993.

45. Ruckley CV, Callam MJ, Dale JJ: Causes of chronic leg ulcer. Lancet ii:615–616, 1982.

46. Cornwall JV, Lewis JD: Leg ulcers: Epidemiology and aetiology. Br J Surg 73:693–696, 1986.

47. Kistner RL: Surgical repair of the incompetent femoral vein valve. Arch Surg 110:1336–1341, 1975.

48. Raju S: Multiple valve reconstruction for venous insufficiency: Indications, optimal technique and results. In Veith FJ (ed): Current Critical Problems in Vascular Surgery. St Louis, Quality Medical Publishing, 1992.

49. Taheri SA, Lazar L, Elias SM, et al: Vein valve transplant. Surgery 91:28–33, 1982.

50. Raju S, Fredericks R: Valve reconstruction procedures for non-obstructive venous insufficiency: Rationale, techniques and results in 107 procedures with 2 to 8 year follow-up. J Vasc Surg 7:301–310, 1988.

51. Halliday P, Harris J, May J: Femoro-femoral crossover grafts (Palma Operation): A long-term follow-up study. In Bergan JF, Yao JST (eds): Surgery of the veins. Orlando, Grune and Stratton, 1985.

18 Upper Limb Venous and Superior Vena Cava Intervention

Endovascular Contributor: Peter Gaines
Surgical Contributors: Fernando E. Kafie and Samuel Eric Wilson

The use of endovascular techniques to intervene on the venous side of the circulation has lagged behind the long strides taken in the arterial system. It is difficult to know why this should be. The initial attempts at minimally invasive treatment by Dotter and subsequent workers were on the arteries, and much interest subsequently was shown by industry when the lucrative coronary market became available. In many ways, venous disease is less well understood than arterial disease, and the tendency of veins to collapse, thrombose, tear, and develop spasm has made them less of an attractive proposition to the endovascular interventionist. Nevertheless, inferior vena cava filters currently are used worldwide, and the explosion in the requirements for permanent and medium term central venous access has pushed many departments into providing venous access services. Given the prevalence of such problems, it is not surprising that, in the upper limb, central line placement and the management of hemodialysis-associated problems should form the bulk of venous work. These subjects are discussed more fully in Chapters 20 and 21. However, there remains the extremely satisfying contribution that interventionists can make to the quality of life of those patients unfortunate enough to be afflicted with superior vena caval occlusion. In addition, there is the more controversial issue of how best to manage patients with Paget–Schroetter syndrome.

SUPERIOR VENA CAVA OBSTRUCTION

Etiology

In 1757, William Hunter described a group of patients with tuberculosis and syphilitic thoracic aneurysms who had superior vena cava obstruction (SVCO).[1] In the late 20th century, when successful inroads have been made into the eradication or management of infectious diseases, the main cause of SVCO is neoplastic disease. In western society, more than 95% of cases of SVCO are caused by malignancy,[2, 3] most due to bronchial carcinoma primarily affecting the right upper lobe bronchus. SVCO complicates up to 15% of cases of bronchial carcinoma[4] and 3 to 8% of cases of lymphoma.[5] Just about any intrathoracic malignancy, either primary or secondary, may result in compression of the central veins. Other causes are listed in Table 18–1.

Clinical Presentation

Patients present with a distressing group of symptoms. Most patients experience facial and arm swelling accompanied by headaches, dysphagia, breathlessness, cognitive impairment, and conjunctival edema. The capacity to generate collateral branches in the thorax is relatively poor, but most patients with occluded central veins achieve some drainage via the azygous, hemiazygous, or intercostal veins. With the gradual progression of disease and poor collateral routes, patients present with increasing severity of their distressing symptoms. Although the 2-year survival rate of patients with bronchial carcinoma presenting with superior venal caval obstruction is only 5%, the successful management of SVCO results in a significant and prompt improvement in the quality of life.

Table 18–1. The Causes of Superior Vena Cava Obstruction

Bronchial carcinoma
Other intrathoracic malignancy can be either mediastinal compression (e.g., lymph nodes) or direct invasion (e.g., mesothelioma)
Fibrosing mediastinitis
Radiotherapy
Chemotherapy
Intravenous devices (e.g., venous access lines, pacemakers, etc.)
Aneurysms
Unknown

Conventional Treatment

SVCO due to intrathoracic malignancy usually is managed by radiotherapy, with or without chemotherapy. Although 80% of patients respond to radiotherapy, this may take up to 3 weeks, and 10 to 20% of patients' symptoms recur.[6–10] In non–small cell carcinoma, less than 50% of patients respond,[11, 12] although higher clinical success has been reported with more aggressive radiotherapy.[13] Not only does radiotherapy take some time to be effective, but it is associated with significant complications, particularly skin burns, malaise, and sickness. Intrathoracic surgery in this group of very ill patients with poor life expectancy clearly should be avoided. Thankfully, with the development of user-friendly, stable, intravascular metallic stents, the 1990s have seen a revolution in the management of these patients.

Endovascular Stents

The year 1986 witnessed the publication of the first paper describing SVCO managed by the placement of an intravascular metallic stent.[14] Since then, there has been considerable expansion in the range of stents available to treat this condition. The Gianturco Z stent was the first to receive widespread attention.[15] It was placed through a 12- to 14-French sheath and was initially available as either a single unit or a double stent, which was simply two single units, linked by a cross-bridge. This stent has excellent radial force, but the single stents were unstable in short stenoses, and disease was able to protrude through the large interstices. The delivery sheath, although inflexible, was of sufficient size to allow effective aspiration of thrombus. The Palmaz Extra Large stent has excellent radial force and is easier to position, but is short, inflexible, and often requires the placement of multiple devices. The Wallstent and Memotherm stents are self-expanding devices, are available up to 16 mm (Wallstent) or 20 mm (Memotherm) in diameter, and are available in longer lengths. Although their radial force is not as high as the Palmaz or Gianturco Z stent, their flexibility offers advantages in cases where the stent is required to take a corner. The choice of stent and technique requires an understanding of the basic pathophysiology of the condition.

The condition known as superior vena caval obstruction is seen when there is either (1) narrowing/occlusion of the superior vena cava (SVC) or (2) stenosis or occlusion of *both* brachiocephalic veins. Symptoms of SVCO are not seen when there is solitary brachiocephalic vein disease. The corollary is that when managing bilateral brachiocephalic occlusions, it is only necessary to recanalize one of the brachiocephalic veins.

When a short stenosis in the main superior vena cava is to be treated, then it makes sense to use a device with high radial force that is easy to place. In this situation, it is entirely appropriate to use the Palmaz Extra Large stent (Fig. 18–1). When the disease involves the brachiocephalic veins, then the segment is either angulated or long and a flexible device of sufficient length is required to manage the full segment of disease. In this situation, either the Memotherm or Wallstent is a good choice (Fig. 18–2).

Technique

Bilateral upper limb venography usually is undertaken via cannulae placed in both antecubital fossae. When venography identifies stenoses without occlusions, it is possible to proceed directly to stent placement.

When venography suggests intrathoracic central vein occlusions, care should be taken in interpreting the images. There may well be severe venous stenoses without thrombosis because of the low flow and poor contrast concentration. In this situation, it is our practice to place catheters from the antecubital fossa into the main central veins and perform direct contrast injections.

When the large veins are thrombosed (Fig. 18–3), this can be managed either by thrombolysis, aspiration, or mechanical thrombectomy. Thrombolysis requires placement of bilateral single or multiple endhole catheters into the proximal veins from the arms. Thrombolytic agents in the same dose as used to manage peripheral arterial occlusions then are infused, and the situation is reassessed after several hours of treatment. Practically, this usually means reimaging the patient later the same day or on the following morning. Mechanical thrombectomy devices have been used successfully in the large veins using both the Amplatz Thrombectomy Device and the Hydrolyser. Mechanical devices require familiarity with their use and are less steerable but do obviate the hemorrhagic risks of thrombolytic drugs. Aspiration of large amounts of thrombus is certainly possible when access has been obtained with a large sheath or guide-catheter.

After either pharmaceutical thrombolysis or mechanical thrombectomy, flow may be achieved even in the presence of large amounts of residual thrombus. It can be difficult to effectively remove all thrombus in a large vein using the currently available thrombectomy devices. When using conventional thrombolytic agents, once flow has been achieved, there is often very little further improvement in the volume of thrombus that is removed presumably because of the effectively reduced concentration of thrombolytic agents in the presence of flow. In this situation, our

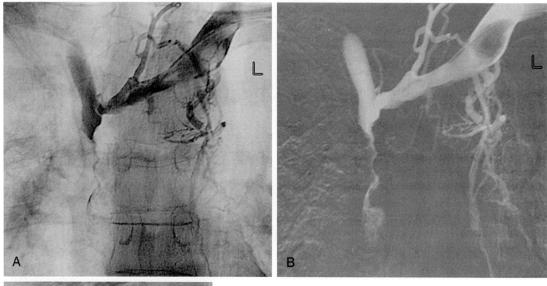

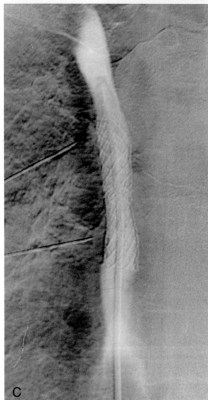

Figure 18–1. *A,* Venogram showing patent brachiocephalic veins with thrombus on the left side, and an irregular superior vena cava (SVC) stenosis. *B,* Same image subtracted to better demonstrate the SVC stenosis. *C,* Successful placement of Palmaz stents within the SVC stenosis.

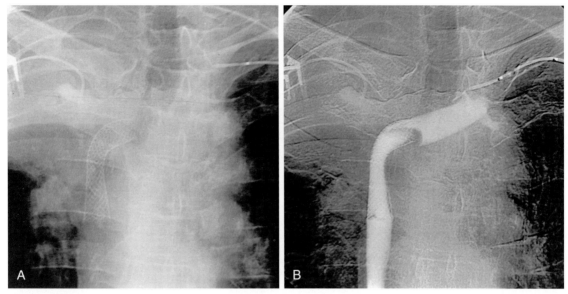

Figure 18–2. *A,* Wallstent taking an acute angulation from the left brachiocephalic vein into superior vena cava (SVC). *B,* Same patient with contrast in the stent. The residual thrombus resolved with heparin treatment.

approach is to aspirate as much thrombus as possible and then place the endovascular stent even when there is a small risk of movement of thrombus through the stent into the lungs.

Stent placement can be achieved from almost any peripheral venous access site. Because radiologists are used to working from the legs, the femoral vein is often the site of choice. When placing stents directly from the arms, spasm is a considerable problem and may completely lock the device in the arm for periods of up to several hours. If it is not possible to place the device from the legs, then the jugular veins are an excellent option.

If the Palmaz stent is chosen, then it is recommended that this be placed through a long sheath because without this, a severe SVC stenosis may displace the stent from the balloon deployment catheter. When a long Wallstent or Memotherm stent is chosen to be placed into the brachiocephalic veins, then the choice of vein would depend on which vein has cleared the best or where the catheter guide wire system is most easily placed. It is recommended that all stents be placed over a heavy-duty wire to prevent prolapse of the device into the right atrium. The Palmaz stent and Memotherm stents are relatively simple devices to place. The Wallstent, although superior in terms of conforming to the vessel curvature, requires a little more practice for reliable deployment. It is often best to partially deploy the stent peripherally in the brachiocephalic vein and then pull the device down into the required position before final deployment. Once the self-expanding stents have been deployed, then they should be balloon-dilated to 12 or 14 mm.

The question of persistent anticoagulation re-mains an unresolved issue. There are no published data to confidently analyze whether long-term anticoagulation improves patency of the stent. In the authors' opinion, it is preferable in this group of ill patients with limited life expectancy not to burden them with oral anticoagulation unless there is a specific indication for this.

Outcome

There have been nearly 50 publications on this subject since the technique was first described. In a review of 24 articles describing 309 patients,[16] complete or partial improvement was recorded in 93.5%. Early occlusion (<1 week) occurred in 6.2% and late occlusion in 7.6%, but these all were successfully managed to achieve a secondary patency rate of 100%. Complications have been described, and these include death from pulmonary embolus, pulmonary emboli without death, major hemorrhage from thrombolysis, shoulder pain, and access site thrombosis. Fortunately, these occur in a small number of patients when thrombolysis is not used (<8%).[16] In our own experience,[15, 17] there is a higher complication rate when using thrombolysis to manage SVC thrombosis. In addition, there is a higher recurrence rate (45%) and a reduced secondary patency rate (85%). Despite this, the patients experience such a dramatic improvement in their symptoms that they still should be offered treatment.

Conclusion

SVC obstruction is a debilitating condition. Radiotherapy is widely available to manage the condition

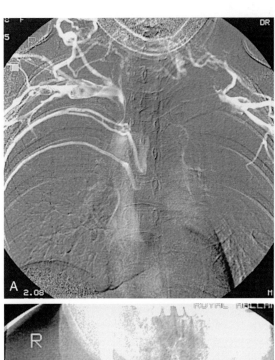

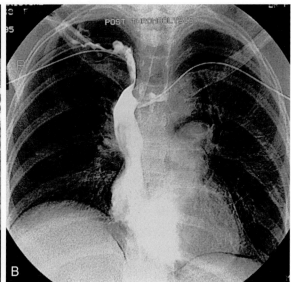

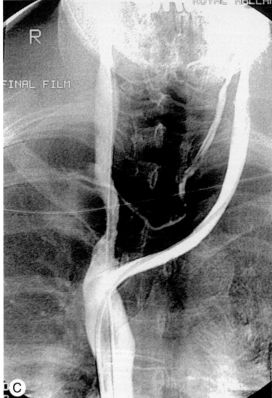

Figure 18–3. *A,* Venogram showing severe stenosis with thrombus of the left brachiocephalic vein and proximal superior vena cava (SVC) and complete occlusion of the left braciocephalic vein. *B,* After thrombolysis most thrombus has cleared and the left brachiocephalic vein is patent. The subclavian veins remain occluded. *C,* Memotherm stents taken into the jugular veins. There is excellent relief of arm and facial symptoms.

but produces significant side effects, is often slow to produce effect, and has a high recurrence rate. However, when radiotherapy is available, costs are usually low, and in many units, this is still the first form of treatment. Stents then are used to manage severe symptoms of SVCO that require urgent decompression or recurrent SVCO after radiotherapy.

Sadly, in many countries, access to the endovascular management of SVCO remains limited. This is a great shame because this form of therapy is more effective than radiotherapy and, in a group of patients with debilitating symptoms, can effect dramatic improvements. SVC stents should be available to any patient with SVCO.

SUBCLAVIAN AND AXILLARY VEIN THROMBOSIS

Subclavian–axillary vein thrombosis (SAVT) is an uncommon condition that produces unpleasant symptoms in the acute phase and has the potential to result in chronic morbidity when left untreated. Primary subclavian and axillary vein thrombosis, commonly known as Paget–Schroetter syndrome, occurs in an otherwise healthy individual and accounts for only 1 to 2% of all venous thromboses.[18] The many causes of secondary SAVT are listed in Table 18–2. Probably the most common causes of secondary SAVT are central venous catheterization and dialysis fistula formation, both of which are becoming more prevalent. Whatever the underlying cause for SAVT, the symptomatology is common and includes swelling and engorgement of the affected arm with cyanosis and pain or discomfort. There is often considerable delay from the onset of symptoms to presentation, and 80% of patients with SAVT have had a previous episode.[19] If left untreated or managed simply with arm elevation and rest, the outcome is poor.[20] Pulmonary embolus has been recorded in approximately 14% of cases.[21]

Unfortunately, because SAVT is uncommon, there are no large series or trials to illuminate the problem

Table 18–2. Causes of Subclavian–Axillary Vein Thrombosis

Primary	Idiopathic/Paget–Schroetter syndrome/effort thrombosis
Secondary	Intravenous catheters or devices
	Dialysis fistula
	Local tumor invasion
	Systemic effects of malignancy
	Local radiotherapy
	Thrombophilia
	Cardiac failure
	Trauma
	Amyloidosis
	Sarcoidosis

and determine the best form of therapy. The management of SAVT can be considered according to whether the clinician is dealing with primary or secondary disease.

Paget–Schroetter Syndrome

Paget Schroetter syndrome most commonly occurs in young men and has a slight preponderance to affect the right arm. The underlying etiology appears to be a combination of an anatomic predisposition and repetitive trauma from strenuous upper body activity. The anatomic peculiarity leading to Paget–Schroetter syndrome is compression of the subclavian vein between the first rib and either the costocoracoid ligament, subclavius muscle, or clavicle.[22] It is thought that with compression of the subclavian vein, the repeated trauma induces endothelial damage with repeated episodes of thrombosis and eventually fibrosis, stenosis, and formation of intrinsic fibrous bands (synechiae). Clearly, the optimal time for intervention is at the initial presentation so that these long-term occlusive effects do not occur.

INVESTIGATION

After the initial clinical diagnosis of SAVT, ultrasound should be used to confirm the diagnosis. Ultrasound is quick and of low cost, and does not involve either ionizing radiation or use of intravascular contrast. In experienced hands, the accuracy is high. Occasionally, however, large collateral branches may be reported incorrectly as patent subclavian veins. Ultrasound has little role to play in defining the underlying cause of venous obstruction. In the appropriate age group, a chest radiograph should be obtained to exclude apical bronchogenic carcinoma, and hematologic advice should be sought for exclusion of the various thrombotic tendencies.

When management by anticoagulation only is the preferred option, there is little reason to continue investigations. If, however, more aggressive intravascular therapy is to be considered, then diagnostic venography from the affected arm is required to carefully delineate the anatomy. After thrombolysis, checking venography may well define the underlying abnormality. Although stress views have been recommended to detect an extrinsic stenosis in those patients in whom venography initially appears normal, it is difficult to interpret the results because 70% of the general population have evidence of venous obstruction when the shoulder is hyperabducted and retracted.[19]

MANAGEMENT

As previously mentioned, conservative therapy in the form of bed rest and arm elevation results in a poor outcome.[20] The effects of anticoagulation are better, and when anticoagulation is introduced early (within 7 days), 80% of patients are recorded as having no residual symptoms.[23, 24] Not all the series reviewing anticoagulation report such good outcome,[25] and, where possible, it is thought advantageous to attend to the underlying compression to restrict future thrombotic episodes.

The use of endovascular techniques, by themselves or as part of a combined approach, to treat Paget–Schroetter syndrome has been described since the mid 1980s.[20] However, few series are large, and many lack long-term follow-up. Locally applied catheter-directed thrombolysis is an obvious solution to the problem of localized venous thrombosis. From 14 studies, 69 patients have had thrombolysis with a total or partial success in 88% of cases.[20] It is unlikely that the choice of thrombolytic agent affects the success: in the United States, the usual drug is urokinase, and in the United Kingdom, recombinant tissue plasminogen activator (rtPA) is preferred. It is our practice to continue from the diagnostic venogram by placing a single end-hole or multiple side-hole 5-French catheter directly into the thrombus. Placement proximal to the thrombus is unlikely to have any effect because the thrombolytic agent will circumvent the occlusion via the collateral branches. It is unlikely that any particular dose regimen is more effective than any other, and the author recommends a delivery of 0.5 mg/hour of rtPA as a constant infusion. Repeat venography is undertaken 4 to 6 hours after the start of treatment or the following morning, whichever is the most appropriate and convenient. Very few complications have been reported during thrombolysis for Paget–Schroetter syndrome, but access site bleeding and pericatheter thrombosis are relatively common. The pericatheter thrombosis is dealt with by retracting the catheter after successful lysis of the intial occlusion. Twelve percent of patients do not respond. Adelman and colleagues[18] report an improved thrombolysis rate in patients with symptoms of less than 2 weeks' duration, and only 33% successful thrombolysis in chronic occlusion.

In those who do respond to thrombolysis, the underlying vein may appear normal or extrinsically compressed, have an intrinsic stenosis, or contain bands and synechiae. Because compression of the subclavian vein is considered a prerequisite for the development of Paget–Schroetter syndrome, when there is no intrinsic stenosis, combining thrombolysis with surgical decompression is a logical approach. Of the 14 patients managed successfully with thrombolysis and undergoing transaxillary thoracic outlet decompression by first rib resection, Adelman and colleagues[18] had a 100% patency rate at a mean follow-up of 21 months. In reviewing 7 years' experience

of the management of Paget–Schroetter syndrome, Beygui and associates[26] had a similar clinical success and high patency rate when thrombolysis was combined with first rib resection and scalenectomy. The timing of thoracic outlet decompression is open to discussion.[27] Some authors recommend immediate decompression to avoid acute rethrombosis, others prefer to wait 6 weeks to allow "healing" of the thrombotic site. A number of current reports confirm the combined approach of thrombolysis and surgical decompression as superior to thrombolysis and endovascular techniques only[18, 26, 28] (Fig. 18–4). This is not surprising given that angioplasty alone does not remove the underlying extrinsic abnormality, and both angioplasty and stent placement incite a restenotic process. After thrombolysis and surgical decompression, some patients continue with symptoms. In these patients, venography is worth considering because many patients have a residual intrinsic abnormality. In this group of patients, angioplasty may be useful in removing the intrinsic stenosis.

When there is intrinsic stenosis after thrombolysis, there are no data to guide whether this should be treated before or after rib resection.[28] From experience with balloon dilatation of venous stenoses in hemodialysis patients, we know that there is a very high recurrence rate. If the patient were to benefit from rib resection alone, then the injury inflicted by balloon dilatation would not benefit the patient in the long term. Conversely, it is not possible to determine which patients with stenosis that appears to be intrinsic do not require balloon dilatation, and it is unlikely that in those patients with a tight intrinsic stenosis, the vein would remain patent with rib resection alone. Until such data are available, either approach is reasonable. Stent placement should be avoided because of the well-reported high fracture rate in this young population.

The upper limb has the potential for extensive and adequate collateral vein formation. Not surprisingly, there is a relatively high success rate after the management of patients with SAVT simply using anticoagulation. With limited available data on the long-term success of endovascular manipulations or surgical decompression in SAVT, a careful decision must be made as to which patients to pursue active intervention above oral anticoagulation. It could be suggested that in patients with very few symptoms, possibly affecting the nondominant arm, oral anticoagulation should be the treatment of choice until more extensive data on active intervention are available.

When a decision is made to pursue aggressive therapy, the patient should be made aware that any intervention is unlikely to totally restore normal physiology and that long-term results are as yet unavailable. Our approach is to initially perform thrombolysis, treat

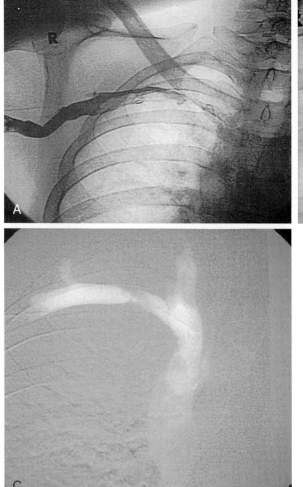

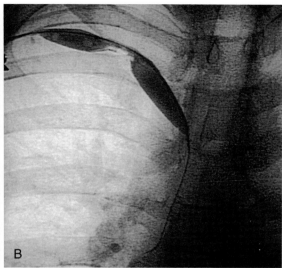

Figure 18–4. *A,* Initial venogram showing thrombotic occlusion of the subclavian vein in a young male patient. *B,* After overnight thrombolysis, there was complete clearance of thrombus. Balloon angioplasty with severe waisting of the percutaneous transluminal angioplasty (PTA) balloon at the typical site in Paget–Schroetter syndrome. *C,* There is considerable luminal irregularity after PTA. The patient went on to have first rib resection with good clinical outcome.

any intrinsic abnormality by balloon angioplasty, and then undertake surgical decompression. As discussed previously, it is probably equally appropriate to undertake rib resection and then treat any venous stenosis that remains and interferes with function. Should intervention subsequent to successful thrombolysis fail, patients treated with oral anticoagulation achieve a high clinical success rate.[26] Thus, it would seem appropriate for patients to continue on oral anticoagulation for some time after primary therapy.

Surgery in Paget–Schroetter Syndrome

Catheter-directed thrombolysis is safe and effectively restores venous patency. Recent studies have shown the value of immediate catheter-directed thrombolytic therapy followed by a period of anticoagulation to allow the acute phlebitic process to subside. Patients then may be considered for first rib resection or sca-

lenectomy to relieve a demonstrated external compression. Patients with long-standing compression may develop fibrosis and stricture formation. This can be relieved after the compressive elements have been removed.

Several methods for correcting intrinsic stenosis have been suggested, including venolysis, patch angioplasty, bypass of the stenotic segment, or percutaneous transluminal angioplasty (PTA) with stent placement. More recently, Lee and associates reported patency in 9 of 11 extremities with subclavian vein thrombosis, but PTA was inferior to first rib resection or scalenectomy.[29] Machleder found poor efficacy of preoperative PTA, with failure of this procedure correlating significantly and adversely with long-term patency rates.[30] This study also noted no additional improvement in long-term patency rates with PTA vs. thrombolytic therapy alone. Unless the extrinsic component is released surgically, PTA has no durable role.

Secondary Subclavian–Axillary Vein Thrombosis

Although thoracic outlet compression can lead to axillosubclavian vein thrombosis, most venous occlusive processes result from trauma or iatrogenic injury (Table 18–2). Long-term intravenous nutrition, upper extremity intravenous access for therapy, or procedures such as central venous pressure monitoring, Swan-Ganz monitoring, or hemodialysis catheters may result in axillosubclavian thrombotic episodes. Chronic axillosubclavian thrombosis may be an indolent and asymptomatic process. The more serious illness for which the patient is under treatment may mask subtle signs of progressive axillosubclavian thrombosis. In these patients, heparin is used to prevent extension of thrombus, thus preserving collateral patency. Thrombolytic therapy is undoubtedly efficacious, but good controlled studies have not been reported. Routine thrombectomy or interposition graft has not been demonstrated to be superior to conservative management in intrinsic venous occlusion, where external compression and arteriovenous fistula-induced venous hypertension are aggravating factors. Thrombosis of axillary–subclavian veins (ASVs) in patients with chronic renal failure undergoing hemodialysis is a consequence of central venous catherization. Catheter-induced thrombosis of the axillary and subclavian veins accounts for most cases of upper extremity deep venous thrombosis. An increase in the overall incidence of SAVT has been noted,[31] probably as a consequence of the increasing use of central catheters. This complication is especially problematic in patients with end-stage renal disease and functioning ipsilateral arteriovenous (AV) grafts or fistulas. In the patient with asymptomatic axillary vein thrombosis who has an ipsilateral AV fistula, early and massive swelling of the entire forearm and brachium can develop such that even superficial venous distension is obscured and skin breakdown is a threat.

The incidence of SAVT after placement of central venous access devices has been studied over the past few years. Deppe and colleagues found an incidence of 3.2% symptomatic SAVT in 154 patients who had peripherally placed central venous port devices between 1991 and 1994.[32] The incidence of asymptomatic SAVT is at least twice that of symptomatic SAVT. For example, of 57 oncology patients who had routine venograms performed after central venous catherization for chemotherapy, 10.5% had silent complete thrombosis of the ASVs, and 46% had incomplete thrombosis. In fact, when counting the 78% who also had fibrin sleeve, only four patients had normal study results.[33] From these data, an incidence of approximately 10% of ASV thrombosis in patients who have had central venous catherization can be predicted. In fact, the incidence of symptomatic SAVT in dialysis patients studied by Criado and associates was 14 of 158 (or 11.5%).[34] All patients had severe arm swelling or dialysis graft thrombosis secondary to previous subclavian vein catheters. The time to SAVT was studied by Horne and colleagues, who found that in 50 oncology patients with silicone venous access device, routine venograms detected partial thrombosis in 30% as early as 6 weeks and complete thrombosis in 6% at 6 weeks.[35] By 12 weeks, 10% of patients already had SAVT. Further, he noted that in another 30 patients who had previous catherization, complete occlusion was noted in 30%, although only 6% had symptoms.[35] The reason SAVT secondary to intrinsic causes is asymptomatic can be found in the development of rich collateral beds in the venous system of the neck and chest wall.

Risk factors for SAVT include the site of the catheter tip, with a site within the ASV being significantly prone to thrombosis (60%) compared with a site in the SVC (21%). The second risk factor for SAVT is placement of the catheter in the subclavian vein as opposed to the jugular vein, the former having a 10% risk of SAVT vs. 2.3% for the internal jugular position. Several other risk factors have been correlated to SAVT, including the use of multiple lumen catheters, insertion technique (multiple vs. single stick), type of catheter used (Silastic having the lowest incidence), and the type of solution infused through the catheter (fluid replacement vs. total parenteral nutrition).

Imaging diagnosis of SAVT has been described earlier in this chapter. Color duplex ultrasound is the investigation of choice for diagnosis of SAVT, followed by venography. With a duplex scanner, the distal subclavian and axillary veins are imaged below the clavicle, and the proximal subclavian and innominate veins are imaged from the supraclavicular fossa. Thrombus can be visualized as a nonechogenic density within the lumen of the vein. The proximal subclavian and innominate veins are often difficult to image, and the SVC cannot be imaged in the chest. However, obstruction in the central veins can be inferred by the absence of the normal respiratory variation of the Doppler examination. Computed tomography (CT) and magnetic resonance imaging (MRI) are noninvasive tests that can help clarify the presence or absence of thrombosis as well as visualize the SVC. Venography is the gold standard for the diagnosis of SAVT but carries the risk of contrast toxicity. Venography is also more accurate than duplex scanning in the diagnosis of stenosis. Criteria considered to show the presence of catheter-related thrombosis include visualization of thrombus, absence of spontaneous flow, absence of phasicity of flow with respiration, incompressibility of the vein with probe pressure, and visualization of increased venous collateral branches. When a thrombus is visualized in the absence of spontaneous flow and respiratory phasicity, the sensitivity rate of the color duplex ultrasound is 94% and the specificity rate is 96% compared with venograms.

While obtaining the SAVT duplex scan, it is also worth determining the flow in the brachial artery preoperatively because higher flow has been linked statistically to prolonged graft patency.

Although less frequent than that of the lower limbs, venous thrombosis of the upper limbs may cause pulmonary embolism. This is usually nonfatal and is facilitated by the delay or absence of anticoagulation therapy. In a prospective study of 86 patients with central venous catheter-related SAVT who had been treated by heparin, a pulmonary embolus confirmed by ventilation perfusion scan and venogram developed in 13 (15%). Two patients died of recurrent pulmonary embolus while being treated with heparin. A polyvinyl or polyethylene catheter was significantly more thrombogenic in this study than a polyurethane or silicone catheter.[36]

Goals of therapy in catheter-induced SAVT are to alleviate the acute symptoms, prevent propagation of clot, and prevent complications. Symptomatic patients should have the catheter removed as soon as possible and have the arm elevated. Systemic anticoagulation should be started to avoid the propagation of clot and to prevent embolization. Oral anticoagulation should be continued for 3 months. Asymptomatic patients require no treatment. If the patient has an asymptomatic SAVT that is recognized preoperatively and another access site is available, it is better to relocate the graft in the extremity with the patent venous outflow system. In some instances, this is simply not possible, and surgical or interventional treatment of the SAVT is necessary (Fig. 18–5). Thrombolytic therapy has been reported as an effective treatment for acute SAVT. Thrombolytic agents provide more rapid resolution and fewer treatment failures than anticoagulation alone. Chang and colleagues[37] reported the use of pulsed-spray injection of tissue plasminogen activator (rtPA) in 12 patients with symptomatic, venogram-confirmed, occlusive thrombi of the subclavian–axillary or jugular veins. Lytic agents were administered via catheters placed directly into the thrombus to optimize drug delivery, limit the necessary dose, and minimize hemorrhagic complications. Veins were treated with one or two 15-minute injections of rtPA delivered directly into the clots with pulse-spray catheters. Twenty-four hours after each treatment, repeated venograms were obtained to assess venous patency. Successful thrombolysis was defined as antegrade flow through the previously occluded segment with minimal collateral venous flow (8 of 12 patients). Continued patency was assessed with repeated venograms obtained after 1 and 2 months of oral anticoagulation. This technique had a high success rate with thrombi less than 2 weeks old regardless of the length of the clot but had limited success with thrombi more than 2 weeks old. Long-term patency, however, was only documented in four of the eight patients (50%).

Surgery for Secondary Subclavian–Axillary Vein Thrombosis

Bhatia and associates[38] previously demonstrated that the 1-year patency rate for simple balloon angioplasty

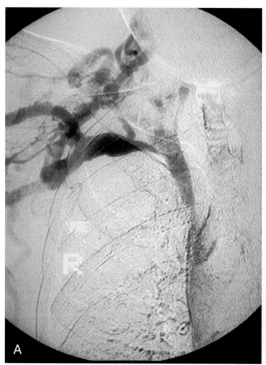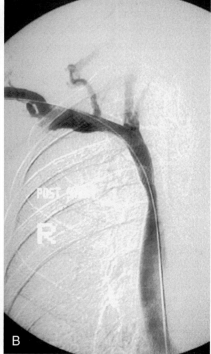

Figure 18–5. *A,* This dialysis patient presented with deteriorating function in his right forearm fistula. There was a past history of bilateral venous cannulation. The preliminary venogram demonstrates stenoses at the confluence of the right subclavian and jugular veins and a further stenosis of the superior vena cava (SVC). Fairly extensive collateral venous flow is seen. *B,* A 14-mm Wallstent has been used to treat the subclavian vein stenosis with immediate improvement in fistula function. In the absence of any symptoms of SVC obstruction, it was decided not to treat the SVC stenosis on this admission.

in patients with SAVT is 10%. These same authors compared the results of surgical treatment vs. percutaneous dilatation with stent placement. Twenty-six patients were studied retrospectively, all with symptomatic thrombosis. Half (13) underwent surgical treatment, which included a bypass procedure (with PTFE of saphenous vein graft). The stent group included 13 patients who underwent percutaneous angioplasty and insertion of a self-expanding rigid stent (n = 6) or balloon-expandable flexible stent (n = 7). No significant complications were reported in each group. The percentages of patients who were symptom free at 6 and 12 months were also similar in the two groups. In their study, surgical bypass and PTA with stent placement were both efficacious in the treatment of central venous obstruction. Reports of successful endoluminal therapy or bypass operation are scant. In Criado and colleagues' study of 14 patients, PTA was attempted in 17 and stents were placed in 13 veins, with a 76% initial success rate.[39] Hemodialysis from 2 to 9 months was achieved in slightly less than half (47%). Restenosis occurred in 12%, and three patients had an early occlusion. Stenotic veins were much more amenable to dilatation and stenting than were occluded veins, in which success was found in only two of eight patients. In a comparison of PTA vs. bypass surgery for SAVT/SVC thrombosis, 13 patients had bypass and 15 had dilatation.[40] Relief of symptoms was 88% at 1 year and 71% at 2 years for those patients having bypass, but these decreased very rapidly to 36% at 1 year and 0% at 2 years for the 15 PTA patients. However, Wisselink and associates noted that repeat angioplasty gave an 86% and 66% success rate at 1 and 2 years, respectively.[41] The success of endovascular techniques in managing stenosis of large central veins appears to be comparable to that of surgical reconstruction, although repeat interventions may be necessary.

Examination of the results of reconstruction of large veins in patients with benign disease can give some indication of the expected success rate in dialysis patients. Gloviczki and colleagues reported on 28 patients who had reconstruction of the SVC (12 patients) or the inferior vena cava and iliac veins (16 patients).[42] Early occlusions were relatively frequent, and in the SVC position, only 50% of patients had relief of symptoms after a mean follow-up of 7 months. In patients with lower extremity venous occlusion, 8 of the 11 patients who had a PTFE graft had construction of a femorofemoral AV fistula, resulting in the majority remaining patent after a mean follow-up of 9 months. The latter experience gives some optimism that a PTFE graft may maintain patency with an AV fistula in place. This, of course, is the situation for dialysis patients.

Management of subclavian vein occlusive disease

in persons with an ipsilateral arteriovenous fistula can be challenging. Gradman and associates[43] reviewed nine patients who underwent exploration and repair of an obstructed subclavian vein after medial claviculectomy. Eight patients had PTFE grafts; one patient had a Brescia-Cimino fistula. Intractable arm edema was the major symptom in five of eight patients. Although the surgical procedures varied from endovenectomy with or without use of patch (PTFE or vein), resection with end-to-end anastomosis, and end-to-end internal jugular to subclavian vein transposition, the results were similar. Postoperative venograms showed patent subclavian veins in all patients. Most grafts (75%) were patent at 8 months postoperatively.

The three bypass procedures available for symptomatic hemodialysis patients with SAVT are:

1. Transposition of the internal jugular to the axillary vein with end-to-side anastomosis ("the jugular turndown" procedure).
2. Axillary to jugular vein PTFE bypass.
3. Crossover PTFE bypass to the opposite axillary vein.

Conclusion

The upper extremities are subject to several unique venous disorders. Upper extremity thrombosis accounts for only 1 to 2% of cases of all deep venous thromboses, but many of these patients will have long-term disabilities if treatment is inadequate.

The treatment of axillosubclavian vein thrombosis is ultimately dependent on the etiologic factors. A multidisciplinary approach between interventional radiology and the vascular surgeon is imperative. "Effort-related" thrombosis is seen in young athletic patients. The treatment should consist of catheter-related thrombolysis followed by surgery.

Catheter-induced axillosubclavian vein thrombosis is seen in association with other medical problems (end-stage renal disease, prolonged intravenous access for antibiotics or total parenteral nutrition, central venous access, and so forth). Initial management should consist of removal of the catheter with institution of anticoagulation. Thrombolysis is performed when the patient is symptomatic (i.e., edema, pain). Surgical or endovascular intervention is reserved for patients for whom medical therapy fails.

REFERENCES

1. Hunter W: History of aneurysm of the aorta with some remarks on aneurysm in general. Med Observations Inquiries 1:323, 1757.
2. Lokich JJ, Goodman R: Superior vena cava syndrome: Clinical management. JAMA 231:58–61, 1975.

3. Davenport D, Ferree C, Blake D, et al: Radiation therapy in the treatment of superior vena caval obstruction. Cancer 42:2600–2603, 1978.
4. Escalante CP: Causes and management of superior vena cava syndrome. Oncology 7:61–68, 1993.
5. Key ST, Kinoshita L, Razavi MK, et al: Superior vena cava syndrome: Treatment with catheter-directed thrombolysis and endovascular stent placement. Radiology 206:187–193, 1998.
6. Perez CA, Presant CA, Van Amburg AL III: Management of superior vena cava syndrome. Semin Oncol 5:123–134, 1978.
7. Lochridge S, Knibbe W, Doty D: Obstruction of superior vena cava. Surgery 85:14–24, 1979.
8. Chen J, Bongard F, Klein S: A contemporary perspective on superior vena cava syndrome. Am J Surg 160:207–211, 1990.
9. Armstrong B, Perez C, Simpson J, et al: Role of irradiation in the management of superior vena cava syndrome. Int J Radiat Oncol Biol Phys 13:531–539, 1987.
10. Kane R, Cohen M: Superior vena cava obstruction due to small-cell anaplastic lung cancer. JAMA 235:1717–1718, 1976.
11. Urban T, Lebeau B, Chatang C, et al: Superior vena cava syndrome in small cell lung cancer. Arch Intern Med 153:384–387, 1993.
12. Wurschmidt F, Bunemann H, Heilmann HP: Small cell lung cancer with and without superior vena cava syndrome: A multi-variate analysis of prognostic factors in 408 cases. Int J Radiat Oncol Biol Phys 33:77–82, 1995.
13. Rodrigues CI, Njo KH, Karim AB: Hypofractionated radiation therapy in the treatment of superior vena cava syndrome. Lung Cancer 10:221–228, 1993.
14. Charnsangavej C, Carrasco CH, Wallace S, et al: Stenosis of the vena cava: Preliminary assessment of treatment with expandable stents. Radiology 161:295–298, 1986.
15. Gaines PA, Belli A-M, Anderson P, et al: Superior vena cava obstruction managed by Gianturco Z stent. Clin Radiol 49:202–208, 1994.
16. Nicholson AA, Ettles DF, Arnold A, et al: Treatment of malignant superior vena cava obstruction: Metal stents or radiation therapy. J Vasc Interv Radiol 8:781–788, 1997.
17. Crow MTI, Davies CH, Gaines PA: Percutaneous management of superior vena cava occlusions. Cardiovasc Intervent Radiol 18:367–372, 1995.
18. Adelman MA, Stone DH, Riles TS, et al: A multidisciplinary approach to the treatment of Paget-Schroetter syndrome. Ann Vasc Surg 11:149–154, 1997.
19. Dunant JH: Effort thrombosis, a complication of thoracic outlet syndrome. Vasa 10:322–324, 1981.
20. Hicken GJ, Ameli FM: CJS: Management of subclavian–axillary vein thrombosis. Can J Surg 41:13–25, 1998.
21. Hurlbert SN, Rutherford RB: Basic underlying clinical decision making—primary subclavian vein thrombosis. Ann Vasc Surg 9:217–223, 1995.
22. Adams JT, DeWeese JA: "Effort" thrombosis of the axillary and subclavian veins. J Trauma 11:923–930 1971.
23. Gloviczki P, Kazmier FJ, Hollier LH: Axillary–subclavian venous occlusion: The morbidity of a nonlethal disease. J Vasc Surg 4:333–337, 1986.
24. Coon WW, Willis PW: Thrombosis of axillary and subclavian veins. Arch Surg 94:657–663, 1967.
25. Sanders RJ, Haug C: Subclavian vein obstruction and thoracic outlet syndrome: A review of the etiology and management. Ann Vasc Surg 4:397–410, 1990.
26. Beygui RE, Olcott C, Dalman RL: Subclavian vein thrombosis: Outcome analysis based on etiology and modality of treatment. Ann Vasc Surg 11:247–255, 1997.
27. Hall LD, Murray JD, Boswell GE: Venous stent placement as an adjunct to the staged, multimodal treatment of Paget Schroetter syndrome. J Vasc Interv Radiol 6:565–570, 1995.
28. Meier GH, Pollak JS, Rosenblatt M, et al: Initial experience with venous stents in exertional axillary-subclavian vein thrombosis. J Vasc Surg 24:974–983, 1996.
29. Lee MC, Grassi CJ, Belkin M, et al: Early operative intervention after thrombolytic therapy for primary subclavian vein thrombosis: An effective treatment approach. J Vasc Surg 27:1101–1108, 1998.
30. Machleder HI: Evaluation of a new treatment strategy for Paget-Schroetter syndrome: Spontaneous thrombosis of the axillary–subclavian vein. J Vasc Surg 17:305–315, 1993.
31. Becker DM, Philbrick JT, Walker FB: Axillary and subclavian venous thrombosis: Prognosis and treatment. Arch Intern Med 151:1934, 1991.
32. Deppe G, Kahn ML, Malviya VK, et al: Experience with the P.A.S.-PORT venous access device in patients with gynecologic malignancies. Gynecol Oncol 62:340–343, 1996.
33. Horne MK III, May DJ, Alexander HR, et al: Venographic surveillance of tunneled venous access devices in adult oncology patients. Ann Surg Oncol 2:174–178, 1995.
34. Criado E, Marston WA, Jaques PF, et al: Proximal venous outflow obstruction in patients with upper extremity arteriovenous dialysis access. Ann Vasc Surg 8:530–535, 1994.
35. Horne MK III, Merryman PK, Mayo DJ, et al: Reductions in tissue plasminogen activator and thrombomodulin in blood draining veins damaged by venous access devices. Thromb Res 79:369–376, 1995.
36. Koksoy C, Kuzu A, Erden I, Akkaya A: The risk factors in central venous catheter-related thrombosis. Aust N Z J Surg 65:796–798, 1995.
37. Chang R, Horne MK III, Mayo DJ, Doppman JL: Pulse-spray treatment of subclavian and jugular venous thrombi with recombinant tissue plasminogen activator. J Vasc Intervent Radiol 7:845–851, 1996.
38. Bhatia DS, Money SR, Ochsner JL, et al: Comparison of surgical bypass and percutaneous balloon dilatation with primary stent placement in the treatment of central venous obstruction in the dialysis patient: One-year follow-up. Ann Vasc Surg 10:452–455, 1996.
39. Lumsden AB, MacDonald MJ, Isiklar H, et al: Central venous stenosis in the hemodialysis patient: Incidence and efficacy of endovascular treatment. Cardiovasc Surg 5:504–509, 1997.
40. Hood DB, Yellin AE, Richman MF, et al: Hemodialysis graft salvage with endoluminal stents. Am Surg 60:733, 1994.
41. Wisselink W, Money SR, Becker MO, et al: Comparison of operative reconstruction and percutaneous balloon dilatation for central venous obstruction. Am J Surg 166:200–204, 1993 (discussion 204–205).
42. Gloviczki P, Bower TC, Toomey BJ: [Prosthetic reconstructions of the inferior vena cava]. Phlebologie 46:479–483, 1993.
43. Gradman WS, Bressman P, Sernaque JD: Subclavian vein repair in patients with an ipsilateral arteriovenous fistula. Ann Vasc Surg 8:549–556, 1994.

Chapter 19 Inferior Vena Cava Filters

Endovascular Contributor: Anthony A. Nicholson

Inferior vena cava (IVC) filters have been available for 20 years, the concept of caval interruption having been suggested by Trouseau in 1868.[1] IVC filters are designed to prevent significant pulmonary emboli in an "at risk" population. The mortality and morbidity caused by pulmonary emboli is difficult to estimate on a worldwide basis, but even in the most medically advanced countries, it is significant, accounting for approximately 200,000 deaths and 570,000 nonlethal episodes annually in the United States. The effectiveness of caval interruption with a filter has never been tested in a randomized controlled trial. This may account for differences in practice within populations and from country to country. For instance, within the United States Medicare population, IVC filter insertion rates vary from 14 to 37 per 100,000,[2] whereas in a single hospital in France, 621 filters were inserted during a 3-year period.[3] This compares to the United Kingdom experience where, in one hospital, for an equivalent size population to the French center, only 60 filters were inserted during a 3-year period.[4] However, we do know that the mortality after one pulmonary embolus in untreated patients is significant. The 48-hour mortality rate in patients with indeterminate ventilation–perfusion scans who were left untreated was 5 to 10% in one study,[5] whereas a meta-analysis of the available literature suggests a 35% mortality rate in the first 12 months if pulmonary embolus is left untreated. Unfortunately, the only attempt at a randomized trial randomized patients to treatment with a filter plus anticoagulants or anticoagulants alone, as if the two treatments were in conflict. Even here, however, the early mortality was very different, with four fatal pulmonary emboli occurring in the group without filters and none occurring in the group with filters.[6]

All the available evidence therefore is in favor of treating pulmonary embolus. Traditionally, anticoagulants have been the treatment of choice, but when these are ineffective or contraindicated, caval interruption with an IVC filter is an effective alternative.

INDICATIONS

Accepted Indications

CONTRAINDICATION TO ANTICOAGULATION

This is the main indication for filtration in our practice (39%). Patients who have had a recent hemorrhagic episode, such as a bleeding peptic ulcer or an intracranial hemorrhage, and patients who recently have undergone major surgery cannot be given anticoagulants. If they suffer a pulmonary embolus or if a significant deep venous thrombosis develops, caval filtration may be their only treatment option. It is also well documented that there is an increased incidence of bleeding complications in anticoagulated patients older than 80 years of age. The use of filters may be the preferred option in this group also. IVC filters have no significant influence on survival in patients who have known malignancy, and they certainly should not be used in terminal malignancies. However, as previously discussed, because of the high early mortality from pulmonary embolus, when there are personal and social reasons for increasing survival time in the cancer patient with coagulopathy due to abnormal liver function, the use of filters is reasonable. In addition, if further treatment is being contemplated in this group, filtration should be considered.

INEFFECTIVE ANTICOAGULATION

Eighteen percent of patients have recurrent pulmonary emboli while adequately anticoagulated. Half of these are fatal.[7, 8] Patients with congestive cardiac failure are at particular risk. Provided that there is no contraindication, patients probably should continue anticoagulant treatment for the prescribed time because there is a higher incidence of both IVC occlusion and postphlebitic syndrome in nonanticoagulated patients who do undergo IVC filtration.[4, 6] In our practice, this is the second most common indication for filter insertion (35%).

COMPLICATIONS OF ANTICOAGULANTS

Patients who have bleeding complications secondary to anticoagulants, such as postoperative bleeding or hemorrhagic stroke, and who have had recent embolic episodes should be considered for filtration. In a small number of patients, hemorrhagic skin rash and platelet dysfunction due to heparin have been observed; because heparin prevents thrombus propagation in deep vein thrombosis (DVT), protection by caval interruption should be considered in such cases.

Such complications are rare indications for filtration, representing only 10% of our practice. However, major bleeding complications secondary to anticoagulants did occur in 9.3% of patients in one series.[4]

Expanded Indications

The following indications are more controversial and are not universally accepted. In the future, temporary filters may provide a less controversial alternative and are discussed later in this chapter.

PROPHYLAXIS IN TRAUMA

DVT was reported in 62% of patients with spinal trauma despite prophylactic heparin in one large series.[9] In addition, in 35 to 60% of patients with pelvic trauma, DVT developed, half of which was in the ileofemoral and deep pelvic veins.[10] Pulmonary embolus was recorded in 2 to 10% and was fatal in 2%. However, in another series,[11] in which 280 high-risk trauma patients were identified, only 12 cases of DVT were identified and 4 had nonfatal pulmonary emboli. Here, the use of prophylactic filtration was not believed to be justified. However, if such patients have a history of DVT or pulmonary emboli and an extended hospital stay greater than 2 weeks, then filtration may be indicated and has been shown to be cost-effective.[12]

PROPHYLAXIS IN PELVIC SURGERY

In a series of 1174 patients, fatal pulmonary embolus was reported in 2.3% who were not given heparin after hip surgery.[13] This incidence decreases to 1% when prophylactic heparin is given, although there are significant bleeding complications associated with this approach,[14] and the incidence increases considerably with age. It is difficult to justify caval interruption in this overall group unless there is a well-documented history of DVT or pulmonary embolus. Even effective temporary filtration may not prove to be cost-effective.

PULMONARY HYPERTENSION

When there is good evidence that pulmonary hypertension is secondary to chronic, recurrent pulmonary emboli, prophylactic filter insertion possibly combined with pulmonary arterial thrombolytic therapy may be indicated. At our own center, we have treated two young females with pulmonary hypertension and documented occult DVT. In both cases, pulmonary arterial pressures have reduced from greater than 80 mm Hg to less than 35 mm Hg within 7 days, and the patients are well at 1-year follow-up. The mortality of pulmonary hypertension from all causes is high, and although most patients die of right heart failure, a significant number do so from single embolic episodes, which they are unable to tolerate. Again, although controversial, on a case-by-case basis, filtration may be indicated.

PROPHYLAXIS IN THE PATIENT WITH ILIOCAVAL THROMBUS

Loose thrombus in the IVC or iliac veins has a high probability of detachment, and anticoagulation is not known to prevent this[15] (Fig. 19–1). However, in some instances, serial follow-up sometimes can show these clots to disappear because of the body's own thrombolytic system. Nevertheless, the decision not to use filters in these patients is potentially disastrous, and few would be prepared to take this course of action.

The intravenous drug abuser occasionally injects thrombotic material into the femoral vein, which can cause massive iliofemoral DVT. The nature of the patient's habit and his or her social circumstances may contraindicate anticoagulants once he or she leaves the hospital. A decision to use filters in such

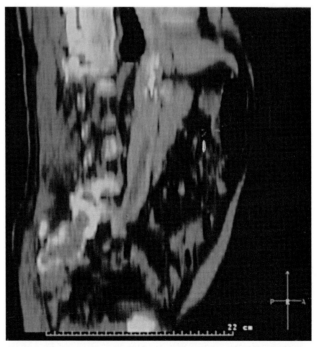

Figure 19–1. Sagittal reconstructed spinal computed tomography (SCT) demonstrating loose thrombus in the inferior vena cava (IVC).

patients may be made after full and rigorous explanation of the problem

MISCELLANEOUS INDICATIONS

Septic thromboemboli probably are treated best by filtration and antibiotics because the only other possible treatment involves tying off the IVC surgically. Patients who have undergone surgical pulmonary thrombectomy should have a filter inserted to prevent recurrence.

Suprarenal Inferior Vena Cava Filter Placement

When possible, IVC filters should be inserted below the renal veins to prevent renal vein thrombosis if IVC occlusion occurs. The suprarenal IVC is shorter and wider than its infrarenal component and is often harder to image because of unopacified blood entering. This makes accurate placement below the hepatic veins difficult, and there are concerns over stability, with the filter being affected by respiratory motion. However, there are situations in which suprarenal insertion is necessary. These include: (1) thrombus in the IVC up to or including the renal veins (see Fig. 19–1); (2) emboli from gonadal vein thrombosis; (3) propagation of thrombus above an existing infrarenal filter; and (4) pregnant patients in whom the gravid uterus is compressing the IVC.

An analysis of available studies revealed 122 patients followed for a mean of 26 months. No increase in prefilter creatinine levels has been reported and filter migration has not been clinically significant, but nonfatal recurrent pulmonary embolus has been reported in 4 to 8%. This also has been the author's experience with suprarenal filters (Figs. 19–2 and 19–3). In the aforementioned rare and limited clinical situations, suprarenal filter placement can be considered. Once a temporary filter with a long retrieval time becomes available, this may be a suitable indication.

CONTRAINDICATIONS

There are no clear contraindications to filter insertion. Even decisions about patients with coagulopathies must be made on a patient-by-patient basis. Clearly, there are many young patients who may require filtration, and decisions must be made with caution. Patients need to be told of their immediate clinical situation and the lack of long-term (>10 year) data on any of the available implanted filters. Even in the pediatric population, filters have proven safe and

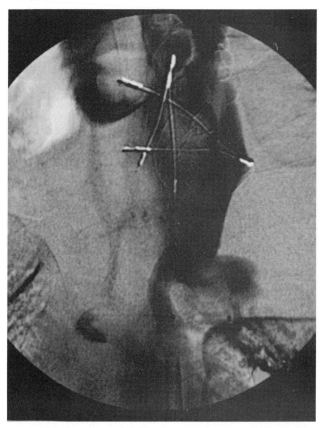

Figure 19–2. Bird's nest filter (BNF) inserted in the suprarenal inferior vena cava (IVC) because of thrombus to the level of the renal veins.

effective at least to 1 year.[16] The complications that we do know about should be made known to the patient.

The megacava is thought by some to be a contraindication to IVC filtration. A megacava is defined as an IVC greater than 2.8 cm in diameter. Certainly

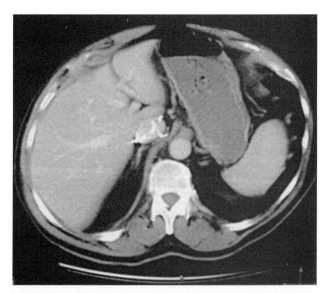

Figure 19–3. Spinal computed tomography (SCT) 2 years after suprarenal filter insertion (see Fig. 19–2) demonstrated no migration, no mechanical failure, and a patent inferior vena cava (IVC).

only the birds nest filter of the currently available devices will fit a cava up to 4 cm. However, because the IVC is elliptical, it appears on contrast cavography to be much bigger than it is. If the two diameters of an ellipse are (x) and (y), then the diameter of the equivalent circle is twice their square root. Thus, for an apparent cava of 2.8 cm, the equivalent circular diameter is 2.54 cm. Because most filters force the cava into a circle (BNF excepted), this is extremely relevant and suggests that the accepted megacava incidence of 2%[17] is probably an overestimate. If a true megacava is encountered, then bilateral common iliac filter insertion is safe and effective.

TECHNICAL ASPECTS OF INFERIOR VENA CAVA FILTER INSERTION

General Considerations

Different filters have different release mechanisms and insertion specifics. It is not the intention of this chapter to describe all the filters available and their technique of insertion. Filters can be inserted from the right or left common femoral vein, the right internal jugular vein or, more recently, the brachial vein in the antecubital fossa (Simon Nitinol Filter). Techniques for puncturing these veins are described elsewhere in this book. Initial cavography should determine the size of the cava and the position in relation to the lumbar vertebral bodies of the two renal veins and the iliac venous bifurcation. It is often best to do this with a cobra-curved catheter. Filter insertion ideally should be below the inferior border of the renal veins and above the bifurcation. The most difficult technical aspect of IVC filter insertion is the unexpected anatomic variant that interferes with what is otherwise a very simple technical procedure.

Anatomic Variants

INTERRUPTED VENA CAVA WITH AZYGOUS OR HEMIAZYGOUS CONTINUATION

This occurs with an incidence of 0.6%. If the azygous or hemiazygous veins are the main routes of venous drainage back to the right heart, they can be selected with appropriate wires and catheters and the filter inserted.

RETROAORTIC LEFT RENAL VEIN

This occurs with an incidence of 2%. Either a filter is inserted above it, risking renal vein thrombosis if the IVC occludes, or below it, which usually means bilateral common iliac vein filters.

LEFT-SIDED INFERIOR VENA CAVA

This occurs with an incidence of 0.5%. The IVC courses along the left side of the lumbar spine and then crosses sharply to the right after receiving the left renal vein. This makes the jugular or arm approach dangerous, especially with rigid systems such as the stainless steel Greenfield. The femoral approach is indicated. If the iliac veins contain thrombus and the system will not negotiate the right angle bend after carefully and gently pushing the system, a suprarenal position may have to be accepted.

CIRCUMAORTIC LEFT RENAL VEIN

This occurs in 8.7% of the population. The left renal vein circles the aorta, the anterior half joining the IVC at the usual level, but the posterior half curves downward and joins at a lower level. Once again, this may leave little choice but to insert bilateral common iliac venous filters.

DOUBLE INFERIOR VENA CAVA

The embryologic persistence of the left and right cardinal veins can be seen in 2% of the population. Sometimes it can be demonstrated only during cavography if the patient is asked to perform Valsalva's maneuver, and it is a good idea to ask the patient to blow into a blood pressure gauge during initial cavography. The failure to diagnose this variant may account for some postfilter embolic episodes because it is usually necessary to interrupt both vessels.

MISCELLANEOUS ABNORMALITIES OF THE INFERIOR VENA CAVA

A thrombosed cava clearly requires a careful internal jugular or arm approach. It also may necessitate the placement of a suprarenal filter. Similarly, intrahepatic caval narrowing requires a femoral approach. The most difficult abnormality to deal with is the presence of an occluded cava and multiple collateral channels. If these are large enough to transport thrombus of a potentially fatal size, they can be filtered. Care has to be taken that venous gangrene does not follow occlusion of all collateral branches.

CHOICE OF INFERIOR VENA CAVA FILTER

General Considerations

It is essential to have available a filter system that can be inserted from the jugular or subclavian route in addition to the more frequently used femoral route.

As temporary filter design improves, it is becoming apparent that a choice of temporary or permanent filtration may have to be made. Choice of filter should depend on the ease of device insertion coupled with device effectiveness and complication rate.

None of the devices available on the market are technically demanding to insert. Some are slightly more complicated than others, but it would be wrong to use a device on this criterion alone. Ultimately, filter effectiveness is based on the ability to prevent death or serious morbidity from large and/or multiple pulmonary emboli. A crucial factor when selecting a filter, therefore, is its efficiency in capturing clinically significant thrombi in vivo. However, clinical follow-up studies are unreliable because there is a high mortality from other causes in this notoriously variable group of patients. It is also difficult to standardize testing conditions in animals whose anatomy and physiology is too different from humans to allow comparison. For this reason, efficiency testing is based on laboratory studies of clottrapping capability. Many different models have been described, and again, the resulting lack of standardization means that available studies demonstrate conflicting results for specific devices. Nevertheless, they are all based on the ability of the filter to trap clots of predetermined and differing diameters and lengths, in tube systems of various diameters and orientations with different flow velocities. A standard testing system currently is available.[18] Filters are also evaluated for their saturation characteristics by single-, double-, and multiple-shot testing. This also influences the positioning of the filter because migration with large thromboembolic loads has been reported.[19] Many of the filters available at the time of writing are conical, relying on the apex of the cone to trap clots. In vitro studies show that the clot-trapping capability of these filters decreases with thrombus load, with subsequent thrombi unable to get into the apex of the cone. When the apex is blocked by thrombus flow, velocities increase around the periphery of the cone, and subsequent clots are pushed through the peripheral wires. In addition, tilting of cone-shaped filters can alter dramatically their clot-trapping ability. A recent study[20] of 12 currently available permanent filters tested, as described previously in the straight (all) and tilted positions (Greenfield and Gunther filters), demonstrated the high single-shot capture capability of conical filters, but confirmed the aforementioned disadvantage with double-shot and multishot testing of this design. Lower capture rates with the Titanium Greenfield and Gunther filters in the tilted position were also confirmed. The highest capture rates in all types of testing were found in those filters that segment the IVC (BNF, Simon Nitinol, and Tulip filters). Prolapse of the BNF filter wires was not found to alter clot-trapping ability at any load.

In another study by the same team,[21] the clot-trapping abilities of temporary filters were found to be inferior to those of permanent filters, and even where high capture rates were demonstrated, cranial movement of temporary filters could be demonstrated with load.

Temporary and Retrievable Filters

A temporary filter is a device that has to be removed within a set time limit. It therefore must be attached to the access site by a catheter or wire that may be left either in an external or subcutaneous position. A retrievable filter is a permanent filter that could be removed within a specified time period (Fig. 19–4).

At the present time, the indications for the use of these devices are not well established. Nevertheless, the potential indications for their use are as follows.

PROPHYLAXIS IN TRAUMA

As previously discussed, patients with spinal and pelvic trauma have a high thromboembolic risk. The main factors inhibiting permanent filter placement are the potential complications, both known and unknown, in the short and long term. There are, however, two encouraging reports[22, 23] of the use of temporary filters, but clearly the relative risks of pulmonary

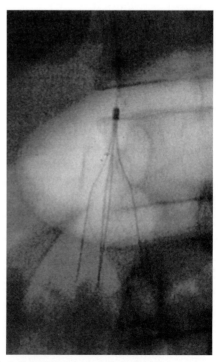

Figure 19–4. Tulip filter inserted 10 days earlier in a patient at risk of pulmonary edema (PE) before surgery. The filter was removed from a jugular approach when the patient was mobile. It contained one small embolus, although a source was not found.

embolus must be compared with the complications of temporary filtration.

PROPHYLAXIS IN WHICH THERE IS A SHORT-TERM CONTRAINDICATION TO ANTICOAGULANTS

This may occur before or after surgery, especially pelvic surgery, or when postoperative DVT develops. However, the filter used would have to have a suitable retrieval time if anticoagulants are to be reintroduced.

PROTECTION OF PATIENTS RECEIVING THROMBOLYTIC THERAPY FOR LOWER LIMB DEEP VEIN THROMBOSIS

Thrombolysis in DVT is a procedure that is gathering momentum in the United States and Europe. In one study of 132 patients, 31% were found to have emboli trapped in a temporary filter, 25% of which were large.[24] However, most do not use filtration. Clearly, if this technique is found to be effective, a randomized trial of filter vs. no filter is required.

PROPHYLAXIS WHEN INFERIOR VENA CAVA THROMBUS IS DEMONSTRATED

Particularly when this is free floating (see Fig. 19–1), patients are at high risk. When the patient is young, the decision to place a permanent filter is not taken lightly. A temporary or retrievable filter may make such management decisions easier.

Currently, there is not enough evidence to recommend these filters in any clinical situation. The lack of literature partly represents the poor technologies available at present. Retrievable filters such as the Gunther Tulip at present have too short a retrieval time and can be awkward to remove. Devices with hooks have the potential for IVC damage on removal. Temporary filters have poor clot-trapping ability and the potential for infection, especially if inserted from the femoral route. Potentially the best of these, the Tempofilter, recently was recalled for modification after it was found to have embolized to the right atrium.

COMPLICATIONS

The major complications relating to the insertion of permanent IVC filters have been documented by Tardy and colleagues[25] as puncture site complications, filter migration, IVC erosion, IVC occlusion, recurrent pulmonary embolism, and lower extremity venous insufficiency.

Puncture Site Complications

Femoral arteriovenous fistulae have been reported after Greenfield filter insertion but are rare and are related to poor vascular access technique. Asymptomatic insertion site thrombosis has been reported in up to 41% of patients[26] and was symptomatic in 1.8% with the Greenfield filter.[27] Most of these thromboses have occurred after jugular insertion. There are those who look for this complication in all patients undergoing filter placement. In our practice, we do not, and a careful review over a 10-year period using mainly the BNF has not revealed a single symptomatic case of insertion site thrombosis.

Filter Migration

Filters can migrate if they are too small for the IVC, if they have inadequate means of fixation or are inserted inexpertly, if they are manipulated excessively at surgery, or if they contain a large thrombus load that causes them to move. In addition, strut fractures can occur (Fig. 19–5), and experience is sufficiently limited with the use of filters that nobody knows what the 10- to 50-year outcome may be in patients who have undergone caval interruption at a young age. For this reason, careful records should be kept and abdominal imaging performed at 5-year intervals. Available rates of migration are indicated in Table 19–1. Our own

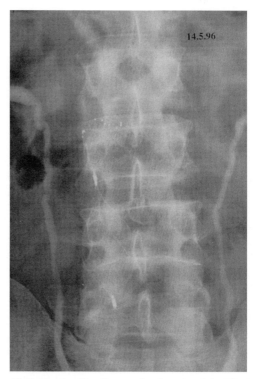

Figure 19–5. Gunther filter 5 years after insertion. It is difficult to see the individual wires because there are multiple fractures.

Table 19–1. Specifications of Five Commonly Used Inferior Vena Cava (IVC) Filters

Filter (Sheath Size)	Maximum IVC Size (mm)	IVC Patency (%)	Migration (%) (Fracture [%])	Recurrent Pulmonary Embolus (%)	Tilting Significant
Greenfield Steel + Titanium (12/14 French)	28	92–95	15 (1)	5	Yes
Simon Nitinol (9 French)	28	91–93	1 (22)	3	No
Gunther Tulip (10 French)	28	92	12 (1)	2	Yes
BNF (14 French)	40	96–98	0–1 (<1)	2.7	No
Vena Tech LGM (12 French)	28	70	18.4 (NA)	3.5–8.4	No

experience with 5- to 10-year follow-up with the BNF is of no migrations and no fractures on follow-up computed tomography (CT) and plain abdominal imaging[4] but migration and strut fracture have been reported.[19, 28] The Antheor filter was removed from the market because of its high rate of migration.[29] The wires on the BNF can migrate upward and lie in the suprarenal IVC (Fig. 19–6). This tendency can be reduced by rotating the introducing catheter at insertion, although as stated earlier, prolapse does not interfere with the filter's efficiency. We have seen these wires in renal (Fig. 19–7) and hepatic veins without any clinical sequelae.[4]

Misplacement of the filter should not be confused with migration. If, on follow-up, an odd filter position is seen, the immediate postinsertion films should be checked. The most common sites for misplacement are the right side of the heart, the right renal vein (Fig. 19–8), and the iliac veins. The right renal vein is particularly susceptible if the kidney is ptotic and the jugular approach is used. If necessary, filters can be retrieved percutaneously[29] using wires and snares but in some clinical circumstances can be left alone.[30]

Inferior Vena Cava Perforation

Perforation of the IVC has been reported with most filter types. In our review, we noted asymptomatic BNF struts outside the caval wall in 85.3% of our patients on CT scanning[4] (Fig. 19–9), and it is probably as high with other devices. There are case reports describing strut erosion causing obstructive uropathy,[31] small bowel volvulus,[32] vertebral body penetration,[33] duodenal perforation,[34] and intractable retroperitoneal pain.[35] However, these are exceptional, and such perforation is nearly always asymptomatic (Fig. 19–10).

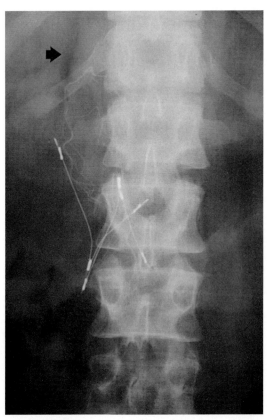

Figure 19–6. Suprarenal wire prolapse (*arrow*) from a well-positioned bird's nest filter (BNF).

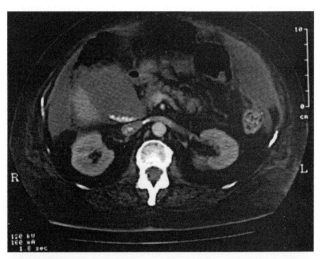

Figure 19–7. Asymptomatic wire prolapse from a bird's nest filter into the left renal vein. The computed tomography (CT) scan was performed 7 years after filter insertion.

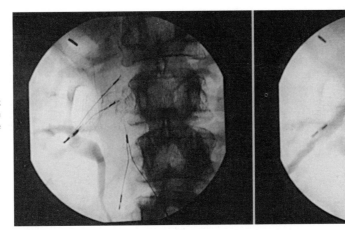

Figure 19–8. Strutts of a bird's nest filter inserted from the jugular vein in a ptotic right renal vein. There were no sequelae after 3 years.

Inferior Vena Cava Occlusion

IVC occlusion by thrombus occurs as a result of the hemodynamic effect of the filter or the sudden trapping by the filter of a massive thromboembolus. Both probably occur in different patients, but again, there appear to be differences between devices (Fig. 19–11; see also Table 19–1). Using the VenaTechLGM filter, Tardy and colleagues[25] reported an 8.9% rate of IVC occlusion. They found no incidence of occlusion with the BNF, although we have found a 4.7% incidence with this filter.[4] Interestingly, these patients all had contraindications to anticoagulants and had documented loose iliofemoral thrombus before filter insertion. It is therefore conceivable that all were the result of massive thromboembolus. Only one was symptomatic, causing bilateral leg swelling that subsided over 3 months as collateral branches opened. The others were identified 5 to 6 years later by previously unrecorded clinical signs (dilated abdominal wall veins) and CT scanning.

The low rate of IVC occlusion reported with the BNF may be due to its design, the fine wires fragmenting and trapping embolus rather than allowing it to remain whole, as in the conical design. These wires also may have less of a hemodynamic effect than other more solid filters.

Recurrent Pulmonary Embolus

Table 19–1 shows the rates of recurrent pulmonary embolism for different caval filters. Overall, recurrence rates are between 2 and 4.8%. Clearly, as discussed, embolus can occur through the filter, especially when there is a thrombus load. This tends to be device specific. In addition, at least some recurrence is via collateral pathways, particularly when the IVC is thrombosed. When there is malignancy, in situ thrombosis can occur in the lungs.

Recurrent Deep Vein Thrombosis and Postphlebitic Syndrome

Decousus and associates,[6] in the only available randomized study, found that at 2 years there was a significantly higher rate of recurrent DVT in a group of patients receiving a filter and anticoagulants compared with a group receiving anticoagulants alone (20.8 vs. 11.6%). However, within this study, different heparin types were also being tested, and different filter types were used, the LGM in 56% of cases. In addition, patients were imaged only for recurrent DVT if they complained of symptoms. It is notoriously difficult to detect recurrent DVT after recent

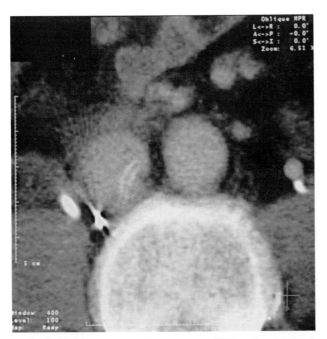

Figure 19–9. Asymptomatic inferior vena cava (IVC) wall perforation by a strutt of a bird's nest filter.

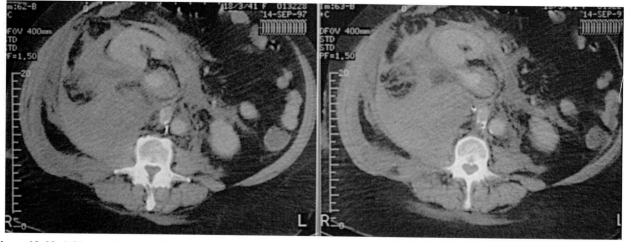

Figure 19–10. A 56-year-old woman admitted with abdominal pain was found to have a large retroperitoneal hematoma and strutt perforation from a bird's nest filter inserted 12 months earlier. The initial surgical diagnosis was of inferior vena cava (IVC) perforation. However, this is a normal finding. The patient's international normalized ratio (INR) was later found to be greater than 10. The hematoma was secondary to anticoagulants and not to the bird's nest filter.

DVT, especially in a population presenting initially with predominantly proximal DVT. It was not stated how many of these recurrences were in the same leg. Presumably, none of these recurrences required treatment because all patients were anticoagulated or had filters inserted. In addition, there is no evidence that a recurrent DVT in the same leg, as opposed to a single episode, leads to an increased incidence of postphlebitic syndrome. The conclusion that the systematic use of IVC filters could not be recommended because of this ignores the early mortality from pulmonary embolism and the excess of symptomatic pulmonary embolism in the anticoagulated group vs. the filtered/anticoagulated group (6.3 vs. 3.4%) at 2 years. The same study also reported an overall rate of major

hemorrhage of 9.8% in patients treated with anticoagulants. In addition, embolus was found within the filter in 16 of 37 patients who had recurrent DVT. Presumably, the filter had prevented this from reaching the pulmonary circulation.

CONCLUSION: ANTICOAGULATION AND INFERIOR VENA CAVA FILTRATION

If not contraindicated, adjunctive anticoagulation after filter insertion is useful to prevent recurrent DVT, IVC occlusion, and insertion site thrombosis. It is probably sensible for any patient in whom recur-

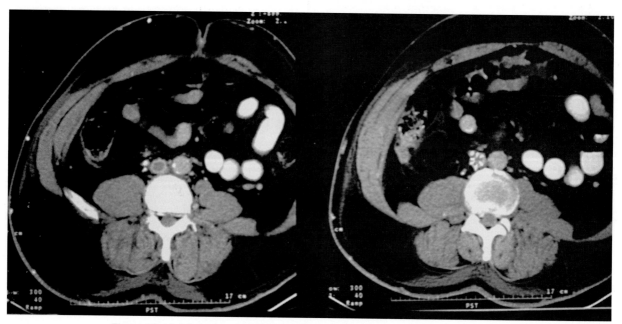

Figure 19–11. Inferior vena cava (IVC) occlusion 4 weeks after Simon nitinol filter insertion.

rent DVT or pulmonary embolus develops after filter insertion and cessation of anticoagulants to continue life-long anticoagulation treatment. However, if anticoagulants are contraindicated, the insertion of an IVC filter is potentially life saving. Despite the lack of a randomized trial, there is enough worldwide experience and literature evidence to suggest that insertion should not be delayed.

REFERENCES

1. Trousseau A: Phlegmasia alba dolens. Clinique Medicale de L'Hotel-Dieu de Paris, 3rd ed., Vol. 3. Paris, JB Bailliere, 1868 pp 652–695.
2. Walsh DB, Birkmeyer JD, Barrett JA, et al: Use of inferior vena cava filters in the medicare population. Ann Vasc Surg 9:483–487, 1995.
3. Bosson JL, Olinic D, Franco G, et al: Partial interruption of the inferior vena cava: 10 year evolution in protocols at Grenoble University Hospital. Study of 621 patients. Vasa 24:34–41, 1995.
4. Nicholson AA, Ettles DF, Dyet JF: Long term follow-up of the Bird's Nest filter (Abstract). CIRSE. 21 (Suppl), Venice, 1998.
5. Rose J: Forty-eight hour mortality in patients with indeterminate V/Q scans not anticoagulated (Abstract). RSNA. 1995.
6. Decousus H, Leizorovicz A, Parent F, et al: A clinical trial of vena caval filters in the prevention of pulmonary embolism in patients with proximal deep vein thrombosis. N Engl J Med 338:409–415, 1998.
7. Mobin-Uddin K, Uttley JR, Bryant LR: The inferior vena cava umbrella filter. Prog Cardiovasc Dis 17:391–399, 1975.
8. Santos GH, Lansman S: Prevention of pulmonary embolism with use of the Mobin-Uddin filter. NY State J Med 82:185, 1982.
9. Jarrel BE, Posuniak E, Roberts J, et al: A new method of management using the Kimray-Greenfield filter for deep venous thrombosis and pulmonary embolism in spinal cord injury. Surg Gynecol Obstet 157:316, 1983.
10. Montgomery KD, Geerts WH, Potter HG, et al: Pulmonary embolus complications in patients with pelvic trauma. Clin Orthop 329:68–87, 1996.
11. Spain DA, Richardson JD, Polk HC, et al: Venous thromboembolism in the high risk trauma patient: Do risks justify aggressive screening and prophylaxis? J Trauma 42:463–467, 1997.
12. Brasel KJ, Borgstrom DC, Weigelt JA: Cost effective prevention of pulmonary embolism in high risk trauma patients. J Trauma 42:456–460, 1997.
13. Johnson R, Green JA, Charnley J: Pulmonary embolism following the Charnley hip replacement and its prophylaxis. Clin Orthop 127:123, 1977.
14. Salzman EW, Harris WH: Prevention of venous thrombo-embolism in orthopaedic patients. J Bone Joint Surg 58A:903, 1976.
15. Stansel MC: Vena cava interruption: Three points of view. Contemp Surg 20:63, 1982.
16. Reed RA, Teitelbaum GP, Stanley P, et al: The use of inferior vena cava filters in paediatric patients with pulmonary embolus prophylaxis. Cardiovasc Intervent Radiol 19:401–405, 1996.
17. Ramchandan ANIP, Zeit RM, Koolpe HA: Bilateral iliac vein filtration. Arch Surg 126:390–393, 1991.
18. Jaeger HJ, Kolb S, Mair T, et al: In vitro model for the evaluation of inferior vena cava filters: Effective experimental parameters on thrombus-capturing efficiency of the Venatec LG filter. J Vasc Intervent Radiol 9:295–304, 1998.
19. White KE, McLean JK: Bird's Nest filter: Inferior strut migration during massive thrombo-embolism. J Vasc Intervent Radiol 7:537–540, 1996.
20. Jaeger HJ, Rotzel K, Eggl P, et al: Comparative in vitro testing of permanent IVC filters in the vena cava physiological model to determine the thrombus-capturing efficiency (Abstract). CIRSE 21 (Suppl), 1998.
21. Jaeger HJ, Breitnfelder M, Mair T, et al: Comparative in vitro testing of temporary IVC filters in the vena cava physiological model to determine the thrombus-capturing efficiency (Abstract). CIRSE 21 (Suppl), 1998.
22. Millward SF, Bormanas J, Burbridge BE, et al: Preliminary clinical experience with the Gunter temporary inferior vena cava filter. J Vasc Intervent Radiol 5:863–868, 1994.
23. Linsenmaier UH, Reiger J, Roc C, et al: Prophylactic use of temporary inferior cava filters: Indications and preliminary results (Abstract). Radiology 201:284, 1996.
24. Thery C, Bauchart JJ, Lesenn EM, et al: Predictive factors of effectiveness of streptokinase in deep venous thrombosis. Am J Cardiol 69:117–122, 1992.
25. Tardy B, Mismetti P, Page Y, et al: Symptomatic inferior vena cava thrombosis: Single study of 30 consecutive cases. Eur Respir J 9:2012–2016, 1996.
26. Dorffman GS, Cronan JJ, Paolella LP, et al: Iatrogenic changes of the venotomy site after percutaneous placement of a Greenfield filter. Radiology 1173:159–162, 1989.
27. Pais SO, Tobin KD, Austin CB, et al: Percutaneous insertion of the Greenfield inferior vena cava filter: Experience with 96 patients. J Vasc Surg 8:460, 1998.
28. Perry JN, Wells IP: Case report: Structural failure of Bird's Nest inferior vena cava filter. Clin Radiol 49:431–432, 1994.
29. Dutsch OS: Percutaneous removal of intra-cardiac Greenfield vena caval filter. AJR Am J Roentgenol 151:677, 1988.
30. Riley P, Mackie G, Taylor S: Migration of an Antheor vena cava filter into the right pulmonary artery. J Intervent Radiol 12:99–101, 1997.
31. Flanagan D, Creasy T, Chataway F, et al: Caval umbrella causing obstructive uropathy. Postgrad Med J 72:235–237, 1996.
32. Lok SY, Adkins J, Asch M: Caval perforation by a Greenfield filter resulting in small bowel volvulus. J Vasc Intervent Radiol 7:95–97, 1996.
33. Wambeek ND, Frazer CK, Kumar A: Penetration of a vertebral body by a limb of the Greenfield filter. Australas Radiol 40:364–366, 1996.
34. Bianchini AU, Mehta SN, Mulder DS, et al: Duodenal perforation by a Greenfield filter: Endoscopic diagnosis. Am J Gastroenterol 92:686–687, 1997.
35. Goldman KA, Adelman MA: Retroperitoneal caval filter as a source of abdominal pain. Cardiovasc Surg 2:85–87, 1994.

Chapter 20 Venous Access

José I. Bilbao, Isabel Vivas, Fermin Urtasun, Beatriz Elduayen, and Antonio Martínez-Cuesta

For a large number of patients who require parenteral nutrition, hemodialysis, or chemotherapy, stable central venous access (CVA) is essential. Traditionally, access devices were placed by surgeons in the operating room and then chest radiography was performed to verify the position of the catheter's distal end. The role of the interventional radiologist was exclusively limited to managing possible complications, such as retrieving fragments, replacing malpositioned catheters, and performing venograms.[1] At present, access devices are mainly inserted by vascular interventional radiologists who use percutaneous techniques.

TYPES OF CATHETER

Catheters have different functions and vary in lumen size, construction, and materials. There are short- and long-term catheters. Generally, the short-term catheter is nontunnelled and should be changed 15 to 20 days after placement because of the high infection risk involved.[2] Such catheter insertion is routine in hospital practice, and, therefore, it is not usually carried out in vascular interventional radiology (VIR) suites. Short-term catheter insertions are low-risk procedures for patients. However, abnormal venous anatomy can complicate their insertion and they can cause venous occlusion. Long-term catheters can be externally tunnelled or have implanted ports.[3, 4] The external catheter is inserted through a subcutaneous route between the skin and the site of the venous puncture. At the proximal end of the subcutaneous tract site, a Dacron cuff allows ingrowth of fibrous tissue to provide mechanical stability and a barrier to infection. Some catheters have a second cuff that serves as a short-term antimicrobial barrier until fibrous tissue is produced (6 weeks). This has silver-impregnated collagen that takes 4 to 6 weeks to dissolve.

External venous catheters may or may not have a valve. Valved catheters, such as the Groshong (Da-

vol), impede the reflux of blood to the interior of the lumen when this is not being used, theoretically decreasing the risk of catheter thrombosis. Nonvalved catheters, such as the Hickman and the Broviac (Bard), differ in number, size, and lumen configuration, as well as in catheter composition. At present, the majority of manufacturers use silicone because of its greater flexibility and low thrombogenicity with respect to other materials. Various types of catheters have round, oval, single, double, or triple lumens. There is even a device (Tesio-Medcom) (Fig. 20–1) that consists of two independent catheters, capable of increased flow rates (up to 400 ml/min). This system has the disadvantage of requiring double tunnelling, which increases infection risk. A more recent development, the Ash (Medcom) catheter, presents the advantages of a Tesio catheter because it has two independent lumens but only one tunnelling route (Fig. 20–2).

The other type of long-term central venous catheter is the implantable port.[5] This is implanted either

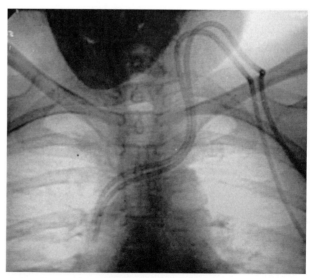

Figure 20–1. Tesio catheter placed from a left internal jugular vein (IJV) approach.

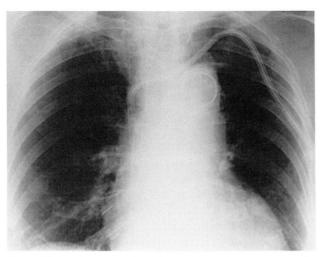

Figure 20–2. Ash catheter placed from a left subclavian vein approach.

in the chest wall or the antecubital fossa.[6, 7] It is made of a silicone or polyurethane catheter that connects with a subcutaneously implanted port. The structure of this port is plastic or titanium; it can be a single- or dual-lumen design and has a silicone membrane that can be easily reached percutaneously with special needles.

Choice of Catheter

The type of catheter to be inserted depends on the indication. The most common applications of long-term CVA are chemotherapy, parenteral nutrition, and hemodialysis. Other applications are transfusion or plasmapheresis, antibiotic therapy, and administration of analgesics. The need to administer various substances simultaneously, especially if these are incompatible, requires a multilumen catheter. This means that the size of each lumen is smaller than the whole and the flow rates are reduced. In addition, a relationship seems to exist between multilumen catheters and an increased incidence of catheter-related infections.

Another factor to bear in mind is frequency of use. If intermittent access is required, implantable ports are preferable, so that skin becomes an antimicrobial barrier during intertreatment periods. On the other hand, an externally tunnelled catheter is indicated in patients who require continuous access or in whom high flow rates are necessary.

VENOUS ACCESS SITES

Subclavian Vein

Traditionally, surgeons have chosen the subclavian vein because of its easy surgical access. Interventional radiologists use this route for the same reason. It remains the most used approach in most centers. However, in patients who require hemodialysis, the risk of developing venous thrombosis that complicates central catheterization from this route means the possible abandonment of this extremity for future graft or fistula access. If this complication occurs, insertion of a self-expandable metal stent may temporarily solve the problem. The internal jugular vein (IJV) is the preferred site for these patients.

ACCESS TECHNIQUES

Standard surgical technique uses anatomic references with no radiologic guidance. An infraclavicular approach is used, located 2 cm under the union of the medial two thirds of the clavicle. The suprasternal cavity is used as a reference point and the needle is advanced toward it at a medial and cephalic angle, following a route that is almost horizontal to the table (Fig. 20–3).

Fluoroscopy can be used in a number of ways. Under direct fluoroscopic control, the subclavian vein is opacified by a peripheral contrast injection in the ipsilateral basilic vein. The patient lies supine, with the head and shoulders in a neutral position and the arms next to the body. Once the entry site in the vein has been chosen as well as the puncture site in the skin (approximately 3 cm lateral to the entry site in the vein), local anesthesia is administered and the needle is advanced toward the vein, which is again opacified with contrast injection. The needle is directed toward the first rib. The vein diameter at this

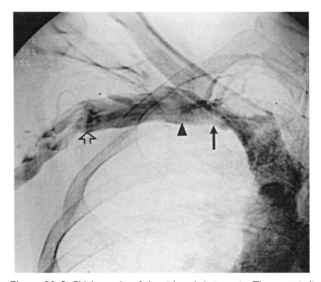

Figure 20–3. Phlebography of the right subclavian vein. The *arrow* indicates the place were the vein is punctured via the standard technique; the *arrowhead* is placed were the vein is punctured by means of fluoroscopy and anatomic landmarks; and finally, the *open arrow* indicates the site were the vein can be punctured by means of fluoroscopy and simultaneous injection of contrast.

level is greatest, and because the vein is between the needle and the lung, the risk of pneumothorax is very low.

Fluoroscopic guidance with use of anatomic landmarks is also acceptable, but as with the surgical approach, there is a risk of catheter entrapment between the clavicle and the first rib, with occurrence of consequent bending or even fracture (pinch off syndrome). Attempting a puncture that is also directed toward the first rib but more laterally decreases this risk (see Fig. 20–3).

The lateral approach also allows better control of possible hemorrhage, and at the same time, the risk of brachial plexus damage and pneumothorax is much reduced (see Fig. 20–3). Once access has been made to the subclavian vein (SCV), a guide wire is introduced and an angiographic catheter is inserted. The guide wire should be placed into the inferior vena cava (IVC), because this allows a stable position for the introduction of catheters, as well as eliminating the risk of arrhythmia caused by manipulations in the right side of the heart.

Ultrasonographic guidance can be used in patients who have a history of allergy to iodine contrast or who have severe renal dysfunction. However, some use it routinely. A high-frequency (5 to 7.5 megahertz [MHz]) transducer is required. The vein can be easily differentiated from the artery because of its lack of pulsation, easy compressibility, and respiratory variation. Ultrasonographic guidance allows more peripheral access to the SCV, reducing significantly the risk of pneumothorax. The vein is imaged transversely and longitudinally, and the needle is advanced into the vein from the lateral edge of the transducer.

Internal Jugular Vein

IJV access has some advantages and specific indications. It is the preferred method for treatment of dialysis patients because the SCV and the arm veins are preserved from possible catheter-related complications. The vein's vertical and superficial route facilitates puncture and allows the catheter to pass easily into the IVC. However, very frequently, it requires slight horizontal tunnelling, and the catheter remains in sight in the inferolateral neck region. Some patients dislike the cosmetic result of this procedure. External jugular venous access is also possible with use of the same route.

ACCESS TECHNIQUES

There are three ways of gaining access to the internal jugular vein (IJV), taking the sternocleidomastoid muscle as a reference.[8] The anterior approach, which is the most used of the three, is carried out anterior to the muscle. The carotid artery is palpated and medially retracted. The puncture is performed in front of the muscle and the needle is advanced toward the ipsilateral nipple from a midpoint in a line traced between the angle of the mandible and the clavicle. With a central approach, the puncture is performed from the apex of a triangle made up of the two heads of the sternocleidomastoid muscle and the clavicle, with the needle also directed toward the ipsilateral nipple. The posterior approach is performed below the sternocleidomastoid muscle, about 3 to 4 cm above the clavicle, with the needle directed toward the suprasternal notch.

Ultrasonographic guidance is useful and, in the majority of cases, makes the puncture successful at first attempt. A 5 to 7.5 MHz transducer is required, and a point midway between the angle of the mandible and clavicle is chosen for the puncture. It is preferable to obtain a projection that shows the vein and the artery in the same plane, so that the vein and not the artery is punctured. Light pressure with the needle is required or the IJV will be compressed, necessitating double-wall puncture.

Thrombosis or stenosis of supra-aortic venous trunks makes it difficult to gain access, even with use of ultrasonography. A transfemoral approach can be used to advance a guide wire and a catheter, which allows selection of the most appropriate jugular access.[9] A loop, or snare, can then be inserted, and the vein is punctured under fluoroscopic guidance, so that the needle crosses the open loop and the guide wire is advanced. When the loop is closed, the guide wire is trapped and thus pulled into the IVC. Once this is done, and the guide wire is firmly trapped, the catheter can be placed in the selected vein.

Inferior Vena Cava

In the past, IVC access was limited exclusively to patients who could not have SCV or IJV access. At present, there are centers where the first option is this access because of the good results described and the cosmetic advantage for the patient of having a concealed catheter.[10]

ACCESS TECHNIQUES

Three routes have been described for IVC access and catheter insertion. Translumbar inferior vena cava access is the most commonly used route. The transhepatic route, with direct access to the IVC through either the hepatic parenchyma or a hepatic vein, and the transfemoral route are also used.

Translumbar access is the most frequently used route to obtain venous access to the IVC. The procedure begins with the patient placed in a supine position to undergo selective catheterization of the femoral vein, through which an angiographic catheter is introduced to the L-3 level. Cavography is performed to check for anatomic variants. The patient is then placed in a prone oblique position with the right side elevated 30 degrees. The puncture site is 3 cm above the right iliac crest and 10 cm lateral to the midline. Under local anesthesia and with contrast roadmapping via the femoral catheter, the needle is advanced toward the IVC following a medial and cephalad angulation. The puncture is made as near as possible to the vertebral bodies. Once IVC access has been confirmed, a guide wire and a catheter are advanced toward the right atrium and the superior vena cava (Fig. 20–4A). In certain thin patients, it is possible to evaluate the IVC with 3 to 3.5 MHz transducers. This allows infrarenal IVC access via direct vision of the needle and without the necessity of a cavography.[1] Computed tomography guidance can also be used if the patient has thrombosis of the femoral, iliac, or upper extremity veins.

Whenever possible, an infrarenal translumbar IVC approach should be attempted. However, if infrarenal IVC occlusion is detected or if there is an absent IVC, a direct IVC approach can be performed through the hepatic parenchyma. The IVC can be accessed directly or through the lumen of a hepatic vein. This is a technique used mainly in children who require maintained parenteral nutrition (e.g., children with short gut syndrome[11]). The main contraindications to this approach are coagulopathies and severe ascites.[12] Direct access to the transhepatic IVC prevents the complication of hepatic vein thrombosis. However, access through a vein allows a more peripheral puncture, decreasing the risk of an accidental lesion to the bile ducts or the branches of the hepatic

artery. The middle hepatic vein is preferred because of its anterior direction, which facilitates puncture and catheterization.

Because these patients are generally young, the procedure is performed under general anesthesia, with ultrasonographic and fluoroscopic guidance. Older patients require mild sedation only. The puncture is similar to that performed for transhepatic cholangiography. The patient lies in a supine position and the puncture is made from a subcostal approach for the middle hepatic vein or from a midaxillary line at the 10th intercostal space for the right hepatic vein. After the administration of local anesthesia, the needle is advanced in a cephalic and medial direction. Repeated contrast injections or, preferably, aspiration and contrast injection, are performed as the needle is removed. Some authors recommend embolization of the hepatic parenchymal tract at the end of the procedure, although this is not necessary.

The third access path for the IVC is the transfemoral route. Given the high infection risk of the inguinal area and the greater tendency for catheters placed in this area to bend, fracture, or break, it is not advisable to attempt permanent access at this site.[13]

Collateral Veins

In patients who have central venous occlusion, large collateral veins can be used for venous access. However, a particular study of each patient should be carried out, because collateral branches can vary greatly. Careful puncture followed by the advancement of hydrophilic guide wires under continuous fluoroscopy with frequent contrast injections, allows the catheter and guide wire to be advanced until a

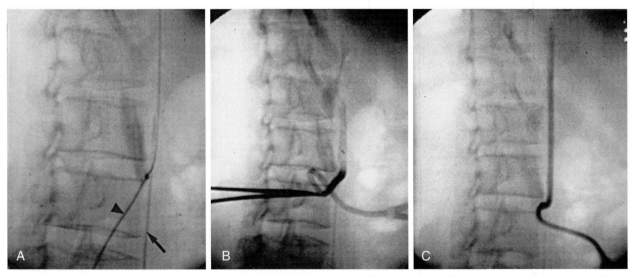

Figure 20–4. Placement of a Hickman catheter in the inferior vena cava. A, A multi–side-hole 5-French (F) catheter *(arrow)* has been placed from the right femoral vein. A hydrophilic guide wire *(arrowheads)* has been advanced through the needle. B, After removal of the dilator, the Hickman catheter is advanced through the peel-away sheath. C, The Hickman catheter is in place.

central vein (e.g., SVC, IVC, innominate trunk) is reached. Once there, a loop snare or any other retrieval system is introduced from the femoral approach to trap and remove the guide (i.e., a through and through technique). Finally, with the guide firmly fixed on both ends, the required catheter is introduced.

CENTRAL TUNNELLED CATHETERS

Central catheters can be tunnelled under the skin, which significantly reduces the infection rate. Tunnelling is usually carried out on the medial side of the chest wall, about 5 cm under the puncture site. At present, there are dual-lumen catheters with preformed angles, which allow tunnelling without producing bends in the catheter. In obese patients and women who have large breasts, the weight of the chest wall causes traction on the catheter so that the distal tip, which should lie at the SCV-right atrial junction, actually lies in the SCV or innominate trunk.[14] In these patients, horizontal tunnelling is preferable, and the distal tip should be left in the right atrium rather than at the SCV-atrial junction.

For IJV access, tunnelling should be directed toward the clavicle and slightly lateral, the second incision being approximately 2 cm above the clavicle. In translumbar access to the IVC, tunnelling is carried out from a lateral and slightly caudal route that allows the patient to have access to the catheter.

Tunnelling technique is similar for all access sites. Once the catheter exit site has been chosen and local anesthesia has been administered, a small incision of 0.5 to 1 cm is made in the subcutaneous tissue; this allows entry of the tunnelling needle, which is directed toward the venous entry point. The catheter is hooked to the distal end of the tunnelling needle in such a way that it is advanced through the subcutaneous tract and then pulled through. Over an Amplatz superstiff guide wire, a peel-away sheath is advanced into the vein. The inner dilator is withdrawn, the catheter is introduced into the vein until the desired location is reached, and the sheath is finally removed (Fig. 20–4 B and C). Occasionally, a hydrophilic wire is needed to avoid collaterals. Tesio catheters require reverse tunnelling (i.e., the tunnelling device is fitted to the distal end of the catheter and the tract is formed from the venous puncture site to the skin exit site). This makes it possible to avoid making a second incision in the skin to introduce the tunnelling device, and the skin acts as an antimicrobial barrier.

SUBCUTANEOUS PORTS

At the beginning of the 1990s the first studies were published describing use of a new port (PAS port) that was specifically designed to be placed in the forearm.[6] Port dimensions (26.7 × 16.5 × 10 mm) and catheter sizes (5.8-French[F]) enabled the port to be implanted peripherally in the forearm, and the catheter in the cephalic or basilic veins. The port was originally made of titanium and the catheter was made of polyurethane. At present, ports are made of polysulphone, a lighter material with increased surface membrane that enables a greater number of punctures to be carried out.

The traditional insertion site for this device was in the infraclavicular fossa. This site has veins of sufficient calibre and adequate subcutaneous tissue caudally. A 5-cm skin incision is made through the dermis into the subcutaneous space, and careful dissection, to create a pocket large enough to insert the port without creating excessive tension, is made. The port may be fixed to the deep fascia with two-three absorbable sutures. Next a subcutaneous tunnel is created to the venous access site, inserting the catheter through the tunnel.

Peripheral ports are now more usually placed in the antecubital fossa where a 2–3 cm incision is made. Dissection is done above the fascia muscle to create a pocket to hold the device. Before this, the vein is punctured and an angiographic catheter is advanced through it. The desired length of the catheter to be implanted is measured with the aid of a special measuring guidewire. Finally, the exact placement of the distal tip of the catheter is done under fluoroscopy. The catheter is tunnelled from the venous puncture site to the subcutaneous pocket where it is connected with the port.

Fluoroscopy is sometimes essential. In patients with very small veins or veins altered by multiple previous punctures, venography from a dorsal vein of the hand can be carried out. The venous map of the extremity obtained allows selective puncture and catheterization of a suitable vessel.

COMPLICATIONS

The percutaneous insertion of CVA devices, with fluoroscopic and ultrasonographic guidance, has several advantages over surgical insertion. Intervention time is considerably reduced because catheters are placed in the majority of patients in less than 30 minutes. Morbidity is decreased because neighbouring structures that could be damaged can be visualized directly. Skin necrosis, especially after extravasation, is a complication specific to subcutaneous skin ports.

Malposition

Malposition of catheters almost never happens with radiologic insertion.[15] McBride, in 1997, presented a study that compared radiologic and surgical insertion of central venous catheters. As with other series, malposition did not occur in the radiology group, but in the surgical group 4.5% of catheters were malpositioned.[16]

Arterial Complications

Accidental puncture of the artery adjacent to the vein can cause local hematoma, hemomediastinum, hemothorax, hemoperitoneum, or hemoretroperitoneum. Pseudoaneurysms or arteriovenous fistulas can also occur. However, firm compression can prevent these complications provided the arterial puncture is recognized and central catheters are not inserted into the artery. Ultrasonographic guidance, contrast injection after puncture, or both confirm the intravenous position of the needle. It is also useful before inserting a thick-sized, peel-away sheath, to insert an angiographic catheter with which to confirm venous catheterization and facilitate the placement of the exchange guide wire in the most adequate site.

Pneumothorax

The use of ultrasonography and fluoroscopy has reduced the risk of pneumothorax. Previously, pneumothorax represented 30% of all complications but now only 0 to 1.6%. Small subclinical pneumothorax that resolves spontaneously is, however, often seen. Significant pneumothorax clearly requires the insertion of a chest drain.

Neural Injury

Neural complications related to venous puncture and CVA can be caused by direct needle trauma, local compression by hematomas, or the use of local anesthesia. The most frequent of these neural complications is brachial plexopathy during SCV access. Horner's syndrome can occur as a result of damage to the sympathetic cervical system.

Ureteral Lesion

In the translumbar approach to IVC, the risk of accidentally puncturing the right ureter can be avoided by advancing the needle very closely to the vertebral body.

Embolization

Catheter fragmentation with distal embolization to the cardiac chambers or the pulmonary artery can occur during CVA. These fragments can be trapped and extracted with the aid of loop snares and other retrieval devices.

The presence of intravenous devices, such as IVC filters, venous stents, and so forth, should be noted, because the catheter can get caught in their metallic mesh, with the consequent risk of mobilization and embolization of the device.

Pinch-off syndrome (POS) is produced by compression of the SCV catheter when it passes between the clavicle and the first rib. This can take the form of a noncompressing kink (grade 1) discovered on chest radiography or a kink that compromises the catheter lumen (grade 2). Grade 3 pinch-off syndrome occurs if the catheter ruptures and embolizes to the RA or pulmonary artery.[17].

Air embolus is an infrequent but very important complication that occurs if the patient takes a deep breath at the moment when the dilator is removed from the peel-away sheath. To avoid this complication, the Trendelenberg position and the Valsalva maneuver should be used at this stage of the procedure.

Cardiac Complications

These complications generally occur during catheter placement and are caused by irritation of the RA wall and the tricuspid valve during guide wire and catheter manipulations. Patients should be monitored during the procedure, although most of these arrhythmias are asymptomatic, disappearing when the stimulus ceases and patients do not require treatment. Sustained supraventricular tachycardia generally reverts with carotid massage, forced breathing, or the Valsalva maneuver. Exceptionally, when it does not revert, medical treatment must be given and even cardioversion considered.

It is also possible to perforate the RA with the wire. It is adviseable to check for signs of cardiac tamponade and look at the heart with ultrasonography of any patient who becomes acutely ill during a procedure. The complication can be dealt with by the simple insertion of a pericardial drain under ultrasonographic guidance.

Infection

Infectious complications make up 0 to 27% of all CVA-related complications. The frequency of catheter-associated infections varies between 10 and 30% or

1.4 per 1000 catheter days. Minor infectious complications can occur at the insertion site. These infections usually appear during the first week and are the result of a contamination produced when the catheter is inserted.[13] With appropriate local treatment, they almost always remit.

Infection can also develop in the skin at the catheter exit site, manifesting itself as a painful reddish area, with edema and, at times, exudation. This can usually be treated with appropriate antibiotics and local antiseptic measures. If infection also affects the subcutaneous tract, only 25% of patients respond to local treatment; the remaining cases may require catheter removal.

Bacteremias, infectious endocarditis, septic thrombophlebitis, and septic pulmonary embolism require catheter removal. About 7% of all patients who have central catheters require catheter removal because of infection.

The skin is the most important source of infection (50 to 70%), which is mainly caused by coagulase negative *Staphylococcus* (20 to 50%). *Staphylococcus aureus* (15 to 25%) and *Candida* (5 to 10%) are the other main infectious agents. The infusate is another source of contamination and distant colonization can also occur secondary to bacteremia from other sources.[18] Catheter removal should not be carried out until clear evidence exists that the catheter is infected or is the source of an infection. When a catheter is removed, a culture of the catheter tip should always be obtained to check for the presence of infection. A new CVA should not be placed until at least 24 hours after the infection has resolved.[13]

Factors predisposing to catheter-related infections include age (infection is more frequent in patients who are younger than 1 year of age, and those over 60 years of age), neutropenia, presence of distant infection, chemotherapy, and bone marrow transplant recipients. A higher incidence of infection is observed in multilumen catheters than in those with a single lumen.

The benefit of administering prophylactic, preprocedure intravenous antibiotics is unproved. It is more important to adopt a careful sterile technique. The postprocedure care of the cathether on the part of the patient and the hospital staff also contributes to infection control.

Catheter-Related Thrombosis

Catheter thrombosis occurs in 3.7 to 10% of patients. It can take the form of pericatheter fibrin sheath, pericatheter venous thrombosis, or intracatheter thrombosis. The presence of a fibrin sheath that envelops the catheter tip is frequently observed a few weeks after catheter insertion and may cause catheter malfunction (Fig. 20–5). The first manifestation of this problem is that blood cannot be aspirated through the catheter. However, this does not mean that the venous flow is obstructed. Cassidy and associates confirmed the presence of a fibrin membrane as the cause of catheter malfunction in 57% of a large population of patients with CVA.[19] Contrast injection shows the presence of this membrane, and the injection may break the membrane proximally by sending it through the venous circulation and re-establishing flow through the catheter. An infusion of heparin given over 20 to 30 minutes can be administered in an attempt to resolve the problem. If this does not dissolve the fibrin sheath, a more interventional procedure may be necessary, such as mobilization of the catheter with the aid of a stiff guide wire or cleaning the catheter with a loop snare introduced through a different venous access. With this loop, the surface of the catheter can be stripped and adherent fibrin fragments can be removed.[20] Sometimes, the inability to aspirate blood from the catheter is caused by the position of the catheter tip against the venous wall, and this should be considered. Contrast injection can be used to differentiate these problems.

Venous occlusion can occur around a catheter that remains patent (Fig. 20–6). If the occlusion is complete, the patient can develop clinical signs of SVC obstruction. However, in 30% of patients, this complication may remain asymptomatic because there are adequate collateral vessels.

Predisposing factors for the development of

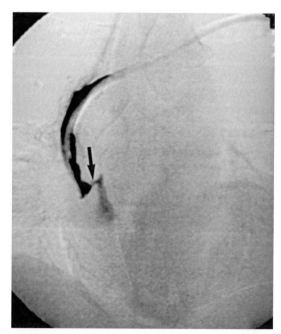

Figure 20–5. The Hickman catheter placed in the left subclavian vein. The tip of the catheter is against the superior vena cava (SVC) vein wall. The contrast is retained around the catheter because of a fibrin sheath. There is a small unobstructed area *(arrow)* from which the contrast enters the right atrium (RA).

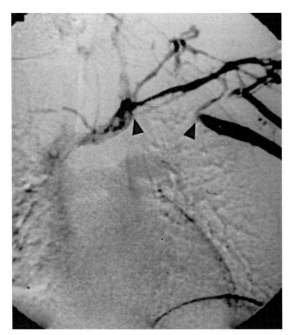

Figure 20–6. The Hickman catheter is placed in the left subclavian vein. A pericatheter thrombus is clearly seen from the venous entry point along the subclavian vein *(arrowheads)*.

thrombosis are coagulopathies, external venous compression, venous stasis, low flow rates, and infusion of sclerosing agents. In the majority of the cases, catheter removal is not necessary, and the thrombosis is resolved by anticoagulation and thrombolysis. Catheter obstruction may also occur as a result of thrombosis of the catheter lumen. Heparinization of the catheter after use can reduce the incidence of this. Full anticoagulation may be necessary in high-risk patients. The obstruction is easily removed by a bolus of thrombolytic, such as urokinase (5000 UI/ml). This is successful in restoring patency in 85 to 90% of cases.

CONCLUSION

CVA performed by vascular radiologists under fluoroscopic guidance is a more effective means of providing long-term venous access with fewer complications and longer patency rates than access performed blindly in operating theaters.

REFERENCES

1. Bjarnason H, Lehmann S: Central venous access. *In* Castañeda-Zuñiga WR (ed): Interventional Radiology, 3rd ed. Baltimore, Williams & Wilkins, 1997, pp 941–966.
2. Dudrick SJ, Wilmore DW: Long-term parental feeding. Hosp Pract 3:65, 1968.
3. Hickman RO, Buckner CD, Clift RA, et al: A modified right atrial catheter for access to the venous system in marrow transplant recipients. Gynaecol Obstet 148:871, 1979.
4. Niederhuber J, Ensminger W, Gyves J, et al: Totally implanted venous and arterial access system to replace external catheters in cancer treatment. Surgery 92:706, 1982.
5. Brothers TE, Von Moll LK, Niederhuber JE, et al: Experience with subcutaneous infusion ports in three hundred patients. Surg Gynaecol Obstet 166:295, 1988.
6. Salem RR, Ward BA, Ravikumar TS: A new peripherally implanted subcutaneous permanent central venous access device for patients requiring chemotherapy. J Clin Oncol 11:2181, 1993.
7. Johnson J, Didlake RH: Peripherally placed central venous access ports: Clinical and laboratory observations. Am Surg 60:915, 1994.
8. Denny DF: Placement and management of long-term central venous access catheters and ports. AJR Am J Roentgenol 161:385, 1993.
9. Kaufman JA, Kazanjian SA, Rivitz M, et al: Long-term central venous catheterization in patients with limited access. AJR Am J Roentgenol 167:1327, 1996.
10. Lund GB, Trerotola SO, Scheel RJ: Percutaneous translumbar inferior vena cava cannulation for hemodialysis. Am J Kidney Dis 25:732, 1995.
11. Somers RJ, Golinko RJ, Mitty HA: Initial experience with percutaneous transhepatic cardiac catheterization in infants and children. Am J Cardiol 75:1289, 1995.
12. Wallace MJ, Hovsepian DM, Balzer CT: Transhepatic venous access for diagnostic and interventional cardiovascular procedures. J Vasc Intervent Radiol 7:579, 1996.
13. Lund GB: Complications from long-term tunnelled venous access catheters. A review. Semin Intervent Radiol 11:340, 1994.
14. Nazarian GK, Bjarnason H, Dietz CA, et al: Changes in tunnelled catheter tip position when a patient is upright. J Vasc Interv Radiol 8:437, 1997.
15. Mauro MA, Jaques PF: Radiologic placement of long-term central venous catheters: A review. J Vasc Intervent Radiol 4:127, 1993.
16. McBride KD, Fisher R, Warnock N, et al: A comparative analysis of radiological and surgical placement of central venous catheters. Cardiovasc Int Radiol 20:17, 1997.
17. Hinke DH, Zandt-Stastny DA, Goodman LR. et al: Pinch-off syndrome: A complication of implantable subclavian venous access devices. Radiology 177:353, 1990.
18. Denny DF: Placement and management of long-term central venous access catheters and ports. AJR Am J Roentgenol 161:385, 1993.
19. Cassidy FP, Zajko AB, Bron KM, et al: Noninfectious complications of long-term central venous catheters. AJR Am J Roentgenol 149:671, 1987.
20. Haskal ZJ, Leen VH, Thomas-Hawkins C, et al: Transvenous removal of fibrin sheaths from tunneled hemodialysis catheters. J Vasc Intervent Radiol 7:513, 1996.

Chapter 21 Interventions in Dialysis Fistulas

Endovascular Contributors: Luc A.E. Turmel-Rodrigues, Alain Raynaud, Marc Sapoval, and Bernard Beyssen

Stenosis is the most frequent complication of hemodialysis access, and it leads to thrombosis. Many mechanisms have been put forward to explain the genesis of these stenoses, but only direct venous trauma and differences in compliance have been proven to date.

Any venous catheterization can induce subsequent stenosis. This is especially true for central veins, where most stenoses result from central catheters placed in intensive care units or from temporary dialysis catheters. Subclavian catheters are particularly damaging, the internal jugular approach less so. Similarly, repeated peripheral venipuncture destroys the veins and precludes the creation of native fistulas for permanent hemodialysis. Turbulence generated by the difference in compliance between prostheses and native veins explains the development of stenosing neointimal hyperplasia at the venous anastomosis of grafts. A similar mechanism explains the juxta-anastomotic stenoses in native fistulas.

More than 70% of U.S. hemodialysis patients have prosthetic grafts whereas 70% of Europeans have native fistulas. This is explained by a higher proportion of diabetics ($> 33\%$ vs. $< 20\%$ in Europe) and African-Americans (40% vs. 1%) in the United States. However, statistics from 1994 show that fewer than 15% of native fistulas were created even in young white nondiabetic U.S. patients. The recent publication of guidelines by the American Kidney Foundation strongly encourages U.S. surgeons to take a step back and to create more native fistulas.[1]

DIAGNOSTIC ANGIOGRAPHY

Angiography must be appropriate to the clinical situation. Stenoses in native fistulas can occur at either anastomosis, whereas stenoses in grafts occur at the venous anastomosis.[2] When there is outflow obstruction (the most frequent situation), antegrade puncture of the fistula or graft is performed some centimeters down from the arteriovenous anastomosis.

In cases of poor inflow or delayed maturation

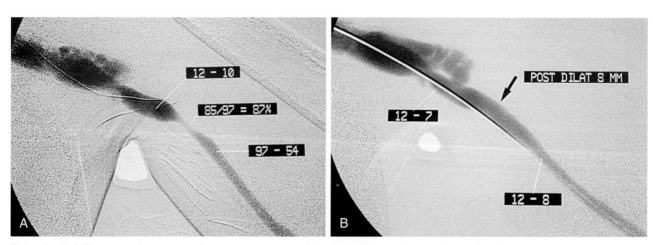

Figure 21–1. *A,* There is a tight stenosis at the venous anastomosis of this 6-mm diameter brachioaxillary graft. Pullback pressure measurement shows 97 mm Hg upstream systolic pressure and 12 mm Hg downstream pressure, corresponding to an 87% systolic pressure loss across the stenosis. Imaging was obtained by injection of CO_2 because the patient had developed a major allergy to iodine after the preoperative upper limb venography performed 4 months earlier. *B,* After dilation to 8 mm and 15 atm with a balloon filled with gadolinium, the result is perfect because it is impossible in retrospect to identify where the initial stenosis was *(arrow).* Pullback pressure measurement confirms the abolition of any gradient through the dilated area.

(mainly native fistulas), subclavian arterial catheterization from the femoral route is recommended to visualize the entire feeding artery and the arteriovenous anastomosis. Retrograde puncture of the brachial artery at the elbow may be necessary when this is not possible, although when there is high outflow or hand ischemia, complete visualization of the arteries of the limb is required.

Stenoses larger than 50% are considered significant. Measurement of the diameter of a stenosis can be impossible in cases of heterogeneity, stricture, or superimposition. In such cases, pullback pressure measurement is more reliable and is not operator dependent (Fig. 21–1). However, pressure gradients, although fully reliable at the venous end of grafts, can underestimate obstruction in native veins if there are collateral branches leaving the fistula before the stenosis, which contribute to reduction in the upstream pressure.

When there is no obvious stenosis on the angiogram despite clinical abnormalities, pullback pressure measurement from the superior vena cava to the arterial anastomosis is indicated. An abrupt, greater than 50% systolic pressure loss indicates a stenosis that was overlooked because of superimposition or inadequate imaging.

A 30 to 50% pressure loss is normal at the arteriovenous anastomosis. In the subclavian vein, definition of a stenosis is angiographically difficult because of the frequent presence of terminal anatomic narrowing and because of the washout flow coming from the internal jugular vein. The presence of collateral branches and a pressure gradient greater than 10 mm Hg are objective signs of stenosis. There is no significant subclavian vein stenosis without upstream collaterals.

ANGIOPLASTY OF PATENT FISTULAS AND GRAFTS

Indications

Stenoses must be treated when they hinder dialysis or threaten patency. Clinically stenoses cause poor inflow with a vacuum phenomenon during dialysis, difficulties in cannulation, venous hyperpressure, arm edema, increased bleeding after needle removal, distal ischemia, aneurysms, pain, or skin necrosis.

There is a tendency to recommend prophylactic dilation of all hemodynamically confirmed stenoses greater than 50% at the venous anastomosis of grafts (dialysis outcomes and quality initiative guidelines).[1] This rule should be enforced for patients with a history of access thrombosis, but not necessarily for patients whose grafts have never thrombosed. Asymptomatic stenosis or occlusion of a brachiocephalic vein

does not have to be treated because such central lesions rarely are the only cause of thrombosis of a peripheral fistula or graft. Similarly, stenoses at the anastomosis of native fistulas must be dilated only in cases of poor inflow because dilatation of a well-functioning fistula could lead to secondary high-flow or steal phenomenon. When repeated dilatation is necessary, it can be performed as an outpatient procedure.

Technique

Hemodialysis fistulas and grafts are made to be punctured and must be used for introduction of dilation catheters. A fistula or graft puncture before dilatation must be performed using local anesthesia in the direction of, but approximately 5 cm from, the stenosis. An antegrade approach should be used for stenoses located far from the arterial anastomosis, and a retrograde approach should be used for stenoses close to the arterial anastomosis. An 18-gauge needle puncture and an 0.035-inch guide wire should be used to insert a 6- to 9-French introducer sheath. A small subcutaneous tunnel between the skin entry point and the fistula or graft entry point facilitates final compression and decreases the risk of pseudoaneurysm formation.

A soft-tip Bentson-type guide wire or angled hydrophilic wire is preferred to cross stenoses. Angulated catheters are helpful for selective catheterization of branches. Once a guide wire has passed through the stenosis, heparin may be given (2000–3000 units), but it is in fact necessary only in small-diameter or low-flow fistulas.

The diameter of the dilatation balloon should be equal to or 1 mm greater than the diameter of the immediate upstream or downstream normal vessel. The dilatation balloon then is inflated slowly to abolish the waist and is left in place for 1 to 3 minutes. Dilatation is often painful, and local anesthesia can help when stenoses are just under the skin.

Hemodialysis access stenoses are often very hard, and high-pressure balloons with bursting pressures greater than 25 atm may be necessary. Balloon rupture during dilatation can cause fragmentation and vessel rupture. However, such complications are rare and balloon bursting is preferable to residual stenoses. Stenoses resistant to 25 bar pressures are infrequent. In our experience, they occur in 2% of grafts, 1% of forearm fistulas, and 4% of the upper arm fistulas (final arch of the cephalic vein).[2] Atherectomy catheters have been reported to be of some value in such cases. Cutting balloons are a more recent and valuable alternative for very tight stenoses, but they are not available in diameters greater than 4 mm.

Immediate postprocedure angiography, with the

guide wire left in place through the dilated area, may show:

1. No residual stenosis and no parietal damage (see Fig. 21–1).
2. Minor parietal damage: 3 to 5 minutes of low-pressure ballooning should be performed to try to smooth the vessel wall.
3. Rupture with clear extravasation of contrast medium and development of a hematoma. The dilatation balloon must be rapidly reinflated to 2 atm for repeated periods of 10 minutes.
4. Recoil causing residual significant stenosis: a new dilatation should be performed with a longer (3 min) inflation time and a balloon that is 1 mm greater in diameter. Oversizing by more than this is not recommended. If this fails, stent insertion is indicated (Fig. 21–2).

Once angioplasty has been performed, the catheters and introducer sheath are removed. The puncture site must be compressed as gently as possible to stop bleeding without stopping flow through the fistula. The outpatient then can get up, and the vascular access is immediately usable for hemodialysis.

Stenosis or occlusion of a central vein are the consequence of previous central catheters (see Fig. 21–2). In cases of chronic occlusion, it may be necessary to use a through-and-through approach by the femoral vein and by the fistula to traverse the occluded lumen successfully. This is necessary when the guide wire passes the stenosis but the obstruction is so severe that the balloon cannot follow.

Complications

Angioplasty-induced rupture can occur at a very low pressure and is not necessarily linked to the balloon bursting (Fig. 21–3). Suspect rupture when the waisting on the balloon suddenly disappears, whatever the level of pressure. The patient often reports a sudden acute pain at the dilated site as soon as the balloon is deflated. If rupture is confirmed, the balloon must be reinflated quickly to 2 atm and left in place for 10 minutes.[3] If previously given, heparin should be neutralized by an injection of protamine sulfate (except in patients being treated with insulin) and the hematoma is compressed manually if clinically accessible. If extravasation continues despite three periods of 10-minute balloon tamponade, a covered stent must be placed.[4] In our experience, rupture during dilatation occurs in 2% of grafts, 10% of Brescia-Cimino fistulas, and 18% of upper arm fistulas.[2] However, the majority were controlled by prolonged balloon inflation, and very few required a stent. The cephalic vein, the axillary outflow of transposed basilic veins, and the postanastomotic area of forearm fistulas at the wrist are the most prone to rupture.

Thrombosis can occur during dilatation if the introducer is occlusive or if the balloon is left inflated for too long a period in a patient who does not undergo anticoagulation. Secondary thrombosis some hours or days after dilatation is vexing and can be explained by excessive final compression, compressive hematoma, overlooked or insufficiently dilated stenoses, secondary clot formation at the dilated site, or stenosis induced at the entry point of the introducer sheath.

Bleeding during dilatation is no longer a problem with the use of introducer sheaths. As after a dialysis session, the cannulation site subsequently can reopen, and control of such bleeding by manual compression is a part of the basic education of hemodialysis patients. When a large introducer sheath has been used (9 French [F]), "U"-shaped suturing can effectively

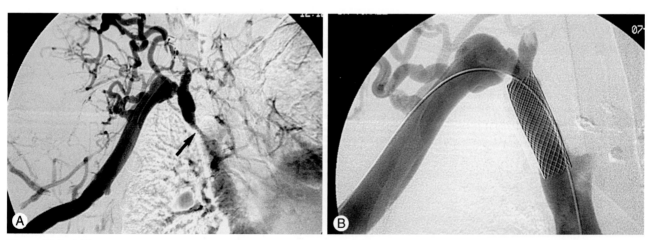

Figure 21–2. *A,* There is a tight stenosis *(arrow)* of the right brachiocephalic trunk in the outflow of a brachioaxillary graft. This caused arm edema despite the development of numerous collateral branches. *B,* There was stenosis recoil despite the absence of any residual waisting on the 14-mm dilation balloon. A short Wallstent was placed that did not overlap either the internal jugular vein or the contralateral innominate trunk. Arm edema disappeared.

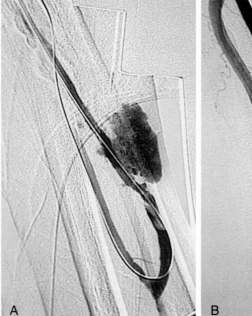
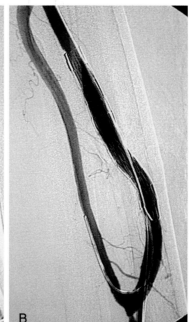

Figure 21–3. A, During the declotting of this 3-month-old radial artery to cephalic native fistula, angioplasty to 5 mm of the immature vein induced a major rupture, which was not controlled after three periods of 10-minute prolonged balloon tamponade. B, Rupture was controlled successfully by placement of a covered stent ("Passager," Boston Scientific Europe), which has since been routinely punctured for hemodialysis during 10 months of follow-up.

prevent such secondary bleeding and pseudoaneurysms.[3]

Infection is a potentially fatal complication and has been reported in all series because hemodialysis patients are immunocompromised. Antistaphylococcal antibiotics are required when a difficult dilation procedure has been prolonged, when several cannulations have been necessary, when clots are present, and above all, in cases of a breach in sterile technique.

Contraindications to Angioplasty

Local infection and severe coagulopathies are absolute contraindications for percutaneous treatment. Dilatation can, however, be planned after correction of these disorders.

Concomitant arterial steal syndrome is also an absolute contraindication for treatment of any stenosis located in the fistula or graft downstream from the arterial anastomosis because its treatment increases flow in the fistula and subsequent steal.

Surgical anastomoses of less than 6 weeks are at high risk of rupture. Gentle dilatation at low pressure with an exactly size-matched diameter balloon, however, can be contemplated at venous anastomoses of grafts because any rupture in this location can be easily controlled by placement of a covered stent.

Immature fistulas—that is, those less than 2 months old—should be sent for surgery if the stenosis is located in the anastomotic area. However, when the underlying stenosis is located on the venous outflow, surgical creation of a new anastomosis downstream from the stenosis would not leave enough vein for

cannulation. In such cases, gentle dilatation is the only possibility to save the fistula, although we know that cannulation and catheterization of an immature fistula also can generate stenosis.

Isolated stenosis within 10 cm of the wrist in a Brescia-Cimino fistula can be dilated, but there is a risk of early restenosis, whereas surgical creation of a new anastomosis downstream from the stenosis is simple, minimally invasive, and lasting.

Long (> 5 cm) stenoses and chronic occlusions can be dilated successfully in forearm fistulas. Radiology also must be the first treatment in central veins because surgical alternatives are technically difficult and invasive. In contrast, dilatation of long stenoses at the venous anastomoses of grafts and in upper arm cephalic veins usually produces poor results, and surgical revision can be contemplated.

STENTS

In contrast to the arterial system, vein diameter increases with the direction of the flow. Therefore, there is a risk of detachment and pulmonary migration of any endoprosthesis that is not large enough or wall adherent. Stents sometimes must be placed in joint spaces (elbow) and must not impair mobility. These anatomic and mechanical constraints mean that flexible self-expandable stents (Wallstent, Craggstent) are preferable to balloon expandable and rigid stents. Stent diameter must be 1 to 2 mm greater than the diameter of the vessel to cling to the intima. When a stent has to be placed in a cannulation area, which is a rare indication, a wide mesh puncturable stent, such as the Craggstent, should be used (see Fig. 21–3). Disappointing results to date for covered stents mean that they can only be recommended for rupture control or elimination of aneurysm (see Fig. 21–3).

Stents must not obviate further surgery and must not compromise the fashioning of new anastomoses. There are four locations where this problem frequently occurs:

1. Stent placement is contraindicated at the venous anastomosis of a forearm graft if the stent would overlap the basilic vein and obviate future creation of a transposed brachiobasilic fistula.
2. A stent placed in the distal cephalic vein must not protrude into the subclavian vein where it could induce stenosis, which would preclude future use of the basilic and axillary veins for a direct fistula or for drainage of an upper arm graft.
3. A stent placed in the subclavian vein must not overlap the ostium of a patent internal jugular vein. This vein is essential for placing a future central catheter or for drainage of a graft running from the axillary vein.
4. A stent placed in the right or left brachiocephalic (innominate) vein must not protrude into the superior vena cava, compromising the flow coming from the contralateral trunk. For stenoses limited to the right brachiocephalic vein, it is also important not to overlap either the subclavian ostium or the internal jugular ostium, that is, to place the stent in the brachiocephalic trunk only (see Fig. 21–2).

Acute dilatation-induced rupture is an emergency in which a stent can save vascular access (see Fig. 21–3). Covered stents are effective in 100% of cases[4] but bare Wallstents frequently work.[5] Stent placement also could prevent the development of a secondary pseudoaneurysm.

Aneurysms can be eliminated by placement of a covered stent across the neck or base. The indication is valuable for aneurysms located in noncannulation areas, where surgery may be difficult. Surgery is preferable in cannulation areas because repeated puncture of the covered stent would reopen connections between flow and aneurysm.

Persistent recoil, where the balloon has inflated fully, should be stented when the residual stenosis is greater than 30%. Before placing the stent, all possibilities with the balloon should be exhausted, as previously described.

There are stenoses whose waisting on the dilatation balloon is not abolished despite the highest pressure presently applicable in the strongest balloons (25 atm). Subsequent residual stenoses are hard stenoses and not soft recoiling stenoses. Stents should not be placed in these cases, which are indications for mechanically more aggressive tools, that is, an atherectomy device or a cutting balloon.

There is no consensus regarding the indications and value of stents to delay restenosis. Some multidisciplinary teams accept redilatating stenoses every 4 months or sooner, if necessary. We do not know whether there is a simple surgical alternative, but we try a stent first. In our experience,[6] stents double the intervals between reinterventions after appropriate use in early recurring stenoses. Stents are, however, valuable only if no residual stenosis has been accepted after insertion. This means that the stenosis previously has been dilated sufficiently and that absolutely no residual waist has been accepted on the inflated balloon. The beneficial effects of stent implantation are explained by the propensity of the stent to achieve a consistently greater increase in luminal diameter than is the case with balloon angioplasty. Stents do not preclude restenosis, but they delay its clinical consequences: starting from a greater diameter, intimal hyperplasia in the stented area takes longer to reduce the vessel lumen to a critical and clinically impairing stage. Accepting a residual stenosis in a stent means a major loss of the advantage of the stent, which probably explains the conflicting results in the literature.[7, 8]

In-stent restenosis usually responds to dilatation. Redilatation can become ineffective if intimal hyperplasia recurs after repeated procedures. This is an indication for surgical revision because attempts to remove intimal hyperplasia by atherectomy devices have not been conclusively successful and because placing a new stent through the original has proved to be ineffective.[6]

Stents also fail when new stenoses occur immediately downstream or upstream. They usually respond well to dilatation. These new stenoses probably can be explained by turbulence caused by the difference in compliance between the stent and the native veins. This impairment of a few centimeters of previously healthy veins means that, in contrast with simple dilatations, stents can reduce the venous capital of the patient.

RESULTS OF ANGIOPLASTY AND STENTING

The essential element in all the literature in the field of vascular access for hemodialysis is that stenoses do recur, sometimes very rapidly, and that redilatations are necessary to avoid subsequent access thrombosis.

The patency rates in the literature must be read with caution because there are few series and the number of patients is low. Also life-table analyses are rare in the later articles, and authors detecting and redilating stenoses before thrombosis have primary patency rates lower than those who have less effective screening programs or those who wait until thrombosis occurs.

Primary patency rates therefore can be misleading if they are not placed in their clinical context.

Secondary patency rates themselves vary from one paper to another, depending on the use of stents and thrombolysis. In consequence, the literature is heterogeneous, and few articles provide all the data for an overall answer.

Primary patency rates after dilatation of prosthetic grafts range from 31 to 63% at 6 months, from 10 to 44% at 1 year, and from 15 to 22% at 2 years.[2, 8–10]

Forearm native fistulas fare better than grafts because, in our experience, they have provided a 43% and 30% patency at 1 year and 2 years, respectively. Conversely, upper arm fistulas have provided results similar to grafts, with 25% at 1 year and 19% at 2 years.[3] Compared with the forearm, these poorer results in the upper arm are the result of difficulties in the management of stenoses in the distal cephalic vein.

Beathard[9] has reported poor patency at 6 months in central veins (29%) after dilatation compared with 52 to 67% for peripheral stenoses. Quinn,[8] however, reported 23% and 12% patency at 6 months and 1 year, respectively, for central veins, results similar to the 31 and 10% in peripheral veins.

Primary patency rates after stent placement range from 17 to 31% at 1 year for grafts compared with 10 to 40% after simple dilatation.[3, 9–12] Rates are poorer in central veins, with 0 to 11% at 1 year compared with 12% after simple dilatation.[9, 12] Rates after stent placements are therefore comparable with those obtained after simple dilatation, leading authors to conclude that stents are of no value in dialysis access. In fact, when stents have been placed to treat only failures and complications of dilatation, which we strongly advocate, the patency rates show that stents are able to provide long-term results in complicated cases equal to those of dilatation in simple cases.

Secondary patency rates after dilatation and stent placement rarely have been reported. In our experience, we have achieved rates for grafts of 92% at 1 year, 83% at 2 years, 68% at 3 years, and 60% at 4 years by reintervening in stents.[3] Vorwerk[12] reported 86% patency at 1 year after Wallstent placement in a heterogeneous series of grafts and native fistulas, with a mean 6.7-month interval between reinterventions. In contrast, Quinn reported a 71% rate at 1 year after simple dilatation of grafts compared with 64% after placement of Gianturco stents, leading to the conclusion that this stent has no value.[8]

In forearm fistulas, reintervention was necessary in our experience every 15 months. Stents were inserted in only 3% of patients to achieve rates of 84%

at 1 year, 83% at 2 years, and 81% at 3 years.[6] Upper arm fistula rates were lower, 77% at 1 year and 71% at 2 years. Furthermore, for grafts, it was necessary to reintervene every 9 months and to use stents in approximately 33% of cases. The poorest results, however, are those achieved in central veins, with 56% at 1 year and 44% at 2 years according to Vesely.[11]

TREATMENT OF THROMBOSED GRAFTS AND FISTULAS

Prosthetic grafts appeared in the 1970s. With acute access thrombosis, it is impossible to continue hemodialysis. A temporary (femoral or jugular) line must be created, or the thrombosed access must be reopened rapidly. Access thrombosis is therefore a relative emergency, which is a curse not only for the patient but also for dialysis nurses, nephrologists, radiologists, and surgeons. It must be avoided and warrants surveillance programs for detection and correction of stenoses, which underlie 90% of thromboses. Because access thrombosis with underlying stenosis frequently occurs during anesthesia performed for general operations (abdominal, parathyroid, carpal tunnel, etc.), the related transient hypotension, dehydration, or hypercoagulability probably maximizes the risk of stenosis-induced thrombosis; also, this probably explains why some patients are prone to access thrombosis and others are not.

Hemodialysis access thrombosis treatment was exclusively surgical until 1985. Radiologists began to dilate stenoses from 1980, with initially disappointing results because of inappropriate equipment. Only patent vessels or thrombosed vessels, which had just been declotted by the surgeon with a Fogarty balloon, were treated.

In the late 1980s, thrombolytic infusion techniques were applied to thrombosed hemodialysis grafts but were rapidly replaced by so-called pharmacomechanical methods. From 1994, purely mechanical methods were used.

Graft Techniques

Before eventual access declotting, the referring nephrologist and the receiving radiologist share the responsibility of deciding whether the patient should be dialyzed through a central line because of hyperhydration or hyperkalemia. The only contraindications to percutaneous declotting are local infection, severe hypocoagulability (patients treated with high-dose warfarin or ticlopidine), grafts of less than 2 weeks, and immature native fistulas.

There are two mandatory stages in the treatment of a thrombosed dialysis access: removal of thrombus and treatment of the cause of the thrombosis, which is, in 90% of cases, an underlying stenosis. Other causes are prolonged hypotension, dehydration, hypercoagulability, and mechanical compression.

Percutaneous declotting of a thrombosed dialysis access is an outpatient procedure. Anticoagulation (at least 3000 units of heparin) and antistaphylococcal antibiotics are mandatory. Regardless of whether thrombolytic agents have been infused previously, the vascular access is cannulated after local anesthesia, and a venous introducer sheath usually is placed with an antegrade approach to treat the venous outflow (Fig. 21–4). A small subcutaneous tunnel between the skin entry point and the vessel entry point is recommended to facilitate final compression and prevent formation of pseudoaneurysms. A 5-French catheter usually is pushed over the wire up to the superior vena cava and then slowly pulled back while contrast medium is injected under fluoroscopy to localize the downstream (central) extension of the thrombosis. The graft is abandoned at this stage if the venous outflow cannot be traversed or recanalized.

A second arterial introducer is placed with a retrograde approach some centimeters downstream from the venous introducer in the direction of the arterial inflow. To avoid hyperpressure caused by re-establishment of arterial flow, thrombi on the venous side usually are removed before thrombi on the arterial side.

Once the thrombus has been removed and the underlying stenoses dilated, the whole fistula or graft must be checked from the feeding artery to the superior vena cava to rule out residual thrombi and stenoses. Incidental arterial embolism should be searched

for and treated, even when the patient is asymptomatic.

Final compression of the entry points of the introducers can be shortened clearly by purse-string suturing,[3] and the fistula is immediately usable for dialysis. Some teams recommend systematic low molecular weight heparin for some days or weeks both to avoid rethrombosis and to treat possible pulmonary embolism.

THROMBOLYSIS

The first thrombolysis technique reported consisted of prolonged urokinase or streptokinase infusions after direct puncture of the occluded graft. Unfortunately, hemorrhagic complications were frequent, and thrombolytic agents alone proved to be too slow. Numerous residual clots still were present after hours, leading to early rethrombosis or necessitating overnight infusions with increased cost and complications and uncertain results.

PHARMACOMECHANICAL TECHNIQUES

Because thrombolytic agents alone were not effective enough, adjunctive mechanical measures such as pulse-spray, balloons, and aspiration catheters currently are used. However, the two methods described subsequently, which originally were described by their proponents with urokinase, have since been used without urokinase by other teams, with similar or better results; this tends to show that the mechanical effect is probably predominant.

The pulse-spray and balloon method has been

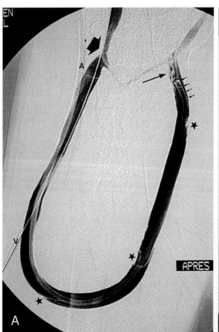
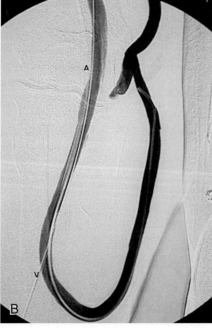

Figure 21–4. *A,* The venous side of this thrombosed forearm loop graft already has been aspirated, unmasking the stenosis of the venous anastomosis, which has not yet been dilated *(wide arrow).* The aspiration catheter *(thin arrows)* is in contact with the arterial plug *(long arrow),* but there are some other residual clots in the loop *(stars). B,* The final angiogram after aspiration and dilatation shows no residual clot, no residual stenosis, and no arterial emboli. A, arterial introducer-sheath; V, venous sheath.

used since 1989, and technical refinements were reported in 1995.[3] Two multiside-holed 5-F catheters are placed in the graft in a criss-cross fashion with their tips at the edge of the thrombus. The active catheter length (segment with the side holes) is selected on the basis of the length of the graft. Tip-occluding wires are placed to obstruct the end holes, and the catheters are fitted with Y-shaped adapters to allow injection in the catheters around the wires.

A 10-ml mixture of 250,000 units of urokinase (or 5 mg recombinant tissue plasminogen activator) and 5000 units of heparin is divided between the two catheters. Rapid forceful pulse-injections of no more than 0.3-ml aliquots then are applied every 30 seconds to each catheter with a tuberculin syringe. After 15 to 20 minutes, careful injection of contrast material evaluates the degree of clot lysis. Thrombolytic injection alone is repeated in cases of a large volume of residual thrombi. The unmasked stenosis of the venous anastomosis then can be dilated. The usual lysis-resistant clot at the arterial anastomosis (the "arterial plug") is detached with a guide wire-directed Fogarty balloon, and residual clots are crushed with a graft matched to the size of the balloon, resulting in hopefully small but inevitable pulmonary embolism. Atherectomy catheters for resistant wall-adherent arterial plugs and stents for suboptimal angioplasty results can be used.

Once the final angiogram and clinical examination are judged to be satisfactory, catheters are removed when the activated clotted time (ACT) is below 200 seconds (which can take several hours).

Pulse-spray with heparinized saline is as effective as pulse-spray with urokinase,[14] which tends to demonstrate that the mechanical effect of clot disruption and embolization is the leading mechanism in Bookstein's technique and that urokinase is just an optional adjunct.

THROMBOEMBOLIZATION AND THROMBOASPIRATION

Thrombolytic infusion with complementary catheter-directed manual thromboaspiration was reported in Europe in 1991 by Poulain.[14] After antegrade and retrograde puncture of the occluded access with 20-gauge needles, a small bolus thrombolytic is injected while the arterial anastomosis is compressed manually to avoid arterial embolism. A thrombolytic agent then is infused with an electric pump for at least 2 hours through each needle. The aim of this initial lysis is to dissolve as much thrombus as possible and to shorten the second phase of mechanical removal of residual clots. The status of the fistula then is checked. Needles are replaced by introducer-sheaths, and residual clots are aspirated with an 8-F large lumen catheter locked to a regular 50-ml syringe. Underlying

stenoses then are dilated. This technique is adapted to very busy radiology departments, where it is impossible to integrate these unplanned patients in the operating program rapidly. The efficacy of thrombolysis is extremely variable but, with complementary thromboaspiration, Poulain demonstrated for the first time that hemodialysis access could be routinely declotted successfully without the help of the Fogarty balloon, now a 40-year old surgical device.

Trerotola and colleagues described intentional embolization of the thrombus into the lungs in 1994.[15] After injection of heparin before any maneuver, the stenosis at the venous anastomosis of the graft is dilated. A Fogarty catheter then is advanced through the introducer sheath placed in the direction of the venous outflow, inflated within the graft, and pushed centrally to clear the clot from the graft. Once the clot is cleared from the venous side of the graft, the Fogarty balloon is pushed from the arterial sheath across the arterial anastomosis. The balloon is inflated, and the firm arterial plug that invariably rests in that location is pulled into the graft. Resistant clots are treated by repeat Fogarty passages or dilation balloons. For arterial plugs resistant to regular Fogarty balloon, Trerotola and colleagues recommend the percutaneous use of the special "Fogarty adherent clot" device. Although the principle of intentional pulmonary embolism was medically shocking, Trerotola and colleagues' arguments for this inexpensive technique were that:

1. The average clot volume in a thrombosed graft is only 3.2 ml and never greater than 8 ml, which represents a minor clot burden (if there is no associated thrombosis of the outflow veins),
2. No complication had been noticed in his initial experience (which is no longer true),
3. Nurses and physicians create thousands of similar small emboli every day when flushing clotted venous lines, and
4. All methods, and especially Bookstein's pulse-spray, induce pulmonary embolism.

This technique must not be used for treatment of rethrombosis within 1 month because of the added burden of pulmonary embolic thrombus.

Balloon-assisted aspiration thrombectomy is a technique of clot mobilization by the Fogarty catheter and is almost identical to Trerotola's method. However, instead of pushing the thrombus into the lungs, the authors try to aspirate as much as possible through the side-arm of the introducer sheaths, but then residual clots still are pushed simply into the outflow.

The Gelbfish Endo Vac device allows thrombi, detached by the Fogarty balloon, to be broken into smaller pieces and removed percutaneously through a metallic introducer by a metallic curette.

Catheter-directed manual thromboaspiration has been used in Europe since 1985. In hemodialysis access, thromboaspiration was first described in 1991 as an adjunct to thrombolytic therapy (see previous section), but thromboaspiration alone since has been reported as a purely mechanical method.[16] Thromboaspiration is a simple concept: a slightly angulated 7- or 8-French catheter with a firm wall, wide inner lumen, and soft tip is pushed through the introducer sheaths over a guide wire (optional in grafts) to make contact with the thrombus. Strong manual aspiration is created through a regular Luer-Lok 50-ml syringe while pulling back the catheter. The syringe and the aspiration catheter are flushed through gauze into a cup, and the procedure can be repeated. Angulated catheters must be used to be able to aspirate clots in aneurysms and curved vessels. The tip of angulated aspiration catheters also can strip the vessel wall and, by occasionally forceful backward-and-forward motion, can detach wall-adherent thrombi, such as the arterial plug.

Clots on the venous side are aspirated first by the venous introducer sheath, but the usual stenosis of the venous anastomosis is dilated later, when the clots of the arterial inflow have been removed (see Fig. 21–4). When a thrombus is trapped in the sheath hemostatic valve, it can be reaspirated with the catheter or the sheath can be removed over a guide wire, flushed, and repositioned. A guide wire or a 5-French catheter then is pushed up to the superior vena cava and left in place through the venous sheath before starting to treat the arterial side through the downstream placed arterial sheath.

The arterial anastomosis is localized by gentle retrograde catheterization with a 5-F catheter over a hydrophilic guide wire. Aspiration of the clots on the arterial side starts from the sheath. The arterial anastomosis must never be crossed: the arterial plug must be the last to be aspirated because restoration of flow pushes loose residual clots into the outflow, although the yet-to-be-dilated stenosis at the venous anastomosis of the graft blocks larger clots. Because the arterial plug is often resistant and needs repeated passes, aspiration occasionally leads to collection of 50 ml of blood and no clots. To avoid blood depletion, this blood is squirted through gauze into a cup, aspirated back into a syringe, and reinjected through the 5-F catheter previously left in the superior vena cava.

After aspiration of the clots on the arterial side, a guide wire is left through the arterial sheath. It is usually necessary to reaspirate the venous side to remove clots that have been pushed by the restored flow and trapped between the introducers, the stenosis, or both at the venous anastomosis. A balloon no smaller than 7 mm (and often 8 mm) is used for dilation of the anastomosis of 6-mm grafts, and stent placement is avoided when possible because of the theoretical increased risk of infection.

Absolutely no residual clot must be accepted on the final angiogram, and complementary aspiration of mural defects must be performed. Pushing the aspiration catheter into the arterial system also treats incidental arterial embolism. Gentle dilation of the entry-points of the introducer-sheaths just before their removal is frequently necessary to avoid induced residual stenoses.

MECHANICAL THROMBECTOMY

The methods described thus far have certain disadvantages. They are time consuming, and lytic agents and pulse-spray catheters are expensive and limited. Concern about pulmonary embolism has led those in litigious societies to reject manual catheter-directed thromboaspiration. Therefore, many teams have placed great hope in mechanical devices. There are two families of declotting devices: those with a direct mechanical stripping action on the thrombus and those based on a vortex or a Venturi effect.

Devices with direct mechanical stripping action include the Arrow-Trerotola Percutaneous Thrombectomy Device (PTD). This is the only device to have been purposely designed for hemodialysis grafts and has been approved by the United States Food and Drug Administration (FDA) since 1997, after having been proven to give results similar to the pulse-spray method.[17] It consists of a motor-driven fragmentation cage made of nitinol that is attached to a drive cable. Both are housed in a 5-French catheter that constrains the self-expandable cage in the closed position, and the cage expands to a diameter of 9 mm in the open position. The open cage is rotated in the graft at 3000 rpm with a separate handheld motor unit. This very flexible (but not over-the-wire) device is advanced past the clot in the closed position, and the cage is deployed by retracting the catheter. The rotator unit is activated to spin the cage, which then is pulled slowly through the clot, macerating as well as stripping the clot from the graft wall. The resultant slurry can be aspirated through the 5-F sheath.

The Cragg thrombolytic brush has a similar action of wall stripping, but the results have not yet been reported.

Devices based on a vortex or on a Venturi effect that pulverize clot are the Amplatz Thrombectomy Device (ATD), the Hydrolyser, the Shredding Embolectomy Thrombectomy (SET) catheter, the Angiojet, and the Trac catheter. The clinical experience published with mechanical thrombolytic devices in hemodialysis grafts currently is limited to several European reports describing the Hydrolyser and a single U.S. report describing the Amplatz device.

The Hydrolyser is a 7-French over-the-wire catheter driven by a conventional angiographic injector. It works best on a fresh thrombus, and wall-adherent residual clots are an Achilles heel, with ancillary procedures required to clear the graft.[18, 19]

The Amplatz Thrombectomy Device is a gas-driven high-speed cam that is FDA approved. Primary patency rates at 1 month (44%) were, however, low in one report,[20] probably because of the residual clots left by the device.

Native Fistula Techniques

The technique of arteriovenous fistula construction at the wrist was described in 1966 by Brescia and Cimino.[21] There are few publications in the literature concerning the treatment of thrombosed native fistulas. There are many reasons for this. It is a far less frequent clinical problem than for grafts, and until now, it was not a U.S. problem. In addition, percutaneous declotting techniques, which have just been validated in grafts, are overall more difficult to perform in native fistulas, whereas surgery remains the technique at the wrist. The consumption of the patient's venous capital by surgical revision appears less prejudicial than in grafts because a thrombosed forearm fistula usually means healthy veins above the elbow for the construction of a new native fistula.

Polytetrafluoroethylene (PTFE) graft declotting is relatively easy because of its easily palpable thick prosthetic wall, graft diameter, average 3.2-ml clot volume, and stenoses located at the venous anastomosis. Thrombosed native fistulas are more difficult. They have a thin wall, which can be difficult to palpate and transfix. Irregular anatomy frequently makes it impossible to localize the anastomosis clinically (Fig. 21–5). Very tight underlying stenoses can occur anywhere and are frequently difficult to traverse. Confusing collaterals are often visible. Sometimes clots are very few but huge. Aneurysms are frequent, often with thick layers of old wall-adherent thrombi. Possible concomitant arterial thrombosis with sharp arteriovenous angulation, which is impossible to traverse from the fistula, often necessitates direct catheterization of the feeding artery.

Only European teams have reported their results after percutaneous treatment of thrombosed fistulas, by low-dose urokinase and thromboaspiration,[14] Hydrolyser,[19, 20] and catheter-directed manual thromboaspiration.[16] Most methods used for grafts are ineffective in cases of huge clots, and they carry a risk of significant pulmonary embolism. This problem can be solved by using the thromboaspiration method.

As for grafts, most fistulas are treated after placement of two introducer sheaths in opposite directions to gain access both to the venous outflow and arterial inflow. Clinical examination is essential to choose the best site for initial catheterization.

Forearm fistulas less than 1 year old or fistulas in obese patients can be impossible to palpate and to cannulate, especially if they are stenosed and have only a few clots. The trick is to place a tourniquet on the upper arm to make the elbow veins swell (see Fig. 21–5). The dilated cephalic or basilic vein at the elbow then can be punctured and catheterized with a retrograde approach. It is then possible to find a way back into the fistula down to the anastomosis. In such cases, this unique retrograde approach is usually sufficient to clear the fistula of thrombi and to dilate underlying stenoses.

When the anastomosis cannot be reached by retrograde approach from the fistula, either because there is a stenosis or because catheter and guide wire are lost in collateral branches, it is helpful to puncture the brachial artery with a 20-gauge needle to image the feeding artery (see Fig. 21–5). This shows where the anastomosis is and helps catheterization by road-mapping. If, however, there is a postanastomotic tight stenosis that cannot be traversed in the retrograde fashion, antegrade catheterization of the feeding artery (usually radial) is feasible. An angulated (4- or 5-F) catheter and a hydrophilic guide wire frequently make it possible to pass the stenosis.

Another trick is to enter the retrogradely inserted introducer with the hydrophilic guide wire. The guide wire then is pushed into the introducer on contact with the hemostatic valve while the introducer is removed. This guide wire inserted via the brachial artery re-emerges from the fistula through the skin above the stenotic area. The introducer sheath is reintroduced over the hydrophilic guide wire, and the stenosis can be dilated with the balloon pushed from the fistula instead of the brachial artery, which limits the size of the hole in the artery.

In cases of concomitant thrombosis of the feeding artery, retrograde catheterization of the thrombosed artery from the fistula is usually possible, and thromboaspiration can be performed with a more flexible 6-F catheter if 7- or 8-F catheters do not pass. If not, aspiration also can be performed after antegrade cannulation of the feeding artery and placement of a 6-French introducer sheath in the brachial artery.

When the fistula is tortuous, with alternating stenoses, sharp angulations, and aneurysms, repeat passes with aspiration catheters or dilatation balloons are likely to be difficult. Similarly, aspiration or dilatation in the anastomotic area can damage the feeding artery (see Fig. 21–5). In such cases, a guide wire is pushed from the introducer sheath into the feeding artery or into the superior vena cava according to the location of the area of concern. After placement of this safety guide wire, a second guide wire is pushed through the same sheath. The sheath then is removed and repositioned only over the second guide wire, leaving the safety guide wire exiting directly through the skin beside the introducer sheath. Although declotting and dilatation maneuvers can be performed through the sheath, the safety guide wire is a fluoro-

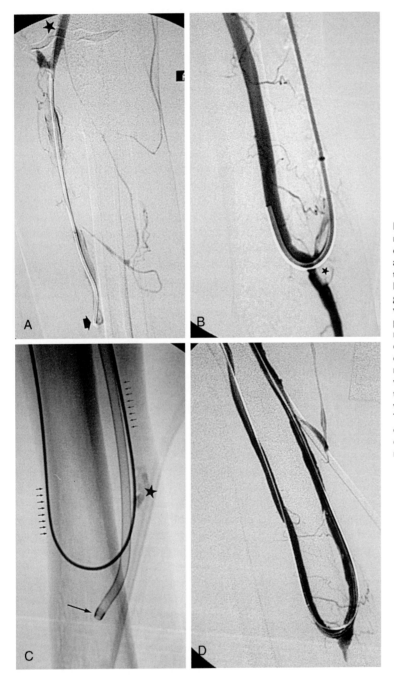

Figure 21–5. *A,* It was impossible to palpate this thrombosed radial fistula, and direct cannulation was impossible. A tourniquet placed on the upper arm made the cephalic vein distend at the elbow. It was possible to cannulate it *(star)* and to find the way back into the fistula with a 5-French catheter *(arrow).* It was, however, impossible to reach the anastomosis, despite guidance by gentle contrast injection. *B,* A 20-gauge needle was placed in the brachial artery at the elbow, and injection permitted localization of the anastomosis, which finally was reached by retrograde catheterization from the fistula. Significant thrombi are seen in this anastomotic area *(star). C,* Because retrograde catheterization was difficult, and to be sure not to compromise the feeding artery during aspiration maneuvers, a safety guide wire was placed from the fistula high into the feeding artery *(thin arrows).* The anastomotic clots then were aspirated with a 7-French angulated catheter *(long arrow).* The small extravasation *(star)* was the result of prior dilatation of a postanastomotic stenosis, which explained the initial difficulties for retrograde catheterization. *D,* Final result after aspiration and angioplasty. The fistula was patent at 8 months.

scopic landmark of the anatomy of the fistula and guarantees rapid reopening of the fistula by dilatation or stent when there are complications.

Old thrombi in aneurysms are usually resistant to lysis or aspiration. These aneurysms are usually large and theoretically should have been preventively revised surgically. However, it is frequently difficult to convince surgeons to operate on a fistula that works well and which patients consider to have an easy access site for dialysis cannulation. Such old thrombi frequently detach during declotting maneuvers and can block the flow intermittently. Because it is not advisable to push such clots into the lungs, the only solution to ensure safety and success of the procedure is to trap them with a stent placed across the aneurysm. A wide mesh puncturable stent can be considered in small aneurysms to enable further cannulation of adjacent segments or in large aneurysms if short-term surgery still is refused by the patient.

TREATMENT OF OCCLUDED CENTRAL VEINS

Concomitant acute thrombosis of central veins is a problem common to native fistulas and grafts. However, like native fistulas, this condition shares the technical problem of occlusion by huge clots. Significant pulmonary emboli can complicate treatment. Catheter-directed thromboaspiration is very effective in thrombosed subclavian and brachiocephalic veins (Fig. 21–6). Underlying stenoses should be stented.

COMPLICATIONS OF PERCUTANEOUS THROMBECTOMY TECHNIQUES

Non–procedure-related deaths are not uncommon during the first month's follow-up in these patients with frequent underlying cardiovascular diseases, which frequently predispose them to access thrombosis.

Pulmonary embolism is an ever-present concern. No declotting technique, even surgical, can claim to avoid emboli, although the majority remain asymptomatic. However, even a small pulmonary embolism can induce bronchospasm, particularly unwelcome in debilitated patients. The risk of bronchospasm can, however, be reduced by injection of heparin before initiation of the thrombectomy procedure. The risks of repeated episodes of embolization in patients who undergo numerous procedures are unknown. Deaths have been reported from pulmonary embolism after pulse-spray and urokinase in two patients with car-

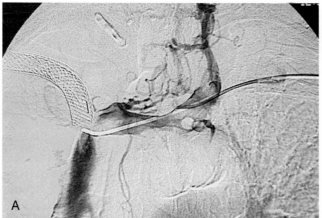

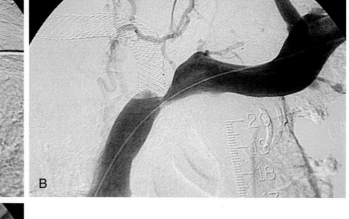

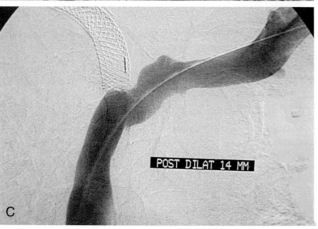

Figure 21–6. *A,* The innominate and the left subclavian veins were thrombosed in the outflow of a brachioaxillary graft in a patient who had numerous dilations to the right side. *B,* All thrombi were aspirated successfully with an 8-French catheter, unmasking a final stenosis of the innominate vein, probably induced by the contralateral stents which, however, did not protrude into the superior vena cava. *C,* After dilatation to 14 mm and 6 atm, the result is perfect, without recoil.

diorespiratory conditions.[22] Also, hemiplegia due to paradoxic embolism, after pulse-spray and urokinase, has been reported in one patient with a patent foramen ovale and a right-to-left shunt.[23] Because all fatal complications probably are not reported in the literature, these reports suggest that techniques recommending intentional embolization of clots are controversial, especially in patients with cardiopulmonary conditions. Our opinion is that catheter-directed manual thromboaspiration of these clots is based on the most satisfactory principle because it aims to remove the thrombus. It has proved to be effective in cases of huge thrombi in central veins. However, the aspiration catheter also occasionally detaches clots, which thus are not aspirated. These must go to the lung. Mechanical devices aiming to pulverize clots would be the ideal, but unfortunately no device to date can claim to be effective on the whole thrombus.

RESULTS

Whatever the method used, mean procedure times from initial puncture to completion of compression range from 90 minutes to 2 hours. Angiography suite occupation time is reduced if initial urokinase infusion is performed in a recovery room.

Immediate success, defined as at least one dialysis treatment via the declotted graft, is reported to range from 71 to 100%.[16]

Many authors do not report primary patency rates but the duration of efficacy of all procedures, including those repeated in the same graft. This produces an overestimation of success because those grafts that rethrombosed within 1 month and were prone to repeated early thromboses underwent surgical revision.

The published primary patency rates after percutaneous graft thrombectomy (or thrombolysis or declotting) range from 44 to 85% at 1 month, 37 to 65% at 3 months, 19 to 39% at 6 months, and 4 to 37% at 1 year.[12–20, 24] A graft that has thrombosed once is therefore at high risk of rethrombosis within 1 year.

Secondary patency rates are reported less frequently, with rates of 52 to 86% at 1 year.[14, 17] Only one article[17] reported the average interval (6 months) between reinterventions (redilatations, stent placements, declotting) performed to maintain or to restore patency.

Few articles have dissociated results in native fistulas from results in grafts.[3, 17, 20] In our experience, the success rate in native fistulas is poorer than in grafts and ranges from 75% (upper arm fistulae) to 89% (forearm fistulae). Failures are due to stenoses that prove impossible to traverse or to the immaturity of the veins. Primary patency rates in the forearm and in the upper arm are 62% and 17% at 6 months,

respectively, and 47% and 9% at 1 year. Secondary patency rates at 1 year are 77% in the forearm and only 40% in the upper arm, with the need for reintervention only every 19 months in the forearm but every 6.4 months in the upper arm. Results are therefore clearly better in the forearm than in the upper arm.

The cost of a procedure is of no value if it is not linked to results. Expensive mechanical devices or truly time-consuming methods could, in fact, be cost-effective if they give superior success and patency rates. Cost-effectiveness calculations also must take into account the frequency and cost of all reinterventions performed to continue hemodialysis, including, for example, the cost of stents and the outcome of patients for whom radiology techniques have failed.

CONCLUSION

Interventional radiology is a proven alternative to surgery for treatment of stenosis and thrombosis in hemodialysis access. It has the overall advantage of being minimally invasive, preserving the patient's venous capital. The abilities and interests of local surgeons and radiologists are important factors; however, where the expertise is available, radiologic treatment should be the method of choice. Ultimately, the choice between surgery and radiology should be debated for each patient and for each lesion.

REFERENCES

1. Schwab S, Besarab A, Beathard G, et al: NKF-DOQI clinical practice guidelines for vascular access. Am J Kidney Dis 30(suppl 4):150–191, 1997.
2. Turmel-Rodrigues L, Blanchard D, Pengloan J, et al: Treatment of failing and failed haemodialysis fistulae and grafts by intervention radiology: Long-term follow-up 1998 (In review).
3. Vorwerk D, Konner K, Schuermann K, Guenther R: A simple trick to facilitate bleeding control after percutaneous haemodialysis fistula and graft interventions. Cardiovasc Intervent Radiol 20:159–160, 1997.
4. Sapoval M, Turmel-Rodrigues L, Raynaud A, et al: Cragg covered stents in haemodialysis access: Initial and midterm results. J Vasc Intervent Radiol 7:335–342, 1996.
5. Raynaud A, Angel C, Sapoval M, et al: Treatment of haemodialysis access rupture during PTA with Wallstent implantation. J Vasc Intervent Radiol 9:437–442, 1998.
6. Turmel-Rodrigues L, Blanchard D, Pengloan J, et al: Wallstents and Craggstents in haemodialysis grafts and fistulae: Results for selective indications. J Vasc Intervent Radiol 8:975–982, 1997.
7. Beathard G: Gianturco self-expanding stents in the treatment of stenosis in dialysis access grafts. Kidney Int 43:872–877, 1993.
8. Quinn S, Schuman E, Demlow T, et al: Percutaneous transluminal angioplasty versus endovascular stent placement in the treatment of venous stenoses in patients undergoing haemodialysis: Intermediate results. J Vasc Intervent Radiol 6:851–855, 1995.
9. Beathard G: Percutaneous transvenous angioplasty in the treatment of vascular access stenosis. Kidney Int 42:1390–1397, 1992.
10. Safa A, Valji K, Roberts A, et al: Detection and treatment of dysfunctional haemodialysis access grafts: Effect of a surveil-

lance program on graft patency and the incidence of thrombosis. Radiology 199:653–657, 1996.

11. Vesely T, Hovsepian D, Pilgram T, et al: Upper extremity central venous obstruction in haemodialysis patients: Treatment with Wallstents. Radiology 204:343–348, 1997.

12. Vorwerk D, Guenther R, Mann H, et al: Venous stenosis and occlusion in haemodialysis shunts: Follow-up results of stent placement in 65 patients. Radiology 195:140–146, 1995.

13. Valji K, Bookstein J, Roberts A, et al: Pulse-spray pharmacomechanical thrombolysis of thrombosed haemodialysis access grafts: Long-term experience and comparison of the original and current techniques. AJR Am J Roentgenol 164:1495–1500, 1995.

14. Poulain F, Raynaud A, Bourquelot P, et al: Local thrombolysis and thromboaspiration in the treatment of acutely thrombosed arteriovenous haemodialysis fistulas. Cardiovasc Intervent Radiol 14:98–101, 1991.

15. Trerotola S, Lund G, Scheel P, et al: Thrombosed haemodialysis access grafts: Percutaneous mechanical declotting without urokinase. Radiology 191:721–726, 1994.

16. Turmel-Rodrigues L, Sapoval M, Pengloan J, et al: Manual thromboaspiration and dilation of thrombosed dialysis access: Mid-term results of a simple concept. J Vasc Intervent Radiol 8:813–824, 1997.

17. Trerotola S, Vesely T, Lund G, et al: Treatment of thrombosed haemodialysis access grafts: Arrow-Trerotola percutaneous thrombolytic device versus pulse-spray thrombolysis. Radiology 206:403–414, 1998.

18. Rousseau H, Sapoval M, Ballini P, et al: Percutaneous recanalization of acutely thrombosed vessels by hydrodynamic thrombectomy (Hydrolyser). Eur Radiol 7:935–941, 1997.

19. Overbosch E, Pattynama P, Aarts H, et al: Occluded haemodialysis shunts: Dutch multicenter experience with the Hydrolyser catheter. Radiology 201:485–488, 1996.

20. Uflacker R, Rajagopalan P, Vujic I, Stutley J: Treatment of thrombosed dialysis grafts: Randomized trial of surgical thrombectomy versus mechanical thrombectomy with the Amplatz device. J Vasc Intervent Radiol 7:185–192, 1996.

21. Brescia MJ, Cimino JE, Appel K, et al: Chronic hemodialysis using venipuncture and a surgically created arteriovenous fistula. N Engl J Med 275:1089–1092, 1966.

22. Swan T, Smyth S, Ruffenach S, et al: Pulmonary embolism following haemodialysis access thrombolysis/thrombectomy. J Vasc Intervent Radiol 6:683–686, 1995.

23. Owens C, Yaghmai B, Aletich V, et al: Fatal paradoxic embolism during percutaneous thrombolysis of a haemodialysis graft. AJR Am J Roentgenol 170:742–744, 1998.

24. Cooper S, Falk A, Sofocleous C, et al: Modified pulse-spray pharmacomechanical thrombolysis technique: Review of 278 procedures. *In* Henry M, Ferguson R (eds): Vascular Access for Haemodialysis V. Chicago, Precept Press, 1997, pp 172–177.

Chapter 22 Transjugular Intrahepatic Portosystemic Shunts

Endovascular Contributors: Anthony A. Watkinson and Jonathan Tibballs
Surgical Contributors: John Craig Collins and I. James Sarfeh

The transjugular intrahepatic portosystemic shunt (TIPS) procedure is a specialized interventional radiologic technique in which a portosystemic shunt is created entirely within the liver via percutaneous venous access from the neck. It is very effective in reducing portal venous pressure, and hence, the portosystemic pressure gradient (PPG) does not compromise subsequent liver transplantation, and produces a unique access to the portal venous system. Its main drawback is limited patency of the shunt because of pseudointimal hyperplasia or thrombosis, necessitating close follow-up and a high reintervention rate.

The first experimental radiologic intrahepatic portosystemic shunt was created in the pig by Rösch and colleagues in 1969.[1] This proved the feasibility of TIPS, but the technique could not progress because of the absence of metallic stents to maintain shunt patency. Colapinto and associates created the first TIPS in a human in 1982[2] using a Gruntzig balloon catheter, but in the absence of a stent, the shunt soon occluded. The technical advances in expandable metal stent technology in the early 1980s once more opened the way for the development of this technique. Several groups, notably those of Palmaz and Rösch, succeeded in creating TIPS in experimental animal studies using a variety of metallic stents, such as the Palmaz and Gianturco Z stent, and subsequently, the Wallstent. Finally, approximately 20 years after the pioneering work of Rösch and colleagues, Richter and associates applied the technique in humans, publishing their pilot series of three patients in 1990.[3] Based on the experience of these early groups, the technique has grown in popularity and now is performed worldwide.

THE CLINICAL PROBLEM

Cirrhosis of the liver produces obstruction of portal venous blood flow at the sinusoidal level and consequently is one of the major causes of portal hypertension. Normal PPG is 12 mm Hg or less, but this may increase to greater than 30 mm Hg in portal hypertension. In an attempt to decompress the portal system, venous collateral vessels (varices) develop, typically affecting the left and short gastric veins, esophageal veins, hemorrhoidal veins, paraumbilical veins, and lienorenal and other retroperitoneal veins.

Of these, esophageal and gastric varices are the most clinically relevant because they have the highest tendency to rupture into either the esophageal or gastric lumen, producing major and often life-threatening hemorrhage.[4] Varices account for 4 to 10% of patients presenting with acute upper gastrointestinal (GI) hemorrhage and are associated with the highest mortality rate of all causes of such hemorrhage, accounting for approximately one-third of deaths of patients with cirrhosis. Esophageal and gastric varices develop in 90% of patients with cirrhosis with an incidence of hemorrhage of at least 30% and an associated mortality rate of 25 to 50% from the first variceal bleed. The risk of recurrent hemorrhage is at least 70%.

The risk of variceal hemorrhage increases with increasing portal pressure, and although the precise relationship between the two is not clear, hemorrhage is rare if the PPG is less than 12 mm Hg.

Conventional medical treatment[4] of acute variceal hemorrhage includes pharmacologic agents such as terlipressin (Glypressin) and octreotide, both of which lower portal venous pressure, and endoscopic sclerotherapy and variceal band ligation, which aim to obliterate the varices, the underlying portal hypertension remaining untreated. Recurrent variceal hemorrhage is treated with beta blockade to lower the PPG and a program of repeated injection sclerotherapy or banding until all visible varices are obliterated. Endoscopic sclerotherapy and banding are associated with an increased incidence of portal gastropathy and nonvariceal upper GI hemorrhage but a low incidence of hepatic encephalopathy. Surgical options in acute variceal hemorrhage include esophageal transection with or without gastric devascularization and portosystemic shunting. These procedures are associated with a high mortality when performed in the emergency setting, especially in patients with severe liver disease (Child's C grade). Even in more elective situations, they can be technically demanding and can compromise future liver transplantation unless expertise is available to perform distal splenorenal or small-diameter prosthetic H-graft portacaval shunts. Surgical portosystemic shunts are associated with deterioration of or new onset of hepatic encephalopathy (as is TIPS), the risk of this being proportional to the diameter and selectivity of the shunt.

The ultimate treatment for chronic liver disease clearly is liver transplantation, but the availability of both donor organs and medical resources are currently insufficient to meet demand, and, in some cases, it is not an appropriate clinical treatment option.

INDICATIONS

The TIPS procedure is very effective at decreasing the PPG and consequently has been applied to most conditions related to or caused by portal hypertension. These are shown in Table 22–1.

Initial enthusiasm for the technique, however, has been tempered somewhat by the incidence of shunt dysfunction related to stent stenosis and occlusion, which renders TIPS in its current form a temporary rather than permanent treatment for portal hypertension. The TIPS procedure initially was regarded as the panacea for treating portal hypertension and in retrospect was employed rather indiscriminately. It is only in the past year or two that the results of controlled trials of TIPS vs. conventional medical and surgical treatments have emerged. Retrospective comparisons of TIPS data to historical medical and surgical treatment data have been hampered by differences in population groups, particularly the severity of liver disease of patients studied, and by different methods of assessing results and complications. This quite rightly has led to a reappraisal of the role of TIPS in

Table 22–1. Indications for Transjugular Intrahepatic Portosystemic Shunt

---

Acute variceal hemorrhage (gastresophageal, gastric, anorectal, parastomal)
Recurrent variceal hemorrhage
Refractory ascites, hepatic hydrothorax
As a "bridge" to liver transplantation
As a trial of shunt surgery
Budd-Chiari syndrome, hepatic veno-occlusive disease
Portal vein thrombosis
Hepatorenal syndrome
Hepatopulmonary syndrome
Protein-losing enteropathy
Treatment of occluded or stenosed surgical portacaval shunts

---

managing complications of portal hypertension and a refinement of indications for its use. Some have argued that given the incidence of shunt dysfunction, such an invasive procedure is very rarely, if ever, indicated. Certainly the number of TIPS creations throughout the United Kingdom varies considerably, even between liver transplantation centers, indicating wide differences in approach.

Conversely, when faced with conditions such as uncontrollable acute variceal hemorrhage and portal vein thrombosis, in which even liver transplantation frequently is not possible, there are often few, if any, useful alternative treatments other than TIPS. The issue in these situations is whether any treatment can improve survival or quality of life. The most accepted indications for TIPS creation at present remain uncontrolled acute variceal hemorrhage and refractory ascites.

Acute Variceal Hemorrhage

TIPS should be reserved for patients with acute variceal bleeding that is not controlled by conventional medical management (pharmacologic agents, mechanical balloon tamponade, endoscopic injection sclerotherapy and banding) (Fig. 22–1). TIPS has been shown to be as effective in controlling hemorrhage from gastric fundal varices as from esophageal varices,[5] unlike endoscopic techniques, which are much less effective in controlling gastric varices than esophageal varices. TIPS has a lower mortality than surgical esophageal transection and gastric devascularization in this setting. Consequently, TIPS is considered at an earlier stage in patients bleeding from gastric varices. Management algorithms indicating the role of TIPS in patients with acute variceal hemorrhage are outlined in Table 22–2.

Although TIPS is very effective at gaining immediate control of acute variceal hemorrhage, these patients still have a very high mortality rate—in the region of 50%—particularly when associated with advanced liver disease, sepsis, and multiorgan failure. This has led to the derivation of prognostic indices[6] that, if validated, will aid in the selection of patients to undergo TIPS in this situation.

Recurrent Variceal Hemorrhage

TIPS also should be considered in patients with recurrent variceal hemorrhage not controlled by medical treatment, and in those patients who are intolerant of repeated sessions of endoscopic sclerotherapy and banding. The alternative treatments in this group of patients are surgical portosystemic shunting or liver transplantation. The only published trial of TIPS vs.

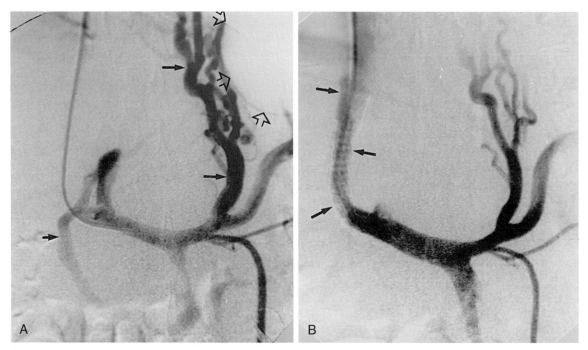

Figure 22–1. Patient with uncontrolled variceal hemorrhage. *A,* Portal venogram after right portal vein branch puncture. Note the left gastric varices *(long arrows)*, recanalized umbilical vein *(short arrows)*, and inflated gastric balloon of the Sengstaken-Blakemore tube *(open arrows)*. *B,* Portal venogram after Memotherm TIPS stent *(arrows)* deployment. Note decreased left portal vein and umbilical vein filling. Left gastric variceal filling also is diminished. The S-B tube has been deflated.

surgical shunting (using small-diameter [8-mm] prosthetic H-graft portacaval shunts) pertains to this group and shows a clear advantage for surgery in terms of rebleeding, reintervention, and mortality rates,[7] although this remains to be corroborated by further larger series.

After the success of TIPS in controlling acute variceal hemorrhage, several controlled trials of TIPS vs. injection sclerotherapy (or variceal band ligation), plus propranolol, in the prevention of recurrent esophageal variceal hemorrhage have been published.[8–10] These show lower rebleeding rates in the

Table 22–2. Management Pathways for Acute Esophageal and Gastric Variceal Hemorrhage

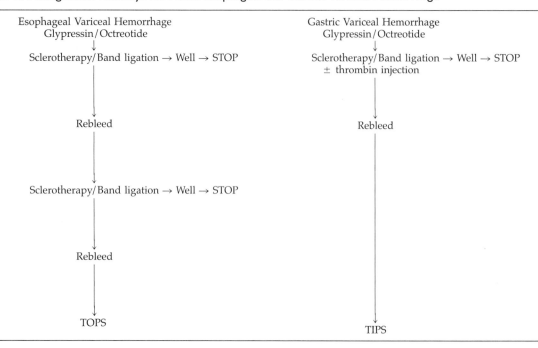

TIPS patients than in the endoscopically managed patients (10 to 20% vs. ~50%, respectively), a higher incidence of worsening or de novo hepatic encephalopathy in the TIPS patients (~35% vs. ~15%), but no overall difference in survival between the two treatments. This suggests that TIPS is a more effective treatment in these patients, but in the absence of a clear survival benefit, it is difficult to justify the intensive follow-up and reintervention rates (~30% at 1 year) that these patients require. Consequently, endoscopic management is likely to prevail for the foreseeable future.

Treatment of bleeding varices at other sites (e.g., anorectal, parastomal) is based on the same rationale of reducing the PPG and can be combined with direct embolization of the varices via the TIPS.

Refractory Ascites

Resolution of ascites after TIPS creation was first noted incidentally in patients treated for variceal hemorrhage. Refractory ascites may be defined as ascites that does not respond to bed rest, salt restriction, and diuretic treatment. It occurs in approximately 10% of ascitic cirrhotics and is associated with more advanced liver disease. Consequently, it is associated with a high mortality of up to 75% if ascites is severe. It has been treated conventionally by large-volume paracentesis with or without albumin infusion, surgical peritovenous shunts, and ultimately, liver transplantation.[11] In some patients, the ascites can reaccumulate so rapidly that weekly paracentesis is required, or the sheer volume of ascites causes discomfort or respiratory embarassment, and it is usually at this stage that TIPS is considered.

TIPS is believed to relieve ascites by reducing sinusoidal portal hypertension and improving renal sodium excretion. It has been suggested that the latter effect is responsible for the improvement in renal function seen in patients with hepatorenal syndrome (HRS) (see subsequent section on HRS). Success also has been reported in using TIPS to treat hepatic hydrothorax. The following indications are more controversial, with evidence for or against TIPS often based on relatively small series of patients.

As a "Bridge" to Liver Transplantation

The aim of TIPS in this situation is to "buy time" before liver transplantation. Reducing portal hypertension decreases the extent of venous collaterals and allows improvement in nutritional and metabolic status. There is some evidence indicating a reduction in hospital stay and blood transfusion requirements in patients pretreated with TIPS, but any overall impact on survival is not yet clear.

The fact that a correctly placed TIPS does not compromise subsequent liver transplantation is one of its main advantages over a surgical portacaval shunt. Even misplaced TIPS stents do not necessarily preclude transplantation, but they certainly can complicate surgery, as any transplant surgeon will testify.

Budd-Chiari Syndrome

Budd-Chiari Syndrome (BCS) results from hepatic vein occlusion, classically due to obstruction of the hepatic vein ostia or inferior vena cava (IVC) by webs or tumors, or by thrombosis of the veins themselves, usually in relation to some form of underlying procoagulant state, although no cause is identified in 60% of cases. Hepatic outflow obstruction results in centrilobular congestion and eventually necrosis, fibrosis, and portal hypertension.

Acute BCS due to venous thrombosis can be treated by thrombolytic infusion directly into the hepatic artery, but results are poor and medical management is associated with a very high mortality. Surgical options include division of membranous webs, portacaval or mesoatrial shunts, or liver transplantation.

Membranous webs can be treated by balloon angioplasty or, preferably, stenting, with good results. Compression of the IVC by caudate lobe hypertrophy also can be treated successfully by metallic stent insertion.

TIPS is a theoretically appealing treatment for BCS because it bypasses the obstructed hepatic venous outflow, increases hepatic perfusion, and reduces portal venous pressure. In subacute and chronic BCS, surgical shunts can be compromised by compression of the intrahepatic IVC by the enlarged caudate lobe. TIPS bypasses the intrahepatic IVC and therefore is unaffected by any caudate lobe compression.

TIPS creation can be technically difficult in the presence of obliterated hepatic veins, although, if necessary, a track can be created between the intrahepatic IVC and portal vein. Underlying procoagulant states should be treated aggressively in an attempt to prevent shunt thrombosis, and systemic anticoagulation may be required.

Portal vein thrombosis coexists with BCS in approximately 20% of cases. Successful thrombolysis via a TIPS of acute BCS with associated extensive portomesenteric thrombosis has been described—a rare situation that nonetheless illustrates the potential of TIPS as a salvage procedure.

The use of TIPS to treat hepatic veno-occlusive disease complicating bone marrow transplantation is based on the same rationale, and several reports of successful cases have been published.

Portal Vein Thrombosis

Despite having long been cited as a contraindication to performing TIPS, successful recanalization of both cavernous and noncavernous portal vein thrombosis (PVT) via TIPS has been reported.[12] The treatment options for PVT are limited. If thrombosis is acute and extensive, there is a risk of intestinal ischemia and infarction, usually compounded by delayed diagnosis. In this situation, the only treatment options are surgical thrombectomy with or without thrombolysis or thrombolytic infusion after percutaneous catheterization of the superior mesenteric artery, but both are associated with low success rates and mortality remains high.

If thrombosis is confined to the main portal vein, the risk is of subsequent portal hypertension and treatment is aimed at avoiding the long-term complications of portal hypertension. Surgical thrombectomy can be performed but is associated with a high rethrombosis rate.

TIPS has the theoretical advantage of permitting early minimally invasive portal vein recanalization, thereby offering the potential to prevent the formation of varices. Having restored portal venous flow, the intrahepatic tract theoretically can be occluded, thereby negating the problems of shunt stenosis and avoiding hepatic encephalopathy (although if the underlying cause of PVT remains, rethrombosis is possible).

Hepatorenal Syndrome

HRS is a common and severe complication of advanced cirrhosis, characterized by renal failure, severe portal hypertension, abnormalities in the arterial circulation, and overactivity of endogenous vasoactive systems. The only treatment previously shown to increase survival in this usually rapidly progressive and fatal condition is liver transplantation, but recent studies[13] suggest that TIPS is effective at improving renal function and may increase survival.

Hepatopulmonary Syndrome

Hepatopulmonary syndrome (HPS) is an uncommon complication of advanced liver disease. It is characterized by the combination of chronic liver disease and pulmonary vascular dilatation, resulting in arterial hypoxaemia. Only three cases of TIPS in HPS have been reported—two describing an improvement in oxygenation after TIPS, and the other no improvement; therefore, the role of TIPS, if any, in this unusual complication of chronic liver disease remains to be proven.

Protein-Losing Enteropathy

Clinical improvement has been reported in a single case, attributed to the effect of reduction in portal pressure.

Treatment of Stenosed Surgical Portacaval Shunts

Surgical portacaval shunts can be accessed via a TIPS, allowing treatment of stenosis or occlusion, but this is achieved much more easily from the IVC via a transfemoral approach. TIPSs have been created in patients with irretrievably occluded surgical shunts.

CONTRAINDICATIONS

Absolute contraindications to TIPS creation include intrahepatic malignancy, polycystic liver disease, liver failure, and right heart failure. Relative contraindications include pre-existing hepatic encephalopathy and PVT. Additional contraindications in patients with refractory ascites include coexisting organic renal impairment and prior hepatic encephalopathy.

TECHNIQUE

Patient Preparation

The degree of patient preparation is dictated to some extent on the urgency with which the procedure is performed. In the emergency setting of uncontrolled variceal hemorrhage, the patients have a Sengstaken-Blakemore tube in place after failed endoscopic treatment and are being transfused actively with blood and blood products. In the elective situation, attempts should be made to correct coagulopathy and renal impairment.

All patients receive intravenous antibiotics, typically 1 g flucloxacillin to protect against contamination by skin organisms.

Most procedures are performed under intravenous sedation (2.5 to 5 mg midazolam or 5 to 10 mg diazepam given as bolus injections, as required) and analgesia (50 mg pethidine given as bolus injections, as required). General anesthesia is used only when there is a significant risk of airway compromise and aspiration, for example, in the presence of a reduced conscious level and active bleeding. Oxygen is administered by facial mask or nasal cannula at 5 L/min, and oxygen saturation is monitored by pulse oximetry. Oropharyngeal suction must be readily available.

Pre-TIPS Imaging

Ideally, all patients should have a Doppler ultrasonographic (US) examination to assess portal vein patency and direction of flow. The portal vein bifurcation can be identified and an attempt made to assess whether it is intra- or extrahepatic. The position and patency of the hepatic veins also can be assessed. Knowledge of the presence of venous collateral branches, particularly the umbilical vein, which sometimes can cause confusing appearances after portal vein puncture, can be helpful, as can an idea of liver size and the presence of focal mass lesions. A contrast enhanced computed tomography (CT) scan to confirm portal vein patency and liver size and shape also can be useful, but it is not essential, and the contrast load may be better avoided if there is renal impairment. Not infrequently, TIPS is performed as an emergency procedure without recent imaging, and a limited Doppler US immediately before the procedure to assess portal vein patency is all that is possible.

Procedure

The basic technique is well described and is summarized schematically in Figure 22–2. The following description is the method used at our institution and is followed by a discussion of variations in technique. The right internal jugular vein is punctured, usually after US localization or under direct US guidance, and a 30-cm long 10-French nylon introducer sheath is introduced. A 7-French Cobra I end-hole catheter and 0.035-inch moveable core 3-mm J wire are introduced and used to catheterize a hepatic vein, preferably the right.

The right and middle hepatic veins can be confused in the anteroposterior (AP) projection but can be distinguished by rotating the fluoroscopic C-arm into the right anterior oblique (RAO) projection. The middle hepatic vein is foreshortened in this projection whereas the right hepatic vein is changed minimally or appears to lengthen. Because the right portal vein branch lies posterior to the middle hepatic vein but anterior to the right hepatic vein, this distinction is clearly of crucial importance when planning the intrahepatic tract. The catheter is advanced as far peripherally into the liver as possible, which usually succeeds in wedging it. If a satisfactorily wedged position cannot be achieved with the Cobra catheter, it is exchanged over a guide wire for a 7-French balloon occlusion catheter. A wedged hepatic venogram then is performed to locate the position of the portal vein. A hand injection of 40 to 50 ml of medical-grade carbon dioxide (CO_2) is made during a 4- to 6-frame/second digital subtraction angiogram (DSA) acquisition in both the AP and lateral projections. This successfully opacifies the portal vein in most patients and is particularly effective if there is reversed portal venous flow (Fig. 22–3).

The 10-French introducer is advanced as far into the hepatic vein as possible, and the Cobra or occlusion catheter is removed.

A Rosch-Uchida transjugular access set then is introduced into the 10-French sheath. This set comprises four parts—a 20-gauge flexible inner puncture needle within a 5-French catheter and a 14-gauge blunt-ended metal cannula within a 10-French outer polytetrafluorethylene (Teflon) catheter, both of which have a 15-degree angle over their distal 4 cm. The puncture needle and 5-French catheter lock together, as do the 14-gauge cannula and 10-French catheter, resulting in a coaxial system of needle/catheter within cannula/catheter. When assembled, the inner needle and catheter project beyond the tip of the outer cannula and catheter by up to 6 cm.

This coaxial system is introduced with the needle tip withdrawn to lie within the tip of the 14-gauge cannula and advanced through the 10-French introducer sheath deep into the hepatic vein. The introducer sheath then is withdrawn to the region of the hepatic vein ostium. With reference to the wedged CO_2 portal venogram images, the needle assembly is withdrawn into a more proximal position within the

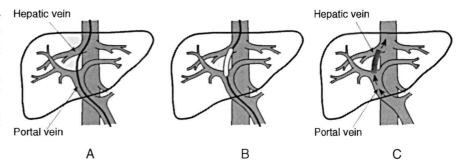

Figure 22–2. Schematic representation of TIPS. A parenchymal tract is created between a hepatic vein and a portal vein branch (A), is dilated with an angioplasty balloon (B), and a metal stent deployed (C). (From Tibballs JM, Watkinson AW, Menu Y: Imaging of the liver and biliary tract. *In* Bircher J, Benhamou J-P, McIntyre N, et al (eds): Oxford Textbook of Clinical Hepatology, 2nd ed. Oxford, Oxford University Press, 1999. By permission of Oxford University Press.)

Hepatic vein

Portal vein

A   B   C

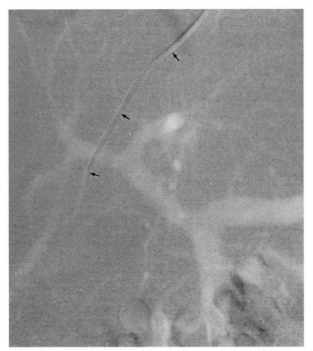

Figure 22–3. Wedged CO_2 venogram via a 7-French end-hole Cobra II catheter *(arrows)*. The intra- and extrahepatic portal vein, splenic vein, and superior mesenteric vein all are clearly shown in a patient with hepatofugal flow.

hepatic vein and rotated to direct its tip toward the right portal vein branch. If the right hepatic vein has been cannulated, anteromedial direction of the needle tip usually is required, which is achieved by rotating the needle assembly in a counterclockwise direction when viewed from the head. The inner needle/catheter then are advanced 3 to 6 cm through the liver parenchyma toward the estimated position of the portal vein branch. Resistance often is felt on puncturing the portal vein wall. The needle is withdrawn, and a contrast-filled syringe is attached to the 5-French catheter, which is withdrawn slowly until blood is aspirated. Contrast is injected to confirm suitable portal vein puncture. If the portal vein is not punctured, the 5-French catheter is withdrawn into the guiding cannula, and the needle is reintroduced. The direction of the parenchymal tract is altered by varying the degree of rotation and the point of exit from the hepatic vein. Occasionally, the coaxial system must be removed and the degree of angulation of the 14-gauge cannula altered. Screening in AP and lateral projections can be helpful in assessing the required degrees of angulation. A second needle pass then is made, and repeated as necessary until the portal vein is punctured successfully.

Having punctured the portal vein, an 0.035-inch angled Terumo wire is used to negotiate from the portal vein branch through the main portal vein and into the splenic or superior mesenteric vein (SMV). If possible, the 10-French catheter also is advanced

through into the portal vein, supported by the 14-gauge cannula if necessary, but the portal vein wall may be too tough to allow this. If the 10-French catheter can be advanced into the portal vein, the puncture is secured and a 0.035-inch Amplatz SuperStiff wire can be inserted directly. If the 10-French catheter cannot be advanced into the portal vein, the 5-French catheter is exchanged carefully over the Terumo guide wire for a 100-cm 4-French Royal Flush straight catheter, which is advanced well into the splenic vein or SMV. This secures the puncture and allows exchange of the Terumo guide wire for an Amplatz SuperStiff guide wire, over which the 10-French catheter can be advanced.

Having established secure portal vein access, an initial portal pressure recording is made, with simultaneous right atrial pressure recording via the introducer sheath to determine the PPG. (The systemic pressure ideally should be measured in the IVC to negate the effect of elevated intra-abdominal pressure, but this would require a second catheter to be placed in the IVC. In practice, there is not usually a large difference between right atrial and IVC pressure, except when there is tense ascites. In this instance, the true residual PPG is measured after TIPS creation.) The catheter is positioned in the proximal splenic vein, and a contrast study using iodinated contrast or CO_2 is performed to delineate the portal venous anatomy and to assess variceal filling.

The liver parenchymal tract then is dilated to 8 mm using an 8 mm × 4 cm Olbert angioplasty balloon. The hepatic and portal vein walls at each end of the liver tract produce waisting of the balloon (Fig. 22–4), and the position of these waists is noted carefully and subsequently used to guide stent placement. This dilatation of the liver tract is painful, and the need for additional analgesia and sedation is reviewed before balloon inflation.

The length of the liver tract is estimated in relation to the opaque markers on the angioplasty balloon, and a stent 1 to 2 cm longer than the estimated tract length is chosen. The superior end of the stent ideally should cover the hepatic vein to the region of the ostium (to prevent hepatic venous stenosis) but must not project into the IVC or right atrium because this could compromise future liver transplantation. The inferior end of the stent should project into the portal vein branch or main portal vein for as short a distance as possible to avoid compromising the portal venous anastomosis at liver transplantation. A 12-mm diameter Memotherm stent of appropriate length is chosen and deployed. The correct position for deployment is estimated with reference to the prior balloon waisting and anatomic landmarks, taking into account respiratory motion. The exact position of the hepatic vein always can be verified by contrast injection through the 10-French sheath. Complete coverage of the liver tract is indicated by flaring of both ends of the stent and can be confirmed by contrast injection. The stent delivery device is removed, and a catheter is reintroduced to measure the resulting portal pressure. In cases of variceal hemorrhage, a PPG of less than 12 to 15 mm Hg is the goal. If this is not achieved initially, the stent is dilated sequentially to 8, 10, or 12 mm until a satisfactory pressure gradient is achieved.

In cases of refractory ascites, the tract and stent are only dilated to 8 mm, regardless of the resulting PPG, in an attempt to minimize the risk of hepatic encephalopathy.[14]

A completion contrast study is performed with a catheter in the splenic vein. Particular attention is made to the degree of variceal filling and intrahepatic portal vein filling. If variceal filling is diminished after TIPS creation and a satisfactory pressure gradient has been achieved, variceal embolization is not performed routinely. If prominent variceal filling persists despite a satisfactory reduction in the PPG, embolization of persistent varices is performed because steal into varices has been implicated in early shunt failure. The threshold for variceal embolization is lower in cases of gastric variceal hemorrhage.

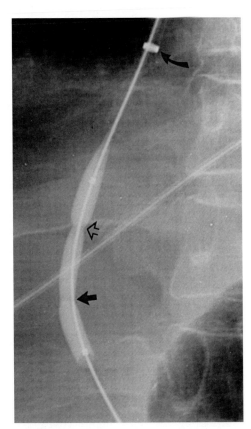

Figure 22–4. Dilatation of the intrahepatic tract. Waisting of the balloon indicates the locations of the hepatic vein *(open arrow)* and portal vein *(solid arrow)* walls. The opaque tip of the 10-French sheath is clearly visible *(curved arrow).*

VARIATIONS IN TECHNIQUE

The main variations in technique are the methods of portal vein localization, the type of needle/catheter assembly used to puncture the portal vein, and the type of stent used.

Portal Vein Localization

Portal vein localization is performed to facilitate portal vein puncture and minimize the risk of capsular perforation.

PREPROCEDURAL TECHNIQUES

Preprocedural assessment of the relationship between the hepatic and portal vein branches using contrast-enhanced spiral CT, magnetic resonance imaging/angiography, and Doppler US has been advocated but is not widely employed. Such imaging frequently is not possible in the emergency setting.

TRANSHEPATIC TECHNIQUES

Transhepatic portal vein catheterization was used in the initial TIPS procedures to outline the position of the portal vein branches and aid their puncture. This inevitably is associated with a risk of potentially fatal intraperitoneal hemorrhage and is not advocated as a routine technique. However, it has re-emerged as a useful technique when performing TIPS for portal vein thrombosis, particularly if the thrombosis is chronic, when other localization techniques cannot be used. Two series report no complications of this technique if the transhepatic tract is embolized at the end of the procedure.

Percutaneous placement of metallic markers adjacent to the right portal vein branch under US or CT guidance before the TIPS procedure has been described. These techniques are safe if fine needles are used, but they add to the complexity of the procedure. They may be of use in patients who have an initial failed TIPS because of inability to puncture the portal vein.

INDIRECT ARTERIOPORTOGRAPHY

Indirect arterioportography via the superior mesenteric or splenic artery in AP and lateral projections may be used to localize the portal vein, assuming that it is patent and flow is hepatopetal. If the splenic artery is catheterized, splenic pulp enhancement can obscure the portal vein on the lateral view; therefore, the superior mesenteric artery is preferred. This technique obviously involves an additional arterial puncture and extends the procedure time a little, but more important, it entails a significant contrast load and therefore is be avoided if possible, particularly if there is renal impairment.

WEDGED HEPATIC VENOGRAPHY

Wedged hepatic venography is usually able to delineate the main intrahepatic portal vein branches and bifurcation. A dedicated balloon occlusion catheter may be used, but frequently a 7-French end-hole angiographic catheter advanced peripherally into a hepatic vein suffices. Contrast is injected by hand or mechanical injector and refluxes through the hepatic sinusoids and into the portal vein. It is particularly effective if there is hepatofugal flow.

Iodinated contrast may be used, but this should be avoided if there is renal impairment. Hepatic laceration requiring embolization has been reported as a complication of this technique.

CO_2 may be used as described previously. This opacifies the portal vein more consistently than iodinated contrast. Extrahepatic extravasation of CO_2 has been documented, but this is less likely than when iodinated contrast is used and appears to be of no clinical consequence. CO_2 embolization to the right heart also has been recorded, but only after the injection of a large volume (120 ml) of CO_2 via an unwedged catheter. This is the technique of choice for portal vein localization and even may be used in the presence of main portal vein thrombosis if some intrahepatic portal vein branches remain patent.

ULTRASOUND

Real-time US can be used to guide portal vein puncture by directly visualizing the needle tip and guiding it toward the portal vein branch. This can, however, be technically difficult because two operators are required, one performing the US and the other controlling the needle. Coordinating the efforts of both operators requires considerable skill. If the US operator scans from an anterior approach, their hands are in the line of the x-ray beam; therefore, simultaneous fluoroscopic screening cannot be used. If the US operator scans from a lateral approach, considerable care must be taken to ensure correct orientation.

In addition, the liver is often small, ascites may be present, and respiratory motion can make reliable visualization of the needle tip difficult.

If multiple needle passes are made, US interpretation becomes increasingly difficult, and if wedged CO_2 venography has been attempted, subsequent US is impossible because retained microbubbles cause a "white-out" effect.

US guidance may be useful in cases of extensive portal vein thrombosis, as described previously.

OTHER TECHNIQUES

Many centers do not attempt to localize the portal vein but rely on anatomic landmarks and the expected relationship between the portal and hepatic veins to aid fluoroscopically guided puncture. Contrast extravasation around the portal vein during attempted puncture can outline the portal vein wall—the "tunnel sign"—and subsequently can be used to target the vein.

Portal vein catheterization via US-guided puncture of paraumbilical venous collateral branches has been described, as has a combined transjugular–transmesenteric technique, in which the superior mesenteric vein is catheterized via a surgical minilaparatomy, under local anesthetic if necessary.

Catheter/Needle Assembly

Various catheter/needle assemblies are available for forming the intrahepatic parenchymal tract. The two most widely used are the Rösch-Uchida coaxial needle and the Colapinto transjugular biopsy needle.

The Rösch-Uchida coaxial needle already has been described. Its main advantages are that a 5-French needle/catheter assembly is used to puncture the portal vein, and consequently, an inadvertent capsular puncture is only 5 French in size. Should capsular puncture occur, the 5-French catheter is in precisely the right point to perform embolization. The 14-gauge metal cannula also provides excellent support within the parenchymal tract and can be used to facilitate catheterization of tough portal vein walls.

The Colapinto transjugular access set includes a 16-gauge metal cutting needle with a distal curve and an outer 9-French catheter. The needle/catheter combination is introduced into the hepatic vein via an introducer sheath. Portal vein puncture then is initiated from the proximal hepatic vein, as described previously. Because a 16-gauge needle is used, capsular punctures are inevitably larger than with the Rösch-Uchida system, with a greater potential for intraperitoneal hemorrhage. If embolization is required, an additional catheter must be introduced, which takes a little extra time and risks losing the precise position of the capsular puncture site. A modification of this system is to use the needle to direct the puncture route, but to make the initial tract with the reverse end of an 0.035-inch Amplatz Super Stiff guide wire. If the operator feels a "give" consistent with portal vein wall puncture, the needle is advanced over the guide wire and portal vein puncture is confirmed by aspiration of blood and contrast injection. The advantage of this system is that it is slightly cheaper than the Rösch-Uchida system.

Both systems allow the direction of the parenchymal tract to be determined by varying the degree of distal angulation of the 14-gauge cannula or the 16-

gauge needle, by varying the degree of rotation and by varying the point of exit from the hepatic vein.

Choice of Stent

The ideal TIPS stent should have high radial strength and radiopacity, should be flexible and mounted on a low-profile delivery system, should be able to be deployed accurately, and should be long enough to cover the entire parenchymal tract.

The first TIPS were created using Palmaz stents, and these continue to be used in some centers. These are balloon-expandable stainless-steel stents that undergo minor, predictable shortening during deployment. They can be placed very accurately, but more than one stent is required to cover all but the shortest parenchymal tracts, increasing the duration and cost of the procedure. They are also relatively inflexible. They can be dilated further if a satisfactory reduction in portal pressure is not achieved initially.

The Wallstent is a self-expanding stainless-steel stent. It is flexible and can be overdilated if necessary. Its main disadvantages are its poor radiopacity and its considerable shortening during and after deployment, which can cause retraction of one end of the stent into the hepatic parenchyma, resulting in shunt failure.

The Memotherm stent is a self-expanding nitinol stent. It has good radiopacity and does not shorten appreciably, although the proximal end does tend to advance during deployment if countertraction is not maintained. Memotherm stents do not feature prominently in the literature, unlike Wallstents, largely because Memotherms were unavailable in the United States, where some of the largest TIPS stents have been performed. There are at least two European centers, including our own, that use the Memotherm and believe that it is the stent of choice.

Other stents such as the Gianturco Z stent and Strecker stent also have been used. The role of covered stents currently is being investigated in response to the suggestion that pseudointimal hyperplasia within stents is stimulated by the presence of bile after bile duct injury during creation of the parenchymal TIPS tract.

Other Variations

Numerous other minor variations of technique have been described, including the following.

VENOUS ACCESS

The right internal jugular vein is the preferred route of access, but the left internal jugular vein can be used, and a TIPS has been created from the femoral vein route.

INTRAHEPATIC TRACT

A right hepatic vein to right portal vein shunt usually is performed, but middle hepatic vein to right or left portal vein or left hepatic vein to left portal vein shunts can be performed. Care must be taken in deploying the stent from the left hepatic vein because its origin is foreshortened in the AP projection, and lateral screening is helpful to avoid deploying the proximal end of the stent within the IVC.

EXTREME INFERIOR VENA CAVA-HEPATIC VEIN ANGULATION

Distortion of hepatic architecture due to cirrhosis is common. In particular, right lobe atrophy can result in the right hepatic vein, assuming a high horizontal position creating an acute angle with the IVC through which the catheter/needle assembly can be too rigid to pass (Fig. 22–5). In such a situation, the 10-French

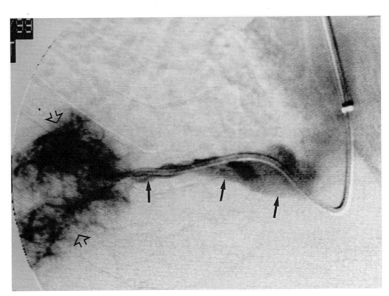

Figure 22–5. Right hepatic venogram (not wedged) via a 7-French Cobra II catheter. The right hepatic vein *(solid arrows)* has assumed a horizontal position bacause of right lobe atrophy characteristic of cirrhosis. The resulting right angle with the inferior vena cava could not be negotiated with the catheter–needle assembly therefore the middle hepatic vein subsequently was selected. Some parenchymal staining with contrast is noted *(open arrows)*.

nylon introducer sheath can be replaced with a 10-French Arrows sheath. This is a flexible articulated metal sheath that cannot be kinked and can provide sufficient support to allow hepatic vein catheterization. Failing this, the middle or left hepatic vein must be used.

VARICEAL EMBOLIZATION

Variceal filling often decreases or disappears after TIPS creation, in which case embolization is not necessary. In some cases, however, prominent variceal filling persists. This can lead to a steal phenomenon, reducing flow through the TIPS and risking early thrombosis, or even to continued hemorrhage. The options in this situation are to further reduce the PPG by dilatation of the TIPS stent or creation of a parallel TIPS, or to embolize the varices. Most embolic agents are suitable, with the combination of coils and absolute ethanol commonly used. The threshold for variceal embolization is lower in patients with gastric variceal hemorrhage and those anticipated to be at risk of hepatic encephalopathy.

TRANSJUGULAR INTRAHEPATIC PORTOSYSTEMIC SHUNT FOR PORTAL VEIN THROMBOSIS

When performing TIPS for PVT, the technical difficulty lies in visualizing the position and confirming puncture of the portal vein branch. Wedged hepatic venography and indirect arterioportography cannot be used. Direct US guidance can be used, but the thrombosed portal vein can be difficult to visualize. There are several reports of using initial transhepatic portal vein localization to guide subsequent portal vein puncture and TIPS creation,[12] and this may be the main indication for this technique. No complications directly attributable to this technique have been reported, but clearly the subsequent use of thrombolysis to clear the portal vein thrombus must be considered very carefully if it has been employed. Having entered the portal vein, it can be impossible to advance a guide wire through the thrombus, particularly if it is chronic, in which case the procedure must be abandoned. If the thrombus can be negotiated, it can be compressed or displaced using a combination of balloon dilatation, mechanical thrombectomy devices, or metal stents. Thrombolysis may be used if no capsular punctures have occurred during attempts to enter the portal vein, with extreme caution if percutaneous portal vein localization has been employed.

"PARALLEL" TRANSJUGULAR INTRAHEPATIC PORTOSYSTEMIC SHUNT

A single TIPS is created in most patients. Very rarely, portal hypertension persists despite a well-functioning stent, or a stent repeatedly occludes because of a mechanical problem, such as kinking at the site of portal vein entry. In either of these situations, a second "parallel" TIPS can be created, usually in the opposite lobe to the existing TIPS (Fig. 22–6).

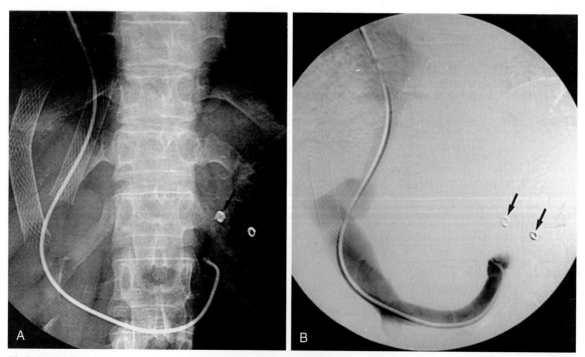

Figure 22–6. Parallel TIPS in a patient with variceal hemorrhage. Despite redilatation and restenting, the initial right-sided TIPS repeatedly occluded; therefore a second TIPS was created within the left hepatic lobe (A). This has required redilatation but remains patent (B). Two embolization coils are present within left gastric varices (arrows).

FOLLOW-UP

TIPS stent stenosis and occlusion are common and typically manifest as recurrent variceal bleeding or recurrence of ascites if undetected. A formal follow-up program is therefore essential to identify and correct TIPS dysfunction before symptoms recur.

A typical follow-up schedule is Doppler US within the first week after TIPS creation to define baseline measurements of flow velocity within the TIPS stent and portal vein, and direction of flow in the hepatic veins and intrahepatic portal vein branches. Repeat Doppler US imaging at 3-month intervals is then performed, proceeding to TIPS venography and pressure measurements if US suggests any deterioration in TIPS function.[15] Some centers also advocate routine portal venography at 6 months.

Portal Venography and Pressure Measurement

The gold standard for evaluating the function of the TIPS remains portal venography with portal pressure measurement. This can be performed via the internal jugular or common femoral venous route. The PPG is the ultimate measure of TIPS function and can be determined directly via the TIPS. Any stenoses found can be treated immediately, and adjunctive treatment such as variceal embolization also may be performed. This is clearly invasive, however, and also expensive.

Doppler Ultrasound

Doppler US (Fig. 22–7) is noninvasive, and several criteria for assessing stent function have been de-

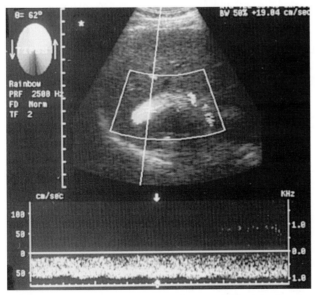

Figure 22–7. Doppler ultrasound of TIPS. The TIPS is clearly patent with a peak velocity of 60–70 cm/sec.

vised. Doppler US assessment of TIPS comprises measurement of flow velocities within the stent and main portal vein below the stent and documentation of flow direction in the intrahepatic portal vein branches and hepatic vein above the TIPS. A patent well-functioning stent is characterized by high velocity (150 to 200 cm/sec) turbulent flow with mild respiratory variation. A wide range of peak velocities may be seen, however; therefore, it is essential that baseline measurements are made soon after TIPS creation. Flow within intrahepatic portal vein branches is assessed easily and is usually hepatofugal. Flow within the hepatic veins above the stent should be toward the IVC, but this can be technically difficult to assess, particularly if the liver is small.

Stent malfunction is indicated by several Doppler US findings. Absence of flow within the TIPS stent identifies stent occlusions in virtually 100% of cases.[16] Stenosis within the stent is indicated by changes in flow velocity, reversal of flow direction within intrahepatic portal vein branches, reaccumulation of ascites, and reappearance of varices.

Velocity changes in stent stenosis depend on the position of the Doppler gate relative to the stenosis. Decreased velocities are found if the gate is placed proximal or distal to the stenosis, but increased velocities may be seen if the gate is placed within or immediately distal to the stenosis. Multiple stenoses or undulating pseudointimal hyperplasia may further complicate the Doppler findings. Early studies reported sensitivity rates of approximately 80% when applying a peak velocity threshold of less than 50 to 60 cm/sec to detect significant stenoses, but more recent studies have reported sensitivities as low as 25%.[15] In view of the complex velocity changes that may be encountered in intrastent stenoses, a change (increase or decrease) in peak stent velocity of 50 cm/sec or greater relative to previous baseline studies has been reported to be more sensitive than a simple maximum flow velocity threshold in detecting both hepatic vein and stent stenoses.[16] Hepatic venous stenosis above the stent causes a decrease in velocity within the stent and, if severe, can cause reversal of flow within the hepatic vein.

Echo-enhanced Doppler US has been reported to increase the accuracy of US in detecting stenoses, but to date it has not been shown to be more accurate than TIPS venography and PPG measurement, which therefore remain the gold standard for detecting TIPS stenoses. If recurrent symptoms develop, TIPS venography and PPG measurement should be performed urgently.

RESULTS

Technical success rates vary from 93 to 100%,[17–20] with usual procedure times of 2 hours or less. The PPG is effectively reduced, on average by 50%, and with appropriate dilatation can be reduced to below the desired level of 12 mm Hg (in cases of variceal hemorrhage) in virtually all cases.

Acute Variceal Hemorrhage

Successful TIPS creation results in immediate cessation of both esophageal and gastric variceal hemorrhage in 95 to 100% of patients. Rebleeding occurs in 10 to 20% of patients and invariably is related to stent stenosis or thrombosis. Fortunately in virtually all such patients, successful percutaneous shunt revision is achieved by balloon angioplasty, further stent deployment, thrombolysis, or mechanical thrombectomy, with subsequent control of bleeding once more.

Occasionally, a single stent does not achieve adequate portal venous decompression and a second "parallel" TIPS is required. It is technically easier to use a different hepatic vein than that used for the initial TIPS. The existing stent marks the position of the portal vein, thereby facilitating its puncture. A parallel stent also may be required if the initial TIPS cannot be revised adequately.

Recurrent Variceal Hemorrhage

When used for prevention of rebleeding esophageal varices, TIPS is associated with a rebleeding rate of 20% compared with 40% for conventional endoscopic injection sclerotherapy or variceal band ligation plus propranolol.[8–10] It is associated with a 35% incidence of hepatic encephalopathy (HE) compared with 15% in the endoscopic group, but this usually is controlled easily by medical means in both groups. No significant difference in survival is seen between the two groups.

Refractory Ascites

Dedicated studies of TIPS for refractory ascites indicate a treatment response in 50 to 80% of patients.[11, 21] Response may be delayed for 1 to 2 weeks after TIPS creation but is usually maximal by 3 months. A subsequent decline in response up to 1 year has been reported, with 1-, 3-, and 12-month response rates of 68%, 48%, and 33%, respectively.[21] A poor response is associated with advanced (Child's C) liver disease, age older than 60 years, and patients with pre-existing organic renal impairment. An accelerated decline in liver function necessitating urgent liver transplantation has been observed in some patients.

Budd-Chiari Syndrome and Hepatic Veno-Occlusive Disease

Despite the theoretical appeal of TIPS in BCS, only small numbers of cases have been reported in the literature, presumably related to the relative rarity of this condition and the technical difficulties alluded to previously. Despite the latter, no technical failures have been reported, although they certainly must have occurred. The largest series includes only 12 patients.[22] Ten of these had either subacute or chronic BCS, and all showed considerable clinical improvement within 1 week of TIPS, although their liver function did not improve significantly. The two patients with fulminant acute BCS died of liver failure due to hepatic necrosis within 10 days.

Portal Vein Thrombosis

The difficulty in performing TIPS for PVT lies in visualizing the position and confirming puncture of the portal vein branch. Consequently, technical success rates of only 60% are achieved.[12] Wedged hepatic venography and indirect arterioportography cannot be used. Direct US guidance can be used, but the thrombosed portal vein can be difficult to visualize. There are several reports of using initial transhepatic portal vein localization to guide subsequent portal vein puncture and TIPS creation, and this may be the main indication for this technique. No complications directly attributable to this technique have been reported, but clearly the subsequent use of thrombolysis to clear the portal vein thrombus must be considered very carefully if it has been employed.

Even having entered the portal vein, it can be impossible to advance a guide wire through the thrombus, particularly if it is chronic, in which case the procedure must be abandoned. If the thrombus can be negotiated, it can be compressed or displaced using a combination of balloon dilatation, mechanical thrombectomy devices, and metal stents. Thrombolysis may be used if no capsular punctures have occurred during attempts to enter the portal vein, with extreme caution if percutaneous portal vein localization has been employed.

Hepatorenal Syndrome

The effect of TIPS on renal function is difficult to assess because the influences of hemodynamic, vasoconstrictor, and antinatriuretic effects are difficult to separate. The evidence, however, does suggest a genuine improvement in renal function in patients with HRS treated with TIPS, as opposed to the deterioration seen in patients with organic renal impairment, although this is based on small numbers of patients.[13]

Hepatopulmonary Syndrome

The three case reports of TIPS in HPS describe conflicting results, with two cases showing improvement. Further studies are awaited.

COMPLICATIONS AND THEIR MANAGEMENT

The TIPS procedure is complex and relatively invasive, and, not surprisingly, a wide range of complications have been described.[23] A few basic principles are employed to reduce complications. Coagulopathies should be corrected using fresh frozen plasma and platelet infusion. Prophylactic antibiotics, including staphylococcal cover, should be given and an aseptic technique employed.

Procedural

MORTALITY

The procedural mortality rate is 0 to 5%, with an average of 1.7% in a survey of 1750 procedures.[20] Higher mortalities can be expected in the emergency setting. There is also a clear learning curve effect, with a procedural mortality averaging 3% if less than 150 procedures have been performed, which is reduced to 1.4% when more than this number have been performed. Procedural mortality usually is related to intraperitoneal hemorrhage, but acute right heart failure also has been described.

INTERNAL JUGULAR VEIN PUNCTURE

Complications related to the venous puncture (common carotid arterial puncture and pneumothorax) can be minimized by using US to locate the vein before puncture, or to puncture under direct US guidance. Some groups advocate the use of micropuncture access sets. Arterial puncture is treated by manual compression and is seldom of consequence. Pneumothorax is treated in the usual way.

HEPATIC CAPSULAR PUNCTURE

This is the most feared complication of TIPS creation because of the risk of fatal intraperitoneal hemorrhage. Its exact frequency is difficult to ascertain, but it has been noted in up to 30% of cases in some series. The rate of intraperitoneal hemorrhage, however, is

only 1 to 6%,[20] therefore, not all capsular punctures result in significant hemorrhage. This may be the result of the subsequent reduction in portal pressure after TIPS creation. Hepatic capsular puncture is related to operator experience and is naturally more likely in small livers.

Confirmed capsular punctures can be embolized with steel coils in an attempt to minimize significant intraperitoneal bleeding, although this has not been proven to do so, and it may be that subsequent TIPS creation and lowering of the PPG is more important. Hepatic arteriography with a view to embolization of a bleeding point may be attempted, but, ultimately, surgery must be considered if bleeding persists.

PUNCTURE OF THE BILE DUCTS AND HEPATIC ARTERIES

Inadvertent puncture of bile ducts and hepatic arterial branches is not uncommon. Postmortem histologic studies of patent TIPS stents have shown a thin, fully endothelialized pseudointima, whereas stenosed or occluded TIPS stents have shown uneven pseudointima with areas of metaplastic biliary proliferation and patent biliary fistulas corresponding to sites of recurrent stenosis or occlusion.[24] This has led to the suggestion that bile extravasation after transection of a bile duct during TIPS creation may result in accelerated pseudointimal hyperplasia, causing shunt stenosis or occlusion, and, consequently, that covered stents may prevent stent dysfunction. However, other histologic studies have not confirmed this strong association between bile duct abnormalities and stent stenosis; therefore, the exact cause of stenosis remains unproven. Hemobilia also has been described as a consequence of bile duct injury. Hepatic arterial punctures are rarely of any clinical significance, although arterioportal fistulas have been implicated as a cause of rapidly deteriorating hepatic function after TIPS creation. These are usually amenable to transhepatic arterial embolization.

EXTRAHEPATIC PUNCTURE OF THE PORTAL VEIN BIFURCATION

If the portal vein puncture site appears to be at to the portal vein bifurcation, the possibility of an extrahepatic portal vein puncture must be considered. The 10-French sheath is advanced as far as possible into the liver tract, and contrast is injected. Intraperitoneal extravasation of contrast indicates an extrahepatic portal vein puncture. This situation is rare, but should it occur, the tract and portal vein wall must not be dilated (because severe intraperitoneal hemorrhage would follow). Two options are available. The first is to continue and deploy a covered stent, if available, which should prevent intraperitoneal hemorrhage.

The alternative is to withdraw the guide wire from the portal vein, withdraw the 5-French catheter into the liver parenchyma, and embolize the tract. The portal vein then is punctured distal to the bifurcation in the hope that subsequent stent deployment and portal decompression will minimize intraperitoneal bleeding.

STENT-RELATED

As in any area of the body, there is the potential for deployment of the stent in the wrong position or of stent migration. The importance of correct stent placement to avoid future liver transplantation compromise already has been emphasized. Stent migration into the right atrium and pulmonary arterial circulation has been described but is rare.

PORTAL VEIN THROMBUS

Nonocclusive portal vein thrombus may be encountered unexpectedly once the portal vein is cannulated and can pose a dilemma about how to proceed. Nonocclusive thrombus often is organized and difficult to disrupt with catheters or guide wires. Thrombolysis is clearly not an option in the setting of variceal hemorrhage. If a large varix is present, it can be catheterized and a partially inflated balloon catheter used to "bulldoze" the thrombus into the varix, thereby clearing the thrombus and embolizing the varix. Alternatively, the stent can be extended to cover the thrombus, with care being taken not to encroach too far down the portal vein and compromise future transplantation (Fig. 22–8). In practice, however, if there is good flow around isolated portal vein thrombus, it can be left and often will lyse spontaneously (Fig. 22–9).

RADIATION BURNS

Long fluoroscopic screening times may accrue if TIPS creation is difficult, and several cases of significant radiation burning with skin necrosis and secondary infection have been described.

Early Complications (Within 30 Days)

MORBIDITY AND MORTALITY

Figures for 30-day mortality vary widely because morbidity and mortality depend on the severity of liver disease (Child's grade), the indication for TIPS, and whether the procedure is performed electively or as an emergency. Direct comparison of reported figures is hampered by variation in the proportion of patients with Child's C disease and active variceal bleeding in different series.

For unselected cases, 4 to 36%, with an average of 10.9%, have been reported[20] (compared with 12 to 20% for elective and 40 to 100% for emergency surgical portacaval shunting), but the 30-day mortality rate for patients with Child's C grade liver disease with uncontrolled variceal hemorrhage is approximately 50%.[6, 17] Prognostic indicators based on markers of liver and renal dysfunction, sepsis, and ventilatory requirement have been developed in an attempt to identify patients with no chance of survival, to avoid unnecessary procedures.[6]

The 30-day mortality rate for elective TIPS for refractory ascites is higher than that for variceal hemorrhage, averaging approximately 20%,[21] compatible with the higher proportion of Child's B and C grade disease in these patients.

Deaths within 30 days of TIPS creation usually are caused by multiorgan failure and sepsis.

HEPATIC ENCEPHALOPATHY

HE after TIPS creation for variceal bleeding occurs twice as frequently as in patients treated with sclerotherapy or variceal band ligation,[8, 10] as frequently as in patients treated with small-diameter H-graft and distal surgical shunts,[7] and less frequently than in patients treated with conventional surgical portacaval shunts. It usually occurs within the first month after TIPS creation, and episodes subsequently decline, presumably related to a degree of stent narrowing due to pseudointimal hyperplasia. HE occurs de novo in 15 to 25% of patients after TIPS, although in 50% of patients with new or worsened HE after TIPS, an underlying medical cause (such as excessive protein intake, hypokalemia, constipation, or hemorrhage) is responsible.[25] Approximately 10% of clinically apparent HE is attributed directly to the TIPS procedure, and this is usually mild and easily controlled medically by conventional means. More severe HE can occur, however, and if uncontrollable, diameter reduction or occlusion of the TIPS stent should be performed.

Risk factors for developing HE post-TIPS include age older than 60 years, advanced Child's C grade disease, and pre-TIPS HE. The absolute portal venous pressure after TIPS recently has been reported to correlate significantly with new or worsened HE, but no significant association with the PPG was found.[25]

HE is more common after TIPS insertion for refractory ascites, although this merely may reflect the higher proportion of patients with advanced liver disease in this group, occurring in up to 67% of patients with a history of HE. Consequently, TIPS should not be used to treat refractory ascites in patients with prior severe HE. The incidence of HE clearly is related to shunt diameter in the context of surgical portacaval shunting, and although a clear

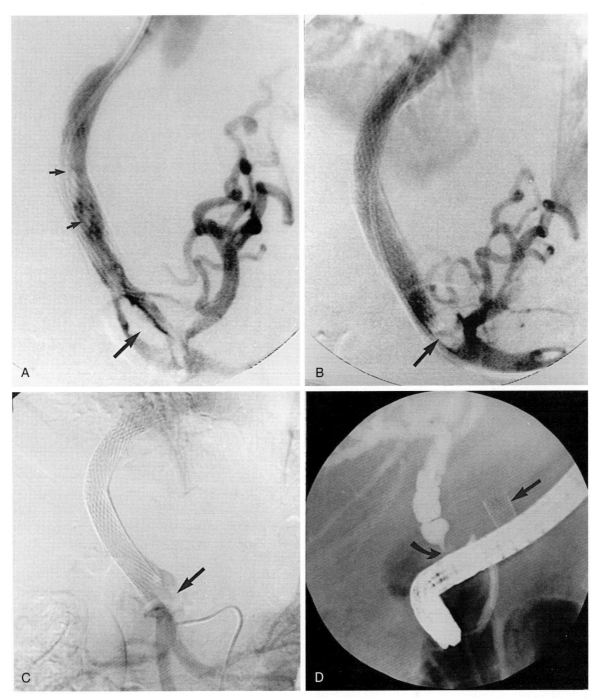

Figure 22–8. TIPS for variceal hemorrhage. *A,* Having deployed the Memotherm stent, there is clearly thrombus within the stent *(small arrows)* and the main portal vein *(large arrow). B,* This could not be cleared; therefore, a second stent was placed. This has improved appearances within the stent, but thrombus persists in the portal vein *(large arrow).* The patient subsequently required liver transplantation. *C,* An indirect arterioportogram shows the lower end of the stent to project almost to the portal vein origin. Thrombus persists within the portal vein *(large arrow). D,* Post-transplant endoscopic retrograde cholangiopancreatography shows an anastomotic stricture *(curved arrow)* with biliary dilatation. Note also the fragment of stent *(large arrow)* within the portal vein—the surgeons had to cut the stent to perform the portal venous anastomosis.

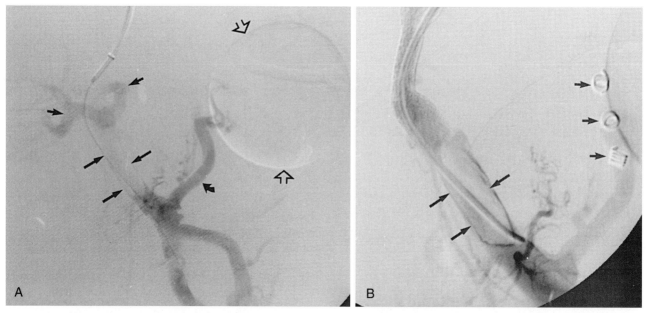

Figure 22–9. TIPS for variceal hemorrhage. *A,* Portal venogram after right portal vein branch puncture. A large thrombus *(long arrows)* is present within the main portal vein. Wedged CO_2 venography had localized the patent intrahepatic portal vein branches *(short arrows)* but had not shown the main portal vein thrombus. Note the inflated S-B tube *(open arrows)* and left gastric varices *(curved arrow). B,* Portal venogram after Memotherm stent deployment and embolization of varices with coils *(short arrows).* Portal vein thrombus persisted *(long arrows)* and could not be dislodged. Despite a pressure decrease across the thrombus, the portosystemic pressure gradient was 15 mm Hg and flow was good. Because the patient was a candidate for future transplantation, further stenting was not pursued. The patient remains symptom free at 4 months.

relationship between TIPS diameter and HE has not been shown, it is recommended that TIPSs for ascites initially are dilated to only 8 mm.[14] Embolization of varices at the time of TIPS insertion may help to reduce the degree of post-TIPS HE.

If medical management fails to control HE, the shunt should be reduced by reducing the internal diameter of the TIPS stent. A dedicated reducing stent was available for use with the Memotherm stent, and although it is no longer produced, it serves to illustrate the principle of this technique. This was a self-expanding device with an outer diameter of up to 14 mm and an internal lumen of 6 mm. Metal filaments surrounding the central lumen promoted thrombosis after deployment, leaving only the central lumen patent (Fig. 22–10). No dedicated devices are available at present, and ingenuity is required in reducing stent diameters. Techniques such as partially uncovering a self-expanding stent, constraining the diameter of its central part with surgical sutures, recovering it, and then deploying it within the existing TIPS stent have been tried (Fig. 22–11*A*). Flaring one or both ends of a balloon expandable stent within the TIPS stent is an alternative approach. Experience is limited, but several successful cases are reported. Alternatively, the TIPS can be occluded totally by means of detachable balloons (Fig. 22–11*B*), or more simply by inflating a latex balloon within the proximal end of the TIPS stent for 12 hours, thereby producing stasis and thrombosis in the distal part of the stent, after which the balloon is removed. The use of diameter reduction

in patients with accelerated liver failure after TIPS creation has been unsuccessful.

SHUNT OCCLUSION

Early shunt occlusion is caused by thrombosis and occurs in 3 to 10% of cases. It usually manifests as recurrent variceal bleeding. It has been associated with mechanical factors, such as prolonged portal vein manipulation or overdilatation, excessive angulation on entering the portal vein, and poor stent placement with incomplete coverage of the parenchymal tract. If two or more stents are used but are not overlapped adequately, slight stent migration can result in exposure of parenchyma between the stents, resulting in thrombosis. Pre-existing portal vein thrombus and underlying procoagulant states also predispose patients to early thrombosis.

Thrombosis is treated by balloon dilatation and thrombolysis or more commonly by deployment of a second stent within the thrombosed stent. Mechanical problems usually require further stent deployment.

Systemic anticoagulation reduces the incidence of acute thrombosis,[26] but because of the low incidence of this complication, its routine use is not advised unless a procoagulant state exists.

REBLEEDING

Early rebleeding raises the possibility of early shunt occlusion (see previous section), but repeat endoscopy is mandatory because it is more often the result of

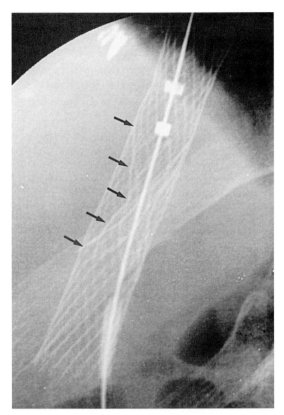

Figure 22–10. The Memotherm reducing stent *(arrows)* deployed within a 12-mm diameter Memotherm stent in a patient with severe hepatic encephalopathy after TIPS.

bleeding from esophageal ulceration after prior injection sclerotherapy or variceal band ligation.[6] These patients are also at risk of gastric and duodenal ulceration.

SEPSIS

Stent-related sepsis has been described but fortunately is uncommon because it can be difficult to eradicate. The stent cannot be removed, and the only treatment option is intensive intravenous antibiotic administration. Consequently, prophylactic antibiotics always should be given before the procedure to prevent sepsis.

LIVER FUNCTION

A transient decrease in liver function, as indicated by an increase in the serum bilirubin level and prolongation of the prothrombin time, is seen in approximately one-third of patients. This usually returns to pre-TIPS levels by 3 weeks, and no significant change in liver function is observed at 6 months.

Accelerated liver failure leading to death or emergency transplantation has been observed in several patients after TIPS insertion for both variceal bleeding and refractory ascites.[11] This dramatic deterioration in liver function has been attributed to diversion of portal blood flow and is almost exclusively seen in patients with advanced (Child's grade C) disease. Occlusion of the TIPS can be performed in an attempt to slow the decline in liver function, but this is seldom successful and urgent liver transplantation is required. The incidence of accelerated liver failure is not precisely known, but some use its occurrence to warn against performing TIPS as a bridge to liver transplantation.

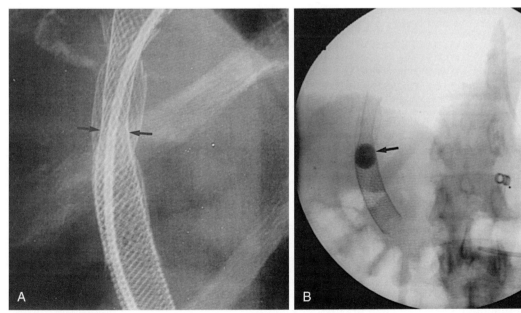

Figure 22–11. Patient with severe hepatic encephalopathy (HE) after TIPS for variceal hemorrhage and ascites. A 12 × 70-mm Wallstent was partially uncovered and its diameter constrained to 6 mm by means of a 5-0 nonabsorbable surgical suture. *A,* The stent was recovered and deployed with the constrained part of the stent *(arrows)* within the hepatic parenchymal tract. *B,* Unfortunately, HE persisted and the TIPS had to be occluded by means of a 14-mm diameter latex detachable balloon.

CARDIOPULMONARY FAILURE

TIPS creation results in increased delivery of blood to the right side of the heart, elevation of right heart and pulmonary artery pressure, and worsening of the already hyperkinetic circulation of portal hypertension. This can result in acute right heart failure, particularly if there is significant pre-existing pulmonary hypertension. This can be rapidly fatal. If not fatal, shunt closure can be performed if medical management fails. Known pre-existing pulmonary artery hypertension is a contraindication to TIPS.

HEMOLYSIS

This rare complication is attributed to mechanical disruption of red blood cells by the metal stent mesh.

Delayed Complications (Beyond 30 Days)

MORTALITY

Overall survival rates range from 75 to 90% at 1 year and approximately 60% at 2 years. Not surprisingly, this is related to the severity of liver disease, with 2-year survival rates for Child's A, B, and C grades of 75%, 55%, and 43%, respectively, reported.[17–20] Deaths occurring more than 30 days after TIPS are usually the result of liver failure, sepsis, or unrelated causes.

STENT STENOSIS AND OCCLUSION

Stent stenosis or occlusion is the most significant problem encountered with TIPS and is the main reason it remains a temporary rather than permanent treatment for portal hypertension. Virtually all cases of recurrent variceal bleeding and ascites are the result of stent stenosis (two thirds) or occlusion (one third).

Primary patency rates are approximately 70% at 6 months, 60% at 1 year, and 20 to 50% at 2 years.[17–20] Most cases of shunt stenosis/occlusion can be remedied with further balloon dilatation and stent deployment, yielding secondary patency rates of approximately 95%. Multiple reinterventions may be required over time.

Stenosis is the result of pseudointimal hyperplasia and occurs most commonly within the hepatic vein proximal to the stent or within the stent itself (Fig. 22–12). Occlusion is caused by excessive hyperplasia or thrombosis superimposed on hyperplasia. Despite reducing the incidence of acute shunt thrombosis, anticoagulation has no significant effect on late stenosis/occlusion.[26] Fortunately, stent patency can be restored by balloon dilatation or further stent deployment in 95% of cases.

In response to the theory that bile extravasation after bile duct injury during TIPS creation may result in accelerated pseudointimal hyperplasia, it has been suggested that covered stents may reduce the incidence of stent dysfunction by sealing the parenchymal tract and preventing bile extravasation. An initial report using the Cragg Endopro System I covered stent in 13 patients shows a primary patency of 76.9% at 6 months,[27] which is encouraging but not dramatically different from other series using uncovered stents; therefore, the results of longer follow-up are awaited.

SURGICAL SHUNTS

The hemodynamic concepts that underpin TIPS were investigated over several decades of portasystemic shunt surgery, and this background contributed to the rapid clinical development of TIPS. Surgical shunts and TIPS share the same mode of action, namely, a lowering of the portal venous pressure with decompression of varices giving a reduced risk of rupture.

Surgically constructed shunts can be classified as total, selective, or partial shunts.

Total Shunts

These were the first to be developed, beginning with Eck and Pavlov's animal studies in the late 19th century. These operations entered clinical use in the 1940s.[28] Total shunts completely divert portal venous blood flow into the vena cava, which deprives the liver of a significant share of nutrient blood flow and compromises first-pass metabolism of gut neurotoxin.[29] For these reasons, total shunts are associated with accelerated liver failure and a heightened risk of HE that ranges between 30 and 70%.[30] These risks are greatest in patients with advanced liver disease but can affect even patients with Child's grade A liver disease. Typical examples of total shunts include the end-to-side and side-to-side portacaval shunts, the proximal splenorenal shunt, and the large-diameter mesocaval interposition graft. Because these techniques are well known to many surgeons, total shunts continue to be employed in some North American centers.

Selective Shunts

The selective shunt, whose prototype is the distal splenorenal shunt, was devised in the 1960s with the aim of minimizing the risk of postoperative encephalopathy.[31] In this complex operation, the cut end of the splenic vein is detached from the pancreas and anastomosed to the left renal vein. Small collateral

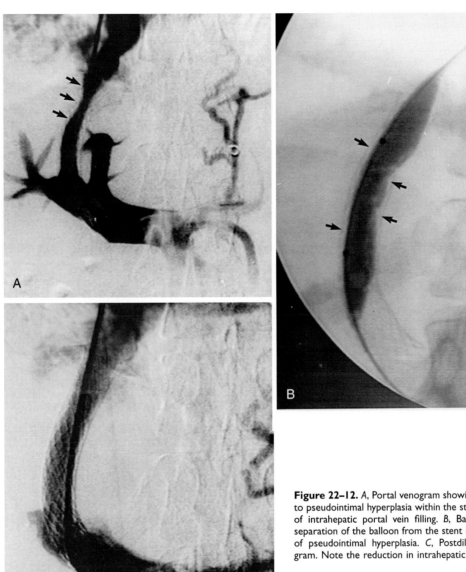

Figure 22–12. *A,* Portal venogram showing stent stenosis due to pseudointimal hyperplasia within the stent. Note the degree of intrahepatic portal vein filling. *B,* Balloon dilatation. The separation of the balloon from the stent is caused by the layer of pseudointimal hyperplasia. *C,* Postdilatation portal venogram. Note the reduction in intrahepatic portal vein filling.

veins are ligated. The left-sided gastrosplenic venous blood flow is shunted systemically while the right-sided portomesenteric hypertension persists. This preserves hepatopedal flow in most patients, at least intially. Early postoperative encephalopathy occurs in less than 10% of patients.[32] Mostly in patients whose portal hypertension is the result of alcoholic cirrhosis, new collateral branches develop over time, and the shunt gradually behaves more like a total shunt.[33] Significant ascites and acute, refractory bleeding are relative contraindications to selective shunting.

Partial Shunts

The partial shunt maintains a moderate degree of portal hypertension, preserving hepatopedal flow in

most cases by diverting a portion of portal venous blood flow through a conduit of fixed resistance and caliber. As was first shown in the 1980s, the portacaval H-graft acts as a partial shunt when constructed with a conduit of suitably small diameter (8 or 10 mm) and combined with the ablation of collateral vessels.[34–36] The procedure is technically straightforward, and long-term patency exceeds 90% at 7 years. Because the pressure gradient across the shunt approximates the critical threshold of 12 torr,[35, 37] variceal rebleeding occurs infrequently (5% after 7 years).[37] Encephalopathy occurs in 10 to 20% but is generally mild and easily controlled.[38] PVT contraindicates partial shunting.

Studies of TIPS compared with portosystemic surgery have been difficult to evaluate because of a lack of agreement on standard terminology. Surgical series are at a disadvantage because strict conventions for reporting deaths, complications, and vascular occlusions are observed. However, extrapolating from the available data, risk-adjusted mortality after TIPS appears to be at least the same or better than in many surgical series (< 10% for elective shunts in patients with Child's grade A and B liver disease).[9, 39] A second source of variability can be found in the definitions of patency that blur the distinction between conventional primary patency and secondary or "assisted" patency. Here, surgical shunts retain a clear advantage because late thrombosis or occlusion of a surgical shunt is a rare event whereas up to 50% of TIPS stents may be expected to require revision within 1 year.[40] This has led to recommendations for frequent US surveillance of TIPS patency. Despite this degree of caution, occlusions may present as variceal rebleeding, which carries a mortality rate of approximately 20%.[41]

The stents used for TIPS are principally 10 or 12 mm in diameter, whereas surgical partial shunts use 8- and 10-mm grafts. Based on previous work, hepatopedal flow is expected 80 to 90% of the time with surgical shunts using 8-mm grafts and 50% of the time with 10-mm grafts.[34, 35] The hemodynamics of a 12-mm TIPS tend to closely approximate those of total shunts.[34, 35] When these larger-diameter shunts are placed, reversal in direction of hepatic portal flow and the expected compromise of nutrient hepatic blood flow predict that postprocedural encephalopathy after TIPS will be at its worst in the early post-treatment period. As the shunt narrows with time, encephalopathy diminishes.[42] If stent occlusion supervenes, mental status reverts to baseline. Thus, it becomes more difficult to quantify encephalopathy accurately after TIPS because of changing flow patterns caused by neointimal hyperplasia and stent revisions.

CONCLUSION

TIPS is a safe and effective technique for creating a portosystemic shunt within the liver, thereby reducing portal venous pressure and the PPG. Its main advantages are that it usually can be performed without general anesthetic and that, if correctly performed, it does not compromise future liver transplantation.

Based on current evidence, it is the treatment of choice for acute esophageal and gastric variceal hemorrhage that cannot be controlled by conventional medical treatment, but despite successful control of hemorrhage in 95 to 100% of cases, this group of patients still has a high 30-day mortality rate of 50 to 60%.

TIPS is superior to conventional endoscopic management plus propranolol in preventing variceal rebleeding but is associated with a higher rate of HE and necessitates close follow-up and reintervention. Consequently, TIPS cannot be recommended for this indication, unless patients are intolerant of endoscopic treatment. At present, portacaval shunt operations confer more durable and effective protection against rebleeding than TIPS. In the setting of well-preserved liver function (Child's grade A and B), patients are best served by a single definitive intervention that minimizes the risk of death from rebleeding. This group should undergo surgical shunting, preferably with procedures that can preserve prograde hepatic portal flow.

TIPS should be used with caution in patients with refractory ascites because although a response can be expected in at least 50% of patients, the risk of HE and need for reintervention may not improve quality of life in these patients with already limited life expectancy. TIPS appears to improve renal function in HRS but causes deterioration if there is pre-existing organic renal impairment.

TIPS may have a role as a salvage procedure in selected cases of BCS, hepatic veno-occlusive disease, and PVT, but further experience is required to formally evaluate its role. The longer-term outlook in these patients also needs to be assessed.

The high rate of restenosis and occlusion is the main limitation of this technique and limits it to a temporizing or salvage technique. The results of using covered stents are awaited with interest. If primary patency rates can be improved, a longer-term role for TIPS may emerge.

REFERENCES

1. Rösch J, Hanafee W, Snow H: Transjugular portal venography and radiological portacaval shunt: An experimental study. Radiology 92:1112–1114, 1969.
2. Colapinto RF, Stonell RD, Birch SJ, et al: Creation of an intrahepatic portosystemic shunt with a Gruntzig balloon catheter. Can Med Assoc J 126:267–268, 1982.
3. Richter GM, Noeldge G, Palmaz JC, et al: Transjugular intrahepatic portocaval stent shunt: Preliminary clinical results. Radiology 174:1027–1030, 1990.
4. Bosch J, Burroughs AK: Clinical manifestations and management of bleeding episodes in cirrhotics. In Bircher J, Benhamou J-P, McIntyre N, et al (eds): Oxford Textbook of Clinical Hepatology, 2nd ed. Oxford, Oxford University Press, 1999, pp 671–693.
5. Chau TN, Patch D, Chan YW, et al: "Salvage" transjugular intrahepatic portosystemic shunts: Gastric fundal compared with esophageal bleeding. Gastroenterology 114:981–987, 1998.
6. Patch D, Nikolopoulou V, McCormick A, et al: Factors related to early mortality after transjugular intrahepatic portosystemic shunt for failed endoscopic therapy in acute variceal bleeding. J Hepatol 28:454–460, 1998.
7. Rosemurgy AS II, Bloomston M, Zervos EE, et al: Transjugular intrahepatic portosystemic shunt versus H-graft portacaval shunt in the management of bleeding varices: A cost–benefit analysis. Surgery 122:794–800, 1997.
8. Sauer P, Theilman L, Stremmel W, et al: Transjugular intrahe-

patic portosystemic stent shunt versus sclerotherapy plus propranolol for variceal bleeding. Gastroenterology 113:1623–1631, 1997.

9. Jalan R, Forrest EH, Stanley AJ, et al: A randomised trial comparing transjugular intrahepatic portosystemic stent-shunt with variceal band ligation in the prevention of rebleeding from oesophageal varices. Hepatology 26:1115–1122, 1997.

10. Rossle M, Diebert P, Haag K, et al: Randomized trial of transjugular intrahepatic portosystemic shunt versus endoscopy plus propranolol for prevention of variceal rebleeding. Lancet 349:1043–1049, 1997.

11. Somberg KA, Lake JR, Tomlanovich SJ, et al: Transjugular intrahepatic portosystemic shunts for refractory ascites: Assessment of clinical and hormonal response and renal function. Hepatology 21:709–716, 1995.

12. Walser EM, McNees SW, DeLa Pena O, et al: Portal venous thrombolysis: Percutaneous therapy and outcome. J Vasc Intervent Radiol 9:119–127, 1998.

13. Guevara M, Gines P, Bandi JC, et al: Transjugular intrahepatic portosystemic shunt in hepatorenal syndrome: Effects on renal function and vasoactive systems. Hepatology 28:416–421, 1998.

14. Somberg KA: Transjugular intrahepatic portosystemic shunt for refractory ascites: Shunt diameter-optimizing risks and benefits. Hepatology 25:254–255, 1997.

15. Murphy TP, Beecham RP, Kim HM, et al: Long-term follow-up after TIPS: Use of Doppler velocity criteria for detecting elevation of the portosystemic gradient. J Vasc Intervent Radiol 9:275–282, 1998.

16. Dodd GD, Zajko AB, Orons PD, et al: Detection of transjugular intrahepatic portosystemic shunt dysfunction: Value of duplex Doppler sonography. AJR Am J Roentgenol 164:1119–1124, 1995.

17. LaBerge JM, Somberg KA, Lake JR, et al: Two-year outcome following transjugular intrahepatic portosystemic shunt for variceal bleeding: Results in 90 patients. Gastroenterology 108:1143–1151, 1995.

18. Stanley AJ, Jalan R, Forrest EH, et al: Long-term follow-up of transjugular intrahepatic portosystemic stent shunt (TIPSS) for the treatment of portal hypertension: Results in 130 patients. Gut 39:479–485, 1996.

19. Kerlan KK, LaBerge JM, Gordon RL, et al: Transjugular intrahepatic portosystemic shunts: Current status. AJR Am J Roentgenol 164:1059–1066, 1995.

20. Keller FS, Rösch J: Results of TIPS (abstract). Presented at the 2nd International Workshop on Interventional Radiology, Prague, June 15–17, 1995.

21. Nazarian GK, Bjarnson H, Dietz CA, et al: Refractory ascites: Midterm results of treatment with a transjugular intrahepatic portosystemic shunt. Radiology 205:173–180, 1997.

22. Blum U, Rossle M, Haag K, et al: Budd-Chiari syndrome: Technical, haemodynamic and clinical results of treatment with transjugular intrahepatic portosystemic shunt. Radiology 197:805–811, 1995.

23. Freedman AM, Sanyal JS: Complications of transjugular intrahepatic portosystemic shunts. Semin Intervent Radiol 11:161–177, 1994.

24. Saxon RR, Mendel-Hartvig J, Corless C, et al: Bile duct injury as a major cause of stenosis and occlusion in transjugular intrahepatic portosystemic shunts: Comparative histopathologic analysis in humans and swine. J Vasc Intervent Radiol 7:487–497, 1996.

25. Zuckerman DA, Darcy MD, Bocchini TP, et al: Encephalopathy after transjugular intrahepatic portosystemic shunting: Analysis of incidence and potential risk factors. AJR Am J Roentgenol 169:1727–1731, 1997.

26. Sauer P, Theilmann L, Herrmann S, et al: Phenprocoumon for prevention of shunt occlusion after TIPSS: A randomized trial. Hepatology 24:1433–1436, 1996.

27. Ferral H, Alcantara-Peraza A, Kimura Y, et al: Creation of transjugular intrahepatic portosystemic shunts with use of the Cragg Endopro System I. J Vasc Intervent Radiol 9:283–287, 1998.

28. Chandler JG: The history of the surgical treatment of portal hypertension. Arch Surg 128:925–940, 1993.

29. Rikkers LF: Portal dynamics, intestinal absorption and postshunt encephalopathy. Surgery 94:126–131, 1983.

30. Langer B, Taylor BR, Greig PD: Selective or total shunts for variceal bleeding. Am J Surg 160:75–79, 1990.

31. Warren WD, Zeppa R, Fomon JJ: Selective transsplenic decompression of gastroesophageal varices by distal splenorenal shunt. Arch Surg 166:437–455, 1967.

32. Rikkers LF, Sorrell T, Gongliang J: Which portosystemic shunt is best? Gastroenterol Clin North Am 21:179–191, 1992.

33. Henderson JM, Millikan WJ, Wright-Bacon L, et al: Haemodynamic differences between alcoholic and nonalcoholic cirrhotics following distal splenorenal shunt: Effect on survival? Ann Surg 198:325–334, 1983.

34. Sarfeh IJ, Rypins EB, Conroy RM, et al: Portacaval H-graft: Relationships of shunt diameter, portal flow patterns and encephalopathy. Ann Surg 197:422–426, 1983.

35. Sarfeh IJ, Rypins EB, Mason GR: A systematic appraisal of portacaval H-graft diameters: Clinical and haemodynamic perspectives. Ann Surg 204:356–363, 1986.

36. Rypins EB, Milne N, Sarfeh IJ, et al: Quantitation and fractionation of nutrient hepatic blood flow in normal persons, in persons with portal hypertensive cirrhosis and after small diameter portacaval H-grafts. Surgery 104:335–342, 1988.

37. Garcia-Tsao G, Groszmann RJ, Fisher RL, et al: Portal pressure, presence of gastroesophageal varices and variceal bleeding. Hepatology 5:419–424, 1985.

38. Sarfeh IJ, Rypins EB: Partial versus total portacaval shunt in alcoholic cirrhosis: Results of a prospective randomised clinical trial. Ann Surg 219:353–361, 1994.

39. La Berge JM, Ring EJ, Stanley AJ, et al: Creation of the transjugular intrahepatic portosystemic shunts with the Wallstent endoprosthesis: Results in 100 patients. Radiology 187:413–420, 1993.

40. Sahagun G, Benner KG, Saxon R, et al: A randomized trial comparing transjugular intrahepatic portosystemic stent-shunt with variceal band ligation in the prevention of rebleeding from esophageal varices. Hepatology 92:1444–1452, 1997.

41. Gschwantler M, Gebauer A, Rohrmoser M, et al: Clinical outcome two years after implantation of a transjugular intrahepatic portosystemic shunt for recurrent variceal bleeding. Eur J Gastroent Hepatol 9:15–20, 1997.

42. Conn HO: *In* Conn HO, Palmaz JC, Rösch J, Rossle M (eds): Transjugular Intrahepatic Portosystemic Shunts: New York, Igaku-Shoin, 1996, pp 281–297.

Chapter *23* Pulmonary Embolism

Endovascular Contributor: Richard D. Edwards
Surgical Contributors: Dan L. Serna and Jeffrey C. Milliken

Pulmonary embolism (PE) is a common condition that, because of its variable clinical expression, remains an underdiagnosed disorder and an important cause of morbidity and mortality. The physiologic effects and clinical outcome of PE are dependent on the size and location of the embolus, the degree of hemodynamic instability, the age of the patient, and the presence of serious coexistent pathology, such as malignant disease, congestive cardiac failure, or chronic lung disease. In most patients, a benign clinical course can be expected with adequate anticoagulation and supportive therapy if there is no evidence of right ventricular dysfunction or systemic arterial hypotension. A minority of patients presenting with major pulmonary embolism pose a more complex therapeutic problem and may require additional measures, such as inotropic support and thrombolytic therapy. If thrombolysis is contraindicated or ineffective, more invasive intervention may be necessary to prevent a fatal outcome. Surgical embolectomy or endovascular techniques, such as clot fragmentation, suction embolectomy, mechanical thrombectomy, or pulmonary artery stenting, may be considered in this situation. Temporary or permanent caval filtration also has an important role to play in the prevention of recurrent embolism. An appropriate therapeutic strategy for the individual patient with major pulmonary embolism is best determined by a multidisciplinary approach involving medical, radiologic, and surgical specialists.

INCIDENCE AND MORTALITY

Dalen and Alpert's landmark paper in 1975 estimated the total number of symptomatic episodes of PE in the United States at 630,000 per year, a figure extrapolated from postmortem data and published mortality data for treated and untreated PE.[1] They estimated that PE was the principal cause of death in 100,000 patients per year and a major contributory factor in a further 100,000, concluding that PE was the third most com-

mon cause of death at that time. The mortality rate in the first hour after the onset of symptoms is approximately 11% and is the result of acute right heart failure. Although the patient may survive the initial embolic event, death caused by recurrent embolism may occur in hours or days. Before the introduction of effective anticoagulant therapy, the mortality rate for untreated PE was estimated at 18 to 30%. A randomized trial published in 1960 showed a clear survival benefit associated with heparin therapy.[2] Estimates of mortality associated with PE vary, but data from the Prospective Investigation of Pulmonary Embolism Diagnosis (PIOPED) project indicated that PE was the principal cause of death in only 2.5% of 399 patients with proven embolism. Although the 12-month mortality rate from all causes was 23.8%, only 10.5% of these were attributable to PE.[3] Cancer, sepsis, and congestive cardiac failure were the primary causes of death in 74% of all fatalities. Recurrent embolism was diagnosed in 8.3% of patients, and this was associated with a 1-year mortality rate of 45%. Ninety percent of deaths due to PE occurred within 2 weeks of entry into the study, supporting the notion that the risk of death is greatest during the early clinical course. More recent data from the International Cooperative Pulmonary Embolism Registry of 2454 patients indicate a less favorable outcome, with a cumulative 3-month mortality rate of 17.5%. Forty-five percent of deaths were causally related to PE,[4] and recurrent embolism was reported in 5.2% in this series. The mortality associated with PE increases with the severity of hemodynamic compromise of the patient. In a multicenter study of 1001 patients with massive pulmonary embolism, the overall in-hospital mortality rate for patients increased from 8% in normotensive patients with evidence of right ventricular (RV) dysfunction or raised pulmonary artery pressure to 25% in patients with cardiogenic shock requiring inotropic support. In more severe cases in which cardiopulmonary resuscitation was required at clinical presentation, the mortality rate increased to 65%.[5]

PATHOPHYSIOLOGY

The severity of hemodynamic changes that occur after major pulmonary embolism depends on the extent of reduction in the cross-sectional area of the pulmonary arterial circulation and the presence or absence of significant cardiovascular pathology. A significant increase in pulmonary artery pressure (PAP) occurs if more than 50% of the pulmonary bed is obstructed, and abrupt elevation can lead to acute RV failure and death within minutes or hours. Hypoxemia due to pulmonary arterial obstruction stimulates pulmonary vasoconstriction with further elevation of PAP. Increased venous return also occurs because of sympathetically mediated systemic vasoconstriction. Cardiac output may be maintained as right atrial pressure and stroke volume increase but progressive RV failure inevitably ensues if 75% of the pulmonary circulation is obstructed. The risk of intracardiac thrombus formation and recurrent PE may be increased in the dilated hypokinetic right heart because of venous stasis.[6] Right-to-left shunting may occur as RV pressure increases, exacerbating the underlying hypoxemia, and paradoxical embolism may occur if there is a patent foramen ovale or atrial septal defect. Patients with cardiorespiratory disease are less able to tolerate elevation of PAP and experience a more pronounced decrease in cardiac output. RV infarction may occur as a result of coronary ischemia associated with increasing wall stress and the physiologic demands of increased RV work. Left ventricular (LV) preload is diminished because of reduction in RV outflow and reduced LV end-diastolic diameter caused by deviation of the interventricular septum toward the left. Reduction in LV preload results in reduced cardiac output and systemic arterial pressure. This can cause a reduction in coronary artery perfusion and result in myocardial ischemia. The consequence of these changes in massive pulmonary embolism, if uncorrected, is circulatory collapse and death.

CLASSIFICATION OF SEVERITY

A classification of severity of PE should be based on its clinical effects rather than purely anatomic considerations because a relatively small embolus may have a disproportionately large physiologic effect in a patient with serious underlying cardiorespiratory disease. Minor PE may remain unrecognized because symptoms are often mild, nonspecific, and transient. Major PE may be subdivided into submassive, massive, and fulminant categories; this clinical stratification mirrors the degree of the pulmonary arterial obstruction in patients without coexistent cardiorespiratory pathology. Various angiographic severity scores, such as those proposed by Miller and Walsh, have been used to provide an objective measure of therapeutic response in pulmonary thrombolysis trials. The Urokinase Pulmonary Embolism Trial (UPET) angiographic severity score (maximum value of 18) is determined by the location of the emboli (central or peripheral) and the degree of obstruction (partial or complete).[7] Massive pulmonary embolism is equivalent to obstruction of two or more lobar arteries, a score of 5 or greater. Many publications emphasize the importance of echocardiographic assessment of RV function in PE, and a recent classification system incorporates these data[8] (Table 23–1).

DIAGNOSIS

Clinical Features

A high index of suspicion, based on the clinical history, assessment of risk factors, and physical examina-

Table 23–1. Classification of Severity of Pulmonary Embolism (PE)

Degree of Severity	I Minor PE	II Submassive PE	III Massive PE	IV Fulminant PE
Symptoms and signs	Transient dyspnea, pleuritic pain, hemoptysis, or fever	Persistent symptoms, sudden dyspnea, pain, tachypnea, tachycardia	Severe dyspnea, tachypnea, cyanosis, tachycardia, syncope	Symptoms as III plus cardiogenic shock, cardiac arrest
Blood pressure	Normal	Normal or slightly reduced	Hypotension	Severe hypotension
PaO₂	Normal	10.6 kPa	< 9.3 kPa	< 8 kPa
Mean PAP	Normal	Normal or slightly elevated	25–30 mm Hg	> 30 mm Hg
Echocardiographic findings	Normal	Normal or minimal signs of RV strain	Signs of RV strain	Signs of right major ventricular strain, acute RV failure
Angiography, % of perfusion defect	< 25%	< 25–50%	> 50%	> 66%

PAP = pulmonary artery pressure; RV = right ventricular.
Modified with permission from Janata-Schwatczek K, Weiss K, Riezinger I, et al: Pulmonary embolism. II. Diagnosis and treatment. Semin Thromb Hemost 22:33–52, 1996.

tion, is the most important factor in the diagnosis of PE. The symptoms and signs of PE may mimic those of other cardiorespiratory diseases, and preliminary investigations such as a chest radiograph, electrocardiograph, and laboratory findings are often nonspecific. The most common symptoms in acute PE are dyspnea, pleuritic pain, apprehension, cough, calf pain, hemoptysis, and syncope. In massive pulmonary embolism, dyspnea, apprehension, and syncope are encountered more frequently. Clinical assessment alone is insufficient to confirm a diagnosis of PE, but the appropriate selection of subsequent diagnostic imaging studies is enhanced by the clinical diagnostic approach.[8] The choice of imaging procedures depends on local availability and the degree of hemodynamic instability of the patient.

Imaging in Pulmonary Embolism

VENTILATION-PERFUSION LUNG SCANNING

Ventilation-perfusion (V/Q) lung scanning is the most frequently used noninvasive method of investigation in suspected PE, and its main role is to stratify patients into high or low probability groups. The PIOPED study compared V/Q scanning with pulmonary arteriography in 933 patients with suspected PE and demonstrated that 87% of patients with high probability scans had positive angiograms.[9] If preliminary clinical assessment indicates a high probability of PE in conjunction with a high probability lung scan, the false-positive rate decreases to 4% and therefore treatment should be instituted without further investigation. Of the 14% of patients who had normal or near normal scans, only 9% had positive angiography re-

sults. Although the V/Q scan may appear normal in some cases of minor embolism, these are unlikely to be of clinical significance. Long-term follow-up of patients with normal V/Q scans has shown no clinical evidence of recurrent emboli.[10] Sixty-three percent of scans in the PIOPED study were of low or intermediate probability, and angiographically proven PE was present in 16% and 33% of these groups, respectively. The likelihood of a positive angiogram result in this category varied from 16% when PE was thought to be a low clinical probability to 66% when there was high degree of clinical suspicion. Patients with an intermediate probability lung scan usually require further investigation to confirm or exclude the diagnosis of PE, although peripheral venous assessment using ultrasound techniques usually precedes pulmonary angiography. The diagnosis of deep vein thrombosis (DVT) may result in the same treatment implications as the diagnosis of PE, and therefore, a preliminary noninvasive investigation is preferred. Management decisions should be determined by the assessing the V/Q scan findings in conjunction with clinical assessment of the patient.

COMPUTED TOMOGRAPHY

Although pulmonary angiography remains the reference standard, technological developments in computed tomography (CT) scanning have led to a wider application of this modality in the investigation of PE. Spiral CT with contrast enhancement can demonstrate emboli in second- to fourth-order pulmonary arteries during a single breath-hold acquisition (Fig. 23–1 A). Occlusive, nonocclusive, and mural thrombus can be differentiated, although small peripheral emboli may

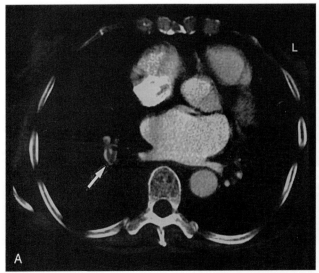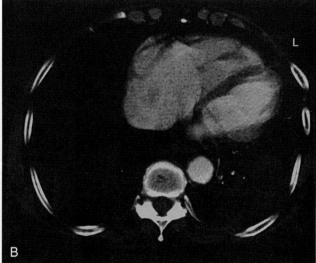

Figure 23–1. *A,* Pulmonary computed tomography (CT) angiogram shows nonocclusive thrombus in the right lower lobe artery *(arrow). B,* Dilatation of right atrium and ventricle secondary raised pulmonary artery pressure (estimated at 50 mm Hg). The patient gave a 7-day history of pleuritic chest pain and had multiple bilateral pulmonary emboli.

be missed. Dilatation of the right heart chambers also may be demonstrated (Fig. 23–1 *B*). A sensitivity rate of 100% and a specificity rate of 96% have been reported,[11] but misinterpretation of intersegmental lymph nodes as embolic filling defects can reduce the diagnostic accuracy. Because CT is noninvasive, it does have an advantage over pulmonary angiography by avoiding the potential complications of puncture site bleeding in patients who receive thrombolytic therapy. Further studies are required to clarify the role of CT angiography in the diagnostic algorithm of PE.

ECHOCARDIOGRAPHY

Echocardiography is emerging as an important noninvasive bedside investigation that can rapidly provide clinically useful information about RV function and PAP in patients with suspected massive PE. Both transesophageal and transthoracic techniques have been employed in this setting, and intra-atrial and central intrapulmonary thrombus can be demonstrated. Echocardiography also can exclude other cardiovascular pathology, such as aortic dissection or pericardial effusion. Echocardiographic criteria of RV dysfunction include RV dilatation (RV end-diastolic dimension > 27 mm, RV hypokinesis, paradoxical septal wall motion, reduced LV size (LV end-diastolic dimension < 36 mm), absence of inspiratory collapse of the inferior vena cava (IVC), increased tricuspid regurgitation jet velocity, and dilatation of the IVC. Estimates of echocardiographic severity of PE have correlated well with angiographic severity scores, and patients with perfusion scan defects of 30% or more have a high incidence of RV hypokinesis and may be at increased risk of recurrent embolism.[6] In critically ill patients with suspected massive or fulminant PE, echocardiography may be the only appropriate investigation, and treatment should be instituted without further diagnostic confirmation if signs of moderate or severe RV dysfunction are present. Echocardiography is readily repeatable, and serial scanning can be useful in assessing the therapeutic response in critically ill patients. The presence or absence of RV dysfunction is important in stratifying patients with massive or submassive PE who have normal systemic arterial pressure into high- or low-risk categories. Although definitive studies are awaited, recent publications suggest that thrombolytic therapy may benefit normotensive patients with massive PE who have evidence of RV dysfunction.[12]

MAGNETIC RESONANCE IMAGING

Magnetic resonance (MR) angiography can demonstrate pulmonary emboli using a variety of sequences, including gradient recalled echo, time-of-flight, cardiac-gated spin-echo, and three-dimensional (3D) cine MR angiography. Although technically feasible, a number of problems, such as cardiac and respiratory motion, flow rate variation in small- and large-caliber vessels, and the spatial orientation of the pulmonary vasculature, limit its clinical application at present.

PULMONARY ANGIOGRAPHY

The definitive diagnostic role of pulmonary angiography has been challenged by the introduction of other modalities such as CT angiography and echocardiography, but it remains an important investigation for confirmation or exclusion of PE in patients who have an intermediate probability V/Q scan. Although it is possible to miss small subsegmental emboli, these may be clinically insignificant and a negative pulmonary angiogram excludes PE for all practical purposes. Selective studies using balloon occlusion techniques can demonstrate subsegmental emboli not visible on conventional angiography. The mortality rate associated with pulmonary angiography in the PIOPED study was 0.5%, with major complications occurring in 1% and minor complications in 5% of patients. Therapeutic intervention, including catheter fragmentation, suction, or mechanical thrombectomy, may be considered immediately after diagnostic angiography if merited by the patient's clinical condition.

Investigation of Deep Venous Thrombosis

Noninvasive assessment of the lower extremity veins by compression ultrasonography or color-flow Doppler ultrasound is an important adjunctive investigation in patients with suspected PE. DVT may be demonstrated by these methods in 40 to 50% of patients with proven PE, and asymptomatic PE may be present in 50% of patients with confirmed DVT.[8] Patients who have an intermediate probability V/Q scan should undergo peripheral venous assessment, and if DVT is diagnosed, they should be treated with anticoagulants. A negative venous study does not exclude PE when this diagnosis is clinically suspected, and further investigations such as CT angiography or pulmonary angiography may be required.

TREATMENT OF PULMONARY EMBOLISM

Supportive Measures

Patients with pulmonary embolism should remain on bed rest, and cardiac monitoring, pulse oximetry, and noninvasive measurement of blood pressure should be performed in patients with major PE. Patients with massive or fulminant PE should be treated in an intensive therapy unit or step-down facility, such as a high-dependency unit. The careful use of narcotic analgesics and low-dose anxiolytics is appropriate for the relief of pain and apprehension. Oxygen should be administered to maintain the oxygen saturation at greater than 90%, and reversal of hypoxemia may reverse pulmonary vasoconstriction associated with major PE. If adequate oxygenation cannot be achieved, endotracheal intubation and ventilatory support may be required. A bolus dose of 5000 to 10,000 units of heparin should be given as soon as the diagnosis of PE is suspected. Invasive procedures such as repeated arterial sampling for blood gas analysis should be avoided if thrombolytic therapy is considered a therapeutic option. Intravenous fluids should be restricted to prevent a further increase in right heart filling pressure and the development of acute RV failure. Patients with deteriorating cardiac output require inotropic support with agents such as dobutamine.

Anticoagulation

Randomized trials in the 1960s conclusively demonstrated the benefit of heparin therapy in patients with PE, with reduction in the mortality rate in untreated patients from 30 to 8%. Heparin accelerates the action of antithrombin III, preventing further clot propagation and thereby enhancing intrinsic fibrinolysis. An intravenous loading dose of 5000 to 10,000 units of unfractionated heparin is recommended, followed by a continuous infusion of 1000 to 1500 units/h in healthy individuals. The partial thromboplastin time should be maintained within the therapeutic range of 60 to 80 seconds, and regular sampling is advised to ensure that effective anticoagulation is sustained. The duration of oral anticoagulation after PE is subject to debate, but a 6-month period usually is advocated. Induction of oral anticoagulation requires 5 days and can be started concomitantly with heparin therapy. The International Standardized Ratio (INR) should be maintained around 3.0 during the crossover period because heparin prolongs the INR by a further 0.5.[13] Recent studies indicate that low-molecular weight heparin regimens are equally effective as conventional intravenous (IV) heparin therapy and that the anticoagulant response to weight-adjusted doses are more predictable.

THROMBOLYTIC THERAPY

Although heparin prevents the further propagation of thrombus, thrombolytic therapy promotes its dissolution and can potentially produce rapid improvement in the hemodynamic status of the patient with PE. Thrombolysis has become standard therapy for myocardial infarction, but its role in hemodynamically stable patients with pulmonary embolism remains controversial. Data from the PIOPED project in the mid-1980s showed that only 6% of 399 patients with pulmonary embolism were treated with a lytic agent,[3] but renewed interest in the use of thrombolytic therapy has occurred because of the favorable results of more recent randomized controlled trials and observational studies. In the future, the indications for thrombolytic therapy may be expanded to include "hemodynamically stable" patients who have evidence of moderate or severe RV dysfunction, although large randomized controlled trials are needed to determine the benefits in terms of clinical outcomes such as death, recurrent PE, and chronic pulmonary hypertension.[6]

Pulmonary Thrombolysis Trials

In a randomized study of 160 patients, the UPET 1 study[14] demonstrated accelerated fibrinolysis in patients treated with urokinase and heparin compared with heparin therapy alone. Superiority of lytic therapy was demonstrated in terms of angiographic evidence of clot lysis, improvement in hemodynamic parameters, and pulmonary capillary perfusion, as measured by radionuclide lung scanning. No difference in mortality at 2 weeks was demonstrated between the treatment groups (9% in heparin group vs. 7% in urokinase group), although a clinical trial with mortality as the primary endpoint would have required a sample size 20 to 40 times greater than the UPET 1 study. The second-phase trial (UPET 2)[15] compared three thrombolytic protocols followed by heparin therapy (streptokinase infusion for 24 hours or urokinase infusion for 12 or 24 hours). Similar 2-week mortality rates were reported, and there were no significant additional benefits of 24-hour infusion of urokinase vs. a 12-hour infusion of urokinase. This trial did not prove or disprove superiority of urokinase over streptokinase, although some benefit was observed in lung perfusion on radionuclide scanning, particularly in patients with massive pulmonary embolism. At long-term follow-up, UPET patients treated with lytic therapy appeared to have less functional disability than those receiving heparin alone.[16]

In the 1980s, Goldhaber and colleagues investigated the efficacy of tissue plasminogen activator (recombinant tissue-type plasminogen activator [rt-PA]) in pulmonary embolism and reported clot lysis in 94% of patients after a 50 to 90 mg infusion over a 2- to 6-hour period.[17] In a subsequent trial comparing IV rt-PA (100 mg/2 h) with urokinase (4400 IU/kg bolus followed by 4400 IU/kg/h for a maximum of

24 hours), clot lysis was demonstrated at 2 hours in 82% of the rt-PA group compared with 48% in the urokinase group.[18] A later trial comparing rt-PA (100 mg/2 h) with short-duration infusion of urokinase (1,000,000 IU/10 min followed by 2,000,000 IU over 2 hours) demonstrated similar safety and efficacy for acute pulmonary embolism.[19] Fixed-dose infusion of lytic agents over a short time period have advantages in terms of simplifying patient management without reducing clinical efficacy or increasing hemorrhagic complications. The effect of lytic therapy on the resolution of echocardiographic features of RV dysfunction was suggested in small case series. In 1993, Goldhaber and colleagues reported the results of randomized trial of the effects of rt-PA vs. heparin on RV function and pulmonary perfusion in patients with acute PE.[20] One hundred one patients with PE were randomized to rt-PA (100 mg/2 h) followed by heparin, or to heparin alone, and RV function was assessed qualitatively and quantitatively by echocardiography at baseline and at 3 and 24 hours. Pretreatment perfusion lung scans were performed and repeated at 24 hours. No patient had systemic hypotension (blood pressure (BP) < 90 mm Hg) before entry into the study, and 36% had evidence of RV dysfunction. Echocardiographic evaluation of RV wall movement showed qualitative improvement in 39% of patients in the rt-PA group and deterioration in 2% ($P = .005$). Quantitative assessment of RV end-diastolic area by planimetry showed a reduction in the rt-PA group during the first 24 hours but no significant change in the heparin group. In the subgroup of patients with baseline RV dysfunction, 89% showed echocardiographic improvement and 6% deteriorated, whereas 44% of the heparin group improved and 28% showed deteriorating function ($P = .03$). The extent of perfusion defects on baseline lung scanning was significantly greater in patients with RV hypokinesis than in those with normal RV wall motion. rt-PA–treated patients showed a significant improvement on serial perfusion lung scanning of 14.6% compared with 1.5% in the heparin group ($P < .0001$). In a 2-week follow-up period, five episodes of recurrent PE occurred in the heparin group, two of which proved fatal. No recurrent embolic events or fatalities occurred in rt-PA group. Data from a multicenter European registry of 719 patients with major PE without hemodynamic impairment at presentation showed a significantly decreased mortality in patients who received thrombolytic therapy compared with those treated with heparin alone.[12] The 30-day mortality rate for the patients treated with lytic therapy was 4.7% compared with 11.1% for the heparin group ($P = .016$), and multivariate analysis showed that only primary thrombolysis was an independent predictor of survival (odds ratio for in-hospital death, 0.46; 95% confidence interval, 0.21 to 1.00). Recurrent PE was

lower in the thrombolysis group compared with the heparin group (8% vs. 19%, $P < .001$), although the bleeding rate was significantly higher in the thrombolysis group (22% vs. 8%, $P < .001$). Although observational data suffer from potential selection bias, these results support the notion that thrombolytic therapy may improve clinical outcomes in hemodynamically stable patients with major PE.

Indications for Thrombolytic Therapy

Although the UPET trials in the 1970s demonstrated the superiority of lytic therapy in over-anticoagulation alone in terms of hemodynamic and angiographic improvement, no mortality difference was demonstrated. Debate about which patients should be treated continues, although acute massive PE associated with arterial hypotension is an accepted indication for lytic therapy (Fig. 23–2). A small randomized trial of streptokinase and heparin vs. heparin alone showed a clear survival benefit in favor of lytic therapy.[21] Four patients with massive PE survived in the thrombolysis group and four patients treated with heparin died of progressive right heart failure. The trial was stopped at this point because of ethical considerations.

The place of lytic therapy in hemodynamically stable patients is more controversial. Patients who have sustained massive PE but who are not hypotensive are deemed to be "hemodynamically stable," but this term is misleading because they may have elevated pulmonary artery pressure or RV dysfunction. This subset of patients may have a worse prognosis than patients with normal PAP and RV function.

Studies in the 1980s showed that resolution of changes of RV dysfunction occur more rapidly with lytic therapy than with heparin alone. Goldhaber suggests that sufficient evidence exists to suggest that normotensive patients with massive PE who have evidence of moderate to severe RV dysfunction should be considered for thrombolytic treatment, provided that there are no significant contraindications.[6]

Contraindications

The decision to start thrombolytic therapy is based on an assessment of the potential risks and benefits of treatment in the individual patient. Hemorrhagic stroke is a catastrophic event for the patient and is associated with significant morbidity and mortality. To minimize hemorrhagic complications, general exclusion criteria for thrombolytic therapy should be observed (Table 23–2).

PE is common in surgical patients within the early postoperative period, but thrombolytic treat-

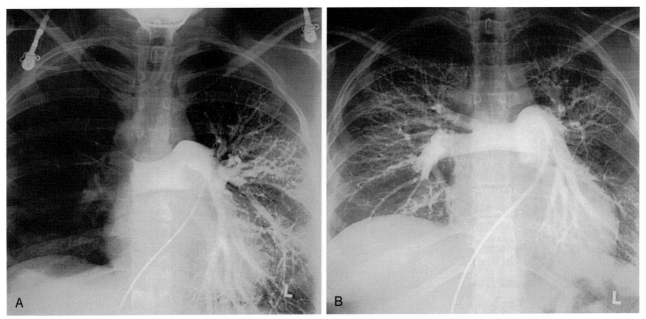

Figure 23–2. *A,* Massive pulmonary embolism with complete occlusion of the right pulmonary artery and multiple left pulmonary emboli. *B,* Marked clinical and angiographic improvement was achieved after 16 hours of lytic therapy.

ment usually is contraindicated within 2 months of major surgery. In the study by Verstraete and associates, four patients who required transfusion of more than 2 units of blood had undergone surgery within the previous 2 weeks.[22] In contrast, Molina and colleagues reported successful lytic therapy in 13 patients with PE within 2 weeks of surgery using a modified low-dose technique.[23] A 2200-IU bolus of urokinase was injected via a pulmonary artery catheter followed by a bolus of 2200 IU/kg/h for up to 24 hours, and the serum fibrinogen level was monitored every 6 hours and maintained above 0.2 g/dl to prevent hemorrhage. Low-dose intrathrombic lytic therapy may be useful in patients with major contraindications to thrombolysis.[24] Because the greatest risk of death is in the first few hours after massive PE, it may be justifiable to accept the risk of major bleeding in patients with contraindications to thrombolysis. In the MAPPET registry of 1001 patients with massive pulmonary embolism, 48% received thrombolytic

therapy and 41% of this subgroup had at least one contraindication to lytic treatment.[5]

Thrombolytic Agents

Thrombolytic agents and regimens approved by the Food and Drug Administration (FDA) and others in current use are listed in Table 23–3. Bolus administration of thrombolytic agents may prevent the development of a prolonged lytic state and reduce the hemorrhagic complications, but further studies are necessary to prove efficacy and safety compared with currently approved regimens. Fixed-dose or weight-adjusted treatment regimens do not require repeated coagulation studies during lytic therapy.

Route of Administration of Thrombolytic Drugs

IV administration of thrombolytic drugs has considerable practical advantages over intrapulmonary or in-

Table 23–2. Contraindications to Thrombolysis

Absolute	Relative (Major)	Relative (Minor)
Active or recent internal bleeding	Major internal bleeding within 3 months	Recent minor trauma including cardiopulmonary resuscitation
Hemorrhagic stroke within 2 months	Major surgery within 10 days	Left heart thrombus (i.e., in mitral valve disease)
Uncorrectable coagulopathy	Severe hypertension (> 200 systolic or > 110 diastolic)	Organ biopsy in previous 10 d
Intracranial neoplasm	Recent arterial puncture	Bacterial endocarditis
Head trauma	Recent obstetric delivery	Pregnancy
	Active peptic ulceration	Proliferative diabetic retinopathy
	Nonhemorrhagic stroke	Advanced age (> 75 y)
	Recent serious trauma	Severe liver or renal failure
	Pericardial effusion	Abdominal aortic aneurysm

Table 23–3. Thrombolytic Agents and Dosage Regimens

Thrombolytic Agent	FDA Approved	Loading Dose	Subsequent Infusion Regimen
Streptokinase	Yes	250,000 IU over 30 min	100,000 IU/h for 24 h
Urokinase	Yes	4400 IU/kg over 10 min	4400 IU/kg/h for 12–24 h
Urokinase		8800 IU/kg over 10 min	8800 IU/kg over 12 h
Urokinase		1,000,000 IU over 10 min	2,000,000 IU over 110 min
Urokinase (bolus lysis)		33,000–44,000 IU/kg over 10 min	
rt-PA	Yes	None	100 mg over 2 h
rt-PA		10 mg bolus	90 mg over 2 h
rt-PA (bolus lysis)		1.32 mg/kg over 2 min	

FDA = Food and Drug Administration; rt-PA = recombinant tissue-type plasminogen activator.

trathrombic drug delivery and simplifies patient management. Treatment can be instituted at the bedside without recourse to the angiographic laboratory and avoids the hemorrhagic complications associated with catheter puncture. A multicenter randomized trial comparing IV with intrapulmonary delivery of rt-PA in 34 patients with acute massive PE showed no significant difference in angiographic or hemodynamic parameters after therapy, and the authors concluded that intrapulmonary delivery confers no additional benefit over the IV route.[22] These findings appear to conflict with the experience of peripheral arterial thrombolysis, in which low-dose intrathrombic delivery of lytic agents is superior to systemic therapy. Experimental models have demonstrated that local high-velocity flow disturbances occur proximal to occlusive emboli, causing rapid washout into the nonoccluded arteries, potentially preventing any enhanced local effect and resulting in systemic dilution of the lytic agent.[25] The authors speculate that this phenomenon may explain the apparent lack of benefit of intrapulmonary delivery of lytic agents over the IV route and suggest that catheter-directed intrathrombic infusion or preliminary mechanical thrombectomy to increase the clot surface area should enhance the effect of lytic therapy. Direct intrathrombic delivery using doses of lytic drugs at 20 to 25% of normal systemic doses has been reported to be effective in patients with massive PE.[24] The technique as described by the authors involves a coaxial system of a guide catheter and infusion catheter (Fig. 23–3). The infusion catheter is advanced into the occluding embolus over a wire and positioned so that the side holes lie within the thrombus. Five of the six patients in the reported series had contraindications to standard thrombolysis, and all improved dramatically with treatment. Notably systemic fibrinogenolysis did not occur, and there were no bleeding complications in this group of patients. Intrathrombic low-dose thrombolysis also may be useful if the response to standard systemic treatment is prolonged or inadequate, but larger studies are required to define its role in relation to other catheter-directed therapies. This technique would seem to be most effective in patients with embolic occlusion of the major pulmonary arteries rather than those with multiple nonocclusive thrombi. Intrathrombic delivery techniques may be used in combination with clot fragmentation, and treatment response may be monitored readily by PAP measurements. Although short-duration systemic thrombolysis is likely to remain the principal route of drug administration, intrathrombic delivery techniques are likely to play a role in selected patients with massive PE.

Complications

The incidence of bleeding complications in the UPET 1 trial was significantly higher in the urokinase group (45% urokinase vs. 27% in heparin group, $P < .05$). This principally was related to invasive procedures associated with data collection (venous or arterial puncture site bleeding). Major bleeding complications in the UKEP study,[26] which compared two dosage regimens of urokinase administered via a pulmonary

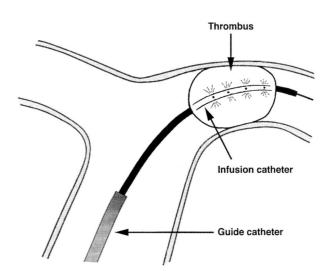

Figure 23–3. Schematic representation of coaxial catheter system for lytic therapy.

artery catheter, were reported in only 43% of cases. In Levine's review of data from published trials of thrombolytic therapy for PE, the reported incidence of major hemorrhage varied from 0 to 45%. Most bleeding complications were catheter related and occurred overall in 20% of patients receiving lytic therapy who had undergone pulmonary angiography. The more recent studies appear to show a reduction in the incidence of major hemorrhage compared with the earlier trials. Although this may be the result of the use of shorter thrombolytic regimens, most of the studies had a small sample size and therefore the true incidence of bleeding complications was difficult to assess. Data derived from the later published studies in this review article suggest an incidence of major hemorrhage of 5 to 10% and a hemorrhage-related mortality rate of 1 to 2%.[27]

MANAGEMENT OF HEMORRHAGIC COMPLICATIONS

Patients receiving lytic therapy should be monitored by staff experienced in the potential complications of this treatment. Simple preventative measures, such as avoidance of arterial puncture for blood gas analysis, intramuscular injections, and reducing patient handling to a minimum, should be observed. In addition to routine monitoring, regular neurologic observations and inspection of arterial or venous puncture sites also should be performed. A careful neurologic history should be elicited because a history of transient ischemic attacks or migraine may be important if neurologic symptoms develop during thrombolytic therapy. In addition to routine biochemical and hematologic investigations (including a coagulation profile), blood should be sent for cross-matching. Administration of thrombolytic therapy should conform to accepted protocols, for example, 100 mg rt-PA infusion over 2 hours, and heparin should not be given concomitantly. Invasive procedures such as pulmonary angiography should be performed by an experienced radiologist, and a single-wall puncture technique should be used. The femoral vein should be punctured below the inguinal ligament to minimize the potential complication of retroperitoneal hemorrhage due to inadvertent puncture of the femoral artery. After pulmonary arteriography, the angiographic sheath should be sutured to the skin to prevent dislodgment. Patients with massive PE requiring lytic therapy despite certain relative contraindications to thrombolysis (e.g., peptic ulceration) should have prophylactic maximal medical therapy specific to that condition to minimize hemorrhagic complications. If major bleeding occurs during treatment, thrombolysis should be discontinued immediately. In the case of a major neurologic event, a CT brain scan should be performed as soon as possible and a neurologic/neu-

rosurgical opinion obtained. Local oozing from puncture sites should be treated by local compression, and persistent femoral venous bleeding around a sheath may be managed by substituting an angiographic sheath of slightly larger caliber. Bleeding from other sources (i.e., gastrointestinal or urinary tract) should be managed conservatively after discontinuation of thrombolysis. If bleeding persists or is potentially life-threatening, an infusion of 10 units of cryoprecipitate will increase the fibrinogen level by 70 mg/dl and increase factor VIII levels by approximately 30% of circulating levels.[28] Two units of fresh frozen plasma, which is a source of factors V and VIII, fibrinogen, and other coagulation factors, also should be given. Replacement transfusion with packed red cells and/or platelets should be considered depending on hematologic parameters. If the patient has received heparin, this may be reversed with protamine. If these measures are ineffective, then endoscopic or surgical control of bleeding may be required. Transcatheter embolization may be appropriate in certain circumstances in which hemorrhage, for example, pelvic arterial bleeding, complicates lytic therapy.

MECHANICAL THROMBECTOMY

Although thrombolysis is indicated for massive PE with hemodynamic compromise, treatment may be prolonged, contraindicated, or ineffective in individual patients. These patients are at greatest risk of death within the first hour of the onset of symptoms, and rapid restoration of pulmonary blood flow and improvement in cardiac output should be the overriding clinical priority. The surgical alternative of emergency thoracotomy and pulmonary embolectomy is associated with a high mortality and is not uniformly available. The cross-sectional area of the peripheral pulmonary circulation is greater than that of the central pulmonary arteries, and therefore, fragmentation and dispersal of an occlusive central thrombus can result in a rapid improvement in blood flow and a decrease in the pulmonary vascular resistance (Fig. 23–4). As a consequence, a variety of catheter-directed techniques have been developed to disperse or remove thrombus in patients with life-threatening PE. The application of these new technologies can result in rapid improvements in angiographic appearances, hemodynamic parameters, and oxygen saturation and emphasizes the therapeutic role of interventional radiology in the management of patients with acute massive PE.

Transvenous Catheter Pulmonary Embolectomy

The concept of transvenous catheter pulmonary embolectomy was first introduced by Greenfield. The

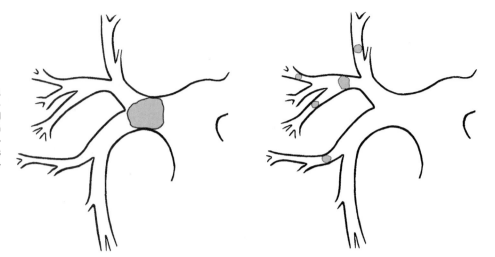

Figure 23–4. The cross-sectional area of the peripheral pulmonary circulation is greater than that of the central pulmonary arteries, and fragmentation and dispersal of central occlusive emboli can result in rapid improvements in blood flow and pulmonary hemodynamics.

initial device consisted of a 12-French dual-lumen catheter with an angulated stainless steel suction cup attached at the distal end. Subsequently the device, was refined by the addition of 10-French steerable catheter and a 7-mm radiopaque plastic suction cup, enabling directional control and access to more lobar branches. The device is introduced by a femoral or preferably jugular venotomy and advanced into the pulmonary circulation under fluoroscopic control using the steerable catheter to negotiate the right heart chambers. The suction cup is advanced into contact with the obstructing embolus, and its position is confirmed by injection of small volumes of contrast media. Suction then is applied by a syringe, and a portion of the embolus is drawn into the cup. Negative pressure is maintained while the catheter and attached thrombus are removed. The process is repeated until a sufficient amount of embolic material is extracted and until hemodynamic improvement occurs. In 1993, Greenfield reported his results in 46 patients from 1970 to 1992.[29] The primary indication for therapy in this group was hypotension despite inotropic support in 91% of cases. The remainder had sustained major PE and required ventilatory support. In an initial group of 10 patients, before device modification, hemodynamic improvement occurred in 90%, but recurrent PE and a mortality rate of 50% prompted routine placement of a vena caval filter. In the total series, successful clot extraction was achieved in 76%, with a 30-day survival rate of 70%. An average reduction in mean pulmonary artery pressure of 8 mm Hg was attained, and mean cardiac output significantly improved from 2.59 L/min to 4.47 L/min ($P < .003$). Mean survival in patients surviving the postoperative period was 89 months (1–237 mo); it was 48 months for the total series. In a subgroup of nine patients with chronic PE, a successful outcome was achieved in only five patients probably because emboli become firmly adherent to the vessel wall after 48 to 72 hours. Complications re-

ported in this series included pulmonary infarction (11%), myocardial infarction (4%), recurrent DVT (6%), pleural effusion (4%), and wound hematoma (15%). Timsit and colleagues[30] reported their 7-year experience of catheter embolectomy in a group of 18 patients, which represented only 1% of 1700 patients referred to their institution with confirmed PE. Embolectomy was successful in 11 of 18 patients, for an overall mortality rate of 28%. They also confirmed that catheter embolectomy is less likely to be successful in patients with chronic PE.

Despite these impressive results, few centers have gained substantial experience with this technique, and the reported series are small. Although the device is bulky and catheter manipulation may be difficult, catheter embolectomy represents an important milestone in the development of the endovascular management of patients with life-threatening PE. More recently, Lang and associates described a modified suction embolectomy technique using a telescopic coaxial catheter system in three patients with massive PE.[31] In two patients, preliminary clot fragmentation was attempted with angiographic or balloon angioplasty catheters followed by intrapulmonary thrombolysis. The technique involves preliminary placement of a 16-French, 40-cm long Check-Flo II Introducer Set in the femoral vein. A 14-French, 90-cm long nontapered Ultrathane catheter is mounted coaxially on a 97-cm long Multipurpose C guiding catheter. The 14-French catheter acts as the main suction catheter, and to prevent clot amputation during withdrawal through the hemostatic valve, a short 14-French peel-away sheath is placed coaxially through the valve. After placing a Glidewire in the relevant pulmonary artery, the 6-French guiding catheter is advanced beyond the embolus. The 14-French suction catheter then is advanced coaxially over it until it comes into contact with the embolus. The clot then is compacted and forced distally until it impacts at a vascular bifurcation. Extraction of thrombus within the peripheral branch is performed with the 6-French catheter after clot capture is confirmed by increasing resistance to aspiration. The authors recommend use of a 30-ml syringe for this part of the procedure to minimize blood loss. The 14-French nontapered suction catheter is used to remove larger fragments after suction is applied with a 50-ml syringe. The device is then removed through the stationary 16-French sheath and withdrawn through the hemostatic valve together with the peel-away sheath. The process then is repeated as necessary according to repeat angiography. Clot aspiration of the 16-French sheath also may be required if blood cannot be aspirated freely after withdrawal of the suction catheter. This can be performed with the 6-French guiding catheter. Thrombi of rubbery consistency, 3 to 8 cm in length, were extracted by this method with a reduction of the clot burden of up to 90%. Procedural blood loss ranged from 60 to 200 ml. Histologic examination showed a mixture of red and white thrombus with cellular appearances consistent with aging clot that embolized from a distal location. The authors speculate that the cohesive structure of the thrombus resists fragmentation, a feature that may favor removal by aspiration techniques. Two of three patients were discharged alive and the third patient died of RV failure, despite two technically successful thrombectomy procedures. Although a larger experience is required before definite conclusions regarding safety and efficacy can be reached, this technique has potential advantages over the larger embolectomy devices as it does not require specialized angiographic skills or surgical venous access and can be performed with any fluoroscopic unit in the emergency situation.

Catheter Fragmentation Techniques

Disruption of centrally located emboli with rapid improvement in cardiopulmonary hemodynamics can be achieved using conventional angiographic catheters and requires no more specialized angiographic skills than pulmonary angiography. Brady and associates[32] reported successful catheter fragmentation of thrombi in three patients with massive PE with significant improvement is systemic and pulmonary arterial pressures and arterial pO_2. Clot fragmentation was performed with 8-French catheters in either a multipurpose or pigtail configuration. After a diagnostic pulmonary angiogram is performed a J-tipped guide wire is advanced together with the catheter to push the thrombus peripherally. The wire then is passed gently beyond the embolus into a distal branch vessel, and the catheter is advanced over it. The wire is withdrawn until the catheter tip resumes its normal configuration, and the clot fragmentation is achieved by pulling the catheter back into the main

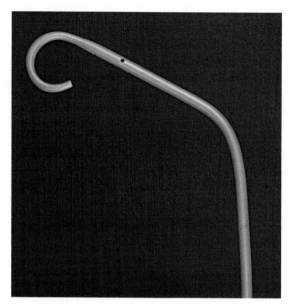

Figure 23–5. Grollman pulmonary pigtail catheter.

pulmonary artery. The process is repeated in one or more vessels until adequate pulmonary blood flow is restored. Clot fragmentation is more likely with the stiffer 7- or 8-French catheters, such as the Grollman pulmonary pigtail catheter (Fig. 23–5), than with standard 5-French angiographic catheters. Two of the three patients received thrombolytic therapy delivered via the catheter placed in the pulmonary trunk. Mechanical fragmentation of thrombus also may reduce the duration of thrombolysis by exposing a greater surface area of thrombus to the lytic agent. Complications related to mechanical fragmentation appear to be very low and tend to be associated with the concomitant use of lytic therapy.

Fava and colleagues treated 16 patients with massive PE using a combination of mechanical fragmentation and thrombolysis.[33] In eight patients, the effects of preliminary mechanical fragmentation were assessed before the initiation of lytic therapy and the mean PAP decreased from 57 mm Hg +/- 9.3 to 39.5 mm Hg +/- 10.9 ($P < .001$). If catheter fragmentation did not result in immediate angiographic improvement, the procedure was repeated with a balloon angioplasty catheter. Balloon diameters were chosen to be equal to or 1 mm less than the diameter of the obstructed artery and varied from 6 to 16 mm. The remaining eight patients had initial PAP < 40 mm Hg and were treated with urokinase delivered directly into the thrombus. If bilateral emboli were present, a second catheter was used to deliver lytic therapy. In this group, mechanical fragmentation was performed at 2 hours if there was no change in PAP or angiographic indices. Complications occurred in three patients (19%) and were restricted to puncture site bleeding, which responded to local compression. In the total group, the initial mean PAP decreased from

48.2 mm Hg +/- 13.4 to 18.5 mm Hg +/- 7.2 ($P <$ .0001). A decrease in the mean UPET angiographic index occurred from a pretreatment value of 13.7 +/- 1.4 to 6.1 +/- 2.2 after therapy ($P <$ .0001). Fourteen of 16 patients (88%) were treated successfully with this combined technique, and one death due to cardiovascular collapse occurred despite improvement in hemodynamic parameters. Lytic therapy was discontinued in one patient because of a reduction in plasma fibrinogen levels below 100 mg/dl, and this patient was treated successfully by surgical embolectomy. This study lends support to the contention that mechanical fragmentation of emboli can produce a rapid improvement in pulmonary blood flow and appears to be without significant complications. It also highlights the value of an intrapulmonary catheter to monitor improvement in angiographic and hemodynamic parameters and allows rapid access for further intervention should the patient's condition deteriorate. The equipment used should be available in most angiographic laboratories, and performance of the technique does not require specialized interventional skills.

Mechanical Thrombectomy Devices

More sophisticated mechanical thrombectomy devices have been developed in recent years to facilitate rapid clot maceration or removal. Although most clinical experience has been accumulated in peripheral arterial or venous thrombotic conditions, there are some published data that suggest that these devices may be of value in patients with massive PE. Mechanical thrombectomy devices can be divided broadly into two categories[34]:

1. Rotational recirculation devices, which macerate thrombus by generating a hydrodynamic vortex produced by high-speed rotating basket or impeller (e.g., Amplatz thrombectomy device [ATD] [Fig. 23–6] or impeller-basket devices).
2. Hydraulic recirculation devices, whose method of action is dependent on the Venturi effect produced

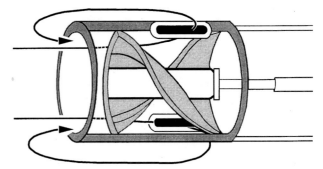

Figure 23–6. Schematic representation of the Amplatz thrombectomy device. A high-speed recessed impeller creates a strong local vortex and draws thrombus into the end hole. The clot then is macerated and recirculated via side holes in the direction of the arrows.

by retrogradely directed high-speed fluid jets. Thrombus is drawn into the aperture of the device, and fragmentation occurs by the high local shear forces (Fig. 23–7). Removal of clot fragments is then possible through a second exhaust channel (Angiojet or Hydrolyser).

In vitro and in vivo studies have demonstrated the feasibility of their use in the pulmonary circulation, but their clinical role is not fully established. They remain experimental devices, and their use should be restricted to use in patients with massive PE, in whom thrombolysis is contraindicated or ineffective. Possible complications associated with these devices include vascular wall damage or perforation, micro- or macroembolization, rethrombosis, hemolysis, and blood loss.

AMPLATZ THROMBECTOMY DEVICE

The ATD is a recirculation device that consists of an 8-French 120-cm long catheter that has an impeller blade recessed within a distal metal capsule to prevent endothelial damage (Fig. 23–8). A compressed air turbine capable of rotational speeds of up to 150,000 rpm powers the impeller drive shaft, and thrombus is drawn into the end hole, macerated, and recirculated via three large side holes in the metal

Figure 23–7. Schematic illustration of the Hydrolyser device. A, The 7-French catheter has inflow B, exhaust channels, and C, a retrogradely directed metal port directs a high-speed saline jet of saline across the suction nozzle. The catheter may be advanced over a guide wire (broken line). Because of the Venturi effect, a pressure gradient is created in the direction of the nozzle and thrombus is drawn into the aperture and fragmented by high shear forces (curved arrows). The mixture of fragmented clot and saline are removed passively via the exhaust channel (open arrows).

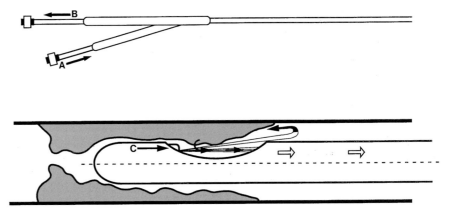

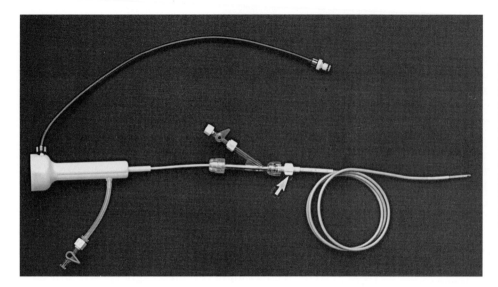

Figure 23–8. The Amplatz thrombectomy device (ATD) consists of an 8-French, 120-cm long catheter with a small impeller recessed within a metal housing at the tip. Compressed air is supplied via the long side arm to a turbine, which powers the drive shaft. The short side arm is used for injection of saline, contrast media or thrombolytic agents. Because the ATD is not an over-the-wire device, an 8-French multipurpose guiding catheter (*arrow*) must be used to direct it within the pulmonary circulation.

housing (Fig. 23–9). A second channel allows injection of thrombolytic drugs, contrast media, or saline. The ATD is not an over-the-wire device and requires a shaped guiding catheter to provide directional control in the pulmonary circulation. In vitro experiments with fresh clot have shown that 95% of particles thus produced are less than 13 microns in diameter.[35] However, others have drawn attention to the fact that such efficiency may not be achievable in flow models, in which the opportunity for thorough recirculation is likely to be diminished.[34]

Uflacker and colleagues described the technique of pulmonary thrombectomy (Fig. 23–10) with the ATD in five patients with massive PE.[36] After pulmonary angiography and pressure measurements, the diagnostic catheter is removed and a 260-cm exchange guide wire is used to advance a 10-French Multipurpose guiding catheter into the target vessel. The ATD then is advanced through a large-caliber hemostatic valve, such as the Morse-Y connector. The ATD is activated in close proximity to the thrombus with a slow to-and-fro motion. The shaped guiding catheter enables a degree of direction control within the pulmonary vessels. After completion, the ATD is withdrawn and the catheter aspirated to remove any re-

sulting slurry. A pulmonary angiogram then is performed, and the process is repeated if thrombotic occlusion persists. In this study, only one patient received lytic therapy during the procedure because the protocol was designed to assess the efficacy of the ATD alone. Angiography and radionuclide scanning demonstrated marked improvement in pulmonary perfusion in one patient, and moderate improvement was observed in three patients. One patient died of a neurologic complication shortly after the procedure, and the remaining four patients showed clinical improvement with resolution of dyspnea, chest pain, and hypotension. Mean PAP increased in three of four patients after thrombectomy. The authors cite various possible causes for this, including improved cardiac output, distal embolization, and pulmonary vasospasm possibly due to neurohumoural mediators or injection of contrast media. Major hemoptysis occurred in one patient, possibly because of a reperfusion syndrome caused by sudden restoration of pulmonary blood flow to an area of infarcted lung tissue. Hemolysis is a recognized complication of thrombectomy with the ATD,[37] and although the resulting elevation of plasma free-hemoglobin can cause intranephric cast formation, this is usually without clinical sequelae. Nevertheless, restriction of activation time to 5 minutes in patients with borderline renal function has been recommended.[36] Although clinical improvement was demonstrated in this small series of patients with massive PE, further experience is necessary to determine its role compared with other therapies. Thrombectomy with the ATD is of limited efficacy when organized thrombus is present.

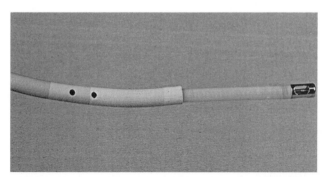

Figure 23–9. Close-up view of the Amplatz thrombectomy device (ATD) emerging from the guiding catheter. Three large side holes facilitate clot expulsion and recirculation.

IMPELLER BASKET DEVICES

Schmitz-Rode and colleagues developed a rotational device consisting of a high-speed impeller centrally positioned within a self-expandable helical basket and

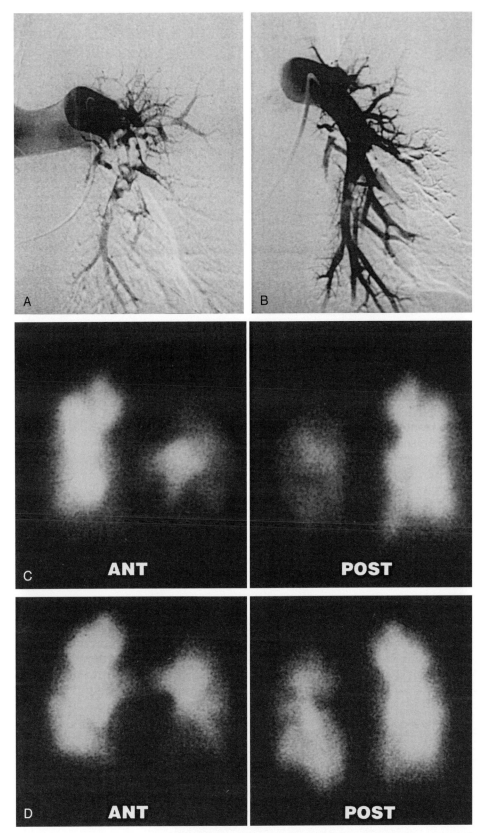

Figure 23–10. A, Left pulmonary angiogram showing extensive emboli in a patient who sustained a massive pulmonary embolism. Lytic therapy was contraindicated because of recent surgery. B, Repeat angiogram after mechanical thrombectomy with the Amplatz thrombectomy device (ATD) shows marked improvement in pulmonary blood flow after an activation time of 20 seconds. C, Perfusion lung scan images before thrombectomy. D, Postthrombectomy scans show improvement in perfusion to the left lung. (From Uflacker R, Strange C, Vujic I: Massive pulmonary embolism: Preliminary results of treatment with the Amplatz thrombectomy device. J Vasc Intervent Radiol 7:519–528, 1996.)

described its use in a canine model.[38] The rotating impeller creates hydrodynamic suction, which draws the thrombus into the basket, where it then is fragmented. The function of the helical basket is to centralize the impeller within the vessel lumen and thus avoid endothelial damage. In vitro testing demonstrated that 90% of the resulting particulate material was smaller than 10 microns in diameter, and animal studies demonstrated complete fragmentation of seven out of nine emboli in the left pulmonary artery within 10 seconds of device activation. No significant hemolysis occurred, but the device had limited steerability, particularly in segmental branches. An over-the-wire variation of this impeller catheter was developed using an 8-French outer guide catheter and a 5-French inner rotating catheter. Longitudinal slits in the distal catheter sections allowed the formation of self-expanding baskets. The outer protection basket remained static while the inner basket rotated at 100,000 to 150,000 rpm. This device was compared with the Thrombolizer, a similar rotational device that lacked an outer protection basket. Animal experiments demonstrated the superiority of the coaxial system in fragmenting of thrombus and a significant decrease in PAP also was demonstrated. The Thrombolizer drive system did not operate consistently, and histology of recanalized pulmonary artery segments showed increased periarterial hemorrhage with this device.[39]

ROTATABLE PIGTAIL CATHETER

Because of the limited steerability of the impeller basket devices, a rotatable high-torque pigtail catheter was designed with an oval side hole at the outer aspect of the pigtail loop in a straight line with the long axis of the catheter. When placed in the pulmonary artery, the movable core guide wire was withdrawn by a few centimeters, stiffened, and then advanced through the modified side hole. This acted as a central axis of rotation when the catheter was rotated with a low-speed electric motor. Steerability was enhanced with this design, and in animal studies, 53% of the occluded arteries were recanalized with a reduction in mean PAP of 73%.[40] Clot fragmentation was coarse compared with the impeller basket design on filtration studies. Perivascular hemorrhage occurred in a minority of animals and appeared to be well circumscribed.

HYDROLYSER

The Hydrolyser recirculation device consists of a 7-French, 65-cm double-lumen catheter (Fig. 23–11) with a 6-mm diameter side hole (suction nozzle) close to the distal tip. The rounded tip has an end hole that allows the catheter to be advanced over a 0.025-inch guide wire. Saline is injected through a supply channel by an angiographic pump at a rate of 3 ml/s at 750 psi. The saline jet is directed retrogradely across the suction nozzle via a small metal end port (Fig. 23–12). The Venturi effect, thus produced, causes a pressure gradient in the direction of the suction nozzle, into which the thrombus is drawn and fragmented. A mixture of clot fragments and saline are removed passively via the exhaust channel into a collection bag. In vitro experiments have determined that the fluid volume removed during thrombectomy is equal to the injected volume plus a 20% increment comprised of clot fragments and blood, and therefore, fluid overload is unlikely to occur. This is of particular importance in patients with massive PE embolism and RV dysfunction in whom IV fluids should be restricted. During device activation, the catheter is

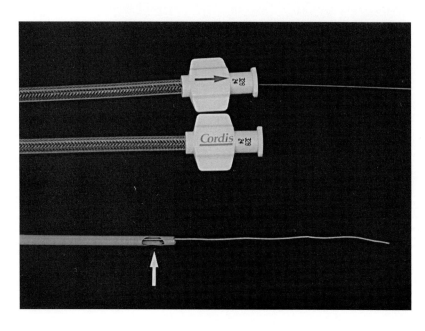

Figure 23–11. The Hydrolyser device consists of a 7-French dual-lumen catheter with a suction nozzle situated close to its distal tip *(arrow)*. Saline is injected through the inflow channel, by an angiographic pump at 3 ml/s at 750 psi. The device can be backloaded over a 0.025-inch guide wire, which exits via the exhaust channel. The wire is removed before activation, and fragmented clot saline mixture is removed passively into a collection bag.

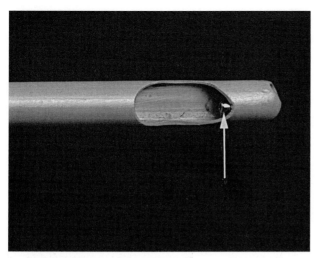

Figure 23–12. Close-up view of the suction nozzle showing the retrogradely directed injection port *(arrow)*.

advanced slowly through the clot, and repeat angiography is performed after 150 ml of saline have been injected. The procedure is repeated depending on the angiographic appearance. The costs of thrombectomy using the Hydrolyser are not prohibitive because specialized equipment is not required, other than a conventional angiographic pump. This device has been effective in peripheral arterial thrombosis,[41] but published experience of its use in PE embolism is limited to two cases.[42] In both cases, a successful outcome was achieved without complications.

RHEOLYTIC THROMBECTOMY CATHETER

The Angiojet rheolytic thrombectomy catheter (RTC) is a 5-French dual-lumen catheter that operates on similar hydrodynamic principles as the Hydrolyser device. The RTC is not an over-the-wire device and requires an 8-French guiding catheter to direct it into the pulmonary circulation. Saline is injected under pressure into a series of retrogradely directed end holes situated in the metal end cap, and the high-velocity jets create the local pressure gradient by the Venturi effect. Thrombus is entrained into the catheter tip, and local shear forces cause clot fragmentation. The resultant particles then are removed via the exhaust lumen with the assistance of an external rotor pump. This device does require a dedicated external drive unit, which contains the injection and exhaust pumps, and this adds considerably to the overall cost. Successful use of the RTC has been reported in two cases of pulmonary embolism in which lytic therapy was contraindicated.[43] Both patients were normotensive but had pulmonary hypertension. One patient had clinical signs of RV failure, but echocardiography data were not included in the report. It was estimated that the other patient's PE had occurred 10 to 15 days previously. The RTC was activated for 30-second

intervals and advanced slowly through the clot under directional control of the guiding catheter. In both cases, procedural time was limited to 30 minutes, and 600 ml of saline/clot mixture was removed from each patient. In one patients, an embolus was left untreated in the right pulmonary artery, and follow-up pulmonary angiography at 1 month showed persistent occlusion in this area. Both patients improved clinically, and PAP had normalized at 1 month.

Experimental studies have demonstrated the feasibility of its use in the pulmonary circulation but the clinical role of the RTC is not fully established. Mechanical thrombectomy is probably best for centrally located occlusive thrombi because the efficacy of thrombolytic therapy may be delayed because of the difficulty in delivering lytic agents to distal thrombus. Caval thrombus should be excluded before pulmonary catheterization from the femoral route. Mechanical thrombectomy techniques have no effect on reducing the incidence of recurrent emboli, and therefore caval filter placement should be considered.

OTHER TECHNIQUES

Pulmonary Artery Stenting

Patients with massive PE who do not respond to thrombolysis or catheter-directed interventions may have firm adherent clot if this has been present for 24 to 48 hours. If conventional endovascular treatment options are exhausted, pulmonary artery stent placement may offer an alternative to surgical embolectomy in critically ill patients. Haskal and colleagues reported a patient who presented with a massive PE, arterial hypotension, and cor pulmonale 12 days after coronary artery surgery.[44] The potential risks of systemic thrombolysis were considered excessive because of recent surgery, and, after a further embolic event, catheter embolectomy and intrapulmonary lysis were attempted. Pulmonary angiography at that time showed bilateral pulmonary emboli, but despite a partial response to this treatment, the patient's clinical condition remained critical. Surgical embolectomy was deemed inappropriate because of the patient's general condition, and therefore, bilateral 10-mm diameter Wallstents were placed in both lower lobar arteries. The patient's condition improved, and survival at 8 months follow-up was reported. Koizumi and associates reported a further case of major PE refractory to lytic therapy that was treated by insertion of 10-mm Wallstents into both pulmonary arterial trunks (Fig. 23–13). In this patient, the systemic arterial pressure improved immediately from 90/60 to 170/90 mm Hg, and survival was documented at 6 months follow-up.[45] Stent placement can effectively relieve pulmonary artery obstruction due to adherent

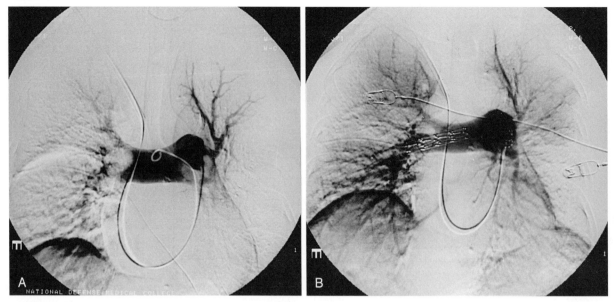

Figure 23–13. *A*, Massive pulmonary embolism associated with hypotension in a patient who failed to respond to thrombolytic therapy and catheter fragmentation. *B*, Angiogram after placement of bilateral Gianturco Z stents. The patient's blood pressure normalized immediately after stent insertion. (From Koizumi J, Kusano S, Akima T, et al: Emergent Z stent placement for treatment of cor pulmonale due to pulmonary embolism after failed treatment: Technical considerations. Cardiovasc Intervent Radiol 21:254–257, 1998.)

pulmonary emboli in critically ill patients and should be considered if other catheter-directed treatments are ineffective and the risks of surgery are considered prohibitive.

Laser Treatment

Although the use of laser energy in the treatment of pulmonary emboli has been investigated in animal experiments,[46] to date clinical use has not been reported. Although partial dissolution of central emboli was demonstrated in four swine, wall perforation was observed in one experiment and the authors concluded that coaxial systems were necessary to centralize the laser tip within the vessel and avoid endothelial damage.

Caval Filtration

Recurrent PE may occur despite adequate anticoagulation in 5 to 19% of patients[4] and usually occurs within 2 weeks of the initial embolic event. Patients receiving thrombolytic therapy appear to have a reduced risk of recurrent emboli.[12, 20] Hemorrhagic complications also may occur as a result of heparin therapy in up to 20% of cases, and a proportion of patients have contraindications to anticoagulation, including active or recent internal bleeding, active peptic ulceration, intracranial disease, coagulopathy, and pregnancy. Prophylactic caval filter placement should be considered in high-risk patients who have: free-floating IVC clot, chronic pulmonary hypertension or significantly impaired cardiorespiratory function, or evidence of DVT before orthopedic surgery. Hemorrhagic complications with anticoagulation therapy are more likely to develop in patients with malignant disease who have DVT or PE, and such patients should be considered for caval filtration. Experimental evidence suggests that septic emboli trapped within a filter can be sterilized with antibiotic treatment.[47] There are no significant contraindications to caval filter placement, but complications, although rare, may include deployment failure, IVC thrombosis, delayed structural failure, device migration or embolism to the heart or pulmonary arteries, and penetration of the caval wall and adjacent structures (see Chapter 19). Recurrent embolism may occur after filter placement, but the incidence of this is less than 5%. Long-term caval patency exceeds 90% with modern devices, and caval occlusion rates of 3 to 10% have been documented with imaging techniques.[48] More recent designs such as the Gunther Tulip filter (Fig. 23–14) are potentially retrievable with a snare device up to 2 weeks after placement. This feature may be considered an advantage in young patients with a long life expectancy. Caval filter placement is employed in up to 10% of cases of PE,[20] but recent publications have questioned the value of prophylactic therapy. Pacouret and colleagues prospectively assessed the embolic risk associated with occlusive and free-floating thrombus in 95 patients with confirmed DVT.[49] They concluded that no higher risk was associated with the presence of free-floating thrombus and that antocoagulant therapy should minimize recurrent PE in such patients. A randomized clinical trial of caval filtration and anticoagulation vs. anticoagulation alone was performed in patients with proven DVT at risk of PE.[50] The rates of recurrent venous thromboembolism, death, and major bleeding were analyzed at day 12 and at 2 years. Recurrent PE (symptomatic or asymptomatic) occurred in 1.1% of patients who received filters compared with 4.7% who were treated with anticoagulants alone. At 2 years, recurrent DVT had occurred in 20.8% of patients in the filter group and 11.6% of patients who did not receive a filter. The authors concluded that an excess of recurrent venous thrombosis offset the initial beneficial effect of caval filtration in high-risk patients with proximal DVT. No difference in mortality or other outcomes was demonstrated in this study.

SURGICAL TREATMENT

The surgical approach to pulmonary embolectomy had its beginnings with Trendelenberg's first description and experimental studies in 1908.[51] The pulmonary artery was exposed directly through a left thoracotomy while a partial occluding clamp was used to control hemorrhage from the opened artery. It was not until years later in 1924 when Kirschner, a former pupil of Trendelenberg, was first able to obtain clini-

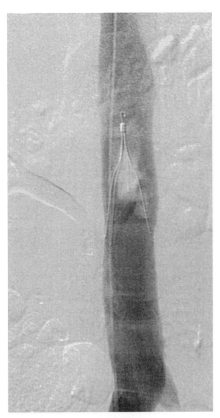

Figure 23–14. Inferior vena cavagram showing a Gunther Tulip retrievable filter containing a trapped embolus.

cal success with surgical pulmonary embolectomy.[52] In 1958, Steenburg and associates accomplished the first successful open embolectomy in the United States.[53] Later, John Gibbons, frustrated by the death of a young woman from a pulmonary embolus, embarked on a remarkable project that would change the course of thoracic surgery. He developed a machine to bypass the circulation from the heart and lungs. Although Dr. Gibbons never had the opportunity to apply his invention to the treatment of PE, Cooley and colleagues reported the first successful use of cardiopulmonary bypass and open thromboembolectomy for acute massive PE in 1961.[54]

Medical and endovascular therapy for pulmonary embolic disease has progressed rapidly over the past generation. Indeed, the standard of care in the treatment of PE is ever changing, reflective of the recent advances in the medical, endovascular, and open techniques for treating this disease. The choice of treatment depends on the nature and severity of the embolism.

Acute Pulmonary Embolism

Surgical intervention in the acute phase is reserved for the most extreme cases and often under the most desperate conditions. This is reflected in the high mortality that is associated with this approach. Accepted indications for open embolectomy include patients who:

1. Require cardiopulmonary resuscitation (CPR) for hypotension;
2. Present with acute massive embolic events who fail thrombolysis and catheter embolectomy[55];
3. Have documented right heart emboli in transit[56];
4. Have chronic pulmonary thromboembolic disease and secondary pulmonary hypertension[57–60];
5. Have a known atrial septal defect or patent foramen ovale.[61]

Boulafendis and associates reported their experience with pulmonary embolectomy in 16 patients with cardiogenic collapse and hypotension unresponsive to vasopressors or CPR.[62] They emphasize early diagnosis and management as important factors in improving the survival of patients requiring heroic measures. These investigators also advocate the use of early cardiopulmonary bypass as a means of support. Partial bypass via the femoral region (venoarterial bypass) may be used to support the patient who is hemodynamically unstable. The common femoral artery and vein are cannulated directly. This may be performed using local anesthetic but does require the presence of a perfusion technician and specialized equipment available in most institutions performing open heart surgery. Venoarterial bypass may be used to support patients during arteriography and in the operating room until the patient is converted to total bypass via a median sternotomy. Gray and colleagues demonstrated that the mortality of patients undergoing emergency open embolectomy is influenced strongly by the preoperative incidence of cardiac arrest.[63] The mortality rate was 11% in patients who had not had cardiac arrest before open embolectomy vs. 64% in patients who had cardiac arrest preoperatively. These results indicate that open embolectomy should be considered early in patients who are too ill for thrombolytic therapy or who fail to show immediate and dramatic improvement with thrombolytic therapy.

Greenfield and colleagues have demonstrated the utility of transvenous embolectomy using either the jugular or femoral approach.[29] A catheter with a suction syringe on the end is used to physically remove clot without opening the chest. This technique achieves best results when the thromboembolism has been present for less than 3 days, after which the clot may become adherent to the vascular endothelium. After 3 days, open embolectomy is recommended for removal of the adherent clot and relieving the strain on the right ventricle.[64] In the setting of acute massive PE, it is accepted to proceed first with thrombolysis. Several dosing regimens using thrombolytic agents have been proposed. Bolus therapy using urokinase or rt-PA have become popular and may be effective even in patients requiring CPR.[65–69] If thrombolysis fails or is contraindicated, embolectomy should be considered early, using either a transcutaneous or open approach.[70] Thrombolytics are very effective at reducing the embolic burden in the patient who is hypotensive and should be strongly considered as initial therapy once the diagnosis is confirmed. If the patient fails attempted thrombolysis and catheter embolectomy is unable to produce hemodynamic improvement, open embolectomy should be performed. The rapid rate by which many patients with acute massive pulmonary embolus deteriorate dictates timely decision making and treatment. Patients who experience an episode of cardiac arrest before open embolectomy have a significantly lower survival rate.[71–73]

Thrombolytic therapy may be contraindicated in the early postoperative patient in whom hemorrhage is a risk, and thus, the clinical scenario must be taken into consideration. A neurosurgical procedure within the previous 10 days should be an absolute contraindication to thrombolysis because this may precipitate dangerous intracranial hemorrhage.[73]

Chronic Pulmonary Embolic Disease

Open embolectomy is the treatment of choice for chronic pulmonary embolic disease (Figs. 23–15 and

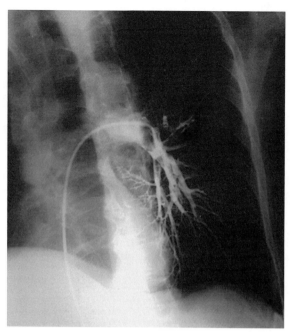

Figure 23–15. Pulmonary angiogram showing large proximal pulmonary embolus with maintained distal perfusion.

23–16). The clinical presentation of chronic embolism is far different from the acute phase, which may be an indication for surgery. These patients are often chronically ill, with persistent shortness of breath and pulmonary hypertension. Allison and associates first performed open thrombectomy for chronic occlusion of the pulmonary arteries in 1958.[74] This technique is useful in patients when occlusion involves the proximal portion of the pulmonary arterial tree and there exists a patent distal pulmonary arterial bed. Jamieson and associates reported their series of 150 patients undergoing open pulmonary thromboendar-

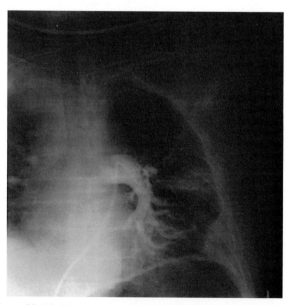

Figure 23–16. Pulmonary angiogram showing large proximal pulmonary embolus with obliterated perfusion to left upper lobe.

terectomy for relief of major vessel thromboembolic pulmonary hypertension.[57] Criteria for surgery in these cases requires (1) a surgically accessible thrombus, (2) no life-threatening concomitant disease, and (3) pulmonary vascular resistance that is greater than 300 dyne-s/cm[5]. Their technique involves a median sternotomy incision, cardiopulmonary bypass, and deep hypothermia with intermittent periods of circulatory arrest. They reported a surgical mortality rate of 8.7% with good hemodynamic and symptomatic results. The authors of this impressive report propose that additional procedures, such as repair of atrial septal defects, coronary artery bypass, or valve replacement, may be performed conveniently during the rewarming period. Although 95% of their patients were in New York Heart Association (NYHA) class III or IV preoperatively, 95% were in class II or I postoperatively. Earlier series from these investigators in similar patients report mortality rates of 16.7% and 12.6%,[58, 59] suggesting that a significant learning curve exists for this unusual and infrequently performed operation.

Moser and associates reported on 42 patients who underwent pulmonary thromboendarterectomy for chronic pulmonary hypertension secondary to chronic thromboembolic obstruction of the pulmonary arteries.[60] Mortality in the postoperative period in this group of patients was 7 of the 42 patients, or 16.7%. All the patients who died postoperatively initially presented with class IV disease. The surviving patients experienced an overall decline in pulmonary hypertension and an improvement of the degree of their heart failure. Daily and colleagues demonstrated a mortality rate of 12.6% with hypothermic circulatory arrest in a similar group of patients.[59] Each of these series represents a technical tour de force in which pulmonary arteries are opened well out into the hilum of the lung with meticulous extraction of chronic, organized thrombus under direct vision.

Echocardiographic evidence of thromboembolism within the chambers of the right heart should be treated by open embolectomy. Although there are no prospective, randomized trials addressing this issue, there is evidence to support early surgical intervention in this group of patients. Farfel and colleagues reported their use of echocardiography in 49 patients with thromboemboli trapped within the right ventricle.[56] The mortality rate was 15% in the group referred for early open thrombectomy, whereas 50% of the patients in the medically treated group died.

CONCLUSION

The diagnosis and management of PE continues to be a difficult problem because of the variable spectrum of clinical presentation, the limitations of diagnostic imaging, and the degree of hemodynamic instability present. The prognosis for most patients with minor PE, with treatment by anticoagulation, is good. Patients with massive PE and hypotension have an associated mortality rate of 25%, which increases to greater than 50% if circulatory collapse is present. Death occurs as a result of right heart failure, and modern thrombolytic therapy and supportive measures can lead to clinical and echocardiographic improvement within hours. Patients in this category who have an absolute contraindication to anticoagulation or who fail to respond to thrombolytic therapy require a more aggressive approach. Catheter-directed treatments, such as clot fragmentation, suction thrombectomy, or mechanical thrombectomy, have a role to play in this situation. If these interventions fail or are not readily available, surgical embolectomy should be considered, although the procedural mortality remains high in critically ill patients. For the patient with chronic pulmonary thromboembolic disease and pulmonary hypertension, surgical therapy remains the treatment of choice. Urgent open embolectomy also should be considered in the patient with echocardiographic evidence of thrombus within the chambers of the right side of the heart, especially in the presence of a communication between the chambers of the right and left heart. The treatment of patients with major PE who are normotensive but who have echocardiographic evidence of RV dysfunction remains controversial. Although large-scale definitive studies are awaited, data emerging from recent trials favor lytic therapy in this intermediate group of patients, provided that there are no major contraindications to thrombolysis.

REFERENCES

1. Dalen JE, Alpert JS: Natural history of pulmonary embolism. Prog Cardiovasc Dis 17:259–270, 1975.
2. Barritt DW, Jordan SC: Anticoagulant drugs in the treatment of pulmonary embolism: A controlled trial. Lancet 1:1309–1312, 1960.
3. Carson JL, Kelley MA, Duff A, et al: The clinical course of pulmonary embolism. N Engl J Med 326:1240–1245, 1992.
4. Goldhaber SZ, De Rosa M, Visani L: International Cooperative Pulmonary Embolism Registry detects high mortality rate (abstract). Circulation 96(Suppl 1):159, 1997.
5. Kasper W, Konstantinides S, Geibel A, et al: Management strategies and determinants of outcome in acute major pulmonary embolism: Results of a multicenter registry. J Am Coll Cardiol 30:1165–1171, 1997.
6. Goldhaber SZ: Thrombolytic therapy in venous thromboembolism: Clinical trials and current indications. Clin Chest Med 16:307–320, 1995.
7. Sasahara AA, Hyers TM, Cole CM, et al: The Urokinase Pulmonary Embolism Trial: A national cooperative study. Circulation 47(Suppl 1):I–1108, 1973.
8. Janata-Schwatczek K, Weiss K, Riezinger I, et al: Pulmonary embolism. II. Diagnosis and treatment. Semin Thromb Hemost 22:33–52, 1996.
9. The PIOPED investigators: Value of the ventilation/perfusion scan in acute pulmonary embolism. JAMA 263:2753–2759, 1990.
10. Kipper MS, Moser KM, Kortman KE, et al: Long term follow-up of patients with suspected pulmonary embolism and a normal lung scan. Chest 82:411–415, 1982.

11. Remy-Jardin M, Remy J, Wattinne L, et al: Central pulmonary thromboembolism: Diagnosis with spiral volumetric CT with the single breath hold technique—Comparison with pulmonary angiography. Radiology 185:381–387, 1992.

12. Konstantinides S, Geibel A, Olschewski M, et al: Association between thrombolytic treatment and the prognosis of hemodynamically stable patients with major pulmonary embolism: Results of a multicenter registry. Circulation 96:882–888, 1997.

13. Goldhaber SZ: Pulmonary embolism. N Engl J Med 339:93–104, 1998.

14. Urokinase pulmonary embolism trial Phase 1 results: A cooperative study. JAMA 214:2163–2172, 1970.

15. Urokinase-streptokinase pulmonary embolism trial Phase 2 results. JAMA 229:1606–1613, 1974.

16. Sharma GVRK, Folland ED, McIntyre KM: Long-term haemodynamic benefit of thrombolytic therapy in pulmonary embolic diseases (abstract). J Am Coll Cardiol 15:65A, 1990.

17. Goldhaber SZ, Vaughn DE, Markis JE, et al: Acute pulmonary embolism treated with tissue plasminogen activator. Lancet 2:886–889, 1986.

18. Goldhaber SZ, Kessler CM, Heit J, et al: Randomised controlled trial of recombinant tissue plasminogen activator versus urokinase in the treatment of acute pulmonary embolism. Lancet 2:293–298, 1988.

19. Goldhaber SZ, Kessler CM, Heit J, et al: Recombinant tissue plasminogen activator versus a novel dosing regime of urokinase in the treatment of acute pulmonary embolism: A randomised controlled multicenter trial. J Am Coll Cardiol 20:24–30, 1992.

20. Goldhaber SZ, Haire WD, Feldstein ML, et al: Alteplase versus heparin in acute pulmonary embolism: Randomised trial assessing right ventricular function and pulmonary perfusion. Lancet 341:507–511, 1993.

21. Jerjes-Sanchez C, Ramirez-Rivera A, Garcia M de L, et al: Streptokinase and heparin versus heparin alone in massive pulmonary embolism: A randomised controlled trial. J Thromb Thrombolys 2:227–229, 1995.

22. Verstraete M, Miller GAH, Bounameaux H, et al: Intravenous and intrapulmonary recombinant tissue-type plasminogen activator in the treatment of acute massive pulmonary embolism. Circulation 77:353–360, 1988.

23. Molina JE, Hunter DW, Yedlicka JW, et al: Thrombolytic therapy for postoperative pulmonary embolism. Am J Surg 163:375–381, 1992.

24. Tapson VF, Whitty LA: Massive pulmonary embolism: Diagnostic and therapeutic strategies. Clin Chest Med 16:329–339, 1995.

25. Schmitz-Rode T, Kilbinger M, Gunther RW: Simulated flow pattern in massive pulmonary embolism: Significance for selective intrapulmonary thrombolysis. Cardiovasc Intervent Radiol 21:199–204, 1998.

26. The UKEP Study: Multicentre trial of two local regimens of urokinase in massive pulmonary embolism. Eur Heart J 8:2–10, 1987.

27. Levine MN: Thrombolytic therapy for venous thromboembolism: Complications and contraindications. Clin Chest Med 16:321–328, 1995.

28. Goldhaber SZ: Thrombolytic therapy for pulmonary embolism. Semin Vasc Surg 5:69–75, 1992.

29. Greenfield L, Proctor MC, Williams DM, et al: Long-term experience with transvenous catheter pulmonary embolectomy. J Vasc Surg 18:450–458, 1993.

30. Timsit J-F, Reynaud P, Meyer G, et al: Pulmonary embolectomy by catheter device in massive pulmonary embolism. Chest 100:655–658, 1991.

31. Lang EV, Barnhart WH, Walton DL, et al: Percutaneous pulmonary thrombectomy. J Vasc Intervent Radiol 8:427–432, 1997.

32. Brady AJB, Crake T, Oakley CM: Percutaneous catheter fragmentation and distal dispersion of proximal pulmonary embolus. Lancet 338:1186–1189, 1991.

33. Fava M, Loyola S, Flores P, et al: Mechanical fragmentation and pharmacologic thrombolysis in massive pulmonary embolism. J Vasc Intervent Radiol 8:261–266, 1997.

34. Sharafuddin MJA, Hicks ME: Current status of percutaneous mechanical thrombectomy: Part I. General principles. J Vasc Intervent Radiol 8:911–921, 1997.

35. Yasui K, Qian Z, Nazarian GK, et al: Recirculation-type Amplatz clot macerator: Determination of particle size and distribution. J Vasc Intervent Radiol 4:275–278, 1993.

36. Uflacker R, Strange C, Vujic I: Massive pulmonary embolism: Preliminary results of treatment with the Amplatz thrombectomy device. J Vasc Intervent Radiol 7:519–528, 1996.

37. Nazarian GK, Qian Z, Coleman CC, et al: Hemolytic effect of the Amplatz thrombectomy device. J Vasc Intervent Radiol 5:155–160, 1994.

38. Schmitz-Rode T, Vorwerk D, Gunther RW, et al: Percutaneous fragmentation of pulmonary emboli in dogs with the impeller-basket catheter. Cardiovasc Intervent Radiol 16:239–242, 1993.

39. Schmitz-Rode T, Adam G, Kilbinger M, et al: Fragmentation of pulmonary emboli: In vivo experimental evaluation of two high-speed rotating catheters. Cardiovasc Intervent Radiol 19:165–169, 1996.

40. Schmitz-Rode T, Gunther RW, Pfeffer J, et al: Acute massive pulmonary embolism: Use of a rotatable pigtail catheter for diagnosis and fragmentation therapy. Radiology 197:157–162, 1995.

41. Reekers JA, Kromhout JG, Spithoven HG, et al: Arterial thrombosis below the inguinal ligament: Percutaneous treatment with a thrombosuction catheter. Radiology 198:49–53, 1996.

42. Henry M, Amor M, Porte J, et al: Percutaneous hydrodynamic thrombectomy with the Hydrolyser catheter in peripheral arteries (abstract). Radiology 201(P):139, 1996.

43. Koning R, Cribier A, Gerber L, et al: A new treatment for severe pulmonary embolism: Percutaneous rheolytic thrombectomy. Circulation 96:2498–2500, 1997.

44. Haskal ZJ, Soulen MC, Huettl EA, et al: Life-threatening pulmonary emboli and cor pulmonale: Treatment with percutaneous pulmonary artery stent placement. Radiology 191:473–475, 1994.

45. Koizumi J, Kusano S, Akima T, et al: Emergent Z stent placement for treatment of cor pulmonale due to pulmonary embolism after failed treatment: Technical considerations. Cardiovasc Intervent Radiol 21:254–257, 1998.

46. Silverman JM, Julien PJ, Adler L, et al: Use of laser energy to treat central pulmonary emboli: A preliminary report. Lasers Surg Med 13:553–558, 1993.

47. Peyton JW, Hylemon MB, Greenfield LJ, et al: Comparison of Greenfield filter and vena caval ligation for experimental septic thromboembolism. Surgery 93:533–537, 1983.

48. Lang W, Schweiger H, Hofmann-Preiss K: Results of long-term venacavography study after placement of a Greenfield vena cava filter. J Cardiovasc Surg 33:573–578, 1992.

49. Pacouret G, Alison D, Pottier J-M, et al: Free-floating thrombus and embolic risk in patients with angiographically confirmed proximal deep venous thrombosis: A prospective study. Arch Intern Med 157:305–308, 1997.

50. Decousus H, Leizorovicz A, Parent F, et al: A clinical trial of vena caval filters in the prevention of pulmonary embolism in patients with proximal deep venous thrombosis. N Engl J Med 338:409–415, 1998.

51. Trendelenburg F: Uber die operative B ehandlung der Embolie Der Lungarterie. Arch Klin Chir 86:686–700, 1908.

52. Kirschner M: Ein durch die Trendelenburgische operation geheiten fall von embolie der art pulmonalis. Archiv fur Klinische Chirurgie 133:312, 1924.

53. Steenburg RW, Warren P, Wilson RE, et al: A new look at pulmonary embolectomy. Surg Gynecol Obstet 107:214, 1958.

54. Cooley DA, Beall AC, Alexander JK: Acute massive pulmonary embolectomy under cardiopulmonary bypass. JAMA 177:283, 1961.

55. Wakefield TW, Greenfield LJ: Diagnostic approaches and surgical treatment of deep venous thrombosis and pulmonary embolism. Hematol Oncol Clin North Am, 7:1251–1267, 1993.

56. Farfel Z, Shechter M, Vered Z, et al: Review of echocardiographically diagnosed right heart entrapment of pulmonary emboli—in transit with emphasis on management. Am Heart J 13:171–178, 1987.

57. Jamieson SW, Auger WR, Fedullo PF, et al: Experience and results with 150 pulmonary thromboendarterectomy operations over a 29-month period. J Thorac Cardiovasc Surg 106:116–126, 1993, discussion 126–127.

58. Daily PO, Dembitsky WP, Peterson KL, et al: Modifications of

techniques and early results of pulmonary thromboendarterectomy for chronic pulmonary embolism. J Thorac Cardiovasc Surg 93:221–233, 1987.

59. Daily PO, Dembitsky WP, Iversen S, et al: Risk factors for pulmonary thromboendarterectomy. J Thorac Cardiovasc Surg 99:670, 1990.

60. Moser KM, Daily PO, Peterson K, et al: Thromboendarterectomy for chronic, major-vessel thromboembolic pulmonary hypertension: Immediate and long-term results in 42 patients. Ann Intern Med 107:560–556, 1987.

61. Bloomfield P, Boon NA, DeBono DP: Indications for pulmonary embolectomy. Lancet 1:329, 1988.

62. Boulafendis D, Bastounis E, Panayiotopoulos YP, Papalambros EL: Pulmonary embolectomy (answered and unanswered questions). Int Angiol 10:187–194, 1991.

63. Gray HH, Morgan JM, Paneth M, et al: Pulmonary embolectomy for acute massive pulmonary embolism: An analysis of 71 cases. Br Heart J 60:196–200, 1988.

64. Uno Y, Horikoshi S, Emoto H, et al: Successful direct embolectomy for acute massive pulmonary thromboembolism. Nippon Kyobu Geka Gakkai Zasshi. 44:1958–1961, 1996.

65. Bottiger BW, Reim SM, Diezel G, et al: High-dose bolus injection of urokinase: Use during cardiopulmonary resuscitation for massive pulmonary embolism. Chest 106:1281–1283, 1994.

66. Langdon RW, Swicegood WR, Schwartz DA: Thrombolytic therapy off massive pulmonary embolism during prolonged cardiac arrest using recombinant tissue-type plasminogen activator. Ann Emerg Med 18:678–680, 1989.

67. Bottiger BW, Reim SM, Diezel G: Erfolgreiche Behandlung einer fulminanten Lungenembolie durch hochdosierte Bolus-injektion von Urokinase wahrend der kardiopulmonalen Reanimation. Anasthesiol Intensivmed Notfallmed Schmerzther 26:29–36, 1991.

68. Scholz KH, Hilmer T, Schuster S, et al: Thrornbolyse bei reanimierten Patienten mit Lungenembolie. Deutsch Med Wschr 115:930–935, 1990.

69. Westhoff Bleck M, Gulba DC, Claus G, et al: Lysetherapie bei protrahierter kardio-pulmonaler Reanimation: Nutzen und Komplikationen. (abstract). Z Kardiol 80(suppl 3):139, 1991.

70. Verstraete M: Thrombolytic therapy of non-cardiac disorders. Baillieres Clin Haematol 8:413–424, 1995.

71. Clarke DB: Pulmonary embolectomy has a well-defined and valuable place. Br J Hosp Med 41:468, 1989.

72. Clarke DB: Pulmonary embolectomy reevaluated. Ann R Coll Surg Engl 63:18, 1987.

73. Hirschl MM, Gwechenberger M, Zehetgruber M, et al: Severe complications following thrombolytic therapy of an acute thrombosis of a prosthetic mitral valve. Clin Invest 72:466–469, 1994.

74. Allison PR, Dunnill MS, Marshall R: Pulmonary embolism. Thorax 15:273–283, 1960.

Section 4

Embolization Procedures

Chapter 24

The Endovascular Approach to Trauma

Endovascular Contributor: David D. Kidney

Endovascular therapy is an integral component in the management of vascular trauma. The availability of a trained interventional radiology team who are capable of diagnostic and therapeutic procedures is of enormous benefit to the trauma patient who has vascular injury. The number and scope of percutaneous endovascular interventions performed in the trauma setting continues to grow.[1] Arterial damage can be difficult to diagnose and treat, particularly in patients who have multiple injuries. Angiography and embolization can prevent prolonged hemorrhage or large hematomas as well as decrease transfusion requirements and obviate the need for surgery. This chapter provides an overview of the subject by looking at the indications, methods, and techniques of embolotherapy and relating them to specific vascular territories and arterial injuries.

GENERAL CONSIDERATIONS

Assessment of the patient with multiple injuries entails a complete and rapid diagnostic evaluation. The identification of vascular trauma from a wound that is actively hemorrhaging is not difficult. However, the same vessel injury in an internal location may be difficult to recognize or diagnose. In the stable patient, abdominal computed tomography (CT) and diagnostic angiography provide an accurate and precise method of documenting the extent of injury. If vascular injury is suspected, diagnostic angiography is indicated unless the patient is in need of immediate surgery.

The location of the injury is important because some anatomic locations are more difficult to access from a surgical point of view. The neck, thigh, and pelvis, areas in which complex anatomy and difficult surgical exploration add a significant risk, make angiography with the potential of embolization an excellent and reasonable alternative.[2]

The goal of the interventional radiologist in the trauma setting is, first, to diagnose or exclude arterial injury and, second, to evaluate the therapeutic op-

tions and perform endovascular procedures when indicated. In trauma patients with arterial injuries, embolization is the most commonly performed endovascular hemostatic intervention.

The introduction of covered stents (stent grafts) has added to the interventional radiologist's armamentarium, expanding the potential of performing endovascular treatment in patients with major vessel injury. Stent grafts can maintain the arterial lumen while the vessel wall injury is repaired; thus the risk of tissue injury or loss is reduced.[1]

TECHNIQUE AND MATERIALS

Diagnosis of vascular injuries is increasingly noninvasive with the use of ultrasonography (US), particularly Doppler and color Doppler imaging (CDI), spiral CT angiography (SCTA), and, to a lesser extent, magnetic resonance angiography (MRA).[3, 4] Contrast arteriography, however, remains the gold standard in the diagnosis of arterial injury, and its unique therapeutic potential makes it the diagnostic method of choice.

Diagnostic angiography is tailored to each individual case, but the technique used must be of high quality, multiplanar, and able to include all potentially injured vascular sites. The study can be carried out with the patient under local anesthesia, although a significant number of trauma patients with multiple injuries are intubated on assisted ventilation at the time of the study. Digital subtraction angiography (DSA) has critical clinical advantages over plain film angiography. Digital subtraction angiography decreases procedure time, contrast load, and radiation dose. Moreover, the availability of rapid sequence imaging, magnification, and roadmapping aid in the performance of rapid and efficient diagnostic and therapeutic examinations.

The principal arteriographic findings in trauma are extravasation, occlusion, intimal irregularity, false aneurysm formation, and early venous filling that indicates arteriovenous fistulas. Diagnostic angiography must be comprehensive, including the whole anatomic area and most document potential sites for collateral flow if embolization is being considered.[2]

The purpose of embolization in the trauma patient is to obtain rapid hemostasis in an actively hemorrhaging artery. Surgery may be avoided, or the surgeon may be presented with a more stable patient. Embolization can also prevent significant hematomas and avoid the complications of prolonged hemorrhage.

In principle, embolization should rapidly occlude the bleeding artery in a selective manner, without putting nonhemorrhaging areas at significant risk of ischemia and infarction. Therefore, the interventional radiologist who performs the procedure must have sound knowledge and experience in working with embolic agents and devices, including their mode of delivery. In addition, the interventional radiologist must understand the individual vascular anatomy of the organ or area of the patient who is being treated, with specific attention to potential tissue loss and collateral flow.

The diagnostic examination of the patient needs to be completed rapidly, with documentation of the bleeding vessel or vascular injury. If the initial angiogram fails to identify a vascular abnormality, selective studies should be performed. An aortogram does not exclude an arterial injury in the internal iliac territory and, therefore, selective internal iliac arteriography is mandatory when there are pelvic fractures and the patient is obviously bleeding. Once contrast extravasation has been seen, a suitable catheter has to be chosen if safe embolization is to be performed. Although a sheath is not absolutely necessary, it can help if a number of catheter exchanges are anticipated. Moreover, when complications occur, such as catheter occlusion or failure of embolic agents to deploy, the ability to remove the catheter and the embolic agent rapidly, without losing access, is vital. For such a procedure, an end-hole catheter is more appropriate than a side-hole catheter because, with the latter device, there is a risk of coils or other embolic agents becoming extruded through side holes at the time of deployment. A catheter with an end shaped similarly to the vessel should be chosen, because the catheter needs to be securely anchored distal to the last branch vessel for secure embolization. The interventionist needs to note the manufacturers' recommendations about the equipment to be used (e.g., polyurethane or polyvinyl catheters are not recommended for use with microcoils). Once a secure catheter position is obtained, embolization can proceed. The use of a coaxial system and microcatheters (e.g., Tracker) allows superselective catheterization and safer embolization. The size of these catheters (3 French [F]) allows superselection of bleeding vessels in solid organs, such as the retroperitoneum or the pelvis. A secure microcatheter position allows the use of Gelfoam particles or microcoils as the embolic agent. However, great care must be taken not to occlude the catheter because of its small caliber. Flushing with saline solution after each embolization is recommended.

Proximal embolization is more likely to occur in certain situations and the use of a dual-lumen balloon catheter for embolization can be helpful. With the balloon inflated proximally, the risk of proximal embolization and nontargeted involvement is much reduced. Forward flow is also reduced, aiding thrombosis and decreasing the risk of inappropriate embolus via fistulas.

The choice of embolic material is dependent on several factors, such as the operator's personal experience, the size of the vessel to be occluded, the extent of the hemorrhage, and the need for temporary vs. permanent occlusion. There are numerous embolic materials available; however, in the setting of trauma, the most commonly used materials have been either the absorbable material, Gelfoam, or vascular coils (stainless steel or platinum). The smaller particulate materials, such as Contour, are occasionally used, and sclerosing-type agents, such as absolute ethanol and isobutyl 2-cyanoacrylate, are contraindicated because of the destructive and necrotic nature of these agents.

Gelfoam is an absorbable substance, which is available in sheets or powder. It is biodegradable and its intra-arterial life is limited; recanalization is common 2 to 3 weeks after insertion. For a trauma patient, Gelfoam can be injected either as single embolic pledgets (or torpedoes), or as a mixture of smaller fragments with a contrast solution. Gelfoam pledgets, which are made up in 50% contrast solution, float. The catheter needs to be flushed with saline solution before embolization. Transparent plastic tubing may be used to connect the syringe to the catheter hub. This tubing enables the Gelfoam pledgets to be identified as they enter the catheter hub. The injection of this solution should be observed fluoroscopically to ensure forward flow of the contrast-Gelfoam mixture. Care should be taken not to inject too rapidly for fear of inducing reflux into more proximal arteries. Once blood flow is significantly reduced, the infusion of Gelfoam should be stopped. If Gelfoam is injected until flow ceases, there is a high risk of causing reflux of material into more proximal vessels with further injection. Gelfoam can be obtained in powdered form also, but this carries the risk of tissue necrosis resulting from distal embolism of tiny fragments and is not suited to the trauma setting. For embolization in the central nervous system, lumbar arteries, external carotids, or vertebral arteries, Gelfoam is also risky because of potential fragmentation and distal embolism via potential collaterals.

A disadvantage of Gelfoam in the urgent trauma setting is that it takes time to prepare, and, sometimes, a number of injections are required to achieve satisfactory embolization. In the hemodynamically unstable patient, permanent coils that can be deployed quickly and lead to more rapid hemostasis and occlusion are indicated. Coils are available in a variety of sizes and shapes and commonly have added fibers to promote thrombogenicity (Fig. 24–1). The available sizes relate to the commonly used catheters and range from .052 inch to .010 inch in various lengths. The most common shapes available are straight and coiled, but more complex spirals are now available (e.g., Tornado). In trauma patients, they are used for permanent occlusion; for rapid control, particularly in larger vessels; in sites where there is a potential for CNS embolization with smaller particles; and for fistula occlusion. The coils are made of stainless steel or platinum and can be deployed via standard diagnostic catheters or microcatheters. Stainless steel coils are less expensive and available in a wide range of sizes, but they are less radiopaque and, because they are ferromagnetic, they have the potential for movement during MR scans. On the other hand, platinum coils do not present any difficulty at MR scanning and are markedly radiopaque, but they are more expensive.

It is of critical importance to choose the correct coil size for both the catheter and the vessel to be occluded. The coil should be able to reform its shape in the vessel lumen without distal embolism or proximal displacement. The coil length is important, because longer coils may not be able to negotiate tortuous vascular anatomy if the catheter has multiple loops and curves. If coils are undersized, there is a risk of the coil's embolizing either proximally or distally. This is of particular importance when an attempt is made to occlude a traumatic arteriovenous fistula. Theoretically, the more complexly shaped coils may have an advantage in promoting thrombosis in larger vessels, fistulas, and vascular malformations. Oversizing causes difficult deployment in backing out of the catheter and potentially partial deployment in more proximal vessels, with associated dangers of nontarget embolization. Both stainless steel and platinum coils are available in either straight or complex configurations and are made more thrombogenic by the addition of synthetic fibers (see Fig. 24–1).

There are two methods of coil deployment: (1) standard push and (2) detachable coils. The latter method employs various ingenious designs that facilitate coil release when they are in the perfect position. The majority of coils used in trauma cases are deployed by means of an appropriate guide wire used as a coil pusher. Occasionally, smaller coils are flushed into position with contrast-saline solution. The coils, which are loaded into coil tubes, are advanced into the proximal end of the catheter by means of the stiff end of a guide wire. The guide wire is then reversed and the coil is advanced under direct fluoroscopic guidance. A floppy-tipped guide wire is appropriate for preventing catheter perforation or catheter pushback. The most critical coil placement is the final one. To prevent proximal migration and resultant nontar-

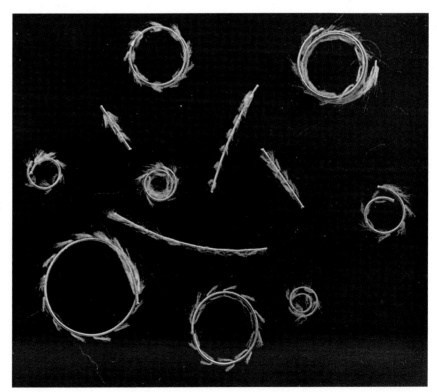

Figure 24–1. Sizes, shapes, and lengths of Hilal platinum embolization coils. (Courtesy of Cook Inc., Bloomington IN.)

get embolization, this final coil must not be placed too close to the arterial ostium. Frequently, the addition of Gelfoam either before or after the placement of coils can complete the procedure.

The great advantage of the detachable coil is that a misplaced or inappropriately sized coil can be retracted and replaced with minimal difficulty. This allows accurate placement and occlusion with use of a minimum number of coils. The GDC coil, which comes in sizes ranging from .018 inch to .010 inch, is deployed with use of an electric current to melt a solder that holds the coil onto an introducer wire. These coils are principally used by interventional neuroradiologists in the treatment of intracranial aneurysms and only rarely used in trauma. They are very expensive. Newer detachable coils are also available, which operate by various mechanical methods (e.g., Jackson detachable coil) and detachable embolization coils of both platinum and stainless steel construction.

In summary, it is vital to choose a coil of correct size and to deploy it distal to the nontarget proximal branching vessels. The appropriate number of coils should be deployed to reduce blood flow; at the same time, proximal embolization should not be risked by overvigorous placement of coils. If a coil is misplaced in a proximal vessel, it can be retrieved by a snare or an intravascular retrieval device. A coil that adheres to the catheter and cannot be safely deployed should be removed with the catheter via a vascular sheath. Further developments in coil technology are proceeding, with new materials and shapes being investigated, and a wider choice of detachable coils becoming available.

COMMON TARGET SITES FOR TRAUMA EMBOLIZATION

Pelvis

There is ample literature supporting the aggressive use of arterial embolization in the treatment of hemorrhage associated with pelvic fractures.[5, 6] The vast majority of patients are hemodynamically stable with pelvic traction,[5] but 60% of deaths that occur in patients after pelvic fractures are the result of uncontrolled hemorrhage. The number of patients who require embolization is small but significant, varying from 2 to 7%. Technical success as high as 100% has been reported.[6] Arterial hemorrhage is related to the specific type of pelvic fracture.[5] Anteroposterior compression fractures and, to a lesser extent, severe lateral compression fractures, are most commonly associated with arterial injury.

The management of these patients is challenging and controversial. Should orthopedic fixation or angi-

ography with embolization be the initial step? In the setting of a positive peritoneal lavage, should angiography pre-empt surgery? Peritoneal lavage can be false-positive in patients who have pelvic fractures caused by either extension of blood through small peritoneal injuries or presence of clinically occult intraperitoneal injuries. Either decision is largely dependent on the availability of experienced personnel in the respective fields. Successful treatment of these patients requires an aggressive and coordinated team approach by the trauma, orthopedic, and radiology services.

Arterial hemorrhage associated with pelvic fracture can be fatal. However, venous injury and bleeding at the site of fracture can also be life threatening. It has been shown that external fixation can significantly decrease hemorrhage from both venous osseous and arterial sources. External fixation is, therefore, mandatory.

Embolization in the management of traumatic pelvic bleeding is more effective than surgical proximal ligation of the injured vessel, because proximal ligation can lead to collateralization and continued hemorrhage. Embolization halts the arterial bleeding, whereas an existing hematoma can tamponade the venous hemorrhage. Technically, the procedure must commence with an abdominal aortogram, with attention paid to both lower lumbar and pelvic arteries. Access should be obtained by a right transfemoral arterial approach, or, if this area is unavailable secondary to hematoma or injury, an approach via the contralateral femoral artery or the left brachial artery can be used. It is likely that most patients who require embolization have hemorrhage that is identifiable by aortic injection. However, if a source of hemorrhage is not identified, selective angiography of both internal and external iliac arteries is indicated. The most likely source of hemorrhage should be considered. If the bony injury is predominantly on the left, the left internal iliac artery should logically be the first target. From a right common femoral approach, a Simmons shaped catheter can be used to enter the contralateral internal iliac artery. The ipsilateral internal iliac artery should also be examined with the same catheter. An oblique internal iliac artery run should be obtained and carefully analyzed for signs of extravasation, aneurysm, or early venous filling. If no source of hemorrhage is identified, it is prudent to proceed with external iliac runs and a midstream aortogram to search for a site of active hemorrhage stemming from either the lumbar artery, the spleen, or other solid organs (Figs. 24–2 and 24–3).

Once a bleeding artery is identified, embolization should proceed to control the site of bleeding quickly (Fig. 24–4). Superselective catheterization is indicated if a single bleeding point is identified. However, speed may be of the essence, particularly in a hemo-

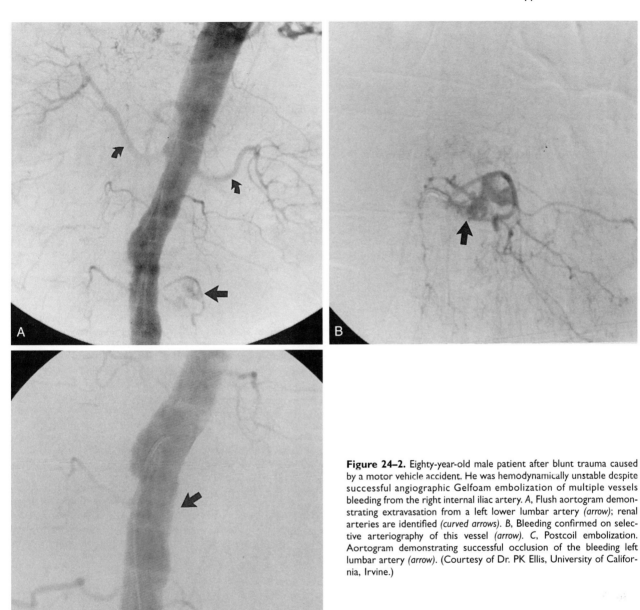

Figure 24–2. Eighty-year-old male patient after blunt trauma caused by a motor vehicle accident. He was hemodynamically unstable despite successful angiographic Gelfoam embolization of multiple vessels bleeding from the right internal iliac artery. *A,* Flush aortogram demonstrating extravasation from a left lower lumbar artery *(arrow);* renal arteries are identified *(curved arrows). B,* Bleeding confirmed on selective arteriography of this vessel *(arrow). C,* Postcoil embolization. Aortogram demonstrating successful occlusion of the bleeding left lumbar artery *(arrow).* (Courtesy of Dr. PK Ellis, University of California, Irvine.)

dynamically unstable patient. If superselective catheterization proves difficult and lengthy, more proximal embolization is acceptable. Once the catheter is securely seated within the bleeding vessel, Gelfoam pledgets can be cut, mixed with dilute contrast, and injected via the catheter. Fluoroscopic guidance is critical if reflux and nontarget embolization are to be avoided, with the decrease in arterial flow identified. It is not uncommon in pelvic injuries to have multiple sites of hemorrhage, and it may be necessary to shower the area with multiple tiny Gelfoam pledgets.

Hemorrhage associated with pelvic fracture most commonly stems from the anterior division of the internal iliac artery. When embolizing a vessel of this size or the proximal internal iliac artery, coils can be used successfully. Patients who have these problems commonly have coagulopathies caused by blood loss, with resultant administration of a large volume of blood products. Hemorrhage may, therefore, persist despite use of coils. In this situation, with coils employed as an underlying mesh or matrix, pledgets of Gelfoam can be added.

If there is active extravasation, the decision to progress to embolization is straightforward. However, if the patient has been aggressively and successfully resuscitated, an actively bleeding vessel may not be identified. Truncated vessels suggestive of transection may be seen. Careful evaluation of these vessels is

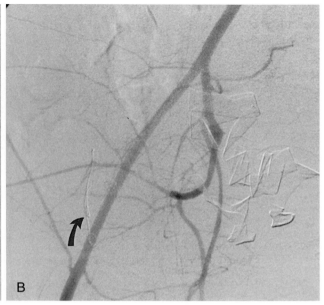

Figure 24–3. Forty-year-old male patient with pelvic fractures after blunt trauma caused by a motor vehicle accident. The patient had successful angiographic Gelfoam embolization of a right internal iliac artery branch; however, he remained hemodynamically unstable. *A,* Right external iliac angiogram *(arrow),* demonstrates extravasation *(outline arrow),* from the inferior epigastric artery *(curved arrow).* *B,* After selective coil embolization of the right inferior epigastric artery *(arrow).* Arteriography demonstrates occlusion with no further extravasation, and the patient became hemodynamically stable. (Courtesy of Dr. L-S Deutsch, University of California, Irvine.)

necessary and, if the suspicion of a transected or injured vessel is high, then prophylactic embolization may be indicated.

A patient who is stable at the time of injury, without clinical evidence of hemorrhage or vascular injury, can months or years later manifest a trauma-related vascular problem. Pseudoaneurysms and fistulas may take months to form and become clinically apparent; therefore, they should be considered in the differential of newly appearing masses in otherwise healthy patients who have a history of trauma (Fig. 24–5).

Penile cavernous arterial injury as a result of blunt peroneal injury can give rise to high-flow priapism. This is a specific entity whose presentation can be delayed by hours or days, and it is best treated by

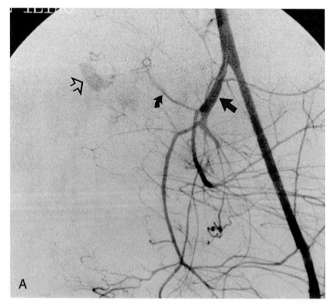
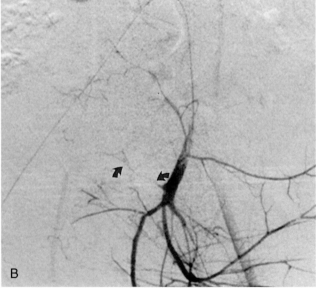

Figure 24–4. Thirty-year-old female patient with multiple pelvic fractures after blunt trauma caused by a motor vehicle accident. *A,* Selective left internal iliac arteriogram with the catheter tip in the proximal internal iliac artery *(arrow)* demonstrates active extravasation *(outline arrow)* from a lateral sacral artery *(curved arrow),* a branch of the anterior division of the internal iliac artery. *B,* Similar projection demonstrates occlusion of the offending branch and no further extravasation *(curved arrows).* The patient stabilized hemodynamically and required no further blood products.

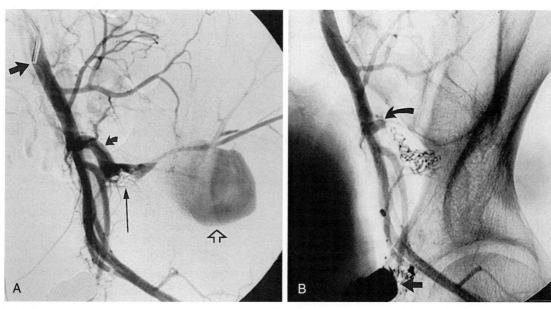

Figure 24–5. Thirty-one-year-old male patient one year after pelvic gunshot wounds demonstrates a left buttock soft tissue mass. Pseudoaneurysm was not considered in the differential. When surgical exploration with biopsy revealed the pseudoaneurysm, urgent angiography was performed. *A*, Angiogram of the left internal iliac artery *(arrow)* demonstrates a pseudoaneurysm *(outline arrow)* of the superior gluteal artery *(curved arrow)*, which remains patent despite a number of coils *(long arrow)*. *B*, After deployment of more stainless steel coils and packing with Gelfoam, hemostasis was finally obtained and the patient stabilized *(curved arrow)*. Note bullet fragments *(arrow)*.

embolotherapy.[7] Embolization with autologous clot or administration of Gelfoam to the ipsilateral common penile artery has a high success rate, with preservation of erectile function.[7]

Complications of embolization in the pelvis are the result of overzealous embolization, overlapping embolizations or, if the patient has underlying vascular disease, embolization of vessels without due consideration of collateral flow. Impotence is a potential complication, and informed consent should include this possibility. As a significant number of these patients have other potential causes for impotence (e.g., urethral rupture, widespread peroneal venous injury, urologic lumbosacral plexus injury), it may not be possible to link later impotence to arterial embolization. In life-threatening hemorrhage, the risk of impotence is a secondary consideration.

Abdomen and Retroperitoneum

Post-traumatic intra-abdominal hemorrhage is most commonly the result of splenic or hepatic injuries, or both.[8] In the past, diagnosis required peritoneal lavage, and surgical treatment with a combination of packing, suturing of the injured organ, or arterial ligation. There is now a positive emphasis on the need for control of hemorrhage and organ preservation. The trend toward conservative nonoperative management of splenic and hepatic injuries goes hand-in-hand with the developments in CT diagnosis and the increased and broadened role of radiology, with both diagnostic and therapeutic interventions.

Hepatic trauma can result in parenchymal hemorrhage, pseudoaneurysms, hemorrhage into the biliary system, or arterial venous fistulas, especially if the injury involves penetrating trauma. Approximately 20% of patients who have blunt abdominal trauma and 25% of patients who have penetrating abdominal wounds have hepatic parenchymal involvement.[8] A number of authors have attempted to grade CT injury and correlate it to management and treatment outcome. Most conclude that CT does competently diagnose patients who have hepatic parenchymal injury but is a poor predictor of patients who develop complications requiring surgery. Becker and associates concluded that the surgical decision to explore the patient must be based on clinical circumstances, including suspicion of other abdominal injuries rather than on a CT grading. Angiography should be reserved for patients who have CT evidence of vascular injury, be it active extravasation, pseudoaneurysm, or fistula formation.[9] Results of a large multicenter study suggest that nonoperative management of blunt hepatic injury is the treatment modality of choice in hemodynamically stable patients regardless of injury grade or size of hemoperitoneum.[10] The study recommends a follow-up CT scan and appropriate intervention if a vascular abnormality is then diagnosed.

Injuries to the liver are divided evenly between penetrating and blunt trauma. If active bleeding is diagnosed by celiac angiography, the portal vein patency and the vascular branching pattern of the hepatic artery must be determined if a decision to embolize is made. Angiographic findings are most typically those of extravasation or pseudoaneurysm formation.

Fistulas may occur between the hepatic artery and either the portal circulation, the hepatic venous radicals, or the biliary radicals. An abnormal vessel with evidence of truncation, transection, or vessel injury, without active extravasation, may also be seen.

As with all trauma embolization, hemostasis must be obtained rapidly, efficiently, and with minimal tissue loss. With the development of microcatheters and the growing experience of a significant number of interventional radiologists in superselective hepatic arterial catheterization for other reasons (e.g., chemoembolization), superselective catheterization and embolization are now more frequent and achievable options. Because the liver has a dual blood supply (two thirds coming from the portal vein), once patency is documented, the hepatic artery is safe to embolize. Surgical management in the past has included main hepatic arterial ligation proximal to the gastroduodenal artery takeoff, and its benefit is most likely the result of the decreased arterial pressure, which can result in hemostasis. Embolization has the advantage of superselection and proximal and distal occlusion. Technically, the catheter tip must be beyond the origin of the cystic artery so that the gallbladder is not rendered ischemic.

The most common embolic agents used are Gelfoam, or, occasionally coils, particularly in the setting of fistulas or larger pseudoaneurysms (Fig. 24–6). Hepatic arterial embolization, in the hands of an experienced interventional radiologist, is a feasible, safe, and realistic alternative to surgery, with a technical success rate of 88%.[8]

The spleen is the most frequently injured solid organ in blunt abdominal trauma. Its surgical removal leads to postsplenectomy sequelae, particularly in children. Nonsurgical conservative management of blunt splenic injury has long been accepted in children and is increasingly used in adults. In theory, CT in the hemodynamically stable patient should be able to select patients who have a high risk of delayed complications. Initial efforts to grade splenic injuries by CT showed poor correlation. Angiographic features of active hemorrhage were advocated as predictors for intervention, whether surgical or endovascular.[11]

Modern spiral CT-based grading systems, which pay particular attention to evidence of vascular injury in the form of extravasation or aneurysm formation, are more specific.[12–14] Studies have concluded that splenic vascular abnormalities seen on spiral CT are associated with clinical failure of conservative management of blunt splenic injuries. A review of 524 patients demonstrated a significant reduction in conservative management failures to 6%, with aggressive angiographic management of CT-diagnosed vascular abnormalities.[12, 13]

Splenic angiography must be performed via a selective end-hole catheter. There are two organ-specific considerations in splenic embolization. The presence of significant collateral flow to the spleen does allow proximal splenic artery embolization with maintenance of flow to the splenic tissue via collateral pathways (e.g., short gastric and pancreatic branches). Theoretically, the decrease in arterial pressure to the spleen as a whole decreases active hemorrhage and causes hemostasis. Care should be taken to note any other vascular injury in the location before embolization so as to ensure that collateral arterial supply is maintained. If main splenic artery embolization is indicated, a single stainless steel coil can be deployed in the main splenic artery, most commonly between the ostia of the pancreatic magna and dorsal pancreatic arteries. More distal deployment is acceptable. The second alternative is superselective embolization to the bleeding point, with use of a coaxial microcatheter. This is particularly indicated if a pseudoaneurysm or hematoma has been identified on a preprocedure CT scan. Once a microcatheter is safely seated at the level of the vascular abnormality, embolization can be performed with use of Gelfoam or platinum microcoils. If diffuse bleeding from the injured spleen is seen, Gelfoam injection distally and proximal coil insertion within the main splenic artery decrease oozing. It has not yet been determined whether these patients retain significant splenic function.

Other intra-abdominal arteries are less frequently injured. Mesenteric or gastric arteries can be injured during blunt or penetrating trauma. These injuries typically have associated hollow viscous injuries that necessitate surgical management. If angiography is requested and significant contrast extravasation is seen from a mesenteric or gastric vessel, temporary occlusion of the injured arteries with a balloon catheter before definitive vascular surgical management may stabilize and improve the patient's chances of survival.

The kidney is the most common major organ injured in the retroperitoneum. Fifty percent of renal vascular injuries are iatrogenic and commonly caused by percutaneous biopsy or nephrostomy. Noniatrogenic trauma is most commonly a penetrating rather than a blunt injury. Most renal injuries are identified and assessed by CT scanning. Many retroperitoneal hematomas are caused by diffuse renal capsule bleeding. This is often self-limiting and, if the patient is stable, can be ignored. However, if intervention is necessary, surgical exploration can be difficult, particularly if a large retroperitoneal hematoma is present, and a significant number of patients who have renal injury go on to have either a heminephrectomy or total nephrectomy. As evidenced by arteriography, the bleeding point is often single and can be treated successfully by embolization (Fig. 24–7).

The goal of embolization in the management of

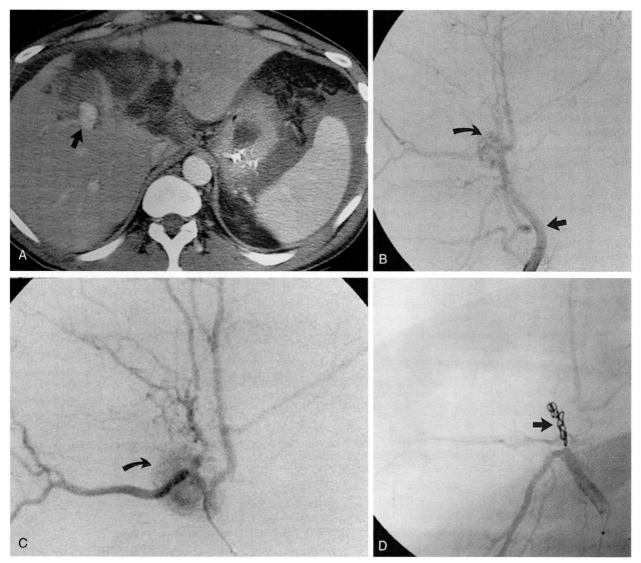

Figure 24–6. Forty-four-year-old male patient 72 hours after a motor vehicle accident. The patient has had blunt abdominal trauma that is being managed conservatively for a liver laceration. An overnight drop in hemoglobin necessitated an emergent contrast computed tomographic (CT) scan. *A,* Axial contrast CT scan of the liver demonstrates a vascular blush in the region of the right hepatic artery *(arrow). B,* Selective right hepatic arteriography *(arrow)* (an aberrant vessel from the superior mesenteric artery) demonstrates active extravasation and pseudoaneurysm formation *(curved arrow). C,* Superselective angiogram with a microcatheter confirms a pseudoaneurysm *(curved arrow). D,* Using a microcatheter and platinum microcoils *(arrow),* the aneurysm was successfully catheterized and embolized without clinically significant tissue loss. Patient did not require surgery or further blood products.

vascular injury in the renal territory is to minimize the amount of tissue and organ loss while obtaining hemostasis. Because the renal arteries are end arteries without potential for collateralization, particular attention and effort must be given to superselect the injured vessel. On selective angiography, the presence of pseudoaneurysm, arteriovenous fistulas, or active extravasation may be identified. The most frequently used embolic materials are Gelfoam and coils. Gelfoam probably minimizes the volume of tissue loss and maximizes the potential for recanalization (see Fig. 24–7).

The next most commonly injured retroperitoneal structures are the lumbar arteries. From a surgical point of view, the identification of bleeding lumbar arteries and their management is difficult when there is an expanding retroperitoneal hematoma. Selective angiography and embolization are feasible and significantly reduce morbidity and mortality for the patient (see Fig. 24–2). The angiographer must always be aware of and consider the possibility of arterial supply to the spinal canal. Care should be taken when performing lumbar artery embolization proximal to L2–L3, where the artery of Adamkiewicz originates. Selective catheterization of the bleeding lumbar artery should be performed, and attention should be paid to the vessel branches. If possible, the catheter should always be advanced distally beyond the origin of any possible spinal branch. This is an ideal vessel to occlude with Gelfoam. However, if the patient is rap-

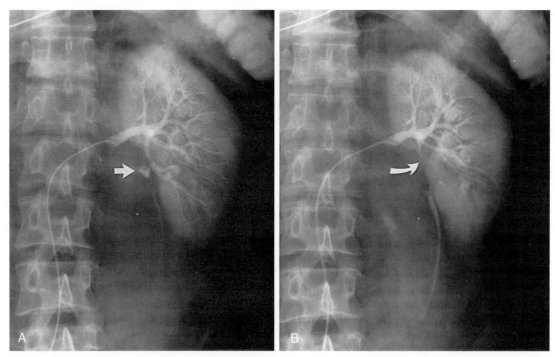

Figure 24–7. Forty-three-year-old male patient after penetrating trauma with screwdriver to left flank. *A*, Selective left renal angiogram demonstrates active extravasation from an inferior pole artery *(arrow)*. *B*, Selective right renal angiogram after coil embolization *(arrow)* demonstrates hemostasis and occlusion of the offending vessel *(curved arrow)*. (Courtesy of Dr. L-S Deutsch, University of California, Irvine.)

idly exsanguinating, a rapidly placed coil may be lifesaving.

Duodenal, pancreatic, and adrenal arteries are rarely angiographically identified as the source of hemorrhage in abdominal trauma. If they are identified, use of basic principles of embolization is a treatment option.

Thorax

Traumatic arterial injury in the thorax can be managed by endovascular techniques. Most reports concern penetrating injury to the internal mammary arteries. There are reports of endovascular treatment for aortic injury, particularly stent graft repair, in which the injury is associated with pseudoaneurysm.[1] Arterial injuries, particularly in penetrating trauma, can involve other vessels, such as the intercostal vessels, but these are difficult to approach and catheterize.

The internal mammary artery has numerous collaterals, and before embolization, an attempt must be made to isolate the abnormal segment to prevent continued bleeding from the collateral flow. Coils are preferred to Gelfoam in this clinical situation because their deployment can be precise, and if there is continued hemorrhage, they can be traversed and other embolic agents can be deployed. The coils should be placed either at the site of injury or both distally and proximally to the bleeding point to isolate the abnormal segment.

Extra caution should be employed if there is embolization of intercostal arteries, because spinal arteries can originate from these vessels. Before embolization it is also advisable to advance the catheter deeply into the intercostal artery. It is advisable to use microcoils rather than Gelfoam or particles to reduce the risk of distal or proximal emboli.

Head and Neck

The majority of vascular neck injuries are penetrating in nature. Both blunt and penetrating injuries can result in vascular trauma and hemorrhage in the face. The anatomy is complex, and surgical exploration is demanding.

Management of patients with such injuries remains controversial. Some surgeons advocate mandatory neck exploration once the platysma has been penetrated. Others advocate a more conservative approach. Angiography remains the gold standard of diagnostic procedures. There is some support for combining physical examination and color Doppler imaging as a method of noninvasive evaluation of patients who have penetrating neck trauma.[3] The balance, however, seems to be tipping toward more liberal use of angiographic assessment of these patients, and the majority of authors now agree with angiographic evaluation, particularly in patients who have zone III penetrating trauma.[15] Zone III is defined as extending from the mandibular angle up to and including the skull base and is an exceptionally difficult surgical area. It is, therefore, well suited to angiographic exploration and treatment. A number of institutions extend the use of angiography to include any hemodynamically stable patients who have penetrating neck injury that has involved the platysma. In a large series of 401 patients, Sclafani and Sclafani found the most commonly injured vessels to be the internal carotid, the vertebral, and the external carotid arteries, respectively.[16]

Diagnostic and therapeutic interventions in the head and neck region, because of proximity to the central nervous system, are challenging and carry significant risk. However, with careful and meticulous attention to detail, a significant number of life-threatening neck and facial vascular injuries can be managed by endovascular means.

Excellent diagnostic angiography is critical before embolization in the territory of the carotid or vertebral arteries. The presence or absence of potential external to internal carotid collaterals and completeness of the circle of Willis must be established. It is rare to perform embolization in the carotid territory. In most situations, an attempt is made to repair the injured internal carotid artery if it is patent. The rare exceptions include a surgically inaccessible lesion (e.g., at the base of the skull), where embolization may become a therapeutic option if a complete circle of Willis has been demonstrated. If antegrade flow is not present in the internal carotid artery and the patient is neurologically intact, embolization can be performed instead of surgical ligation.

In the external carotid artery, embolization can play a major role in the treatment of intractable oronasal and craniofacial bleeding (Fig. 24–8). Embolization

is well established as a definitive treatment in spontaneous intractable nasal bleeding and is just as effective in treatment of traumatic oronasal bleeding.[17] In patients who have severe craniofacial injury, the typical indication for angiography is continued active hemorrhage, an expanding hematoma, or both. Before embolization, potentially dangerous anastomoses between the external and internal carotid arteries must be demonstrated. Accurate positioning of the catheter is critical to prevent any possibility of reflux of embolic material. There is excellent collateralization between the left and right external carotid arterial territories. Proximal and distal occlusion are vital, although bilateral embolizations may be necessary to ensure complete hemostasis. Again, the most common embolic materials are Gelfoam and coils, although polyvinyl alcohol particles have been used successfully.

When vertebral arterial injury is identified as a pseudoaneurysm, an arteriovenous fistula, or a contrast extravasation, complete evaluation of the posterior cerebral circulation is necessary before embolization. In a small number of patients, the contralateral vertebral artery may be hypoplastic or absent, or it may terminate in the posterior inferior cerebellar artery. This precludes the option of sacrificing the injured vessel. Atresia and hypoplasia of the vertebral artery occur in approximately 3% and 2% of patients (left and right side, respectively). Vertebral artery injuries are difficult to access surgically. In the presence of a normal contralateral vertebral artery and normal vertebrobasilar vasculature, it is rare for embolization of a single vertebral artery to result in any significant neurologic deficit.[18] Given the continuity of the vertebral artery to the vertebrobasilar system, Gelfoam and

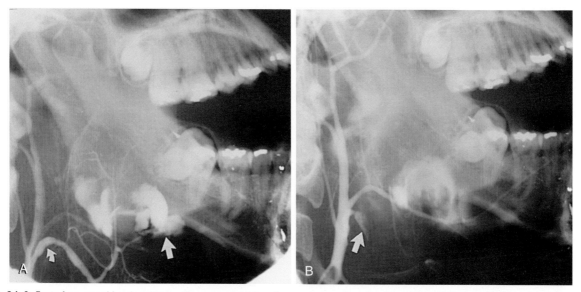

Figure 24–8. Forty-four-year-old male patient with penetrating injury from stab wound to the right neck, with an expanding hematoma in zone III. *A,* Selective external carotid arteriography demonstrates active hemorrhage *(arrow)* from the lingual artery *(curved arrow). B,* After Gelfoam embolization, arteriography demonstrates occlusion of the target vessel *(arrow).*

other particulate materials are contraindicated. Coils are the embolic agents of choice (Fig. 24–9). An attempt should be made to isolate the injured segment by embolizing proximally and distally to the bleeding point, thus preventing the distal ipsilateral vertebral artery from filling retrogradely from the contralateral vertebral artery, which would result in further hemorrhage. If the lesion cannot be traversed for placement of coils distal to the injury and there is persisting hemorrhage from the contralateral vertebral artery, the choice is between surgical distal ligation or a somewhat technically challenging embolization from the contralateral vertebral artery via the basilar artery. Fortunately, this is rarely necessary, because it is usually possible to traverse the injured segment, insert coils, and prevent any focal continued hemorrhage.

The use of angiography and embolization in penetrating neck injuries, particularly in patients with zone III injuries, has a low morbidity and high success rate.[15–18]

Extremities

In the extremities, arterial injury typically results from penetrating trauma. The axilla and thigh are excellent sites for endovascular diagnosis and management. In the lower extremity, a number of reports have documented the usefulness of embolization in the treatment of active bleeding from the profunda femoris artery. A contralateral approach to the injured extremity is advantageous and selective diagnostic angiography is mandatory. Given the excellent collateral circulation, it is also advisable to attempt to isolate the focal bleeding point to prevent rebleeding from collateral flow. This can be done either by proxi-

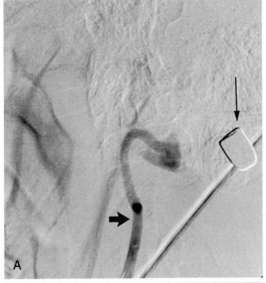

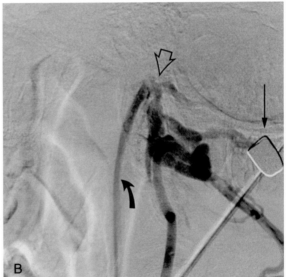

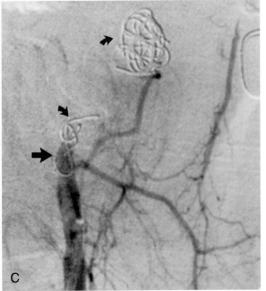

Figure 24–9. Fourteen-year-old male patient post-gunshot wound to the left neck with expanding hematoma without neurologic deficit. *A, B,* Selective left vertebral arteriography *(arrow)* demonstrates a high-flow arteriovenous fistula from the vertebral to the internal jugular vein *(curved arrow).* Note bullet fragments *(long arrow).* After confirmation of right vertebral artery patency and adequate filling of the left posteroinferior cerebellar artery, coil embolization was performed *(outline arrow). C,* After embolization with coils *(curved arrows)* arteriogram demonstrates complete occlusion of the vertebral artery *(arrow)* without collateral filling of the aneurysm. Patient stabilized and no further surgical intervention was needed. (Courtesy of Dr. H. Pribram, University of California, Irvine.)

mal and distal coil deployment or by coil deployment at the level of the abnormality. More distal vascular injury can be managed with embolization and sacrifice of the vessel (Fig. 24–10). The clinician must also remember that occasional vascular abnormalities stemming from trauma may not appear for days or weeks after the initial episode.

Advances in stent graft technology allow treatment of damaged larger vessels, occluding arteriovenous fistulas, and pseudoaneurysms. With a stent graft, arterial lumen patency can be maintained while the vessel wall injury is repaired. An attempt to fill a large aneurysm sac with coils demands a significant volume of embolic material and may cause a physical deformity. Therefore, if stent grafting is not used, a single, well-placed proximal coil can thrombose the feeding vessel rather than large numbers of coils within the pseudoaneurysm (Fig. 24–11).

In the upper extremity, most vascular injuries are the result of penetrating trauma, predominantly stab and gunshot wounds. There is a large collateral circulation around the shoulder from the axillary and subclavian arteries. Transcatheter embolization of small branch vessels is relatively safe (Figs. 24–11 and 24–12). The importance of secure anchoring of the catheter and slow speed of embolization cannot be overemphasized if Gelfoam is used, particularly in the extremities, where reflux and nontarget embolization can lead to disastrous consequences.

COMPLICATIONS OF EMBOLIZATION

The major complication of embolization is tissue or organ loss distal to the embolized vessel. Nontarget tissue embolization from reflux of embolic material, coil misplacement, or coil loss are preventable by meticulous attention to technique. To prevent these complications, an appreciation of the target vascular anatomy is vital before proceeding with embolization. In the presence of multiple vascular injuries or in patients who have had previous vascular surgery, particular attention must be paid to the potential collateral flow. Sacrificing the profunda femoris artery in a 20-year-old with pristine vessels may be a reasonable decision to save the patient's life; however, in a 70-year-old with peripheral vascular disease, it may not be. It is rarely acceptable to perform embolization in areas where there is no collateral flow. Embolizing in overlapping vascular territories is also contraindicated because of the increased risk of ischemic necrosis. An attempt must always be made to be as superselective as possible. However, in critical situations, where there are multiple bleeding sites, this can be difficult. For example, in pelvic fractures, where there are multiple bleeding sites from the internal iliac arteries causing profound hemodynamic instability, it may be an option to embolize the proximal internal iliac artery or, alternately, to attempt multiple super-

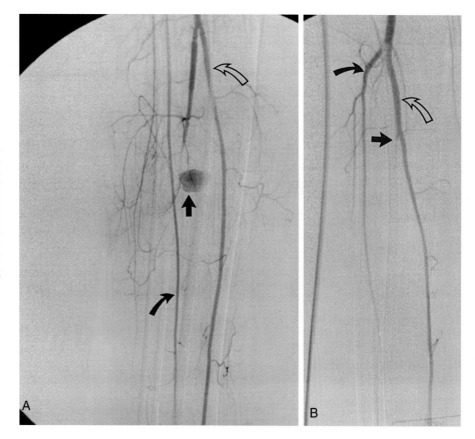

Figure 24–10. Thirty-two-year-old fireman two weeks after explosive injury to the right lower extremity, who came to the hospital with active bleeding. *A,* Right lower extremity arteriogram demonstrates pseudoaneurysm of the peroneal artery *(arrow)* with wide patency of the anterior *(curved arrow)* and posterior tibial arteries *(outline arrow). B,* After embolization with Gelfoam, there was complete occlusion of the peroneal artery *(arrow).* (Courtesy of Dr. R Malek, University of California, Irvine.)

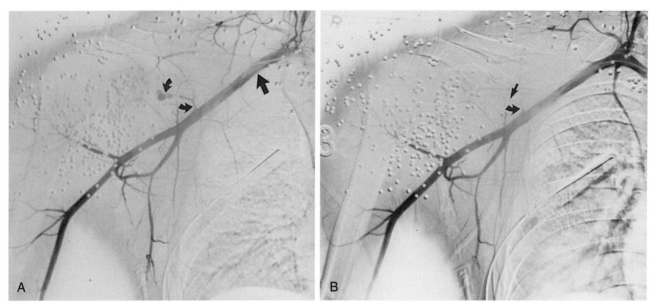

Figure 24–11. Thirty-three-year-old male patient after gunshot wound with birdshot. *A,* Selective right subclavian arteriogram *(arrow)* demonstrates active extravasation from the dorsal scapular artery *(curved arrows). B,* After coil angiogram *(arrow),* there was occlusion of the bleeding vessel *(curved arrow).* (Courtesy of Dr. L-S Deutsch, University of California, Irvine.)

selective embolizations. Both procedures may well be lifesaving. Given patent contralateral internal iliac vessels and common femoral arterial patency, speedy proximal embolization and stabilization of the patient may be the best choice, because it is unlikely to result in significant tissue loss.

The second principal complication is nontarget embolization. This is most commonly a technical error and, therefore, extreme care is always warranted, with mandatory meticulous attention to detail. Safe, stable positioning of the catheter must be achieved before attempted embolization. Whether using Gelfoam or

coils, the aim of embolization is to significantly decrease forward arterial flow initially, and the temptation to pack the artery too rapidly or vigorously must be avoided. Vigorous packing of the bleeding artery with embolic agents can lead to flushing of this material into more proximal vessels, with potentially disastrous results. When traumatic arteriovenous fistulas are being treated, the embolic material size is critical because of the potential of venous through-flow to the systemic venous system. When coils are used, appropriate coil sizing is critical. A coil too small for the arterial lumen can be backflushed into the more

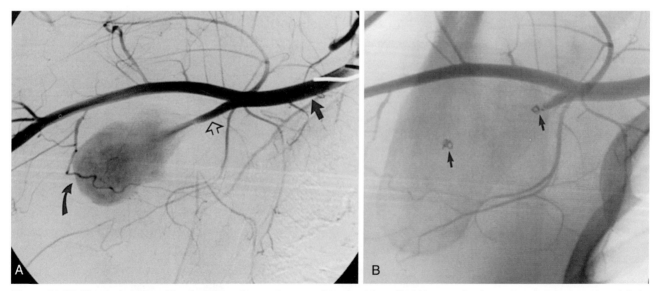

Figure 24–12. Twenty-three-year-old male patient after gunshot wound to the right axilla with expanding hematoma. *A,* Selective right subclavian arteriogram *(arrow)* demonstrates active extravasation and pseudoaneurysm *(curved arrow)* formation from the right subscapular artery *(outline arrow). B,* Selective embolization with coils demonstrates occlusion of the target vessel *(arrows).*

proximal vessels or be carried distally. If the coil chosen is too large, there is potential for the proximal end of the coil segment to cover the arterial orifice and risk thrombosis in more proximal vessels. At the end of the procedure, careful angiography should be performed, because too forceful an injection of contrast can also result in reflux of embolic material.

There is hope that the future availability and wider variety of detachable coils will facilitate more accurate placement, decrease a number of complications, and reduce overall procedure times.

Pain, fever, nausea, and vomiting can occur as part of a postembolization syndrome and are managed symptomatically.

CONCLUSION

There is little doubt of the important contribution made by diagnostic angiography and therapeutic embolization in the treatment of patients who have traumatic vascular injuries. Embolization is not the ultimate or definitive therapy for trauma patients with vascular injury. However, it can occasionally replace surgery or become a presurgical aid in the stabilization of the patient. The availability of an interventional radiologist to perform these techniques on an emergency basis is vital. In addition, pseudoaneurysms and fistulas often appear weeks to months after the initial injury, and surgical procedures can then be avoided.

In summary, embolization can play a critical role in the management of the patient who has vascular trauma. This role continues to expand as technical advances, such as microcatheters, stents, and stent grafts, become available and further extend the territory and injuries that can be treated.

REFERENCES

1. Ohki T, Veith FJ, Marin ML, et al: Endovascular approaches for traumatic arterial lesions. Semin Vasc Surg 10:272–285, 1995.
2. Ben-Menachem Y: Bleeding from trauma. Interventional Radiology. New York, Thieme Medical Publishers, Inc., 1990, pp 378–395.
3. Demetriades D, Theodorou D, Cornwell E III, et al: Penetrating injuries of the neck in patients in stable condition. Arch Surg 130:971–975, 1995.
4. Nunez D Jr, Rivas L, McKenney K, et al: Helical CT of traumatic arterial injuries. AJR Am J Roentgenol 170:1621–1626, 1998.
5. Ben-Menachem Y, Coldwell DM, Young JWR, et al: Haemorrhage associated with pelvic fractures: Causes, diagnosis, and emergent management. AJR Am J Roentgenol 157:1005–1014, 1991.
6. Agolini SF, Shah K, Jaffe J, et al: Arterial embolization is a rapid and effective technique for controlling pelvic fracture haemorrhage. J Trauma Injury Infect Crit Care XX:395–399, 1997.
7. Bastuba MD, Saenz de Tejada I, Dinlenc CZ, et al: Arterial priapism: Diagnosis, treatment and long-term follow-up. J Urol 181:1231–1236, 1994.
8. Schwartz RA, Teitelbaum GP, Katz MD, et al: Effectiveness of transcatheter embolization in the control of hepatic vascular injuries. J Vasc Intervent Radiol 4:359–365, 1993.
9. Becker CD, Gal I, Baer HU, et al: Blunt hepatic trauma in adults: Correlation of CT injury grading with outcome. Radiology 201:215–220, 1996.
10. Pachter HL, Knudson MM, Esrig B, et al: Status of nonoperative management of blunt hepatic injuries in 1995: A multicenter experience with 404 patients. J Trauma Injury Infect Crit Care 40:31–38, 1996.
11. Becker CD, Spring P, Glotti A, et al: Blunt splenic trauma in adults: Can CT findings be used to determine the need for surgery? AJR Am J Roentgenol 162:343–347, 1994.
12. Cocanour CS, Moore FA, Ware DN, et al: Delayed complications of nonoperative management of blunt adult splenic trauma. Arch Surg 133:619–625, 1998.
13. Gavant ML, Schurr M, Flick PA, et al: Predicting clinical outcome of nonsurgical management of blunt splenic injury: Using CT to reveal abnormalities of splenic vasculature. AJR Am J Roentgenol 168:207–212, 1997.
14. Davis KA, Fabian TC, Croce MA, et al: Improved success in nonoperative management of blunt splenic injuries: Embolization of splenic artery pseudoaneurysms. J Trauma Injury Infect Crit Care 44:1008–1015, 1998.
15. Demetriades D, Chahwan S, Gomez H, et al: Initial evaluation and management of gunshot wounds to the face. J Trauma Injury Infect Crit Care 45:39–41, 1998.
16. Sclafani AP, Sclafani SJA: Angiography and transcatheter arterial embolization of vascular injuries of the face and neck. Laryngoscope 106: 168–173, 1996.
17. Komiyama M, Nishikawa M, Kan M, et al: Endovascular treatment of intractable oronasal bleeding associated with severe craniofacial injury. J Trauma Injury Infect Crit Care 44:330–334, 1998.
18. Yee LF, Olcott EW, Knudson MM, et al: Extraluminal, transluminal, and observational treatment for vertebral artery injuries. J Trauma Injury Infect Crit Care 39:480–486, 1995.

Chapter 25 Visceral Embolization

Endovascular Contributor: James E. Jackson
Surgical Contributor: *Bruce Stabile*

The success of endovascular therapy of acute gastrointestinal (GI) hemorrhage depends on three main factors: the ability to define the bleeding site; the source of hemorrhage; and the experience of the angiographer.

The only direct angiographic sign of GI hemorrhage is contrast extravasation into the bowel lumen (Fig. 25–1), and this may be absent on initial selective angiograms because of the intermittent nature of acute GI bleeding. Superselective studies may provoke bleeding, but in many cases one must rely on other "indirect" angiographic signs, such as the presence of an aneurysm or the demonstration of early venous return, vascular irregularity, vascular truncation, neovascularity, or varices. Very rarely, no abnormality is detected in a patient with a proven endo-

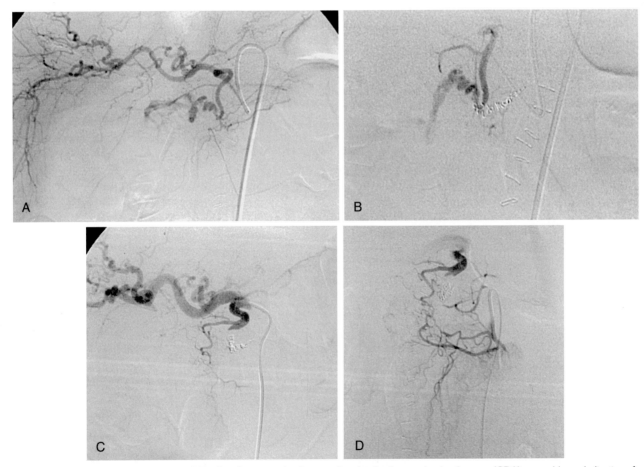

Figure 25–1. Massive upper gastrointestinal bleeding due to peptic ulcer eroding the distal gastroduodenal artery (GDA) treated by embolization after failed endoscopic therapy. *A,* Common hepatic arteriogram demonstrates massive contrast medium extravasation from the distal gastroduodenal artery. *B,* The right gastroepiploic artery has been occluded with microcoils beyond the point of contrast medium extravasation. *C,* Coils have been placed within the GDA immediately proximal to the point of hemorrhage, thus isolating the defect in the arterial wall from the circulation. *D,* A selective inferior pancreaticoduodenal artery angiogram performed after embolization confirms the complete isolation of the distal GDA from the circulation.

scopic source of hemorrhage, and in such cases, "prophylactic" embolization of the apparently normal vessels supplying the vascular territory in question may be justified.

The role of digital subtraction angiography (DSA) in patients with acute GI bleeding is worth discussing at this point. The superior contrast resolution of DSA when compared with conventional film in most cases makes the detection of contrast extravasation into the bowel lumen much easier, although care must be taken to ensure that movement is kept to a minimum to avoid the generation of confusing DSA artifacts. Bowel peristalsis is abolished easily by the use of antiperistaltic agents, but patient respiration may be more difficult to control, especially in a group of individuals who are often unwell. A useful technique in such patients is the acquisition of images during normal respiration with multiple masks being obtained before the injection of contrast. A suitable mask then is available for most of the images acquired after a subsequent contrast injection. Subtle vascular irregularity may be missed because of the inferior spatial resolution of DSA, but this is rarely a significant problem as long as magnified selective images are obtained.

DSA becomes even more important and is almost mandatory during embolization procedures because it allows rapid angiography to be performed with immediate review. There is no doubt that DSA has made embolization considerably safer both for this reason and because it allows the use of smaller quantities of contrast agent in patients who are often very unwell.

When contrast extravasation is seen, the vessel from which it originates may not be obvious on the initial study. This is particularly true when the bleeding source overlies the epigastrium because branches of the pancreaticoduodenal arcade, the right and middle colic arteries, and occasionally the jejunal arteries all may be superimposed at this site. In such cases, superselective studies of these vessels will be required to define accurately the hemorrhaging vessel.

When the source of hemorrhage is a large vessel such as the main trunk of the gastroduodenal artery owing to, for example, its direct erosion by an adjacent duodenal ulcer (see Fig. 25–1) or a pancreatic pseudocyst, curative embolization should be relatively straightforward because embolization coils (or detachable balloons) can be placed on either side of the arterial defect, thus completely isolating it from the circulation. When bleeding is from numerous small bleeding points, however, as occurs with hemorrhagic gastritis, treatment by embolization is less likely to be successful because it may be difficult to reduce the perfusion pressure in all the vessels from which the bleeding is occurring because of the presence of a very rich collateral arterial supply to the upper GI tract.[1]

The angiographer performing embolization should be experienced in selective and superselective catheterization and also have a sound knowledge of the normal vascular anatomy of the territory that is being occluded. By way of a simple example, a pseudoaneurysm of the gastroduodenal artery causing GI bleeding should be treated (as mentioned previously) by isolating it entirely from the circulation, and this may be best performed by placing coils on either side of its neck. If however, only the proximal gastroduodenal artery is occluded, then the pseudoaneurysm continues to fill, usually via the inferior pancreaticoduodenal artery arising from the superior mesenteric artery, but other sources may include the left gastroepiploic artery arising from the distal splenic artery and the transverse pancreatic artery arising from the dorsal pancreatic artery. If these potential collateral supplies are not appreciated by the angiographer, it is easy to see how such a lesion, which is often only visible on the celiac axis (and not the superior mesenteric) arteriogram, might be treated inappropriately and unsuccessfully by proximal occlusion of the gastroduodenal artery alone. The neglect of simple attention to anatomic considerations such as these is probably the most common cause of failure to control bleeding by embolization.

INDICATIONS

Embolization is undoubtedly the procedure of choice for traumatic (accidental and iatrogenic) arterial bleeding from the liver and also should be the procedure of choice for aneurysmal disease of the visceral arteries in the upper GI tract.[2, 3] The surgical treatment of many of these lesions is associated with considerable morbidity and mortality, although embolization can be performed successfully in most patients under local anesthetic.

Severe bleeding from benign duodenal or gastric ulcers usually is managed successfully by a combination of endoscopic methods and medical therapy, but the occasional patient continues to bleed. The choice between embolization and surgery in these individuals often depends on the expertise that is available. There is no doubt, however, that embolization controls hemorrhage in most of these individuals if it is performed correctly. If surgical oversewing is attempted first and bleeding continues, then embolization still may be successful.

CONTRAINDICATIONS

There are few, if any, absolute contraindications to embolization of acute upper GI hemorrhage, other than those related to angiography itself, such as an uncorrectable, severe bleeding diathesis or history of a severe reaction to contrast medium. Particular care should be exercised, however, in those patients who have severe visceral arterial atheromatous disease, in those who have undergone (failed) vasopressin therapy, or in those who have a history of upper GI surgery involving the ligation of normal branches supplying the stomach. These individuals are at an increased risk of gastric infarction after embolization.

TECHNIQUE

Following are certain general principles that are common to all embolization procedures.

The operator should:

1. Have a thorough knowledge of the normal and variant anatomy;
2. Always ensure a secure catheter position before injection of embolic material;
3. Always perform good quality angiograms of the vascular territory to be embolized so that the anatomy is appreciated fully;
4. Choose the right embolic agent for the lesion being embolized;
5. Always mix nonradiopaque embolic material with contrast medium before injection;
6. Inject embolic material in small aliquots and under continuous fluoroscopy to ensure that it is passing only into those vessels that need to be embolized;
7. Perform diagnostic angiograms at various times during embolization to assess the progress of the vascular occlusion, being careful not to overinject embolic material to obviate the possibility of embolic material refluxing around the catheter into normal vessels;
8. Always stop in case of uncertainty and perform a check arteriogram.

Liver

Persistent, severe hemobilia, whether secondary to liver biopsy, percutaneous biliary intervention, or accidental trauma, is almost always from an intrahepatic arterial source. Arteriography often shows arterial irregularity or aneurysm formation (Fig. 25–2), and there may be active contrast extravasation into the biliary tree. Other angiographic signs include the presence of arterioportal shunting (see Fig. 25–2), and, in the case of liver biopsy or biliary intervention, needle tracks may be visible as linear opacities.

Conventional surgical therapy of hemobilia consists of the ligation of extrahepatic arterial branches, and this may be successful in some individuals be-

cause it decreases perfusion pressure to the site of the arterial injury. In a significant number of patients, however, bleeding persists because of the rapid development of an intrahepatic arterial collateral supply, and this is the principal reason why embolization should be considered as the first-line treatment in these individuals.

Embolization has a higher success rate and a lower morbidity than surgery for the control of an arterial source of hemobilia because of the technique's ability to identify and then superselectively catheterize and occlude the abnormal intrahepatic vessel(s) while preserving the surrounding normal hepatic arterial supply. The hepatic arterial branches are not end-arteries and occlusion must, therefore, be performed *across* the vascular abnormality (aneurysm, arterioportal communication) to prevent its continued supply *via* more distal intrahepatic collateral branches. In some cases, this requires the use of a coaxial catheter (see Fig. 25–2).

The choice of embolic agent depends partly on operator preference and partly on the anatomy of the abnormality being occluded. A pseudoaneurysm of a small peripheral intrahepatic artery can be treated very successfully by placing metallic microcoils on either side of its neck. Alternatively, the vessel can be "packed" with small particulate embolic material such as polyvinyl alcohol or absorbable gelatin sponge. This has the same effect as distal and proximal embolization with coils but is perhaps more likely to produce localized liver ischemia and embolization of adjacent normal hepatic arterial branches because of the inadvertent reflux of embolic material.

Stomach and Duodenum

Causes of gastric and duodenal bleeding include peptic ulcers, pancreaticoduodenal arcade aneurysms (duodenum), neoplasms (usually gastric, duodenal, or pancreatic in origin) and iatrogenic causes such as biopsy and surgery. Although the extensive vascular supply to this portion of the bowel makes embolization safer, it also means that the successful control of hemorrhage is more difficult because an occlusion created in one vessel supplying a bleeding point is bypassed rapidly through collateral channels that may be difficult or impossible to catheterize. The treatment of gastric or duodenal bleeding, therefore, often requires the use of small particulate embolic material to achieve a relatively distal block.

Persistent bleeding from gastric or duodenal peptic ulceration that does not respond to local transendoscopic therapy often is caused by erosion of the ulcer into an adjacent large artery, usually a branch of the left gastric artery, the main trunk of the gastroduodenal artery (see Fig. 25–1), or the retroduodenal

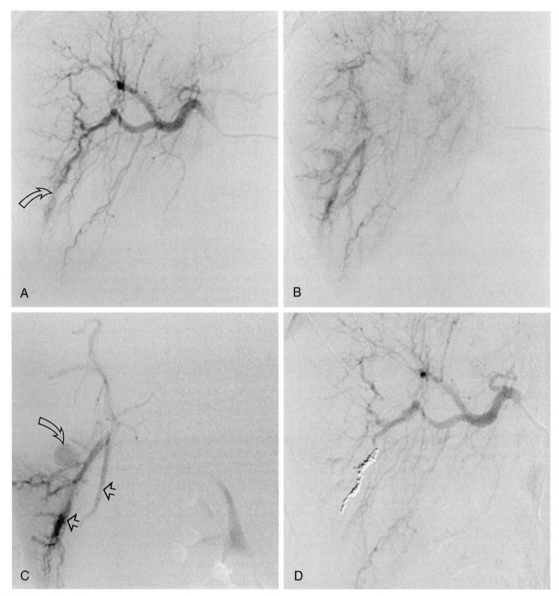

Figure 25–2. Hemobilia after liver biopsy treated by embolization. *A, B,* A selective right hepatic arteriogram demonstrates an area of arterioportal shunting in the periphery of the right lobe of the liver *(arrow). C,* A coaxial catheter has been introduced into the distal right hepatic arterial branch immediately proximal to the arterioportal fistula. Portal venous filling *(straight arrows)* and an arterial pseudoaneurysm *(curved arrow)* are seen. *D,* Microcoils have been placed within the peripheral arterial branch beyond and proximal to the arterioportal communication. A postembolization right hepatic arteriogram demonstrates occlusion of the fistula. (From Coley SC, Jackson JE: Pulmonary arteriovenous malformation. Clin Radiol 53:396, 1998.)

(posterior superior pancreaticoduodenal) artery. Such patients can be successfully treated operatively, and this may be combined usefully, in certain individuals, with a more definitive antiulcer surgical procedure (e.g., highly selective vagotomy).

Alternatively, and particularly in those patients who are poor candidates for general anesthesia because of old age, poor lung function, severe hypovolemia, and so forth, angiography and embolization can be performed.[4]

The method of embolization performed depends on the angiographic findings. When a defect is demonstrated within the wall of a large artery with brisk contrast extravasation, occlusion is performed on ei-

ther side of the abnormality, usually with metallic coils in the manner described previously under the management of hemobilia (see Fig. 25–1). The results of this form of treatment in terms of arresting bleeding are likely to be extremely good.

More difficulty is experienced when the source of bleeding is seen to be a small peripheral branch of the left gastric artery or pancreaticoduodenal arcade or when no angiographic abnormality is visualized. In such cases, an attempt should be made to reduce the perfusion pressure to the vascular territory around the ulcer while avoiding the occlusion of normal visceral vessels; the superior mesenteric artery is at particular risk during occlusion of the pancreatico-

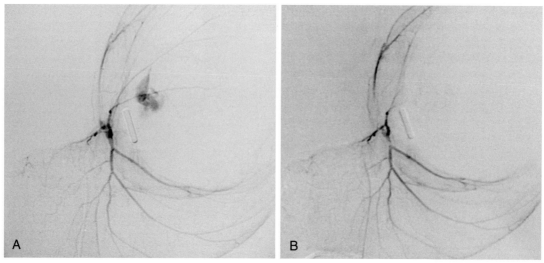

Figure 25–3. Bleeding from left gastric artery caused by acute ulcer treated by selective embolization. A, Selective left gastric arteriogram demonstrates active contrast medium extravasation from a branch of the left gastric artery. The bleeding vessel was catheterized selectively and embolized with polyvinyl alcohol. B, Selective left gastric arteriogram postembolization demonstrates complete occlusion of the bleeding vessel.

duodenal arcade. Embolization of duodenal bleeding, therefore, may involve occlusion of the distal anterior superior pancreaticoduodenal artery, the distal retroduodenal artery, and the proximal right gastroepiploic artery with metallic coils (to protect normal vessels) before the injection of small particulate polyvinyl alcohol into the gastroduodenal artery.

During embolization of a small branch of the left gastric artery, highly selective catherization is desirable so that small particulate emboli can be introduced directly into the bleeding vessel (Fig. 25–3). If this is not performed, rebleeding is not uncommon because of collateral supply from the short gastric arteries (which are usually extremely difficult or impossible to catheterize selectively), the right gastric artery, or the right and left gastroepiploic arteries.

Aneurysmal disease of the pancreaticoduodenal arcade may be associated with acute or chronic pancreatitis (which is discussed subsequently) or may be secondary to atheromatous disease. The latter combination of atheromatous disease and aneurysm formation often is associated with hypertrophy of the pancreaticoduodenal vessels either as a result of atheromatous stenosis of the celiac axis or, more commonly, compression of the celiac axis origin by the median arcuate ligament of the hemidiaphragm. Whatever the cause, embolization is the procedure of choice because the aneurysm can be isolated successfully from the circulation in most cases. When there is associated arterial hypertrophy of the pancreaticoduodenal arcade, embolization usually is performed most easily via the inferior pancreaticoduodenal artery arising from the proximal superior mesenteric or first jejeunal arteries.

The stomach and duodenum may be involved by primary tumors (e.g., carcinoma, stromal cell), by

neoplasms in adjacent viscera (e.g., pancreas, gallbladder), or by secondary deposits (e.g., breast, melanoma). The treatment of choice must be surgical resection, but this may be neither possible nor in the patient's best interest because of tumor size or the presence of extensive metastatic disease, in which case embolization may be attempted.

Those tumors most commonly referred for embolization because of severe, unremitting bleeding are inoperable primary leiomyosarcomas and large vascular pancreatic neuroendocrine tumors.

In the authors' experience, one is more likely to find a focal arterial abnormality on angiography in patients with a history of intermittent severe bleeds rather than those who have a persistent slow or moderate "ooze." When a focal lesion is seen, particularly if contrast extravasation also is demonstrated, embolization can be directed toward this abnormality even if there is a large amount of surrounding neovascularity. In many patients, however, the only angiographic abnormality visualized is that of extensive neovascularity, often with evidence of venous occlusion and resultant variceal formation. In such cases, one can only aim to try and reduce perfusion pressure to the site of bleeding by occlusion of the tumor vessels. Great care must be taken to avoid the embolization of adjacent normal structures that may be infiltrated by the tumor.

The results in this group of patients are not good, and although some improvement may be obtained, this is usually short lived.

Pancreas

Acute and chronic pancreatitis may be associated with severe GI bleeding because of the involvement of adjacent vessels.[2-6] The splenic vein commonly is occluded with resultant segmental portal hypertension, causing splenomegaly and gastric varices. If this causes GI bleeding, a cure can be achieved by splenectomy, and this operation often can be combined with pancreatic surgery if this is indicated. A "medical splenectomy," performed by embolization of the splenic artery, has been reported with successful results in some patients with segmental portal hypertension. This procedure is not without risk because of the possible complications of splenic abscess formation or splenic rupture, and the likely subsequent growth of the spleen could cause rebleeding. Beneficially, however, if a subtotal splenic embolization is performed, some functioning splenic parenchyma are left in situ, and the patient's susceptibility to infection, especially by *Pneumococcus* species, should not be increased.

Arterial erosion, either by pancreatic enzymes during an episode of acute pancreatitis or by pressure from an adjacent pseudocyst in chronic pancreatitis, may cause life-threatening hemorrhage. This may occur into the pancreatic duct (hemosuccus pancreaticus) (Figs. 25–4 and 25–5), in which case each episode of bleeding usually is associated with severe epigastric pain, directly into the duodenum or into the retroperitoneum. The surgical treatment of acutely bleeding peripancreatic pseudoaneurysms is associated with mortality rates of 16% for lesions around the pancreatic tail and up to 50% for those around the pancreatic head. The results of embolization are much better than this, and there is little doubt, therefore, that this method of treatment should be the procedure of choice, with surgery reserved for those patients in whom embolization is not possible.

Embolization should, once again, be aimed at isolating the involved vessel from the circulation, and this is usually possible by placing metallic coils on either side of its neck (see Figs. 25–4 and 25–5). Filling the pseudoaneurysm with metallic coils should be avoided, if possible, for several reasons. First, the cavity is likely to expand during embolization because of the radial force of the coils (owing to the presence of intraluminal thrombus and the lack of a true wall), with the potential risk of rupture; coils subsequently may migrate from the pseudoaneurysm

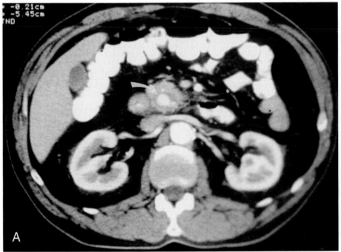

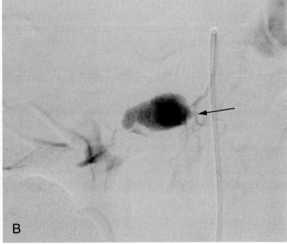

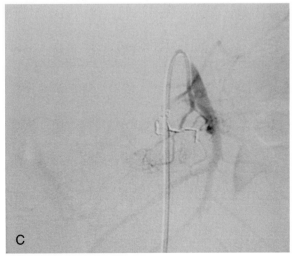

Figure 25–4. A 53-year-old man with a history of chronic pancreatitis and several episodes of acute upper gastrointestinal bleeding associated with severe epigastric pain radiating through to his back. *A,* Contrast-enhanced axial computed tomography (CT) scan through the abdomen demonstrates a brightly enhancing cavity within the uncinate process of the pancreas consistent with a pseudoaneurysm *(arrow)*. *B,* A selective inferior pancreaticoduodenal artery (IPDA) angiogram demonstrates contrast opacification of the pseudoaneurysm contrast medium extravasation into the pancreatic duct, through the ampulla, and into the duodenum. The origin of the pseudoaneurysm from a branch of the IPDA has been "arrowed." *C,* No further contrast medium extravasation is seen after embolization across the neck of the pseudoaneurysm with platinum microcoils. (From Coley SC, Jackson JE: Pulmonary arteriovenous malformation. Clin Radiol 53:396, 1998.)

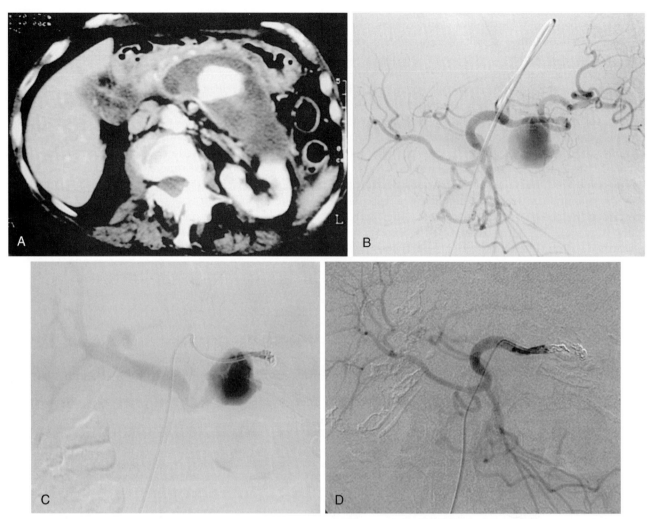

Figure 25–5. A 66-year-old woman with episode of acute pancreatitis complicated by massive upper gastrointestinal bleeding via the pancreatic duct. *A,* A contrast-enhanced axial CT scan demonstrates an enhancing cavity within a large peripancreatic fluid collection consistent with a pseudoaneurysm within a pancreatic pseudocyst. *B,* Celiac axis arteriogram demonstrates the pseudoaneurysm arising from the proximal splenic artery. Later images in the same run showed that this aneurysmal cavity also communicated directly with the splenic vein as shown in *C.* The splenic artery immediately beyond the pseudoaneurysm has been occluded with metallic coils. A check arteriogram to confirm occlusion of the "back door" shows the communication of the pseudoaneurysm with the portal venous system. *D,* Coils have now been placed immediately proximal to the pseudoaneurysm, thus isolating it from the circulation. Splenic supply was preserved via the left gastric artery. (From Beard JD, Gaines PA: Vascular and Endovascular Surgery: A Volume in a Companion to Specialist Surgical Practice. London, WB Saunders, 1998.)

cavity into the gut or pancreatic duct; and satisfactory control of hemorrhage is less likely because the coils often change their position as the surrounding thrombus resolves.

Bleeding Beyond the Ligament of Treitz

In most individuals, angiography is used to localize the source of GI hemorrhage in this part of the bowel and treatment is then surgical. One of the major reasons for this is that the finding of contrast extravasation on angiography is very nonspecific and the underlying cause of the bleeding often is not known. Thus, an acutely bleeding small bowel angiodysplastic lesion may have the same appearance as an actively bleeding avascular small bowel tumor or an area of ulceration caused by vasculitis or inflammatory bowel disease. In some patients, however, the use of arterial embolization or the localized infusion of vasopressin may be useful, either as a definitive treatment in patients in whom there is a confident diagnosis or as a means of stabilizing the patient before later surgery. Although embolization in the upper GI tract is generally very safe, beyond the ligament of Treitz there is a higher risk of gut infarction because of the presence of a poor collateral circulation. The vasa recta are those branches arising from the marginal artery that supply the gut, and these vessels do not anastomose with one another. After piercing the intestinal wall, they become mural trunks and then subdivide into numerous vessels that freely anastomose with one another along the length of the intestine and across the antimesenteric border. These anastomoses are relatively large in the jejunum and become smaller, although more numerous, in the ileum and are even less well developed in the colon.

The aim of embolization should be to reduce the perfusion pressure to the area of contrast extravasation, thus allowing hemostasis while preserving the collateral circulation to the gut wall. Some interventionists believe that embolic occlusion should be performed at a point proximal to the vasa recta because the transmural anastomoses are not sufficiently large to definitely maintain gut viability. Others believe that the vasa recta may be occluded safely with microcoils.[7] What is certain, however, is that small particles that pass into the mural trunks must be avoided because gut infarction almost certainly will ensue. For this reason, if particles are to be used, a size of 355 to 500 μm polyvinyl alcohol is most commonly used. Great care must be taken to inject only a small quantity of particles at any one time because occlusion may occur rapidly, with resultant spill of further particles into important adjacent collateral vessels. This may be difficult to judge, and for this reason, the authors prefer to use platinum microcoils positioned within the final intestinal arcade or the vasa recta (because these devices can be placed accurately) as long as a sufficiently distal catheterization can be achieved with a coaxial catheter (Fig. 25–6).

VASOPRESSIN

The use of intra-arterial vasopressin for acute upper or lower GI hemorrhage gained widespread accep-

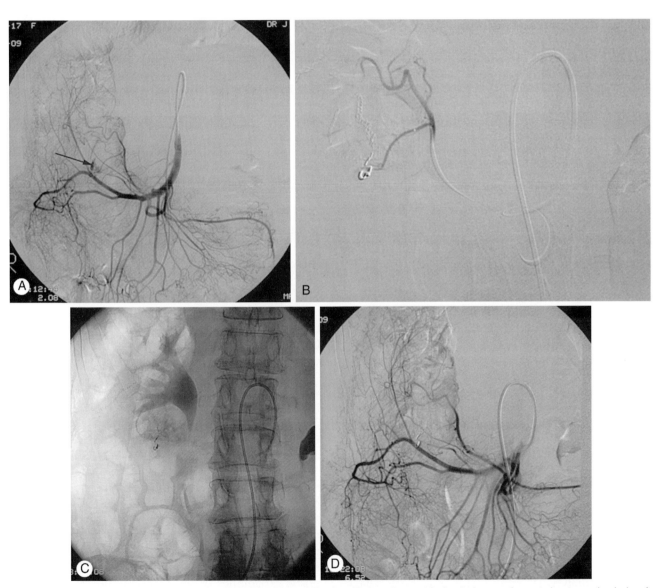

Figure 25–6. A 66-year-old woman presenting with brisk perirectal bleeding 10 days after a right hemicolectomy for an ischemic cecal volvulus. *A,* Main superior mesenteric arteriogram demonstrates brisk contrast medium extravasation *(arrow)* from the region of the ileocolic anastomosis. *B,* A distal branch of the right colic artery supplying the anastomotic bleeding point has been catheterized selectively and embolized with platinum microcoils. *C,* Control film after embolization demonstrates the microcoils adjacent to the surgical staples at the ileocolic anastomosis. *D,* Postembolization superior mesentric arteriogram shows no further bleeding and preservation of adjacent gut vessels. The patient had no further bleeding and was discharged home 3 days later. (From Beard JD, Gaines PA: Vascular and Endovascular Surgery: A Volume in a Companion to Specialist Surgical Practice. London, WB Saunders, 1998.)

tance in the United States in the 1970s and 1980s but was never as popular in the United Kingdom and Europe. Although it often successfully controls hemorrhage during the infusion itself, rebleeding is common when the agent is discontinued, and there are a number of serious side effects associated with its use. Cardiovascular complications of arrhythmia, bradycardia, hypertension, cardiac arrest, myocardial infarction, visceral infarction[8, 9] and vascular occlusion at the puncture site have all been reported and may occur in up to 43% of patients. In addition to these complications, there is the problem of maintaining the selective catheter position during the infusion. For these reasons, the use of vasopressin has fallen out of favor in many centers. In the authors' own institution, if the patient is not a surgical candidate, intra-arterial vasopressin no longer is used, and embolization is performed as the procedure of first choice.

COMPLICATIONS

The possible complications of angiography and selective catheterization include puncture site hematoma, contrast medium reaction, and arterial dissection, and there is a higher incidence of such problems in patients undergoing complex interventional procedures than in those undergoing simple diagnostic studies. The reasons for this are obvious and include the fact that patients are usually unwell and are often not very cooperative; they also may be hypovolemic and have abnormal clotting mechanisms as a result of repeated transfusions.

Complications specific to the embolization procedure are those of inadvertent occlusion of a normal vascular territory (which should be avoidable if one adheres to the general principles of embolization outlined previously), bowel infarction, and persistent bleeding.

Arterial embolization above the ligament of Treitz is associated with a low risk of ischemic complications because of the extensive collateral vascular supply to this area. Occlusion of the left gastric arterial branches can be performed with fairly small-caliber particulate materials in the treatment of localized or diffuse gastric hemorrhage, with little fear of causing necrosis of the stomach unless there has been previous surgery in the upper abdomen, which might interfere with the potential collateral vascular supply (e.g., gastric surgery or splenectomy), or when there is severe atheromatous disease. Similarly, small branches of the pancreatico-duodenal arcades may be occluded safely when treating duodenal hemorrhage.

Poor embolization technique in which proximal arterial occlusion is performed without distal occlusion is a common cause of recurrent bleeding. This lapse in technique usually results in continued retro-grade perfusion of the bleeding site via collateral vessels and makes subsequent treatment by further embolization extremely difficult or impossible because of a lack of direct vascular access to the lesion.

CONCLUSIONS

Embolization should be the procedure of choice for arterial bleeding that occurs from the liver and for peripancreatic aneurysmal disease. The results of this procedure for these indications are extremely good, provided that the embolization is performed with a meticulous technique. Embolization of other bleeding sites in the upper GI tract usually is reserved for those patients who are not candidates for surgery. Despite the fact that these patients are often in poor condition, embolization may prove very useful, either by providing definitive treatment or by stopping bleeding for a short time, thus allowing the patient's condition to improve before later surgery. Embolization below the ligament of Treitz is performed most commonly as a life-saving procedure in those individuals who are unfit for surgery. It is associated with an increased risk of gut ischemia and infarction but is often successful in this group of sick patients. It may be a curative procedure or may allow stabilization of the patient for subsequent definitive surgery.

SURGICAL PERSPECTIVE

Introduction

Much progress has been achieved in the management of GI bleeding since its first clinical descriptions more than 5000 years ago. Definition of the anatomy of the GI tract and the vascular system and the elucidation of the pathophysiology of hemorrhagic shock allowed the development of strategies to resuscitate the hypovolemic patient and surgically correct the bleeding lesion. Barium contrast radiography and general anesthesia were important contributions that enabled physicians and surgeons to more effectively localize and treat the wide variety of causes of GI bleeding.

More recently, new and sophisticated invasive techniques have been introduced that not only allow direct demonstration of bleeding sites and vessels, but also provide opportunities for immediate, targeted therapeutic intervention to control bleeding. Both upper and lower GI fiberoptic endoscopy and visceral angiography have expanded dramatically the diagnostic capabilities of the clinician and improved patient outcomes. Although the overall mortality rate from GI bleeding has been in the range of 8% to 10%, a recent survey of more than 1200 cases documented fatal outcomes in only 2.1%.[10] Approximately three fourths of the patients had upper GI bleeding sites, with duodenal and gastric ulcers being the most common sources. Among lower GI bleeders, diverticula were the most frequent cause. Almost one half of all patients received endoscopic therapy consisting of injection sclerotherapy, electrocoagulation, heater probe, rubber band ligation, or laser phototherapy. Visceral arteriography and transcatheter hemostatic therapies were used in only a minority of cases, but the overall impact of nonsurgical therapy was such that only 7.1% of patients required surgery.

Upper Gastrointestinal Hemorrhage

Whenever GI hemorrhage is believed to be emanating from proximal to the ligament of Treitz, or whenever the issue is in doubt, flexible esophagogastroduodenoscopy should be the initial invasive diagnostic procedure. The accuracy rate of the technique is approximately 95%, and the overall complication rate is less than 1%.[11] Upper endoscopy has the capability of not only identifying the site of bleeding but also the underlying pathologic lesion, such as peptic ulceration, neoplasm, mucosal tears and erosions, and vascular malformations. Endoscopy also permits estimation of bleeding rate and rebleeding potential, and offers a variety of therapeutic interventions appropriate for specific lesions.[12]

The role of visceral arteriography in upper GI bleeding is relatively limited. In the uncommon circumstance in which upper endoscopy is unavailable or inconclusive and the bleeding lesion is believed to be proximal to the ligament of Treitz, celiac and superior mesenteric arteriography can be extremely helpful. However, the patient most likely to be diagnosed by this technique is one who is actively bleeding. Therefore, adequate volume resuscitation, red blood cell replacement, and hemodynamic monitoring must be assured before and throughout the patient's stay in the angiography suite. With an active bleeding rate of 0.5 ml/min or greater, extravasated angiographic contrast is likely to be seen. Lower rates of bleeding and intermittent bleeding decreases the sensitivity of the study.[13] Despite these limitations, angiodysplastic lesions, particularly arteriovenous malformations, often can be detected in the absence of active bleeding by virtue of their characteristic vascular architecture and premature venous filling. Most importantly, whether active bleeding is present or not, arteriography has the capability for immediate therapeutic embolization of the feeding vessel.[14]

Because of its ready availability, effectiveness, low risk, and low cost, therapeutic upper endoscopy is the first-line treatment for most patients with upper GI hemorrhage. Angiographic transcatheter embolization plays a secondary therapeutic role and is best reserved for instances of arterial bleeding in which endoscopic intervention has failed or is not available. Angiographic embolization should not, however, be attempted if there is persisting hemodynamic instability after appropriate resuscitation efforts and failed endoscopic therapy. Unstable patients with ongoing upper GI hemorrhage should be taken promptly to the operating room for surgical exploration and direct suture control or excision of the bleeding lesion.

Peptic ulceration of the stomach and duodenum remains the most common cause of upper GI bleeding. In most instances, ulcer bleeding is self-limited. Endoscopic control has proven efficacy and cost-effectiveness in patients with severe hemorrhage and high likelihood of recurrent hemorrhage.[15, 16] Angiographic transcatheter embolization of the bleeding artery has been used in ulcer hemorrhage with a success rate of greater than 50%, whereas intra-arterial infusion of vasopressin has been distinctly less effective.[17] Because the collateral blood supply to the stomach and duodenum is very rich, embolization rarely is complicated by ischemia.

With the recognition that most peptic ulcers are caused by either *Helicobacter pylori* infection or the use of nonsteroidal anti-inflammatory drugs, the necessity for definitive ulcer surgery has come into question. Because most ulcers can be cured by medical means, a more aggressive nonoperative approach to bleeding ulcers may be justified. Embolization of actively bleeding gastroduodenal or gastric arteries resistant to endoscopic control may become employed more frequently as an alternative to salvage surgery for life-threatening ulcer hemorrhage.

Gastric hemorrhage from diffuse mucosal inflammation and superficial erosions is rarely severe, but life-threatening hemorrhagic erosive gastroduodenitis associated with shock, sepsis, multiple trauma, major burn, or head injury still occurs as a component of the multiple-organ failure syndrome. In such cases, selective intra-arterial infusion of vasopressin has been reported to stop the bleeding in up to 80% of patients, but recent experience is limited[18] for the reasons stated previously. Operative gastric devascularization has been used as an alternative to total or near-total gastrectomy in the most severe cases, with anecdotal success.[19] One could speculate that similar results might be expected with extensive angiographic embolization of the stomach combined with aggressive endoscopic intervention and gastric antisecretory therapy.

A variety of relatively uncommon causes of major upper GI hemorrhage are occasionally amenable to angiographic embolization. Bleeding gastroduodenal tumors should be treated by surgical excision whenever possible. Profusely bleeding very advanced malignancies, such as adenocarcinoma, lymphoma, or malignant stromal tumors not amenable to resection, can be controlled well by embolization of the major artery feeding the tumor. Because tumor vessels are incapable of vasospasm, intra-arterial infusion of vasopressin is ineffective.[19] Angiodysplasic lesions of the upper GI tract, such as telangiectasias and arteriovenous malformations, are typically small and multiple in approximately two thirds of patients.[19, 21] Most are amenable to endoscopic ablation, but embolization of solitary large lesions, particularly in elderly poor-risk patients, can be an effective alternative to surgical excision. In contrast to the more common vascular malformations, Dieulafoy's lesion is an abnormally large submucosal artery of the proximal stomach that is prone to very brisk and potentially exsanguinating hemorrhage when eroded. Endoscopic attempts at bleeding control are typically ineffective, and surgical excision or ligation of the lesion is required.[22] Angiographic embolization might be as effective as ligation, provided that thrombosis could be accomplished both proximal and distal to the bleeding site.

Hemobilia is a rare cause of upper GI bleeding that typically results from blunt or penetrating hepatic trauma with fistula formation between a branch of the hepatic artery and the biliary ductal system. When active bleeding from the ampulla of Vater is present, hepatic arteriography can localize the fistula, and selective embolization of the feeding artery is usually curative.[23] Hepatic resection should be reserved for cases of repetitive angiographic failure and those caused by neoplasm or severe intrahepatic calculus disease not treatable by conservative measures.

A group of bleeding lesions ideally suited to angiographic embolization are the pseudoaneurysms and pseudocyst hemorrhages consequent to pancreatitis. Upper GI hemorrhage results when the pseudoaneurysm or pseudocyst ruptures and decompresses either into the stomach or duodenum. Less commonly, bleeding is into the pancreatic duct and thus into the duodenum via the ampulla of Vater (hemosuccus pancreaticus). The splenic artery is by far the most frequently involved vessel, but virtually every major upper abdominal vessel has been implicated.[24] Once the diagnosis is suspected based on clinical presentation or endoscopic findings, emergency celiac axis and superior mesenteric arteriography is mandatory because safe operative exposure for vascular ligation or pancreatic resection is often impossible in the face of phlegmonous pancreatitis. After arteriographic delineation of the bleeding lesion, transcatheter embolization should be performed both proximal and distal to the point of arterial rupture to protect against rebleeding via collateral flow. Only rarely has splenic infarction, pancreatic necrosis, or bowel ischemia complicated embolization, and the failure and mortality rates for the procedure are 24% and 10%, respectively.[24] By comparison, the mortality rate for operative control of bleeding pseudoaneurysms and pseudocysts is 19%, whereas that for medical therapy alone is a prohibitive 74%.[24] These figures reflect the extraordinarily high lethality of the disease and the extreme difficulty typically encountered in obtaining operative control of the bleeding vessel.[9] Postoperative visceral arteriography and transcatheter embolization or residual bleeding is a particularly effective salvage procedure when phlegmonous inflammation has precluded curative vascular ligation or pancreatic resection.[9, 25]

Lower Gastrointestinal Hemorrhage

Because of the broad expanse of the small bowel, colon, and rectum and the antegrade flow of shed blood, endoscopic visualization of lower GI bleeding lesions is often difficult or impossible. This is most particularly true of acute massive bleeding, which constitutes some 10 to 20% of all hemodynamically significant lower GI bleeding episodes. Nevertheless, the initial diagnostic intervention in such cases (after upper GI hemorrhage has been ruled out) is anoscopy or rigid proctosigmoidoscopy. Once anorectal bleeding from hemorrhoids, ulcers, neoplasms, and diffuse mucosal disease have been eliminated as etiologies, major hemorrhage from the small or large bowel should be evaluated next by either selective visceral arteriography or nuclear scintigraphy. The latter technique is preferable for patients with ongoing significant bleeding who respond readily to resuscitative measures. The bleeding scans are noninvasive and nontoxic and may detect bleeding as slow as 0.1 ml/min, as well as intermittent bleeding not appreciated by arteriography.[26] Disadvantages of the scans include lack of specificity, absence of therapeutic potential, and the possibility of therapeutic delay. Although the reported accuracy of nuclear scintigraphy has varied widely, its use as a screening test for active bleeding before arteriography is to be encouraged.[27]

Either with or without antecedent nuclear scintigraphy, angiographic study of actively bleeding patients should proceed without undue delay. Bleeding sources with rates as low as 0.5 ml/min can be detected, and the technique allows the immediate therapeutic use of intra-arterial infusion of vasopressin or transcatheter embolization.[27, 28] Because of the much greater likelihood of ischemic infarction in the lower vs. the upper GI tract, transcatheter embolization has, until recently, been used infrequently to control intra-arterial bleeding from the small and large bowels. Thus, selective vasopressin infusion has been the mainstay of angiographic treatment for severe lower GI hemorrhage. However, the high complication rate and limited success of vasopressin, described previously, together with advances in catheter and wire design and increasingly sophisticated embolic agents, have made embolization the procedure of choice

Diverticulosis of the colon is present in more than 50% of the population older than 60 years of age in western society and is the most common cause of massive lower GI hemorrhage.[10, 17, 27, 29] Although involvement of the right colon by diverticula is distinctly less common than involvement of the left or sigmoid colon, bleeding is thought to be more frequent from right-sided lesions, but this is not well substantiated.[27] Most patients settle conservatively, but approximately 5% require intervention for continued hemostatically significant bleeding. Thus, arteriographic localization of the bleeding diverticulum can permit restriction of bowel resection to hemicolectomy rather than subtotal colectomy. In elderly or debilitated patients, unfortunately, the risk of rebleeding after initial control with vasopressin may be as high as 50%.[30] Embolization is therefore the best treatment option.

Arteriovenous malformations are for the most part acquired lesions of the cecum, ascending colon, and ileum in elderly patients that can cause brisk but usually self-limited episodic bleeding. Angiography and colonoscopy have increased dramatically the recognition of these lesions as important causes of lower GI hemorrhage. The angiographic criteria for identification of nonbleeding arteriovenous malformations include early and prolonged filling of the draining vein, clusters of small arteries, and visualization of a vascular tuft. Intra-arterial infusion of vasopressin is useful for control of bleeding, but embolization seldom is indicated. Rather, the temporary period of hemostasis afforded by vasopressin should be used to prepare the colon for colonoscopic confirmation and treatment of the lesion.[31]

In general, arteriography and transcatheter embolization have little or no role in inflammatory bowel disease or tumors of the lower GI tract. Massive bleeding is very rare in these conditions and, when present, is best managed by surgical resection. Likewise, Meckel's diverticulum complicated by bleeding peptic ulceration is exclusively a surgically treated entity. In instances of obscure lower GI bleeding due to small bowel vascular malformations, diverticula, or other lesions, visceral arteriography can be highly elucidating with regard to both bleeding site and etiology. Although embolization is used infrequently as primary treatment, preoperative superselective placement of a catheter into the bleeding vessel can serve as an extremely useful guide for the surgeon performing a targeted local bowel resection that encompasses the bleeding site.

CONCLUSION

The optimal management of potentially lethal GI hemorrhage demands a highly coordinated and coop-

erative effort using endoscopic, radiologic, and surgical techniques. Visceral angiography and transcatheter embolization of a specific bleeding site provide an important therapeutic capability in the selected patient that can relieve the surgeon of the burden of responsibility for a high-risk operative procedure. The efficacy of embolization in certain clinical circumstances currently is unquestioned because it most rapidly secures control of hemorrhage and maximizes the potential for patient survival. It is anticipated that the indications for, and application of, angiographic transcatheter embolization will continue to expand.

REFERENCES

1. Athanasoulis CA, Waltman AC, Novelline RA, et al: Angiography: Its contribution to the emergency management of gastrointestinal haemorrhage. Radiol Clin North Am 14:265–280, 1976.
2. Mandel SR, Jaques PF, Mauro M, et al: Nonoperative management of peripancreatic arterial aneurysms: A 10-year experience. Ann Surg 205:126, 1987.
3. Baker KS, Tisnado J, Cho S-R, Beachley MC: Splanchnic artery aneurysms and pseudoaneurysms: Transcatheter embolization. Radiology 163:135, 1987.
4. Keller FS, Barton RE, Rösch J: Angiographic diagnosis and therapy of gastrointestinal tract bleeding. In Freeny PC, Stevenson GW (eds): Margulis and Burhenne's Alimentary Tract Radiology, 5th ed. Mosby, St. Louis, 1994, pp 994.
5. Stanley JC, Frey CF, Miller TA, et al: Major arterial haemorrhage: A complication of pancreatic pseudocysts and chronic pancreatitis. Arch Surg 111:435, 1976.
6. Eckhauser FE, Stanley JC, Zelenock GB, et al: Gastroduodenal and pancreaticoduodenal artery aneurysms: A complication of pancreatitis causing spontaneous gastrointestinal haemorrhage. Surgery 88:335, 1980.
7. Nicholson AA, Ettles DF, Hartley J, et al: Coil embolotherapy for colonic haemorrhage. Gut 43:79, 1998.
8. Kiviluoto T, Kivisaari L, Kivilaakso E, et al: Pseudocysts in chronic pancreatitis: Surgical results in 102 consecutive patients. Arch Surg 124:240, 1989.
9. Stabile BE, Wilson SE, Debas H: Reduced mortality from bleeding pseudocysts and pseudoaneurysms caused by pancreatitis. Arch Surg 118:45, 1983.
10 Peura DA, Lanza FL, Gostout CJ, et al: The American College of Gastroenterology Bleeding Registry: Preliminary findings. Am J Gastroenterol 92:924, 1997.
11. Sugawa C, Steffes CP, Nakamura R, et al: Upper GI bleeding in an urban hospital. Ann Surg 212:521, 1990.
12. Fleischner D: Endoscopic therapy of upper GI bleeding in humans. Gastroenterology 90:217, 1986.
13. Baum S: Angiography and the GI bleeder. Radiology 143:569, 1982.
14. Walker TG, Waltman AC: Angiographic diagnosis and therapy of upper GI hemorrhage. In Bennett JR, Hunt RH (eds): Therapeutic Endoscopy and Radiology of the Gut. Baltimore, Williams and Wilkins, 1990, pp 167–177.
15. NIH Consensus Conference: Therapeutic endoscopy and bleeding ulcers. JAMA 262:1269, 1989.
16. Ralph-Edwards A, Himal HS: Bleeding gastric and duodenal ulcers: Endoscopic versus surgery. Can J Surg 35:177, 1992.
17. Peterson WL, Laine L: Gastrointestinal bleeding. In Sleisenger MH, Fordtran JS (eds): Gastrointestinal Disease, 5th ed. Philadelphia, WB Saunders Company, 1993, pp 162–192.
18. Johnson WC, Widrich WC: Efficacy of selective splanchnic arteriography and vasopressin perfusion in diagnosis and treatment of gastrointestinal hemorrhage. Am J Surg 131:481, 1976.
19. Steffes C, Fromm D: The current diagnosis and management of upper gastrointestinal bleeding. Adv Surg 25:31, 1992.
20. Allum WH, Brearly S, Wheatley KE, et al: Acute hemorrhage from gastric malignancy. Br J Surg 77:19, 1990.

21. Gilmore PR: Angiodysplasia of the upper gastrointestinal tract. J Clin Gastroenterol 10:386, 1988.
22. Bech-Knudsen F, Toftgaard C: Exulceratio simplex Dieulafoy. Surg Gynecol Obstet 176:139, 1993.
23. Rosch J, Peterson BD, Hall LD, et al: Interventional treatment of hepatic arterial and venous pathology: A commentary. Cardiovasc Intervent Radiol 13:183, 1990.
24. Stabile BE: Hemorrhagic complications of pancreatitis and pancreatic pseudocysts. *In* Beger HG, Warshaw AL, Buchler MW, et al (eds): The Pancreas: A Clinical Textbook. Oxford, Blackwell Scientific Publications, 1997, pp 606–613.
25. Boudghene F, L'Hermine C, Bigot J-M: Arterial complications of pancreatitis: Diagnostic and therapeutic aspects in 104 cases. J Vasc Interv Radiol 4:551, 1993.
26. Alavi A, Ring EJ: Localization of gastrointestinal bleeding: Superiority of ^{99m}Tc sulfur colloid compared with angiography. Am J Radiol 137:741, 1981.
27. Stabile BE, Stamos MJ: Gastrointestinal bleeding. *In* Zinner MF, Schwartz SI, Ellis H (eds): Maingot's Abdominal Operations, 10th ed. Stamford, Appleton and Lange, 1997, pp 289–313.
28. Ure T, Vernava AM, Longo WE: Diverticular bleeding. Semin Colon Rect Surg 5:32, 1994.
29. Leitman IM, Paull DE, Shires GT: Evaluation and management of massive lower gastrointestinal hemorrhage. Ann Surg 209:175, 1989.
30. Browder W, Cerise EJ, Litwin WS: Impact of emergency angiography in massive lower gastrointestinal hemorrhage. Ann Surg 204:530, 1986.
31. Church JM: Angiodysplasia. Semin Colon Rect Surg 5:43, 1994.

Chapter 26 Varicocele Embolization

Endovascular Contributors: Irving P. Wells and Inge B. Nockler
Surgical Contributor: William F. Hendry

A varicocele can be defined as a dilatation of the veins of the pampiniform plexus within the scrotum. This dilatation is caused by an increase in pressure of the venous blood flow as a result of incompetence of the valves of the testicular (internal spermatic) vein, allowing transmission of high-pressure blood flow from the renal vein and the inferior vena cava downward to the pampiniform plexus. Over time, the increased pressure of blood flow within the veins of the pampiniform plexus leads to their dilatation. This dilatation is most marked when the transmitted pressure is highest, as in the erect position or during a Valsalva maneuver. In some cases, partial obstruction of renal venous drainage on the left by a tumor or pressure from the superior mesenteric artery as it crosses the left renal vein may initiate the varicocele. This latter occurrence is known as the nutcracker phenomenon. Approximately 90% of testicular veins contain one or more valves, and these are usually at or close to their orifices. In the presence of a varicocele, these valves can usually be shown by venography to be absent or only partially competent (Figs. 26–1*A* and *B*).

Varicoceles occur on the left in nearly all cases. This has been associated with the way in which the left testicular vein enters the renal vein at a right angle, which may predispose to reflux more than the oblique entry of the right testicular vein into the inferior vena cava. There is, however, an incidence of bilateral varicoceles, which may be approximately 10%, depending on how the diagnosis is made. Unilateral right-sided varicoceles are very rare.

All methods of treating varicoceles depend on stopping the testicular venous reflux. Since the 1890s, surgeons have known that tying the left testicular vein is an effective form of treatment for men who have left-sided varicoceles. Since then, surgical techniques have been refined and there are several operations available that differ in where the vein is ligated and, more recently, by the introduction of a laparoscopic approach. Since the 1970's, it has become apparent that occluding the testicular vein by emboliza-

tion is also effective, and that this procedure offers minimal morbidity and cost, with results comparable to those of surgery.

VARICOCELES AND SUBFERTILITY

A survey of 9038 male partners in infertile marriages showed that of those with abnormal semen, as defined by abnormality of sperm count, morphology, or motility, 25.4% had varicoceles, whereas of those with normal semen, only 11.7% had varicoceles.[1] There is doubt about the definition of semen normality and the influence of it on conception.[2] There is, however, no doubt that varicoceles have an effect on testicular function. Several theories as to why this may be have been postulated: alteration of the hypothalamic-pituitary-gonadal axis, reflux of adrenal and renal metabolites, elevated scrotal temperature, and stagnation of blood, which causes hypoxia. Because of the association of varicoceles with testicular dysfunction, it has become widely accepted that subfertile men with abnormal semen should undergo treatment of their varicocele. In the United Kingdom, this treatment is largely confined to clinically evident left-sided varicoceles, although in the United States it is commonplace to offer embolization for subclinical varicoceles diagnosed by ultrasonography on the left or right side. Kondoh and associates[3] found that failing to treat a subclinical right-sided varicocele at the same time as a clinical left-sided varicocele led to a suboptimal outcome in terms of semen characteristics. It has yet to be shown clearly, however, that the treatment of subclinical right-sided varicoceles has any effect on subsequent pregnancy rates. Indeed, given the variable conception rate of subfertile couples, the influence of treatment of any varicocele on conception rates is difficult to define.

ANATOMY

Successful treatment of varicoceles, particularly with the use of embolization, requires a thorough under-

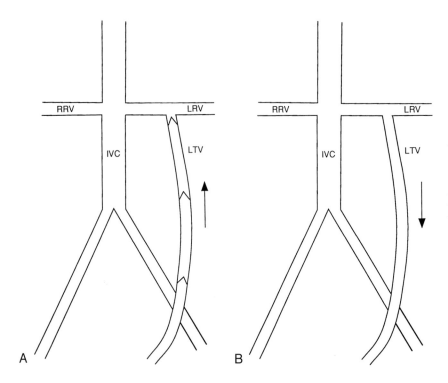

Figure 26–1. *A,* In the normal testicular vein, there are one or more valves that ensure that blood flow is toward the heart. *B,* In the presence of a varicocele, valves in the testicular vein are usually absent. The direction of blood flow is toward the scrotum, particularly in the erect position. Transmission of high pressure from the renal vein and IVC leads in time to dilatation of the pampiniform plexus. IVC = inferior vena cava; RRV = right renal vein; LRV = left renal vein; LTV = left testicular vein.

standing of the anatomy of the testicular (internal spermatic) veins.

The deep veins draining the testis and epididymis pass through the inguinal canal. The external spermatic veins then drain into the femoral vein via the inferior epigastric vein. The ductus deferens vein drains into the internal iliac vein via the vesicle veins. The testicular vein, which parallels the testicular artery and drains superiorly into the renal vein on the left and the IVC on the right, is responsible for the high-pressure venous reflux that causes the varicocele (Fig. 26–2). This vein can be occluded at different levels, depending on the mode of treatment employed, whether radiologic or surgical, and it is essential to be aware of the anatomic variations in this vein if the outcome of embolization is to be optimized.

The left testicular vein in its most simple form represents a single channel running from the inguinal canal up to the left renal vein; in the presence of a varicocele, it usually contains no competent valves (Fig. 26–3A). In this situation, it does not matter at what level the vein is occluded. In fact, most testicular veins show communication with other veins in the lumbar and retroperitoneal compartments, which may or may not contain valves (Fig. 26–3B). Because of these potential collaterals, which may be difficult to demonstrate adequately, it is always good practice to embolize the testicular vein over as long a length as possible. There is a high incidence of partial duplication of the testicular vein leading to so-called parallel collaterals. These have been characterized by Murray and associates.[4] In the presence of high parallel collaterals (Fig. 26–3C), it is essential to ensure that

adequate embolization has been performed below the level of the distal junction of the veins if recurrence is to be avoided. With middle collaterals (Fig. 26–3D), it is often possible to occlude both veins and also

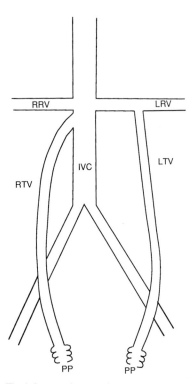

Figure 26–2. The left testicular vein drains to the left renal vein and the right testicular vein to the inferior vena cava just below the right renal vein. IVC = inferior vena cava; RRV = right renal vein; RTV = right testicular vein; LRV = left renal vein; LTV = left testicular vein; PP = pampiniform plexus.

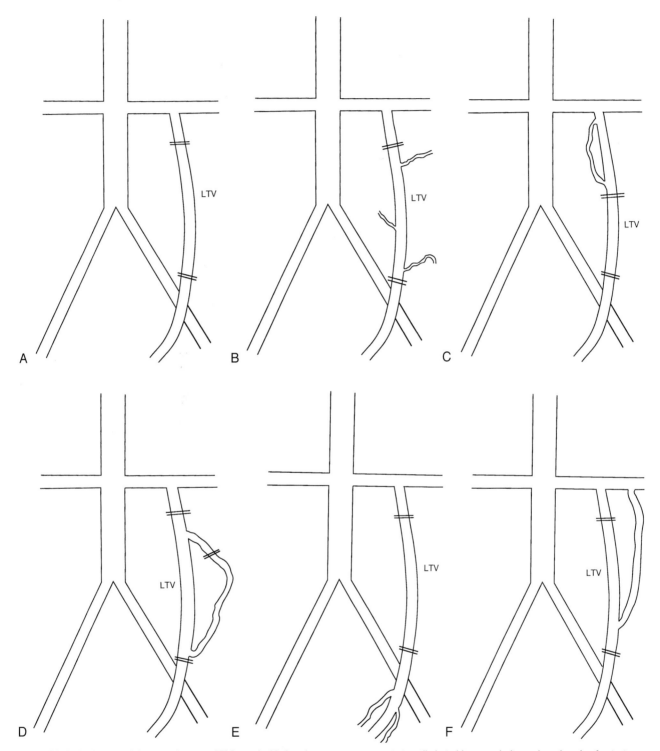

Figure 26–3. *A*, A single left testicular vein (LTV) trunk. Under these circumstances it is still desirable to embolize a long length of vein in case collaterals or side branches are not filling. Coils should be placed between the two marks *//*. *B*, Many testicular veins have several side branches. These may form subsequent collateral flow and embolization should ideally be performed over sufficient length to exclude them. *C*, In the presence of high parallel collaterals, it is essential to occlude the common distal vein trunk. *D*, In the presence of middle collaterals, either the common distal trunk or both proximal veins should be embolized. *E*, Low parallel collaterals are very common, and as long as the long common trunk above them is embolized adequately, they should not cause recurrence. *F*, In the presence of a second testicular vein branch draining into the renal vein, it is necessary to embolize below their junction. It is not usually possible to cannulate both veins separately because the second vein often joins the renal veins in the renal hilum. It is failure to identify this anatomic feature that probably leads to most poor results of embolization.

the distal or proximal common channel. Low parallel collaterals (Fig. 26–3E) are very common and can be dealt with by adequate occlusion of the proximal common channel, which should be embolized distally. There is also the possibility of a high duplication persisting up to the renal vein, with insertion at more than one site into the more proximal renal vein or the renal hilum (Fig. 26–3F). This is the variation that is probably most responsible for recurrence after embolization, because the second communication with the renal vein may go undetected. Ensuring that embolization of the testicular vein takes place as distally as possible is the best approach. Occasionally, there is no main testicular vein joining the renal vein, but instead there is a leash of small tortuous veins. This type of anatomy may preclude embolization.

There are much rarer variants of normal left testicular venous drainage that may occasionally be encountered. In approximately 1% of men, the left testicular vein drains directly into the inferior vena cava (IVC), usually just below the renal vein in a similar fashion to that seen on the right side. In some patients, there are two left renal veins. The upper vein passes normally in front of the aorta, whereas the lower one passes behind the aorta to form a circumaortic venous ring. In the presence of a circumaortic left renal venous ring, the testicular vein usually joins the lower limb but may join either the preaortic or retroaortic component or may even drain via branches into both (Fig. 26–4). If no testicular vein can be identified draining into the left renal vein, this may either be due to a competent valve at the ostium of the testicular vein or variant anatomy. It is always worth searching the IVC below the renal vein in this situation, either to find the orifice of a directly draining testicular vein or the lower component of a renal venous ring. In the presence of duplication of the IVC below the renal veins, the left testicular vein usually drains into the left IVC.

On the right side, the variation in anatomy of the testicular venous drainage has been given less attention because of a much lower incidence of right-sided varicoceles. The ostium of the right testicular vein is usually located just below the renal vein where it enters directly into the IVC. It may, however, join the IVC at a common ostium with the renal vein, or it may drain either exclusively or via a branch or branches into the right renal vein. Some examples of testicular vein anatomy as demonstrated by venography are shown in Figs. 26–5 to 26–13.

TECHNIQUE

Patient Preparation

A great deal has been written about the technique of embolization of varicoceles. The procedure can be-

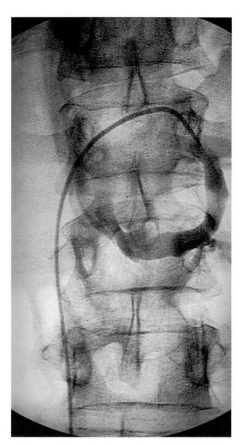

Figure 26–4. The catheter has been placed in the upper component of a left renal venous ring. Its tip has entered the lower retroaortic component along which contrast medium is seen flowing back to the inferior vena cava (IVC). In this case, a testicular vein was never identified.

come very protracted and complicated if all of the refinements and recommendations of some operators are incorporated. There is much to be said for a technique that is as simple and speedy as possible, bearing in mind the need for optimal results. This type of approach is favored in the description that follows.

Embolization of the testicular vein can be carried out as a one-day procedure. It is practical to admit the patient in the morning, perform the procedure in the middle of the day, and discharge the patient in the early evening, after 4 hours of rest and observation. A full informed consent is obtained. The procedure is performed under local anesthetic in the radiology department, with use of standard angiographic equipment. Some operators like to use a tipping tabletop, but this has not been found necessary by most and is not required if embolization is carried out with use of coils. Premedication is often recommended, but embolization of a varicocele should not be a painful technique, and it is not routinely necessary. If the patient finds the procedure uncomfortable, intravenous analgesia or a sedative can always be given in the radiology suite. Of more importance is the tendency for a fit young man to undergo a vasovagal reaction more frequently than in the case with the

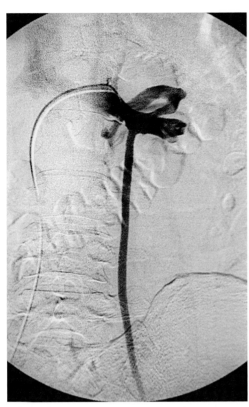

Figure 26–5. Left renal venogram showing free reflux down a left testicular vein that contains no valves. No collaterals or branches are seen.

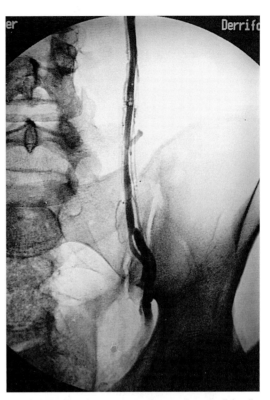

Figure 26–6. Left testicular venogram showing low parallel collaterals. In addition, there are fine, long, parallel collaterals and one lateral side branch. The vein should be embolized over its length from just above the junction of the low collaterals.

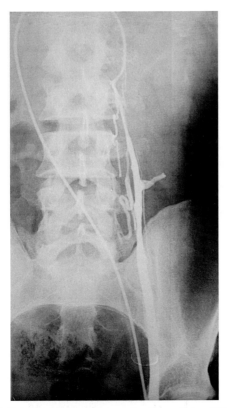

Figure 26–7. Left testicular venogram showing multiple middle parallel collaterals and a large lateral side branch. Embolization needs to cover all the side branch collaterals.

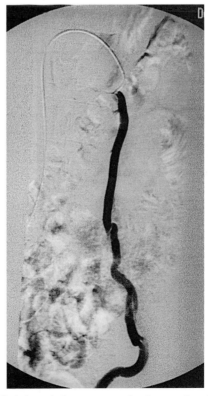

Figure 26–8. Left testicular venogram showing two branches arising laterally in the distal vein. Embolization should cover these.

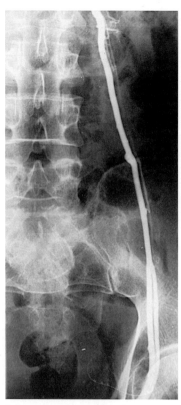

Figure 26–9. Left testicular venogram showing division of the vein distally. Embolization must include the common proximal trunk.

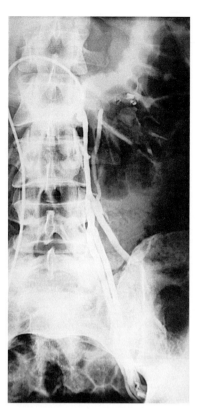

Figure 26–10. Left testicular venogram showing multiple parallel collaterals at all levels.

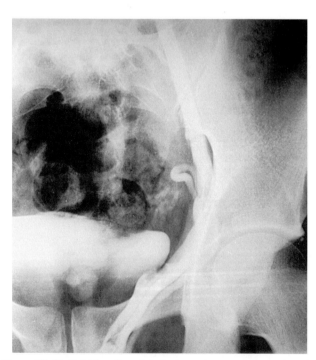

Figure 26–11. Multiple collaterals in the low pelvis into the inguinal canal are often present. They can be ignored and the vein above embolized.

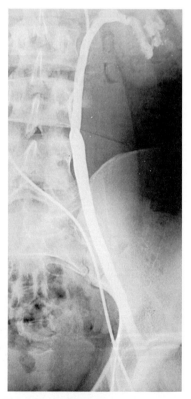

Figure 26–12. The catheter seen at the top of the radiograph is entering the testicular vein at its usual position. Contrast medium has opacified a second communication of the testicular vein and the renal vein more laterally. It is important to be sure that embolization is carried out below the juncture of these two veins.

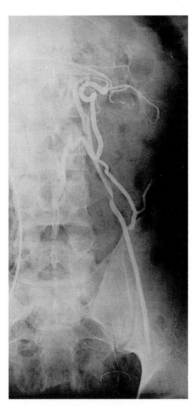

Figure 26–13. Left testicular venogram showing multiple tortuous branches communicating with the lumbar venous plexus and renal vein. It proved impossible to achieve a satisfactory position of the catheter to perform embolization in this case.

unfit, elderly patient who is usually encountered in the angiography suite. Because of this, some operators routinely premedicate with atropine. Patients should not eat solid food for 6 hours before the procedure but should remain well hydrated. This is best achieved by allowing patients to drink rather than setting up an intravenous infusion, because the former option saves money and veins. Good hydration ensures adequate venous distention and reduces the sensitivity of the kidneys to contrast medium administration. Use of nonionic contrast medium improves patient comfort and reduces the incidence of side effects related to the contrast medium employed.

It is essential to have regard for the need of minimizing radiation dose during embolization of varicoceles. It is rarely, if ever, necessary to delineate the vascular anatomy within the scrotum. Indeed, it should be routine practice to protect the gonads with a lead shield. At all stages throughout the procedure, attention should be given to tight coning of the X-ray beam, and screening times should be kept to a minimum.

Venous Access

Access to the venous system can be made via the femoral or right internal jugular routes. The jugular route has the single advantage that the direction of catheterization favors passage of the catheter down the testicular vein to achieve distal embolization. It was often the preferred technique in early descriptions of the procedure. It is also easier, on occasion, to catheterize the right testicular vein from the jugular approach, and if many right-sided cases are performed, it may prove advantageous to be familiar with the technique. Most radiologists are, however, more familiar with femoral puncture, and the femoral approach is usually more comfortable for the patient. The difficulty that the early operators experienced in achieving distal catheterization of the testicular veins has largely been overcome by the development of refinements, such as narrower catheters, coaxial systems, and hydrophilic coating of guide wires and catheters. For these reasons, the femoral approach is generally preferred, with the right femoral vein being preferable to the left because of its much straighter course through the iliac veins to the IVC.

Following skin cleansing and local anesthetic infiltration, catheterization of the right femoral vein is performed. A one-part needle is used, and flow of venous blood through it may be augmented by asking the patient to perform a Valsalva maneuver during the puncture. It may be helpful to mark the skin along the femoral arterial pulsation. This gives a visual guide to the position of the femoral vein just medial to the artery. Inadvertent puncture of the artery should be avoided because this may contribute to a hematoma, and if a hematoma does occur, adequate compression should be applied before proceeding to further attempts at venous puncture. A J-guide wire is passed through the needle up to the mid-IVC. This has less tendency to pass inadvertently up the ascending lumbar branches of the iliac veins than a straight wire, but either may be used. A vascular sheath of sufficient size is then inserted to accommodate the catheter being used. It is always wise to use a vascular sheath when embolization is performed, so that if the catheter occludes, it can be withdrawn without losing vascular access.

Catheterizing a Testicular Vein

Assuming the left testicular vein is being sought, a cobra-shaped catheter is passed over the wire and used to select the left renal vein, which joins the IVC on its left lateral side at the level of L1/L2. The exact choice of catheter for selection of the left renal vein and then the testicular vein depends on personal preference. The cobra shape is widely available and is made in most French sizes. It is also available with a hydrophilic coating and in various degrees of stiffness. Other catheter designs may be used, usually based on a double right-angle type of configuration designed to facilitate cannulation of the testicular vein without displacement of the catheter from the renal vein. Different manufacturers have different names for these types of catheters, and it is wise to keep a selection within the radiology department. The Hopkins curve is a standard example. With experience, however, the simple cobra catheter, with its wide specification, usually proves sufficient to carry out the procedure on most occasions.

A 5-French (F) cobra catheter with a hydrophilic coating is recommended. Its relatively narrow diameter and slipperiness facilitate passage down the testicular vein without causing spasm. The cobra Slip Cath or the Glide Cath are good choices. The orifice of the left renal vein is wide and can usually be entered easily. It may, however, prove less easy to advance the catheter along the renal vein toward the hilum for performing the initial renal venogram. This difficulty may be overcome by passing a floppy wire out to the renal hilum through the catheter and then following it with the catheter while anchoring or gently retracting the wire. A Bentson-type wire is ideal for this maneuver and also, subsequently, for passage down the testicular vein.

Once the catheter is placed distally within the renal vein, a venogram is performed by injecting 20 ml of contrast medium by hard hand injection during a Valsalva maneuver. If the testicular vein is incompetent, there is usually a flow of contrast into it that shows its location for catheterization. If, during the passage of the catheter or wire out to the renal hilum, the testicular vein is entered on the inferior border of the renal vein, it is not necessary to perform the renal venogram; rather, proceed straight to a testicular venogram. The testicular vein orifice should be sought by probing the inferior border of the renal vein along its length. A degree of anticlockwise torque on the catheter often facilitates entry into the vein. Once the catheter has entered the testicular vein, a venogram can be performed to show the anatomy of the testicular vein. A hand injection of 10 ml of contrast medium during a Valsalva maneuver is used and the distribution of collaterals can be defined. As previously discussed, it is essential to embolize in such a way that the potential for recurrence of the varicocele by residual patent collateral pathways is minimized. Once the anatomy is demonstrated, a plan of action can be formulated. In the great majority of cases, however, the ideal embolization involves occluding the testicular vein from deep in the pelvis up to near its insertion into the renal vein. In so doing, it is likely that most parallel channels are excluded. The most important factor in successful embolization, therefore, is achieving distal passage of the catheter within the testicular vein. If the Bentson wire does not pass distally down the testicular vein, a hydrophilic wire, such as the glide-wire or the roadrunner,

is often successful. Once the wire is in position, the catheter is passed over it. It is important to realize that the catheter does not pass over the wire unless the wire is gently retracted as the catheter is advanced, so that the catheter and wire do not form redundant loops. It is particularly important to visualize the catheter curve as it passes from the IVC through the renal vein into the testicular vein orifice. There is a tendency to advance the catheter up the IVC, with the result that it pulls out of the testicular vein. If this starts to happen, the catheter should be withdrawn slightly to re-establish a tight curve over the renal vein into the testicular vein. If the catheter still refuses to follow the wire but rather pushes up into the IVC, the use of a guiding catheter may be found very helpful. It should be stressed that the need to resort to the use of a guiding catheter should be very infrequent if proper control of catheter and wire are adopted, but on occasion it can save the procedure. An 8-F hockey stick guiding catheter (Fig. 26–14) is recommended. This is inserted through an appropriately sized sheath and can be advanced over a wire to the orifice of the renal vein. The cobra catheter can then be advanced through the guiding catheter and over the wire down the testicular vein.

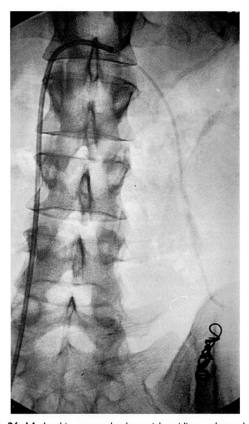

Figure 26–14. In this case, a hockey stick guiding catheter has been placed in the proximal renal vein to overcome the tendency of the cobra catheter to pass up the IVC rather than follow the wire down the testicular vein. The cobra catheter can be seen in the distal testicular vein with multiple coils below it.

The tendency of the cobra to advance up the IVC is overcome by the guiding catheter.

If the jugular route is chosen, cerebral catheters of the headhunter type are usually best, and, as with the femoral route, a vascular sheath should be employed. The same catheter usually suffices for both left and right sides, if required.

Catheterization of the right testicular vein is often less easy than catheterization of the left, because of the anatomy and because in many centers the procedure is attempted much less commonly than is the left. The cobra catheter is often the catheter of choice, but sometimes a Simmons curve is preferable. The orifice of the vein can often be demonstrated by performing a venogram during a Valsalva maneuver, with the catheter tip at the junction of the IVC and right renal vein. Probing the right lateral border of the IVC just below the renal vein and at the ostium of the renal vein may be required. Once the catheter has entered the vein, the same considerations as to passage of the wire and catheter distally apply as they did on the left side. It may not, however, be possible to gain distal placement, particularly, if it has been necessary to use a Simmons curve catheter to cannulate the vein. The same embolizing agents as used on the left are employed.

The exact positioning of the catheter depends on the anatomy and the type of embolic agent used, but on almost all occasions, regardless of which side is being embolized, the catheter must be passed distally into the pelvic portion of the testicular vein. A great hindrance to this is the tendency of the testicular vein to go into intense spasm.

TESTICULAR VEIN SPASM

Spasm may completely prevent onward passage of the catheter and may even, on occasion, render the vein so narrow as to prevent withdrawal of the catheter. The best way to prevent spasm is to perform as little manipulation as possible by using atraumatic wires and narrow catheters that have hydrophilic coatings. Once spasm has occurred, antispasmodic agents given either systemically or through the catheter do not usually produce any improvement, and the only course of action may be to wait until the spasm passes (Fig. 26–15). This may take some time, and the procedure may have to be abandoned. Alternatively, it may sometimes be possible to proceed with a coaxial system using either a 2.5- or 3-F inner catheter through the 5-F catheter. There are several proprietary coaxial embolization systems available that are very nice to use but also very expensive. In this setting, a cheaper alternative using a straight 3-F catheter over a 0.025 inch wire through the 0.038 inch lumen of the 5-F catheter often suffices. This combination allows the placement of 5-mm diameter stainless steel coils

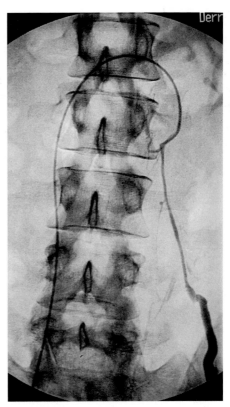

Figure 26–15. Passage of the cobra catheter into the renal vein has caused intense spasm. The normal caliber of the testicular vein can be seen below the segment of spasm.

through the 3-F catheter and often achieves satisfactory distal embolization if the 5-F catheter fails to advance (Fig. 26–16A and B). The 5-F cobra catheter is left in the proximal testicular vein and the wire is removed. The 3-F straight catheter is preloaded with the 0.025-inch wire, so that about 3 cm of wire protrude from the end of the catheter. This combination is then passed through the cobra catheter until the wire exits from its tip. The 3-F catheter is then held while the wire is advanced down the testicular vein. Once the wire has passed distally, the 3-F catheter can be passed over the wire while both the cobra catheter and the wire are anchored. Although small tungsten coils are available, these are difficult to handle and 5-mm stainless steel coils are recommended for use through the coaxial system described. It should be stressed that multiple coils are required to achieve embolization over the length of the vein from the distal location in the pelvis up to within 5 cm of the renal vein. Platinum coils are available in larger sizes but are expensive. Spasm occurs less often as operator experience increases, and using the techniques described should very seldom lead to a failed procedure.

CHOICE OF EMBOLIC AGENT

Most commonly used types of embolic agent have been used in the testicular veins, and each tends

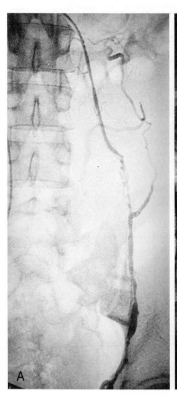
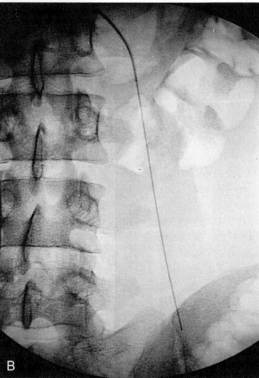

Figure 26–16. *A*, Left testicular venogram showing spasm around and beyond the cobra catheter. *B*, A 3-French (F) straight catheter has been passed distally over an 0.025-inch wire through the 5-F cobra catheter. This allows distal embolization in cases of spasm or difficult anatomy.

to have its advantages and disadvantages. Different operators describe why their choice is best, but there is little evidence that outcomes are significantly different depending on choice of agent. All the options are described briefly, making a clear preference for tungsten coils.

Liquid Sclerosants

Sclerosing agents are widely used for varicocele embolization, particularly in mainland Europe, where Varicocid is popular. This is a mixture of sodium morrhuate (a fatty acid) and benzyl alcohol. Other agents used have included hot contrast medium,[5] hypertonic glucose, and ethanol. The advantage of using a sclerosing agent is that it flows along the testicular vein, extending into side branches and producing embolization over a large part of the testicular venous drainage. The disadvantage of this is that the sclerosing agent may travel too distally and cause a painful pampiniform phlebitis. Although this is usually of limited duration, it may cause a long-standing hard lump and may even lead to testicular atrophy. A device to externally compress the testicular vein at the level of the superior pubic ramus has been described,[6] which prevents flow of the sclerosing agent into the scrotum. Others have described the use of a distal detachable balloon to prevent this complication.[7] Care must also be taken to prevent flow of the sclerosing

agent proximally into the renal vein. Careful observation of flow characteristics and use of contrast medium before administering sclerosant are necessary. Injection of the sclerosant during performance of the Valsalva maneuver produces distal flow, and table tilting may help to control flow.

Detachable Balloons

These are expensive and require larger diameter catheters for guidance than do coils. Their placement is rather more complicated than that of coils, and the particular advantages that detachable balloons have in other vascular territories, such as the arteries of the head, are less evident in the testicular vein. Pollak and associates[7] have described a technique in which a balloon is detached distally and proximally within the testicular vein with a sandwich of sclerosing agent (70% dextrose) between. Makita and associates[8] have described a method of using guide–wire-directed detachable balloons. There is no evidence that these relatively complex and expensive techniques are superior in outcome to a simpler and less expensive technique using coils.

Coils

The advantages of coils are that they are much cheaper than balloons, do not produce pampiniform phlebitis, and are usually easy to place. It is also probably true to say that most vascular radiologists are familiar with their use in other vascular territories. Coils can be delivered through relatively narrow 5-F catheters, reducing the chance of creating spasm. A potential disadvantage of coils is the limited segment of embolization. This can be overcome by using multiple coils at levels in the testicular vein from distal to proximal. The development of long, relatively soft, highly radiopaque tungsten coils that cause rapid thrombosis has further improved the performance of coils. Spirale tungsten coils can be placed rapidly over a long length of the testicular vein. They are easy to place through the 5-F hydrophilic catheter and can be cut to the required length. The tungsten coil comes as a long length that can be cut shorter. It is possible to use long lengths distally in the testicular vein to achieve rapid embolization, but care must be taken not to use too long a length of coil in the proximal vein, or inadvertent protrusion of coil into the renal vein or IVC may occur. Whatever type of coil is used, a floppy wire, such as the Bentson, is used to advance the coil through the catheter. When using the Spirale coils, it is necessary to flush the catheter with saline solution and deploy the coil quite speedily to prevent thrombosis in the catheter. Careful observation of the catheter during deployment prevents inadvertent misplacement. Multiple stainless steel coils can also be used easily and successfully,[9] including through the 3-F coaxial catheter, if required. Coil diameter should be chosen to be just larger than the vein. Measurement of the vein diameter should take place during performance of the Valsalva maneuver to ensure that the maximum vein diameter is seen. Coils or balloons should not be deployed when the testicular vein is in spasm.

After embolization, a final testicular venogram may be performed. Thrombosis of the vein may take 20 minutes or so to occur if coils have been used, and if the embolization has covered the vein from distal to proximal ends, it may not always be deemed worthwhile waiting to observe the final appearance. Once again, the rapid thrombotic effect of the Spirale coils is an advantage in this situation. Figures 26–17 to 26–21 show some examples of coil embolization.

COMPLICATIONS

In the majority of cases using the preferred method described, the hydrophilic 5-F catheter passes distally down the testicular vein with ease. The coils can be deployed along the length of the vein safely and speedily, and the need to worry about complex anatomic considerations are minimal. The whole procedure can be accomplished in less than 30 minutes and there are unlikely to be complications. However, all

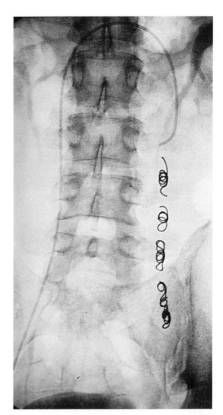

Figure 26–17. Multiple tungsten coils have been placed along the length of the testicular vein.

does not always go so smoothly, and an understanding of the anatomic variations and technical options ensures success in the maximum number of cases. It is also vital to understand the potential for complications, so that their incidence, although already low, can be kept to a minimum.

Complications of testicular vein embolization are infrequently of a serious nature. The reported overall frequency of complications varies between 1 and 30%, with the majority being minor hematomas. It is worth considering each potential complication in more detail.

Groin Hematoma

Small amounts of bruising after femoral vein cannulation are often seen. The incidence of larger hematomas worthy of comment is very small. Seyferth[10] reported only 1 in 580 cases of patients undergoing testicular vein cannulation. Zuckermann and associates[11] in a more recent report describe 5 hematomas occurring in a series of 182 patients. It would seem likely that the incidence of hematomas will tend to decline with the use of smaller catheters and sheaths. There are no reports of groin hematomas requiring surgical intervention.

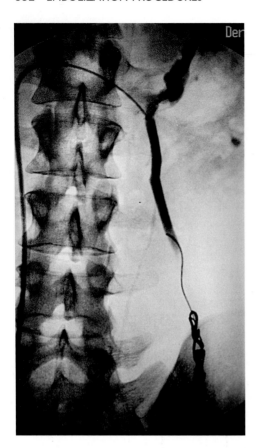

Figure 26–18. Left testicular venogram shows occlusion of the vein immediately after coil placement. Note that the uppermost tungsten coil has failed to coil, leaving a length of straight wire. This shows why embolization should not be performed too close to the renal vein and why shorter lengths of coil should be used more proximally.

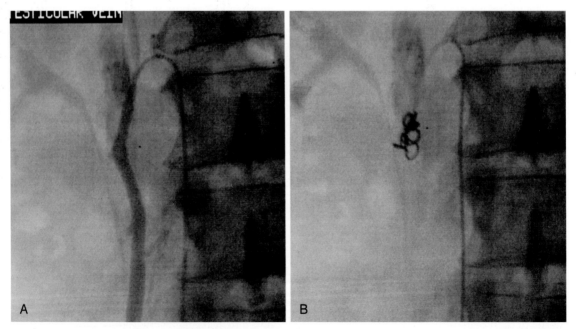

Figure 26–19. *A*, Right testicular venogram showing free reflux. *B*, The acute angle of the right testicular vein junction with the inferior vena cava (IVC) often makes distal passage of the femorally placed catheter difficult. In this case, coils have been placed proximally with a good clinical result.

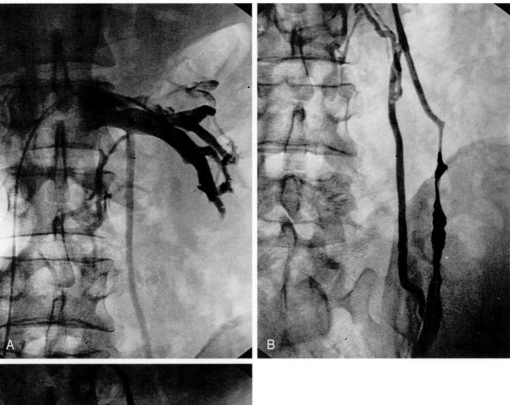

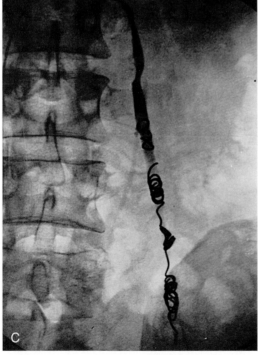

Figure 26–20. *A,* Left renal venogram showing reflux down the left testicular vein. There is a branch at the orifice communicating with the lumbar venous plexus that is unlikely to be of significance. There are no other branches shown. *B,* Following embolization with tungsten coils distally, a large parallel collateral has become evident, joining the testicular vein at the level of L3. *C,* Coils have been placed across the orifice of the parallel collateral and it no longer fills.

Venous Damage

Occlusion of the femoral vein is potentially possible after any procedure involving percutaneous access to it, but this complication is not reported specifically as a complication of varicocele embolization. Extravasation of contrast from the testicular vein is encountered during testicular vein catheterization, but is not always reported as a complication. Dissection or perforation of the testicular vein was reported to occur in

36 out of 580 patients in one series.[10] Perforation may lead to transient lumbar pain and may necessitate abandoning the procedure, but it very seldom leads to serious sequelae. There is one report of venous bleeding leading to ureteric obstruction. Perforation or dissection is usually seen when there is an attempt to pass catheters in a vein that has gone into spasm or when an attempt is made to cross a competent valve. If this complication is encountered, it is worth waiting for a few minutes and trying once again to

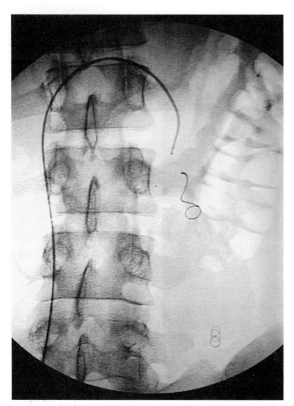

Figure 26–21. In this case, 5-mm steel coils have been placed distally through a 3-French (F) coaxial catheter followed by 8-mm steel coils more proximally through the 5-F cobra catheter.

cross the segment of vein involved with a hydrophilic guide wire. It is often possible to pass the wire beyond the perforation and complete a successful procedure.

Pampiniform Phlebitis

This occurs as a specific complication of embolization with use of liquid sclerosing agents. Distal passage of the agent into the veins of the pampiniform plexus causes chemical phlebitis, which may produce scrotal pain that is usually self-limiting between 1 and 5 days. Whether or not pain is encountered, there may be a subsequent thrombosis of the plexus leading to a hard nodule. Sigmund and associates[12] found an incidence of 14% of these complications in their series of 554 cases, and Seyferth[10] described an incidence of 3%. It is difficult to avoid phlebitis in some patients, even with the most meticulous technique, but the use of vein compression with the special device described by Hunter and associates[6] seems to be effective. Potentially, it would be even more effective not to use sclerosing agents in the first place.

Migration of Embolic Material

Migration of coils or balloons out of the testicular vein may occur and result in embolization to the pulmonary circulation. In all reported cases, this has not led to serious clinical consequences but did lead to one young pilot's being denied clearance to fly jet aircraft.[13] In all but one reported case, the migration has been of detachable balloons rather than coils. There are about half a dozen cases alluded to in the literature of balloons embolizing to the lungs. It has been suggested that migration may be caused by deploying a balloon into a testicular vein in spasm. It is believed that when the spasm resolves the vein diameter increases, allowing migration of the balloon upward. There is one report of coil migration to the lung.[14] The patient, a 19-year-old, complained of chest discomfort and reduced stamina at follow-up, but the authors concluded that these complaints were not genuine. It is recommended that balloons or coils are not deployed within 5 cm of the testicular vein insertion into the renal vein (see Fig. 26–18). If coils are placed too proximally, it is possible that if there is inadequate coil up, a length of uncoiled wire may extend up into the renal vein. If this complication does occur, it may be possible to grab the coil with a snare and remove it through the femoral sheath. The diameter of balloons or coils chosen should be larger than the testicular vein to ensure good anchorage.

RESULTS

The results of embolization of varicoceles have been remarkably consistent over the years, regardless of the technique employed. Technical success as defined by ability to occlude the testicular vein averages approximately 90%. Zuckermann and associates[11] in a large series of 582 cases achieved a technical success rate of 95.7%. Causes of technical failure are largely related to difficult anatomy, with failure to identify the testicular vein and spasm making a small contribution. Reyes and associates[15] found similar technical success rates (90%) in a large series of adolescents who had varicoceles.

After a technically successful embolization, a clinically obvious varicocele disappears or diminishes in size in 85 to 95% of cases. Thus, the overall success rate should be described as 85 to 95% in 90 to 95% of technically successful cases (i.e., an average of 83%). This is most clear in those patients who are treated for symptomatic varicoceles for which the outcome is easily assessed. More difficult to assess are those men who are treated for subfertility, who make up the great majority of cases in most series. Improvement in parameters of sperm function can be seen in nearly all men after technically successful embolization. This improvement is most significant in sperm motility.[10] However, it is less clear what influence this change in sperm characteristics has on conception. This is because so many subfertile couples have other concurrent treatment, and the conception rate in such couples is variable anyway. Zuckermann and associates[11] separated a group of couples who had had no other treatment and found a pregnancy rate of 60% after successful embolization. They concluded that this was greater than could be attributed to chance alone.

Many series have demonstrated that embolization can be effective in treating varicocele recurrence, after either previous embolization or surgical treatment. The surgical recurrences are often necessitated by low parallel collaterals that respond well to high embolization. Murray and associates[4] found that they could successfully treat 25 out of 26 surgical recurrences with embolization. Postembolization recurrences are more usually caused by collaterals at the proximal end of the testicular vein and are less amenable to re-embolization. Murray and associates[4] found a 61% success rate of re-embolization in this group.

SURGICAL ALTERNATIVES

Ligation of Varicocele

The internal spermatic vein can be divided above, within, or below the inguinal canal. The suprainguinal approach requires general anesthesia and good muscle relaxation. An incision is made in the skin crease centered on the midpoint of the inguinal ligament, and the peritoneum is rolled medially to expose the retroperitoneal tissues.

After careful dissection, the testicular vessels are identified and the internal spermatic vein or veins are divided. The testicular artery is preserved whenever possible. However, this is not essential because the testicle derives its blood supply from three sources; namely, the testicular artery, the cremasteric artery, and the artery to the vas, which anastomose freely around the testis. After antibiotic powder has been insufflated, the wound is closed in layers. The inguinal approach is similar to that used for inguinal hernia repair. Once the spermatic cord is identified, its coverings are opened and the internal spermatic vein is divided. If the cremasteric vein is obviously dilated, it is also divided. A scrotal approach to varicoceles has been used in the past but is not recommended because the dilated veins have divided into the multiple channels of the pampiniform plexus, which require individual ligation. In the course of this ligation, the arterial supply to the testis may be interrupted.

COMPLICATIONS OF VARICOCELE LIGATION

Few complications occur if the veins are ligated at or above the internal ring, although hydrocele formation is occasionally seen. Testicular atrophy is very uncommon with this approach but occurs in up to 10% of cases following multiple scrotal ligation or scrotal excision.[16]

Recurrence of varicoceles is observed in approximately 10% of patients treated by high ligation and is invariably caused by opening of persistent small venous collaterals draining into the internal spermatic vein, which are unrecognized at the time of operation. Murray and associates found that recurrence after ligation was caused by midperitoneal or inguinal parallel collaterals, whereas after embolization, high retroperitoneal or renal vein collaterals were responsible.[4] Recurrence of varicoceles occasionally demands further treatment by reoperation or embolization, which should be preceded by venography to define any anomalies in the venous anatomy.

Laparoscopic Ligation of Varicocele

Laparoscopic ligation or clipping offers another approach to the treatment of varicocele and has yielded good results.[17-19] The technique is, however, time consuming and has become less popular as experience with embolization has increased.

CONCLUSION

This chapter was written in early 1998 and describes the use of the Tungsten "Spirale" coil as an embolic agent. Recent reports suggest that these coils dissolve very slowly *in vivo* and though no case of tungsten toxicity has been reported they have been withdrawn from use. If coils are to be used for varicocele embolization, steel coils are recommended. In centers where there are appropriately trained interventional radiologists, embolization is a very effective alternative to surgical ligation of varicoceles. Performed under local anesthesia as an outpatient procedure, it is cost effective, associated with minimal morbidity, and allows most patients to return to normal activity immediately.

REFERENCES

1. World Health Organization: The influence of varicocele on parameters of fertility in a large group of men prescribing to infertility clinics. Fertil Steril 57:1289–1293, 1992.
2. Hargreave TB: Varicocele—a clinical enigma. Br J Urol 73:401–408, 1993.
3. Kondoh N, McGuro N, Matsumiya K, et al: Significance of subclinical varicocele detected by scrotal sonography in male infertility: A preliminary report. J Urol 150:1158–1160, 1993.
4. Murray RR, Mitchell SE, Kadir S, et al: Comparison of recurrent varicocele anatomy following surgery and percutaneous balloon occlusion. J Urol 135:286–289, 1986.
5. Hunter DW, King NJ, Aeppli DM, et al: Spermatic vein occlusion with hot contrast material: Angiographic results. J Vasc Intervent Radiol 2:507–515, 1991.

6. Hunter DW, Bildsoe MC, and Amplatz K: Aid for safer sclero-therapy of the internal spermatic vein. Radiology 173:282, 1989.

7. Pollak JS, Egglin TK, Rosenblatt MM, et al: Clinical results of transvenous systemic embolotherapy with a neuroradiologic detachable balloon. Radiology 191:477–482, 1994.

8. Makita K, Furui S, Tsuchiya K, et al: Guidewire directed detachable balloon: Clinic application in treatment of varicoceles. Radiology 183:575–577, 1992.

9. Ferguson JM, Gillespie IN, Chalmers N, et al: Percutaneous varicocele embolisation in the treatment of infertility. Br J Radiol 68:700–703, 1985.

10. Seyferth W, Jecht E, and Zeitler E: Percutaneous sclerotherapy of varicocele. Radiology 139:335–340, 1981.

11. Zuckermann AM, Mitchell SE, Venbrux AC, et al: Percutaneous varicocele occlusion: Long term follow-up. J Vasc Intervent Radiol 5:315–319, 1994.

12. Sigmund G, Bahren W, Gall H, et al: Idiopathic varicoceles: Feasibility of percutaneous sclerotherapy. Radiology 164:161–168, 1987.

13. Matthews RD, Roberts J, Walker WA, et al: Migration of intra-vascular balloon after percutaneous embolotherapy of varicocele. Urology 39:373–375, 1992.

14. Verhagen P, Blom JMH, Van Rijk PP, et al: Pulmonary embolism after percutaneous embolisation of left spermatic vein. Eur J Radiol 15:1990–1992, 1992.

15. Reyes BL, Trerotola SO, Venbrus AC, et al: Percutaneous embolotherapy of adolescent varicocele: Results and long term follow-up. J Vas Intervent Radiol 5:131–134, 1994.

16. Fritjofsson A, Ahlberg NE, Bartlley O, Chidekel N. Treatment of varicocele by division of the internal spermatic vein. Acta Chir Scand 132:200–210, 1966.

17. Ralph DJ, Timoney EG, Parker C, et al: Laparoscopic varicocele ligation. Br J Urol 72:230–233, 1993.

18. Lenk S, Fahlenkamp D, Gliech V, et al: Comparison of different methods of treating varicocele. J Andrology 15(Suppl):34S–37S, 1994.

19. Lynch WJ, Badenoch DF, McAnena OJ: Comparison of laparoscopic and open ligation of the testicular vein. Br J Urol 72:796–798, 1993.

Chapter 27 Embolization in the Female Pelvis

Endovascular Contributors: John Reidy and Lindsay Machan
Surgical Contributor: Stephen Killick

FIBROID EMBOLIZATION

Uterine fibroids, or leiomyomas, are benign tumors and are the most common tumors occurring in the female reproductive tract. Their etiology is not known, but they are sensitive to estrogen and tend to involute at the time of the menopause. The current fashion for hormone replacement therapy thus has a tendency to potentiate fibroids beyond menopause. Fibroids increase in size and frequency with age, and they are more common in nulliparous women. They are approximately three to nine times more common in African-Caribbean women, in whom they tend to be larger and to occur at an earlier age. It has been estimated that approximately 40% of all women who are menstruating at 50 years of age have uterine fibroids.

Probably about half of all fibroids are asymptomatic, but in the remainder, the most common presenting symptoms are dysmenorrhea and menorrhagia. Menstrual periods may be prolonged and heavy, with flooding and clots. Anemia may occur, and very rarely, fibroids may present with severe bleeding. The other symptoms of fibroids all are related to the mass effect of the fibroids and the enlarged uterus. They may press on the bladder, causing a variety of urinary symptoms and even ureteric obstruction. Neurologic symptoms such as sciatica occur rarely. When fibroids are large, the enlarged uterus can result in abdominal distension, and this can be quite marked so that the woman appears to be pregnant.

Fibroids very commonly are found in women attending fertility clinics, but their role in infertility is not clear. It is thought that they are more likely to cause late miscarriages, rather than prevent pregnancy.

On abdominal examination, the uterus may be enlarged and may even approach the size of a full-term pregnancy. Although the diagnosis usually does not present a problem, a particular concern expressed regarding embolization of fibroids is that because pathology is not obtained (unlike hysterectomy or myo-

mectomy), a uterine sarcoma could simulate fibroid disease. This condition is, however, extremely rare, and the more rapid clinical progress of a solitary lesion should alert the clinician to the diagnosis.

Development of Uterine Artery Embolization

Considering that embolization has been used in the pelvis for a variety of conditions since the early 1980s, it is somewhat surprising that it was not until 1995 that embolization was reported as a primary treatment for fibroid disease. Ravina and colleagues first described embolization as a preoperative adjunct to surgery in 31 patients.[1] One year later, the same group reported on 16 patients, all considered candidates for surgery, who had embolization as the primary treatment.[2] They selectively catheterized both uterine arteries, which they embolized with polyvinyl alcohol (PVA) particles to the point of complete occlusion. At a mean follow-up of 20 months, 11 of their patients had a good clinical result, with three partial improvements and only two failures who went subsequently to surgery. Since this report, there has been considerable interest in this procedure, and although long-term results are still not available, there are generally good short- and medium-term results with a low risk of complications. Although the number of reports in the world literature are few, there is an ever-increasing clinical experience of this procedure.[1-5]

Technique of Fibroid Embolization

Before consenting to fibroid embolization, women should be given a clear account of realistic expectations of the procedure. Unlike an established procedure, such as a hysterectomy, where the patient's understanding and expectations of the procedure are fairly well established, it is important to explain what uterine embolization entails. It is particularly important to explain that the procedure inevitably results in severe pain and the postembolization syndrome and to discuss the management of these side effects. It has been suggested that uterine embolization could be done as a 1-day outpatient procedure, but the postprocedure pain really makes an overnight admission necessary. Radiologists must work closely with their gynecologic colleagues. A gynecologist must have recently assessed the woman before the procedure and must agree to observe her for follow-up afterward.

Radiologists should only attempt fibroid embolization when they are very experienced with arteriography and embolization techniques. It is also important to have state-of-the-art angiographic equipment that keeps the X-ray dose to a minimum. Both uterine arteries are catheterized selectively and then embolized to the point of complete occlusion. No attempt is made to superselectively catheterize these arteries or selectively embolize the fibroids, as opposed to the remainder of the uterus. Coaxial catheterization has been advocated, but we do not believe that this is necessary because it increases the time, complexity, and cost of the procedure and is not necessary when small catheters and hydrophilic guide wires are used. Others have advocated catheterizing both femoral arteries with a contralateral approach to each uterine artery. We have found that it is only necessary to access via the right femoral artery, with very rare exceptions. With this approach, an initial attempt is made to catheterize the right internal iliac artery. Usually this is either straightforward or the angle is too acute and it is not easily possible. When this occurs, the contralateral uterine artery is catheterized and embolized first, and then the right internal iliac is catheterized with a reversed-loop catheter technique formed from the left side. Our approach is to selectively catheterize each internal iliac artery with a 4-French cobra-type catheter and then attempt to get the hydrophilic guide wire to go into the uterine artery without any selective contrast injections and filming. Often, and particularly when the uterine artery is of good size, it is very straightforward to get the guide wire into the uterine artery and the catheter then easily follows. The uterine artery has a characteristic tortuous course, being fairly low in the pelvis and coursing medially. If a test injection shows that the uterine artery has been catheterized satisfactorily, some confirmatory images should be obtained to demonstrate that the artery has been catheterized and to show the extent of the vascular supply to the fibroid. If the uterine artery is not easily catheterized, then it is sometimes necessary to do some imaging of the internal iliac artery to demonstrate its origin and course. This can take the form of a road map or an oblique imaging sequence. When the uterine artery has been demonstrated clearly, it is usually easier to selectively catheterize it.

The blood supply to the uterus is by paired uterine arteries, and in fibroid disease, no other arteries need to be considered. They are often of equal size, but there may be some asymmetry. In fibroid disease, they usually give rise to abnormal vessels that have a corkscrew-like appearance with marked hypervascularity, and often the shape of a fibroid is outlined by the abnormal vascularity. The aim of the embolization is to totally occlude the vascular bed and the main uterine artery to the point of complete occlusion. This is achieved by injecting particles mixed with contrast until the forward flow in the uterine artery has been abolished and there is a tendency to reflux in the main artery. PVA particles mainly have been used, with the most popular size between 300 and 500 particles. Large quantities sometimes may be needed to effect complete occlusion in large fibroid disease, and it is not unusual for 6 bottles (6 $\times$ 100 mg) of PVA to be needed. This is usually followed by a suspension of Gelfoam that results in complete stasis in the uterine artery (Fig. 27–1 A and B). Using these particulate emboli, both clear ischemia results and clinical results appear to be very good. Using smaller particles would increase the effectiveness of the embolization and possibly increase the risk of complications. Generally, the nonbiodegradable PVA has been the particulate embolization material of choice, but some assessments are taking place about whether Gelfoam alone would be as effective because this would have significant cost implications. Gelfoam costs much less than the PVA.

There is a concern in uterine embolization, particularly in younger women, that the ovaries are in the direct X-ray beam. Thus, every possible measure should be used to decrease the amount of radiation. State-of-the-art angiographic equipment with dose-reduction features and pulsed fluoroscopy is important. The skill of the operator should enable the fluoroscopy times to be kept to a reasonable level. Limited filming should be obtained, and it is only necessary to demonstrate selective catheterization of the uterine artery and the angiographic details of the fibroid disease. Short fluorographic sequences with low frame rates (1/s) are all that is necessary. It is not necessary to obtain postembolization filming. Careful collimation techniques also restrict the primary beam and avoid some direct exposure to the ovaries. This is particularly important if fluoroscopy is needed to control the embolization procedure when the image field only needs to include the tip of the catheter and the proximal uterine artery.

Before starting up a uterine embolization program, it is essential to establish a pain-relief protocol for these patients. At the beginning of the procedure, sedation usually is given. Pain will not occur until

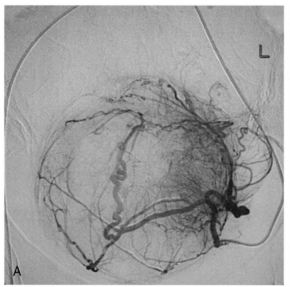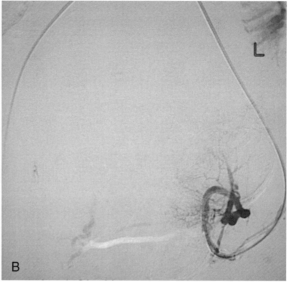

Figure 27–1. *A,* Uterine artery embolization. A Sim 2 catheter has been passed over the aortic bifurcation from the right common femoral artery and the uterine artery selectively catheterized. *B,* 350- to 550-micron polyvinyl alcohol (PVA) injection has effectively occluded the artery.

the second uterine artery is embolized, and strong analgesics should be given just before this stage. Our practice is to give an intramuscular injection of 10 mg morphine and then set up a patient-controlled analgesia (PCA) system set to give 1-mg boluses of morphine with 6-minute lockouts. This results in a maximum self-administered dose of 12 mg/h. The postembolization syndrome and the morphine are likely to result in some nausea and vomiting, and it is also important to prescribe antiemetics. We do not routinely give antibiotics. With rare exceptions, women are able to go home the next day. They should be given a supply of analgesics because some less severe pain may persist for 2 to 3 weeks. They should be advised to take about 2 weeks off from work, but some women are able to go back to work sooner.

Complications

Our current best assessment of this technique is that bilateral complete occlusion of both uterine arteries must occur for it to be effective. Thus, the mechanism of the improvement in symptoms and the shrinkage of the fibroids are clearly the result of ischemia, and we have demonstrated fibrosis on follow-up magnetic resonance imaging (MRI) studies. It is not surprising that the acute ischemic insult to the uterus and fibroids results in severe pain. Although not invariable, most women experience pain, and this may be very severe, such that strong analgesics are needed for the first 12 to 18 hours. This should be managed effectively by warning the patient to expect pain after the procedure and by establishing an effective pain-relief protocol. Pain is part of the postembolization syn-

drome that also consists of general malaise and sometimes nausea and vomiting. Most women are discharged the following day but need some oral analgesics to cover the recovery period. Occasionally, severe pain has necessitated re-admission for further episodes of pain not controlled with oral analgesics. Less severe degrees of pain may last for 2 weeks or so, sometimes associated with malaise and fever. Also to be expected for a few weeks after the procedure is the presence of an intermittent nonpurulent discharge, and sometimes fragments of fibroids may be passed. This spontaneous extrusion of fibroids per vaginum probably occurs in up to about 10% of the women. This is particularly likely with submucous fibroids, which may have a stalk. Larger fibroids may be expelled and may be associated with some dilatation of the cervix. Occasionally, submucosal fibroids may present by protruding through and dilating the cervix. Sometimes, the stalk can be ligated via a hystoscope, but if it is broad, then this is not possible. Embolization is a suitable treatment in these situations because the avascular fibroid may be expelled subsequently and easily detached with no bleeding.

The potential of the women to become pregnant after bilateral uterine embolization is of some concern. Reports after embolization for bleeding and for gestational trophoblastic tumors suggest that the potential to get pregnant may not be affected greatly by bilateral uterine artery embolization. In our experience, with an average patient age of about 41 years, not many women presenting for embolization are trying to get pregnant. The more common situation is that they do not want to exclude the possibility that they may want to get pregnant in the future. The Paris group has reported pregnancies after embolization for fibroids, and one of our patients became pregnant one cycle after the procedure. Aside from pain, serious complications appear to be very rare.

Amenorrhea developed after the procedure in one of our patients 42 years of age, although she had a previously normal follicle-stimulating hormone (FSH) level 1 year earlier. Amenorrhea after this procedure rarely has been described, and patients usually recover (Fig. 27–2 A and B). We believe that this may be a rare problem, but further follow-up data are needed. It is recommended that FSH levels be obtained routinely before uterine embolizations, but sometimes the FSH levels in older women are elevated, indicating the onset of menopause.

There is concern that after the complete embolization of both uterine arteries, more serious consequences than pain and subsequent fibrosis may occur. Hysterectomy would appear to be very rarely necessary. Four months after embolization of very large fibroids, a necrotic uterus associated with a marked discharge and anaerobic infection developed in one of our patients, who subsequently needed a hysterectomy. Another with a complex gynecologic history who had previous surgery presented with a large pyosalpinx 4 months postembolization; she had a hysterectomy and a salpingo-oophorectomy.

Results

Only 4 years have passed since uterine embolization for fibroids first was reported, and currently, there are only five reported series with a total of 90 cases. Despite this and the absence of any long-term results,

there has been a general acceptance of this technique, so that large numbers of procedures are being performed. In the absence of any controlled or long-term data, this largely relates to the great low risk of serious complications from this procedure and to encouraging short- and medium-term results. In the original study, Ravina and his group reported complete resolution of the symptoms in 11 of 16 patients, 3 with partial improvement and only 2 failures.[2] They subsequently have reported but not yet published their 5-year data, suggesting that recurrences do not seem to occur. McLucas and his group at UCLA reported on 11 patients, with improvement in 8 and a 40% reduction of the uterine size, as shown on ultrasound.[3] More recently, Worthington-Kirsch reported on 53 patients, with an improvement in abnormal bleeding in 88% and a 94% improvement in the bulk-related symptoms.[5] They reported three significant complications. One patient had a hysterectomy on day 12 for severe abdominal pain. Another patient had some upper gastrointestinal bleeding that resolved with no specific therapy, and a third patient was re-admitted with severe pain that required analgesia only. We have performed uterine embolization in 166 women with fibroids (age range 29–53, mean 41 years). In those patients for whom a 6-month follow-up is available, significant clinical improvement has occurred in the majority. We have shown in a small group of patients using pre- and 3-month postembolization MRI studies that the overall volume reduction rate is approximately 50%.[4] This is in keeping with other reports. We have noted that this volume reduction often is associated with a high degree of patient satisfaction in terms of abdominal distension.

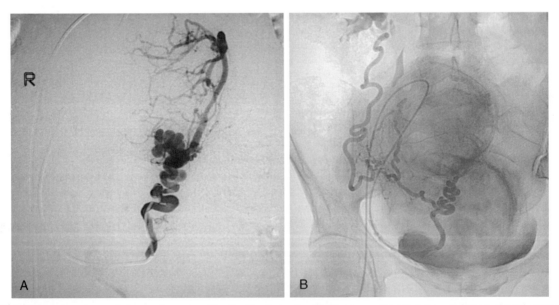

Figure 27–2. A, Late appearance of the ovarian artery. The Sim 2 catheter is withdrawn over the bifurcation, and the ipsilateral uterine artery is catheterized. B, After effective embolization, there is reversed flow of the ovarian artery that was not seen at the initial injection.

Conclusion

There currently do not appear to be any contraindications to uterine embolization. Patients generally are being considered when they express a reluctance to undergo a hysterectomy or myomectomy or when the gynecologist does not consider them to be suitable candidates. Criticisms have been raised that there is no randomized controlled trial comparing embolization with conventional treatments. This presents major problems in comparing a hysterectomy with embolization; the more realistic study would involve myomectomy vs. embolization. Clearly more data and longer term follow-up are needed before the place of this very promising technique can be established.

OVARIAN VEIN EMBOLIZATION

Chronic pelvic pain is one of the most frustrating and common problems encountered in gynecology. Chronic pain is defined as "pain that is present for at least 6 months."[6] In laparoscopic studies, approximately one third of patients with chronic pelvic pain have endometriosis, one third have other structural abnormalities, and one third have no obvious findings.[7] Because of the nature and chronicity of the pain, the symptom complex becomes intertwined with alterations in daily function and interpersonal relationships, and there is often a significant psychological overlay. Therefore, chronic pelvic pain is a difficult problem for the clinician to manage and is often refractory to surgical therapy.

Indications for ovarian venography and embolization include:

1. Unexplained chronic pelvic pain. All women must have a laparoscopy and pelvic ultrasound to exclude other pathologies. Lack of abnormal vasculature at either of these studies does not preclude the possibility of ovarian vein reflux on venography.
2. Lower extremity varicose veins immediately recurrent after adequate surgical treatment.
3. Severe labial/perineal varicosities. These are very difficult to treat, and conservative therapy always should be contemplated. If intervention is undertaken and the patient has ovarian vein reflux, like lower extremity varicose veins, these veins will recur immediately after sclerosis unless the ovarian vein "pressure column" is interrupted surgically or under radiologic guidance.

Varicosities in the pelvis secondary to retrograde flow in the ovarian vein are a recognized cause of chronic pelvic pain.[8] Although the syndrome is appreciated less than the corresponding entity in men,

it has been termed *pelvic congestion syndrome.* The resulting symptom complex includes varying degrees of pelvic pain typically worsening after long periods of standing or at the end of the day, labial varicosities, and dyspareunia (at the time of sexual intercourse or, more typically, immediately afterward). Many women note varicose veins in their legs that may recur after recurrent surgical procedures.

As with retrograde flow in the gonadal vein in men, critical analysis of both the disorder and its treatment is difficult because pelvic varicosities are seen in many asymptomatic women and because there are numerous causes of chronic pelvic pain. In addition, it is unusual for pelvic venous ectasia to develop after pregnancy; however, in "physiologic" venous ectasia, blood flow is antegrade. Any patient considered to possibly have this disorder should have the benefit of gynecologic examination, pelvic ultrasound, and laparoscopy to exclude pelvic infectious disease, tumors, or endometriosis before ovarian venography.

Ovarian venography is performed in the same manner as venography of the spermatic veins, except that if the patient has reflux sufficient to cause pelvic pain, it is obvious on left renal vein or proximal right ovarian vein injection. There is no need to overcome competent valves. If ovarian vein reflux is confirmed in a patient with the appropriate clinical symptoms, retrograde flow can be interrupted by surgical ligation[9] or by embolization,[10] with cure and symptomatic improvement rates of 73% and 78%, respectively, being reported. This compares with reported improvement of 66% in women with pelvic congestion syndrome after bilateral oophorectomy and hysterectomy with subsequent hormone replacement.[11] Preprocedure diagnosis with ultrasound has been reported[12] (Fig. 27–3 A); however, in this author's hands, this has been disappointing in prospectively predicting patients with ovarian vein reflux. Computed tomography (CT) and MRI also can aid diagnosis (Fig. 27–3 B and C), but ovarian venography is definitive (Figs. 27–4 and 27–5).

Technique of Ovarian Venography and Embolization

TRANSFEMORAL ROUTE

A catheter is introduced into the right femoral vein via the Seldinger technique and directed into the peripheral left renal vein. This can be a 5-French straight catheter with tip-deflecting wire or a preshaped catheter such as a cobra catheter. A left renal venogram is performed by hand injection with the patient on a tilt table in the upright position, and a Valsalva maneuver

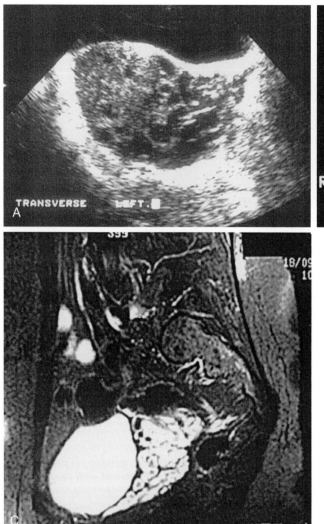

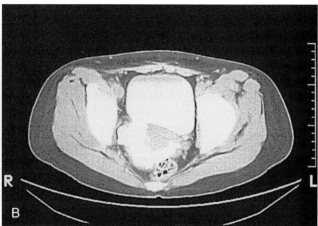

Figure 27–3. Ovarian varicosities: *A*, Ultrasonographic; *B*, Axial computed tomography (CT); *C*, T2-weighted fat-suppressed magnetic resonance imaging (MRI) scan.

is performed. If there is no reflux into the ovarian vein, and it clearly arises from the renal vein, this is considered a negative study. Selective ovarian venography to detect reflux in nondilated veins is not necessary in our experience. If there is ovarian vein reflux, the catheter then is advanced into the distal portion of the left ovarian vein and forceful injection is performed to identify all collateral channels. The catheter then is directed as far caudal as possible into each of the major branches, and embolization of the main ovarian vein and all visible collateral channels with glue, tetradecyl sulfate, or Gianturco coils is performed, extending back to within 2 cm of the ovarian vein origin. The catheter then is exchanged for a Simmons II catheter or its equivalent and is directed into the right ovarian vein. A right ovarian venogram and, if needed, embolization are performed in the same fashion as described for the left (Fig. 27–6).

TRANSJUGULAR ROUTE

Under ultrasound guidance, a sheath is introduced into the left internal jugular vein. The sheath is used for patient comfort during the procedure. A catheter, usually of multipurpose shape, is positioned into the peripheral portion of the left renal vein, and a diagnostic renal venogram is performed. Selective ovarian venography and embolization are performed using the same diagnostic criteria and methods described for the transfemoral route. The multipurpose-shaped catheter is used to perform the right ovarian venogram with no catheter exchange required. If the ovarian venograms are negative, then bilateral internal iliac venograms are performed because rarely, isolated pudendal vein reflux causes symptomatic pelvic varicosities.

SURGICAL PERSPECTIVE

Arterial embolization has an established role in postpartum hemorrhage and may have a future role in the treatment of uterine fibroids and ovarian venous abnormalities. Following is a description of these conditions as seen by the gynecologist and a discussion

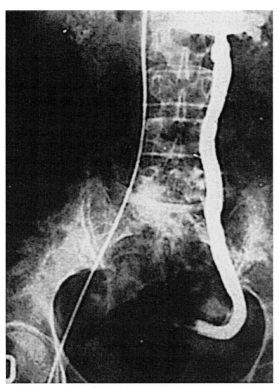

Figure 27–4. Normal ovarian vein. A left renal vein injection demonstrates reflux into an ectatic left ovarian vein. However, there is an intact vein in the pelvis and no varicosities fill.

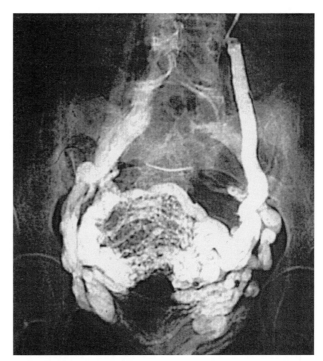

Figure 27–5. Pelvic congestion syndrome. Selective injection of the left ovarian vein results in opacification of an extensive network of varicose pelvic veins.

of the difficulties and problems with current therapies.

Fibroids

Current ideas about fibroids (leiomyoma, myoma) are that they arise as the result of an estrogenic influence on the myometrium. They are the most common tumor in women of reproductive age and probably in humans in general. Their reported incidence depends on the method of detection. Postmortem examinations have shown an incidence of up to 50%, but if hysterectomy specimens are sectioned into 2-mm slices, 77% are found to contain fibroids. The reason for their growth to a size capable of causing symptoms, which is particularly common in African-Caribbean women, is unclear but is not the result of an increased mitotic rate.

If a woman can accept the loss of her uterus, the treatment of symptomatic fibroids is usually a straightforward hysterectomy, but a number of surgical and medical treatments are used for women for whom this is undesirable or inappropriate (Table 27–1).

THE SYMPTOMATOLOGY OF FIBROIDS

Women do not complain of fibroids. They report a huge number of gynecologic symptoms, which in-

clude menorrhagia, recurrent miscarriage, pelvic pain, a pelvic mass, urinary symptoms, and even things like bloatedness (Table 27–2). The gynecologist makes the diagnosis of uterine fibroids, a diagnosis that has

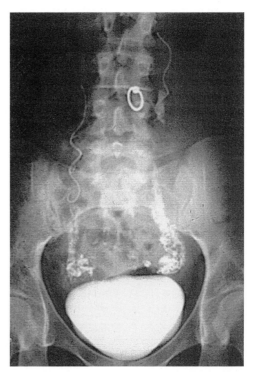

Figure 27–6. Postembolization image demonstrates opacified glue in the peripheral ovarian vein branches and coils occluding the proximal ovarian veins bilaterally. Elongated coils are believed to be less likely to recanalize.

Table 27–1. Problems Encountered With Traditional Treatments for Fibroids

There is doubt that the presenting symptoms are caused by the fibroids.
Patient may wish for future fertility.
Patient is a high risk for surgery.
Major surgery is undesirable because of extended convalescence.
Fibroids in different locations need different approaches.
Medical treatments are of transient benefit or are ineffective.
Fibroid may be sarcomatous.

become more frequent in parallel with the increasing resolving power of vaginal ultrasound machines. The leap of faith is that the symptoms that the woman reports are the consequence of her fibroid uterus. This is tempting because the gynecologist can treat fibroids extremely effectively by surgery. It is also an entirely reasonable assumption when a woman with a 20-week-sized uterus reports menorrhagia. In patients in whom the symptoms are more nebulous and the fibroids are small, the association is much less clear.

In one study, fibroids were not detected in hysterectomy specimens any more frequently if the presence of fibroids was stated preoperatively to be the reason for the hysterectomy. It also has been shown that women with higher education are more likely to have the diagnosis of fibroids. These findings suggest that treatment is performed for symptoms and the diagnosis of fibroids is used when a justification is required.

Hysterectomy obviously cures menorrhagia and dysmenorrhea even when they are not caused by incidental fibroids. A treatment such as arterial embolization, which only removes the fibroids, may not be as effective.

FUTURE FERTILITY

Public opinion is moving away from the acceptability of hysterectomy, and there is a strong call for alternatives. Gynecologists have been criticized by a very vocal feminist lobby who view the uterus as a symbol of femininity, the preservation of which, it is claimed, is not given appropriate importance by predominantly male gynecologists.

Childbearing is being delayed by an increasing number of women in the developed world, and this

increases the chances of fibroid development. Nulliparous women are twice as likely to have fibroids as women who have had children, and fibroids are a common diagnosis in the one in six of all couples that are referred for fertility investigations.

It is not difficult to imagine how some fibroids can cause subfertility if they impinge on the intramural part of the fallopian tube. There also are claims that implantation can be impaired over a submucous fibroid and that recurrent miscarriage can result. Therefore, myomectomy is advocated to increase both fecundity and live birth rates, but prospective randomized studies to prove the efficacy of this treatment are lacking. What is certain is that pregnancy after myomectomy can be complicated by uterine rupture, particularly if the fibroid was large enough for the endometrial cavity to be opened at the time of surgery. Elective cesarean section is advisable if this is the case or if an extensive myometrial dissection is performed.

Arterial embolization would have advantages if it did not weaken the uterine wall to the same extent as myomectomy. There is the concern that after bilateral uterine artery embolization, uterine blood flow during a subsequent pregnancy might not always be sufficient for adequate placental perfusion.

FITNESS FOR SURGERY

Fibroids usually decrease in size after menopause; thus, women with symptomatic fibroids are almost exclusively of reproductive age. Incidental disease affecting fitness for surgery is therefore less common than in other surgical groups.

Obesity can be a problem. The incidence of fibroids increases by 21% for every 10-kg increase in weight, presumably because of the conversion of circulating androgens into estrogens by the aromatase enzyme present in the excess adipose tissue. Conversely, smoking is recognized as a hypoestrogenic state. Therefore, the heavy smoker, with her consequent anesthetic risk, is less likely to need an operation for fibroids.

The overall mortality of total abdominal hysterectomy for nonmalignant disease is reported as 8 in 10,000 in Australia and 5 in 10,000 in the United States. Morbidity is much higher, and incidence rates between 18% and 47% have been recorded. Hysterectomy usually requires a 5-day hospital stay and at least a 6-week convalescence. Three months off work after surgery is not uncommon. Long-term complications are of greatest concern and are probably more frequent than commonly appreciated (Table 27–3).

Hysteroscopic myomectomy can remove submucous fibroids in obese women, but this still usually requires general anesthetic. Anesthetic techniques

Table 27–2. Symptoms Associated With Uterine Fibroids

Fibroids Likely to Be the Cause	Fibroids Less Likely to Be the Cause
Menorrhagia	Urinary frequency
Pelvic mass	Pelvic pain
Dysmenorrhea	Recurrent miscarriage
	Subfertility

Table 27–3. Complications of Hysterectomy

Short Term	Long Term
Complications of anesthesia	Psychological
Postoperative hemorrhage	Bowel dysfunction
Surgical injury to incidental structures	Urinary dysfunction
Infection and fever	Abdominal pain
Urinary retention	Sexual dysfunction
	Earlier menopausal symptoms

used for arterial embolization may have an advantage for patients at increased risk from general anesthetic.

CONVALESCENCE

A greater proportion of women currently contribute to family income; they have careers for which, in the age group when fibroids are common, a 3-month absence as a consequence of major surgery would be detrimental. Minimal access surgery is a major advance in reducing the duration of convalescence. Hysteroscopic or laparoscopic myomectomy may only require a few days off work, and consequently, these operations are quickly becoming more popular. Postoperative recovery after arterial embolization is unlikely to be quicker than after minimal access surgery.

FIBROIDS IN DIFFERENT LOCATIONS

Fibroids can grow to occupy different sites within the myometrium or even, rarely, undergo torsion and sever their myometrial connection and seed elsewhere in the peritoneal cavity. The position of a fibroid determines which symptoms it causes and also which surgical or medical approach is most useful.

Subserous fibroids are more likely to cause pressure symptoms and can be approached laparoscopically if they are pedunculated. Submucous fibroids are more likely to cause menorrhagia or dysmenorrhea and can be treated hysteroscopically. The most difficult fibroids to deal with surgically are those located in the middle of the myometrium, particularly if they are small and multiple. In these cases, hysterectomy may be the only treatment option, although there may be an argument for medical therapy if the main symptom is menorrhagia. Arterial embolization may hold the greatest benefit for these cases.

MEDICAL TREATMENTS

The desire to avoid surgery has led to a search for medical agents to treat fibroids. Combined oral contraception reduces the risk of fibroids developing. It has been calculated that for every 5 years of oral contraceptive (pill) use, the incidence of fibroids decreases by 17%. Oral contraception also treats the most common presenting symptom associated with fibroids, menorrhagia, and it is safe to give to women in this age group who do not have other risk factors for pill use.

Other medical treatments for menorrhagia are less effective for large fibroid uteri. Prostaglandin synthetase inhibitors are unlikely to reduce blood loss to acceptable levels, and the danazol-like drugs usually are associated with unacceptable side effects, particularly nausea and weight gain.

Gonadotropin-releasing hormone (GnRH) agonists have been used extensively in the treatment of fibroids, either as a prelude to surgery or as sole therapy. Their mode of action is to induce a hypoestrogenic state and therefore reduce both fibroid size and uterine artery blood flow. Fibroid volume commonly is reduced by 50% after 3 months of therapy, and studies have shown a reduction in virtually all fibroid-induced symptoms. However, side effects of therapy include severe hot flashes and a loss of bone mineral density, so this type of therapy cannot be maintained. Add-back estrogen and progestogen therapy reduces these side effects without restimulating fibroid growth but is not usually prescribed long term.

The reduction in uterine artery blood flow reduces blood loss at subsequent surgery and is particularly useful before hysteroscopic myomectomy. Sequelae of uterine artery embolization also are rarely seen with GnRH agonist therapy. These include ischemic pain, tenderness, pyrexia, elevated white cell count, and even fibroid expulsion.

SARCOMATOUS CHANGE

Sarcomatous change in a fibroid is rare, probably no more than 1 in 1000 cases. Nevertheless, differentiating a uterine sarcoma from a fibroid is vitally important and can be difficult. Imaging techniques, particularly MRI, may show a less well-defined outline, and the tumor may have grown rapidly over a period of a few months, but both of these characteristics can be seen in a benign fibroid. In practice, it is not until the histologic report is obtained that many uterine sarcomas are suspected, and even then the correlation between histologic features and clinical outcome is poor. Arterial embolization does not allow for histologic examination, and there is the concern that some uterine sarcomas might be missed.

THE ROLE OF ARTERIAL EMBOLIZATION IN TREATING FIBROIDS

Arterial embolization has the potential to improve the options for treatment of uterine fibroids. The main

Table 27–4. Risk Factors for Postpartum Hemorrhage

Uterine overdistension (e.g., big baby, twins, polyhydramnios)
Previous postpartum hemorrhage—increases risk by 20%
Antepartum hemorrhage (e.g., abruption, placenta previa)
Prolonged labor
Grand multiparity

advantage appears to be that the uterus can be retained even in the case of multiple small fibroids situated deep within the myometrium. Further reassurance needs to be gained, particularly with regard to subsequent pregnancy and postoperative complications.

Postpartum Hemorrhage

All childbirth is accompanied by some degree of hemorrhage, and, to a certain extent, the hemodynamic changes of pregnancy lessen the consequences of blood loss so that hematologic instability is less likely at the time of birth. Postpartum hemorrhage (PPH) is defined as bleeding after the birth of the baby that is enough to cause hematologic instability; generally, this is regarded as 500 ml or more. Approximately 3% of all deliveries are accompanied by PPH.

Conventional therapy is based on prevention by predicting those cases in which PPH is likely and by actively managing the third stage. Risk factors for PPH are shown in Table 27–4. Active management of the third stage includes the administration of an oxytocic drug as the baby is born, which reduces the risk of PPH by 40%.

Once PPH occurs, the clinical maxim for treatment is that an empty, contracted, uninjured uterus does not bleed. Once the uterus is known to be empty, various pharmacologic agents are used to initiate contractions. If the uterus contracts but the bleeding continues, the assumption is that the uterus is ruptured and the cavity needs to be explored to exclude retained pieces of placenta and confirm the diagnosis before laparotomy. Problems encountered in the treatment of PPH are listed in Table 27–5.

PROBLEMS WITH CONVENTIONAL TREATMENT

PPH is a major cause of maternal morbidity, although the confidential enquiries into maternal deaths in the United Kingdom reveal a very small number of deaths from PPH each year (Table 27–6). Most of these deaths are deemed to be the result of substandard care or an unusual factor, such as the patient refusing a blood transfusion. They would not, therefore, be prevented by an alternative treatment such as arterial embolization.

The diagnosis of excessive bleeding can be delayed because a young woman may lose 15% of her blood volume before showing signs of tachycardia and hypotension. Alternatively, obstetric hemorrhage can be particularly brisk and the situation can become extremely stressful with a young previously healthy woman who is bleeding profusely, often with attendant husband and relatives.

Acquired coagulation problems need to be treated hematologically, and physical damage to the uterus or cervix needs appropriate surgical repair, which can be technically difficult. As always, hysterectomy is a final alternative.

Rarely, the uterus fails to respond to all pharmacologic efforts to induce contractions. In these cases, once uterine damage has been excluded, hysterectomy may be advocated. Bilateral ligation of the uterine or internal iliac arteries is an alternative. These procedures are said to be 95 to 97% successful, with a 10% complication rate. However, the potential for preserving uterine function and the selectivity of embolization make this the procedure of choice if transfer to the appropriate catheter laboratory can be organized quickly and efficiently. The main place for uterine artery embolization in cases of PPH appears to be when uterine atony cannot be rectified by drugs and the situation allows adequate time for transfer to an appropriately equipped catheter laboratory.

CONCLUSION

The role of embolization in the female pelvis is developing. Embolization is the treatment of choice for PPH and has been for at least 10 years. Embolization is not, therefore, an experimental technique when it

Table 27–5. Problems Encountered in the Treatment of Postpartum Hemorrhage

Substandard medical care
Patient refuses blood transfusion
Diagnosis is delayed
Structural damage to the uterus or cervix
Coagulation problems such as hypofibrinogenemia supervene
Uterus does not respond to pharmacologic efforts to induce
  contraction

Table 27–6. Deaths From Postpartum Hemorrhage (PPH) in the United Kingdom, 1985–1996

Triennium	Deaths From PPH	Rate per Million Maternities
1985–1987	6	2.7
1988–1990	11	4.6
1991–1993	8	3.4
1994–1996	5	2.3

is used to treat symptomatic fibroids, but its precise role alongside other treatments has yet to be determined. Ovarian vein embolization offers a viable alternative to surgery in the treatment of pelvic congestion syndrome.

REFERENCES

1. Ravina JH, Merland JJ, Herbreteau D, et al: Embolisation pre-operatoire des fibromes uterins. Presse Med 23:1540, 1994.
2. Ravina JH, Herbreteau D, Ciraru-Vigneron N, et al: Arterial embolisation to treat uterine myomata. Lancet 346:671–672, 1995.
3. Goodwin SC, Vedantham S, McLucas B, et al: Preliminary experience with uterine artery embolisation for fibroids. J Vasc Intervent Radiol 8:517–526, 1997.
4. Bradley EA, Reidy JF, Forman RG, et al: Transcatheter uterine artery embolisation to treat large uterine fibroids. Br J Obstet Gynaecol 105:235–240, 1998.
5. Worthington-Kirsch R, Popky G, Hutchins F: Uterine arterial embolisation for management of leiomyomas: Quality of life assessment and clinical response. Vasc Intervent Radiol 208:625–629, 1998.
6. Robinson JC: Chronic pelvic pain. Curr Opin Obstet Gynecol 5:740–743, 1993.
7. Kames LD, Rapkin AJ, Naliboff BD, et al: Effectiveness of an interdisciplinary pain management program for the treatment of chronic pelvic pain. Pain 41:41–46, 1990.
8. Hobbs JT: The pelvic congestion syndrome. Practitioner 216:529–540, 1976.
9. Rundqvist F, Sandhold IE, Larsson G: Treatment of pelvic varicosities causing lower abdominal pain with extraperitoneal resection of the left ovarian vein. Ann Chir Gynaecol 2:946–951, 1984.
10. Machan LS, Fry PF, Doyle DL: Treatment of the pelvic congestion syndrome by ovarian vein embolization. In Press.
11. Beard RW, Kennedy RG, Gangar KF, et al: Bilateral oophorectomy and hysterectomy in the treatment of intractable pelvic pain associated with pelvic congestion. Br J Obstet Gynaecol 98:988–992, 1991.
12. Juhasz B, Kurjak A, Lampe LG: Pelvic varices simulating bilateral adnexal masses: Differential diagnosis by transvaginal color doppler. J Clin Ultrasound 20:81–84, 1992.

Chapter 28 Embolization of Congenital Lesions

Endovascular Contributor: *James E. Jackson*
Surgical Contributor: *Bruce M. Achauer*

On the basis of cell kinetics, Mulliken[1] and his co-workers[1] have demonstrated two major types of vascular birthmark that are histologically distinct. *Hemangiomas* are acquired vascular tumors (hence the suffix "-oma") of infancy, which enlarge by rapid cellular proliferation and always undergo involution (sometimes incomplete); these demonstrate endothelial hyperplasia, have an increased mast cell count, and have a multilaminated basement membrane. *Malformations*, on the other hand, are true congenital birthmarks that never show spontaneous involution. These lesions exhibit a normal rate of endothelial cell turnover, a normal mast cell count, and a normal thin basement membrane. This biologic classification is now the official nomenclature used by the International Workshop of Vascular Anomalies. Incorrect terminology is still commonly used, however, both in clinical practice and in many peer-reviewed journals, and this makes review of these two distinct vascular lesions and their reported response to treatment difficult. If this is to change, it is important that a single classification system is used. In particular, the term *hemangioma* should be reserved for the tumor of infancy and not for true vascular malformations. A short discussion of the use of laser therapy in treating hemangioma is included later in the chapter.

The cause of vascular malformations is unknown. It is generally held that arrest or misdirection of the normal development of the vascular tree takes place during one of the three stages of vasculogenesis outlined by Woolard,[2] which gives rise to anomalous vascular structures.[3] They are truly inborn errors of vascular morphogenesis, which are subclassified into high- or low-flow types, depending upon the presence or absence of arteriovenous shunting, with the low-flow category further subdivided into capillary, venous, lymphatic, or mixed lesions, according to the type of vessel that is predominantly involved[1] (Fig. 28–1). They are present at birth and are usually evident at that time, although they may occasionally only become obvious many years later as a result of progressive vascular ectasia. They grow commensu-

rately with the child, although a sudden increase in size is not uncommon during adolescence or pregnancy or as a response to trauma.

Pulmonary and systemic arteriovenous malformations differ considerably in their appearance and treatment and are, therefore, discussed separately.

PULMONARY ARTERIOVENOUS MALFORMATIONS

Clinical Features

Although the majority (80 to 90%) of pulmonary arteriovenous malformations (PAVMs) occur in association with hereditary hemorrhagic telangectasia (HHT), they may also occur in individuals without this condition when they are more commonly single. They represent a direct communication between pulmonary arteries and pulmonary veins, and affected individuals are, therefore, at risk of paradoxical embolization, the most severe consequences of which include transient ischemic attacks, strokes, and cerebral abscesses. Such neurologic complications are a major cause of morbidity and mortality and are the main reason why treatment is mandatory, even in the asymptomatic patient.

On direct questioning, two thirds of patients admit to exertional dyspnea resulting from the presence of the right-to-left shunt through the malformations and the associated hypoxemia. Nevertheless, the exercise capacity of these individuals is often remarkably well preserved for their level of cyanosis, a finding almost certainly related to their low pulmonary vascular resistance and low pulmonary artery pressure.[4]

Large numbers of patients are asymptomatic at the time of diagnosis and are identified on routine chest radiography. Associated clinical features, such as epistaxis and gastrointestinal bleeding, may be present and should raise the suspicion of associated HHT. Screening of relatives of patients with known

369

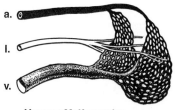

Venous Malformation

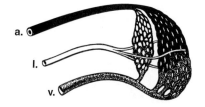

Capillary Malformation

Figure 28–1. Diagrammatic representation of the vascular malformations. a = artery; v = vein; l = lymph vessel.

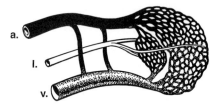

Arteriovenous Malformation

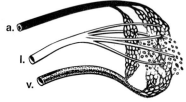

Lymphatic Malformation

HHT is an important aspect of care that allows early diagnosis and treatment of PAVMs in some individuals before they become symptomatic.

On examination, abnormal physical signs are present in the majority of patients. Cyanosis and digital clubbing are found in some patients, and a pulmonary bruit may be audible over a large PAVM when it lies close to the lung surface. Telangiectasia of the skin and mucous membranes is obvious in the majority of individuals with associated HHT.

Investigation

The chest radiograph is usually abnormal, although the characteristic findings of a peripheral, well-circumscribed, and noncalcified opacity connected by blood vessels to the hilum is not always seen.

Helical computerized tomography may beautifully delineate PAVMs and is a useful investigation to demonstrate the number and distribution of lesions.

The size of the right-to-left shunt through the malformations may be easily and accurately measured by pulmonary scintigraphy with use of an intravenous injection of radiolabeled albumin microspheres or macroaggregates. Such particles are usually trapped within the normal pulmonary capillary bed on their first pass through the lungs. In the presence of large-caliber shunt vessels, however, the labeled particles pass through into the systemic circulation and are distributed according to regional blood flow. The size of the right-to-left shunt can be accurately calculated by measuring the radioactive counts over the right kidney (which is assumed to receive 10% of the cardiac output at rest) and comparing these with the radioactive counts in the injected dose.[5]

Pulmonary angiography is essential in patients suspected of having PAVMs, not only to confirm the diagnosis but also to define the number and morphology of the lesions so that treatment can be planned appropriately. Lesions may be classified into three main types on the basis of their angiographic appearances. The first and most common type of AVM (~80%) consists of a single pulmonary artery-to-pulmonary vein communication, with the venous component being aneurysmal and nonseptated (Figs. 28–2 and 28–3). The second type has multiple feeding arteries and draining veins, with the proximal venous component being aneurysmal and septated (Fig. 28–4). The third type consists of numerous communications between small arteries and veins (such that it is difficult to actually define the site of arteriovenous shunting) without a large aneurysmal venous component (Fig. 28–5).

Embolization of some or all of the PAVMs may be performed at the time of the initial diagnostic angiogram. Lesions are frequently demonstrated during angiography that are not visible on the plain chest radiograph.

Angiography and Embolization

Consent is obtained from all patients after careful explanation of the procedure, its likely benefits, and its possible complications. Each patient receives a mild sedative and analgesic preparation and a loading dose of intravenous antibiotics (vancomycin 500 mg) an hour before the procedure. In the angiography suite, an ear oximeter and electrocardiographic monitor are attached to the patient before angiography is performed.

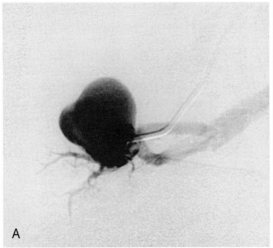

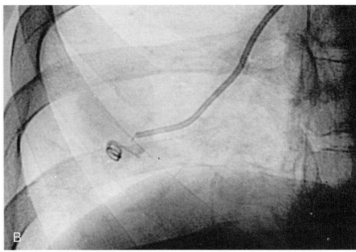

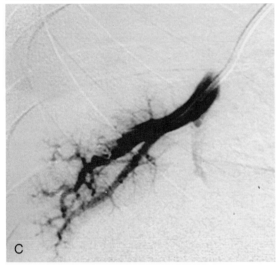

Figure 28–2. Embolization of simple pulmonary arteriovenous malformation (PAVM). *A,* Right basal pulmonary arteriovenous malformation (PAVM) with single feeding artery and single draining vein showing the catheter position at the neck of the malformation prior to embolization. *B* and *C,* Control film and post-embolization arteriogram demonstrate complete occlusion of the malformation by a single coil with preservation of normal pulmonary arterial branches.

Using a femoral venous approach, selective right and left diagnostic pulmonary angiograms are performed via an angled pigtail catheter in frontal and oblique projections with use of a digital subtraction technique (see Figs. 28–4*A* and *B* and 28–5*A*) after measurement of pulmonary arterial pressure. The pigtail catheter is then exchanged for a 7-French (F), end hole only headhunter catheter, which is used selectively to catheterize the arterial feeding vessel to an arteriovenous malformation (AVM). A 7-F catheter is preferred because it affords more stability than catheters of smaller size and is consequently more secure and less likely to become displaced from the neck of the malformation during subsequent embolization. Digital subtraction angiography is performed to establish the precise vascular anatomy of the malformation to be embolized (see Fig. 28–3*A*), and multiple projections may be required to fully define its neck. It is important not to inject any air during arteriography because this is likely to pass through the arteriovenous communication that is being studied and may cause angina with (ST) depression, as demonstrated by electrocardiography, or cerebral ischemia. The former is common even if very small amounts of air are injected.

Before the insertion of an embolization device, the catheter tip is placed at a site distal to any identifiable branches supplying normal lung and as close as possible to the neck of the AVM (see Fig. 28–2*A*).

The only safe agents to use when embolizing a pulmonary AVM are steel coils (see Fig. 28–4*C*) or detachable balloons, because the size of these devices can be predetermined by the operator. Particulate agents, such as polyvinyl alcohol or absorbable gelatin sponge, should obviously not be used because these pass through the malformation into the systemic circulation with potentially disastrous consequences.

Proponents of balloon embolization favor this occlusion device because of the ability to position the balloon precisely before detachment. Additionally, they claim that balloons can be placed more distally in the feeding vessel of a PAVM than can coils, thus preventing, or at least reducing, the incidence of occlusion of normal vessels arising from the feeding artery. Coils are preferred to balloons by this author for several reasons. Using the technique described

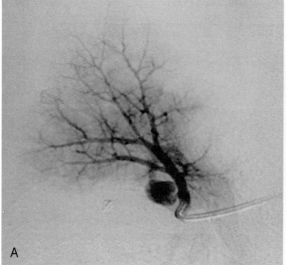

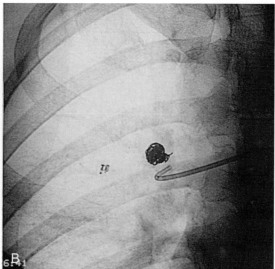

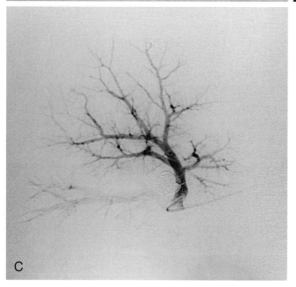

Figure 28–3. Embolization of simple pulmonary arteriovenous malformation (PAVM) by filling of the venous sac. A, Selective arteriogram of right upper lobe pulmonary branch demonstrates a small PAVM with a short single feeding artery. B and C, Control film and postembolization arteriogram demonstrate complete occlusion of the PAVM achieved by packing of the venous sac coils with preservation of the main trunk supplying a large portion of the upper lobe.

below, it has been found that often only a single catheter need be used for the embolization of all PAVMs, thus avoiding the need for the multiple catheter exchanges that are required with most detachable balloons. With the selection of an appropriately sized coil, very distal embolization of the vessel can be achieved. Indeed, in the smaller PAVMs, in which occlusion can be performed with only one or two tiny coils, there is less likelihood of occluding proximal normal vessels than is the case with a balloon, because of the length of the latter when inflated.

The choice of coil size is critical and depends upon the diameter of the feeding artery to the PAVM. If too large a coil is chosen, it lies along too great a length of the feeding vessel without forming a tight spiral; consequently, there is a risk of occluding proximal vessels to normal lung. If it is too small, the coil may pass through the AVM into the systemic circulation. The choice of an ideal coil size and its exact positioning within the feeding vessel to a PAVM

have been made much easier since the introduction of detachable steel coils. These can be simply removed from the catheter if the size is wrong, or partially withdrawn and reinserted if they are poorly positioned initially, making the procedure both easier and safer.[6]

Before introducing the coil, a straight 0.035-inch wire is passed through the catheter to ensure that its tip position is stable. The coil is advanced carefully along the catheter to ensure that there is no displacement of the catheter tip, and is then placed within the feeding vessel. A coil of ideal size for the vessel being occluded can be seen as it exits the catheter to form a slightly distorted first loop when it grips the vessel wall. The catheter tip is then pushed back a short distance as the coil is advanced further before returning to its original position as the second loop exits. A tight figure of eight is thus formed. Further appropriately sized coils are then positioned as required so as to produce a very tight nest until the

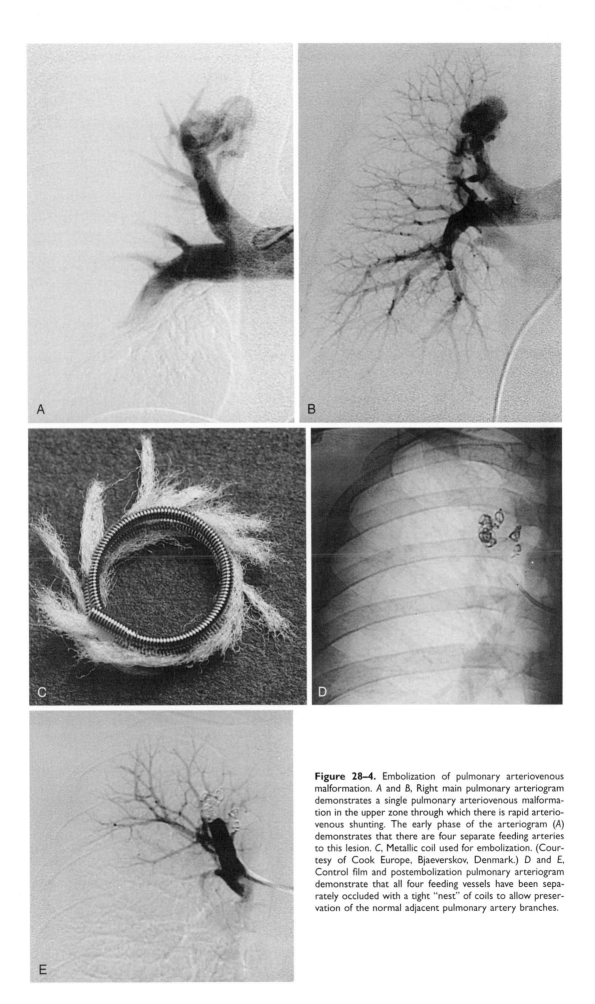

Figure 28–4. Embolization of pulmonary arteriovenous malformation. *A* and *B*, Right main pulmonary arteriogram demonstrates a single pulmonary arteriovenous malformation in the upper zone through which there is rapid arteriovenous shunting. The early phase of the arteriogram (*A*) demonstrates that there are four separate feeding arteries to this lesion. *C*, Metallic coil used for embolization. (Courtesy of Cook Europe, Bjaeverskov, Denmark.) *D* and *E*, Control film and postembolization pulmonary arteriogram demonstrate that all four feeding vessels have been separately occluded with a tight "nest" of coils to allow preservation of the normal adjacent pulmonary artery branches.

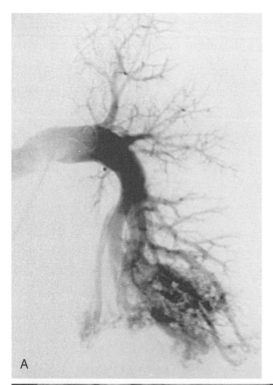

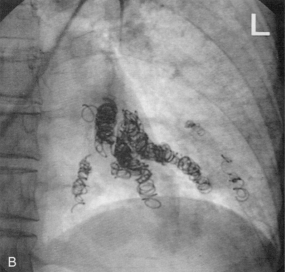

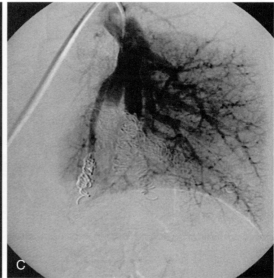

Figure 28–5. Embolization of complex arteriovenous malformation. *A,* Left pulmonary arteriogram demonstrates a large diffuse pulmonary arteriovenous malformation (PAVM) involving the left lower lobe supplied by numerous pulmonary artery branches. *B* and *C,* Control film and postembolization arteriogram demonstrate numerous coils packing the length of these feeding vessels, with complete obliteration of arteriovenous shunting.

vessel is completely occluded (see Figs. 28–2*B* and *C,* 28–4*D* and *E,* 28–5*B* and *C*). A tight nest is critical for several reasons: first, to avoid occlusion of proximal vessels; second, to prevent recanalization of the main vessel; and third, to prevent continued perfusion of the malformation via the bronchial arteries.

The procedure is then repeated for further arterial feeding vessels. Catheterization and embolization of practically all malformations can be achieved with the same angiographic catheter.

Certain PAVMs have too short a neck for successful embolization using the technique described without the risk of occlusion of a large segment of normal lung. In such circumstances, obliteration of arteriove-

nous shunting may still be achieved by packing the aneurysmal venous sac of the malformation itself with coils (see Fig. 28–3*B* and *C*), although this technique is theoretically associated with more potential risks than is conventional embolization, including systemic migration of a coil or thrombus and venous sac rupture. Diffuse PAVMs consisting of numerous feeding vessels, numerous draining veins, and no proximal dilated venous component may require many coils placed along the length of the feeding arteries to achieve complete occlusion (see Fig. 28–5).

Each embolization session usually lasts about 2 to 3 hours, the length of the procedure being determined by the number and complexity of the malformations requiring embolization, the safe dosage of contrast medium permissible in that particular individual, and the patient's tolerance of the procedure. A further dose of antibiotics (vancomycin 500 mg) is given 8 hours after the procedure.

Subsequent embolizations are performed as required until all significant malformations have been occluded. Several embolization sessions may be required in some patients who have extensive disease. The sessions are usually separated by a period of several weeks, allowing full respiratory function tests to be performed when the patient has recovered from his or her hospital stay. This ensures that the benefit obtained from each embolization can be fully assessed.

Results

Most patients report a considerable increase in their sense of well-being, and the physiologic improvements that are obtained are impressive.[7, 8] A residual right-to-left shunt can remain in some patients even when all macroscopic arteriovenous malformations have been successfully occluded. This is due to the presence of small PAVMs (with feeding vessels of 2 mm or less) that are often present in patients with HHT. Whether the obliteration of the larger PAVMs can reduce the risk of neurologic complications in patients with a residual, but smaller, shunt is a question that can only be answered by long-term follow-up.

Complications

Complications related to embolization of PAVMs are uncommon. Chest pain may occur several days after embolization when especially large malformations have been occluded. The cause of this is not clear but may be due to pleural inflammation adjacent to the thrombus within the large venous sac or to a localized area of pulmonary infarction. Should pleuritic pain occur, it rarely lasts more than a few days, and oral analgesic medication is usually all that is required.

Migration of an embolic device through the PAVM should be a rare complication in experienced hands. Should it occur, however, percutaneous retrieval of the device should be relatively straightforward unless it has migrated into the internal carotid territory. With the introduction of detachable embolization coils, this complication is even less likely to occur than it was previously.

When detachable balloons are used, there is a theoretical risk of balloon deflation and subsequent migration into the systemic circulation after the patient has left the angiography suite. Although this is unlikely with the detachable balloons that are currently available commercially, the possibility of its occurrence has been one of the factors influencing the choice of coils as embolic agents in this disorder.

Neurologic deficits have occurred during embolization with full recovery in two reported cases. There are several possible reasons for these episodes, including displacement of thrombus by the catheter tip within one of the malformations, migration of thrombus that had formed on the coils, or a gas embolus introduced via the angiographic catheter.

The polycythemia that is present in some patients increases their risk of developing a deep venous thrombosis, especially if the embolization procedure has been particularly prolonged. It is, therefore, important to avoid dehydration, to restrict the procedure to between 2 and 3 hours, and to encourage early mobilization.

As already mentioned, some patients have a persistent right-to-left shunt despite embolization of all macroscopic PAVMs because of the presence of residual microscopic shunts. Such patients obviously remain at risk of neurologic complications (albeit a lower risk than before embolization), and it is important that they are aware of the need for antibiotic prophylaxis before undergoing dental treatment or minor surgery.

SYSTEMIC VASCULAR MALFORMATIONS

Clinical Features

All malformations are present on the day of birth, although they may not be evident at that time. If there is a dermal component, it is easily visible, although it is important to remember that the clinically obvious cutaneous mark may represent only a small part of the total lesion. Large, deep-seated malformations may also be visible at an early stage because of associated deformity, such as localized swelling or limb hypertrophy, although it is sometimes surprising how extensive a lesion can be without being clinically obvious. The nature of the symptoms caused by a particular malformation depend to some extent upon its site, its size, and the type of vessel that it predominantly involves.

LOW-FLOW LESIONS

Capillary malformations, which are often the least impressive in terms of findings on clinical examination, are not uncommonly the cause of severe symptoms, particularly pain, especially when there is involvement of muscle. Examination may be unremarkable other than perhaps some minor soft-tissue swelling, with or without an overlying dermal stain, despite extensive diffuse involvement of deep tissues as evidenced by magnetic resonance imaging (MRI). Local hyperhidrosis is common; ulceration and bleeding rarely occur.

Venous lesions, when large, are often the cause of severe cosmetic deformity, and they may change considerably in size when the part of the body that is involved is held dependent. They not infrequently cause a large amount of pain, which may be due to venous engorgement when held dependent, or to spontaneous thrombosis, which is common. A mild consumptive coagulopathy may be evident on testing, but this is rarely of clinical significance. Overlying varicose eczema and skin ulceration may occur, particularly when there is lower limb involvement, because of unremitting venous hypertension, and this is often very difficult to heal once it has developed. Limb soft tissue and skeletal overgrowth is also a common problem, with large lesions, especially when sited around the growth plates of the long bones; lower limb overgrowth causes a limp, and a painful scoliosis may develop if the leg length discrepancy is not recognized and corrected.

An increase in pain often associated with swelling is frequently reported after exercise of the affected part of the body, and this is presumably related to an increase in blood flow through the lesion. Such discomfort may last for only a few hours or for several days.

Lymphatic lesions are often large and may be associated with dermal vesicles. They commonly appear because of deformity, weeping of lymphatic fluid, or secondary infection.

HIGH-FLOW LESIONS

These may be asymptomatic, but many patients complain of pain (which may be severe), local hyperhidrosis, ulceration, and bleeding. These last two complications may occur with a malformation involving any superficial site, but they are a particular problem when the lesion involves a digit, which is probably caused by a combination of local severe venous hypertension and distal tissue ischemia resulting from a steal effect through the high-flow shunts. If they are massive, they may cause high-output cardiac failure, although this is, fortunately, rare and occurs with only the most extensive AVMs.

Diagnosis

In the majority of individuals, the diagnosis of a vascular malformation is simple and requires nothing more than a good clinical history and clinical examination. Many patients will come for treatment during early puberty with a history of an increase in the size of—or the development of symptoms related to—a soft tissue mass that has been present for many years (perhaps noted at the time of birth). Presentation is equally common, however, in patients in their second or third decades, although once again, these individuals are often aware that there was a pre-existing abnormality that had caused them little, if any, symptoms in the past.

Findings on clinical examination vary from no abnormality to a massive lesion affecting a large part of the body. A cutaneous stain may be the full extent of a malformation, or it may be the sign of a much larger, deep-seated abnormality. A soft-tissue mass should be carefully examined, and its various characteristics should be recorded, including size, consistency, presence or absence of tenderness and pulsation, and possibility of transillumination. Soft, compressible lesions that fill rapidly when compression is released and that swell more when the part of the body they involve is held dependent are characteristic of venous malformations. Phleboliths are often palpable within these lesions. Firm, non-, or poorly compressible lesions, which are pulsatile and over which a bruit may be heard, are characteristic of AVMs. A hand-held Doppler probe is one of the most useful instruments to have available in an outpatient clinic at which patients with vascular malformations are being assessed, because this tool allows demonstration of arteriovenous shunting in some lesions in which pulsation cannot be detected clinically. Other signs may be present, which indicate that a particular lesion is long standing, such as soft tissue hypertrophy, skeletal hypertrophy, or both.

There are occasions, however, when the diagnosis may be less clear-cut. In the neonate who has been noted to have a soft-tissue swelling at or soon after birth, it may be very difficult to be sure at the initial examination whether this represents a vascular malformation or a hemangioma. A history of development a few days or perhaps weeks after birth accompanied by early rapid growth strongly favors the latter diagnosis, but such a clear-cut history is not always available. In such cases, the true diagnosis only becomes apparent on follow-up after a few months.

Post-traumatic arteriovenous fistulas may occasionally mimic a high-flow vascular malformation, particularly if they are of long standing. There is usually a history of significant trauma, and the diagnosis can generally be easily confirmed by selective arteriography.

It is obviously critically important that a malignant soft-tissue neoplasm is not labeled as being a benign arteriovenous malformation and if there is any concern about the nature of the lesion because of an atypical history or clinical examination, then further investigation and in many cases a biopsy are mandatory. Certain lesions may mimic high-flow vascular malformations, and these include primary lesions, such as angiosarcomas and alveolar soft-part sarcomas, and metastatic vascular deposits typically originating from renal or thyroid neoplasms. Such metastatic deposits may appear many years after treatment of a primary tumor, and this, again, reiterates the need to obtain a good history at the time of first appearance.

A biopsy, when necessary, may be performed surgically as an open procedure. Suitable tissue may be obtained in most instances, however, by using a percutaneous cutting biopsy needle, although image guidance is recommended when taking a core from the more vascular lesions. Ultrasonography (U/S), computed tomography (CT), or MRI scanning may usefully demonstrate portions of the "tumor" to be biopsied that are less vascular than others. Alternatively, the biopsy can be performed during angiography. This is a useful technique, not only because it allows optimal placement of the biopsy needle in the lesion away from the largest vessels, but it also allows embolization of the "tumor" after biopsy as a primary treatment or if bleeding does occur.

Investigation

Because of their rarity, it is not uncommon for patients with vascular malformations to have been referred to several different specialties and hospitals before the diagnosis is even suspected, and such individuals will often have undergone a variety of different investigations, and sometimes even a biopsy. By the time they are referred to a clinician with a good knowledge of these lesions, they are greatly relieved to be informed of the benign nature of the malformation, and many of them require nothing more than discussion about their condition and reassurance that the malformation is a birthmark and not cancerous. These individuals often have a lump that is not associated with any symptoms, and these do not require further investigation.

For patients in whom the diagnosis is in doubt, or for those who are being considered for treatment, the best investigation depends to some extent on the type of malformation and on the form of therapy that is proposed. In practically all cases, however, an MRI scan provides the most useful information and is often the only radiologic investigation that is required.

Plain films are rarely necessary but may be useful when assessing associated bony abnormalities. Marked bony deformities may result from long-standing compression by an adjacent malformation (particularly venous lesions). These deformities are often especially notable when they involve the facial bones because extensive facial asymmetry may result. Full-length films of the lower extremities are seldom necessary when assessing leg length discrepancy because an accurate measurement can usually obtained by careful clinical examination with the use of blocks of varying height positioned beneath the shorter leg. If a radiologic measurement is required, however, this is best obtained by performing a CT tomogram. Calcified phleboliths are commonly seen in venous malformations.

Color Doppler U/S clearly differentiates high-flow from low-flow lesions and may indicate the extent of the abnormality. When the malformation has a single arteriovenous communication (truncal AVM), the site of this may be clearly delineated, and this may be helpful during treatment. It is also a useful, noninvasive tool for follow-up examinations, particularly of high-flow lesions.

Certain low-flow malformations may be associated with deep venous anomalies, including aplasia or hypoplasia, and duplex U/S represents the most accurate method of assessing these vessels. The association between deep and superficial venous abnormalities is extremely important to appreciate; the stripping of superficial varicosities in the presence of deep venous aplasia is likely to make matters worse rather than better.

CT has been largely replaced by MRI scanning when vascular malformations are investigated because of the latter's considerably better soft-tissue delineation. Helical CT with three-dimensional reconstructions may, however, be very useful, either when assessing bony deformity if corrective surgery is being considered or when an MRI scan is contraindicated.

MRI is the most useful investigation for both initial assessment and follow-up. The full extent of high- and low-flow vascular malformations, including soft-tissue and bone involvement is beautifully delineated with use of this modality, and images may be performed in any plane, which is helpful to both the surgeon and the radiologist when they are planning therapy (Fig. 28–6A). A fat suppression sequence usually provides the best contrast between the malformation and the surrounding normal tissue.

Angiography is only required for lesions that have been shown to be of high-flow type by clinical examination and Doppler scan and that are being considered for treatment. Pure low-flow lesions may not show any angiographic abnormality or they may be demonstrated as an increased capillary stain without arteriovenous shunting, by some punctate staining of abnormal veins, or both, and these findings are not useful for planning therapy.

Those low-flow lesions with an abnormal venous component as demonstrated by clinical examination,

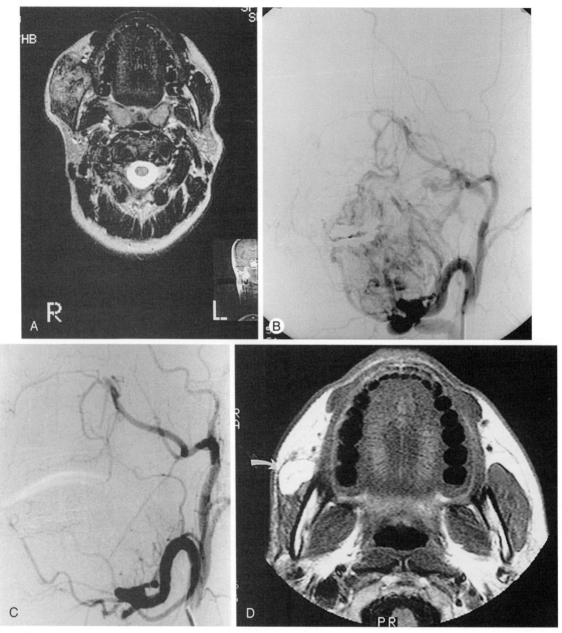

Figure 28–6. Treatment of facial vascular malformation by a combination of embolization and surgical excision. *A,* Axial magnetic resonance imaging (MRI) scan demonstrates a mass of mixed signal intensity involving the right cheek and distorting the adjacent masseter muscle. *B,* Lateral view of a right external carotid arteriogram demonstrates a large high flow vascular malformation deriving its principal supply from a markedly dilated facial artery. There is also some supply from branches of the maxillary artery. *C,* Right external carotid arteriogram after embolization of the facial and maxillary arterial supplies show devascularization of the arteriovenous malformation (AVM). *D,* Axial MRI scan after surgical excision demonstrates complete removal of the AVM with part of the masseter muscle. An area of high signal intensity at the site of surgery *(arrow)* represents fat which has been inserted in order to maintain cheek symmetry.

Doppler U/S, and (or) MRI scanning may be delineated by direct puncture venography, and the deep veins may be separately studied at this time if there is still doubt as to their involvement despite previous imaging using other modalities. Diagnostic direct puncture venography of these venous malformations is often combined with percutaneous sclerotherapy (see later discussion).

Arteriography for high-flow lesions is principally performed to assess the type of arteriovenous communications present within the malformation that determine the best approach for treatment by embolization (see later discussion). The diagnostic angiogram is often combined with therapy. Occasionally, the decision will have been made by this time that surgical excision offers the patient the best chance of long-term palliation or cure, and arterial embolization is performed at this first procedure before planned surgery, which should be performed within 24 to 48 hours.

Approach to Treatment

In 1976, Szilagyi and associates[9] commented in their report on congenital AVMS of the limbs that "with few exceptions, their radical cure by surgical means is impossible; and the large majority of patients do well on a carefully supervised conservative regimen, with surgical intervention reserved for individually defined instances." These comments are still true today, although the last sentence would now read "with embolization, surgical intervention, or both reserved for individually defined instances." Having said this, there have been major advances since that time both in our understanding of these lesions and in our ability to treat them by embolization, and there can be little doubt that there are now a greater number of individuals who can be treated satisfactorily with this technique.

It should be stressed again, however, that not all patients require treatment. In fact, in a tertiary referral center for vascular malformations, fewer than 50% of individuals who are seen need any active therapy other than supportive measures, such as the prescription of a compression stocking for a patient with lower limb swelling and varicosities related to a venous malformation. It is equally important to mention that the treatment of these rare vascular birthmarks should be restricted to major referral centers and should only be performed by individuals who have a proper understanding of the various malformations that occur. A patient who has a lesion treated incorrectly, either by surgery or embolization, is not only unlikely to experience any improvement in symptoms, but may suffer considerable harm, and such a patient may be much more difficult to treat later. For malformations that are considered suitable for treatment, the different therapeutic options can be divided into embolization alone and surgery with or without preoperative embolization. Surgical and other approaches are discussed at the end of this chapter.

Embolization

LOW-FLOW MALFORMATIONS

Venous malformations are best treated by direct puncture sclerotherapy, and this should always be performed under imaging control. The technique involves a direct puncture of one of the dilated varicosities (that forms part of the malformation) along with venography to delineate its anatomy. Particular note should be made of the amount of contrast medium required to fill the abnormal vascular spaces and the opacification of normal draining veins. Before administering the injection of liquid sclerosant, it is preferable to decompress the lesion, if possible, so as to increase the total surface area of the abnormal vein walls that come into immediate contact with the sclerosant. This cannot always be achieved, however, either because the outflow from the lesion is extremely sluggish or because there is a risk of displacing the needle or cannula from the malformation. The amount of sclerosant used should be similar to the quantity of contrast medium used, produces filling of the malformation on the diagnostic venogram, and this should be injected during compression of normal venous outflow, if this is significant. The needle or cannula is then removed and the malformation is immediately compressed.

There are a variety of agents that may be used for venous sclerotherapy. The three most commonly employed agents are absolute alcohol, 3% sodium tetradecyl sulfate (STD), and Ethibloc (a vegetable protein, predominantly composed of prolamine or corn amino acids, which is mixed with amidotrizoic acid [for radiopacity], oleum, and then with ethanol). The first of these causes extreme pain when injected into the patient, and although the previous instillation of a local anesthetic into the venous sac may relieve the discomfort, the procedure is usually best performed under a short general anesthetic. STD does not produce the same degree of discomfort, and most patients can easily tolerate the procedure with a local anesthetic alone. For this reason, STD is the agent preferred by this author. Ethibloc produces an intensely inflammatory reaction that may last several weeks, and although it is resorbed, this may take many months, prior to which it may be discharged through the skin. All three agents produce similar results. Complete eradication of the lesion is seldom, if ever, achieved, but good, long-lasting symptomatic improvement can be expected in terms of reduction in size, swelling, and pain. Recurrent symptoms can be treated by further procedures.

Lymphatic lesions may be treated by percutaneous sclerotherapy, and this may be usefully combined with surgery in certain individuals. Good results have been reported with the embolic agent Ethibloc and with the other sclerosants mentioned previously. After puncture and drainage of the lymphatic malformation, contrast medium is injected to delineate the anatomy and to assess the volume of the abnormal cavity. The lesion is again drained and sufficient Ethibloc or other sclerosant (absolute alcohol, 3% STD, tetracycline) is injected to coat the walls of the sac. Compression is then applied. This may produce a satisfactory result in itself, but some authors prefer to combine Ethibloc sclerosis with surgical excision.

HIGH-FLOW VASCULAR MALFORMATIONS

Embolization provides the mainstay of treatment for most patients who have high-flow vascular malformations, but, although excellent palliation may be afforded by use of this technique, a cure is unlikely. Relatively new technology in the form of coaxial catheters and the use of liquid embolic agents, such as absolute alcohol or N-butyl-2-cyanoacrylate ("glue"), has allowed the trans-arterial embolization of lesions that were previously considered untreatable, with good clinical and radiologic outcomes.[10] There are still some patients, however, who have lesions that make treatment either extremely hazardous or impossible to access via an arterial approach because of one or more of the following reasons: there may be multiple small feeding arteries supplying the lesion; important normal arterial branches may arise in very close proximity to a malformation; extreme arterial tortuosity may preclude successful catheterization; or previous therapy (embolization or surgery) may have occluded arterial access to the central portion of the malformation. In such circumstances, direct puncture or transvenous embolization techniques may be helpful. One of these two techniques may, in fact, be the best method of embolization for some high-flow lesions even in the absence of one of the relative contraindications to an arterial embolization listed previously, and this is discussed later.

A knowledge of the different anatomic configurations of high-flow malformations is essential to understand how best to approach any particular lesion and obtain the best results from embolization. Houdart and associates[11] have proposed a classification of *intracranial* arteriovenous malformations, which is based entirely on the angiographic appearances of these lesions and which can be usefully applied to peripheral AVMs. It is important to point out that this classification applies only to high-flow lesions and does not contradict the classification proposed by Mulliken, which was described earlier. Rather, it is complementary to Mulliken's classification in that it can be used to plan the best route for embolization.

Houdart and associates reviewed 99 intracranial AVMs in 98 patients and distinguished three types of fistula within them. These they termed:

1. *Arteriovenous*, in which there are no more than three separate arteries supplying a single initial venous component
2. *Arteriolovenous*, in which multiple arteries shunt into a single, central, dilated venous component
3. *Arteriolovenulous*, in which there are multiple shunts between arterioles and venules. In this type, the first identifiable normal venous component is separate from the shunts.

Of these types of fistula, the authors suggested that types 1) and 2) can be treated by an arterial or a venous approach, whereas type 3) can only be treated from the arterial side (although this is perhaps not true for peripheral arteriovenous malformations [see later discussion]). The choice of approach in types 1) and 2) depends upon several factors, including the number of arterial feeders, their accessibility to catheterization, and the vulnerability of adjacent normal vessels to inadvertent occlusion if an arterial embolization is attempted. Whichever route is employed, embolization must be performed as near as possible to, or across, the arteriovenous communications themselves. Unduly proximal embolization of feeding arteries is to be deplored because—as is the case with surgical ligation—recurrence is invariable and subsequent access to the lesion to provide more definitive treatment for the patient is severely compromised. The three different approaches to embolization are best discussed by considering in turn the different anatomic configurations of arteriovenous malformation described earlier, although it is important to note that not all occurrences of any one lesion necessarily conform to one particular type of anatomic configuration throughout, and it is not uncommon to find two or three of these different arteriovenous communications in one malformation.

Arteriovenous (Fig. 28–7) lesions include the rare congenital truncal arteriovenous malformation in which there is a single communication between an artery and a vein. This communication is also seen, however, within other lesions that at first sight appear more diffuse, although this may only be appreciated by superselective arterial catheterization. As mentioned previously, embolization of this form of arteriovenous communication can be performed via an arterial approach or via a direct puncture (or retrograde venous catheterization) of the dilated venous component immediately beyond the fistula (see Fig. 28–7E). When the communications are large, they are often most easily occluded from the arterial side, although the embolic material must bridge the communication itself (i.e., lie partly within the venous component) and not lie proximal to it within the feeding vessel. If an arterial approach is used, therefore, a liquid embolic agent is necessary, with absolute alcohol or glue being the most commonly used agents. If suitable control of arterial inflow and venous outflow cannot be achieved during embolization, glue is probably the agent of first choice because it can be timed to polymerize at the site of the fistula, whereas absolute alcohol is likely to be rapidly washed through and diluted without achieving an occlusion.

Patients who have *arteriolovenous* (Fig. 28–8) lesions can similarly be treated from the arterial or venous sides, although the latter approaches are likely to be considerably simpler because of the numerous arterial feeding vessels that are usually present. As has been mentioned, a venous embolization can be performed via a puncture directly into the aneurysmally dilated venous component of the lesion or retrogradely via a suitable draining vein, if one is pres-

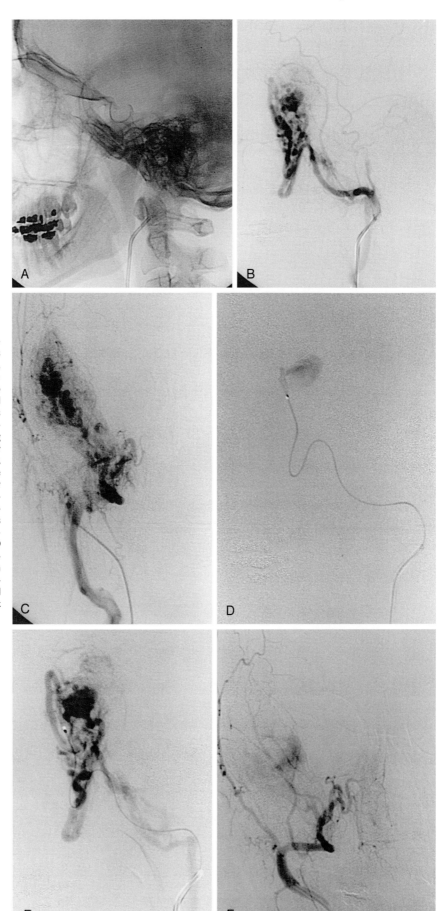

Figure 28–7. Right infratemporal fossa arteriovenous malformation (AVM) with arteriovenous anatomy treated by arterial embolization. *A*, Control film of right external carotid arteriogram with catheter immediately proximal to the bifurcation into the superficial temporal and maxillary arteries. *B*, The maxillary artery is hypertrophied and deep temporal arteries supply a high-flow vascular malformation involving the right infratemporal fossa. *C*, Frontal view with the catheter in the same position as *B*. *D*, A coaxial catheter has been introduced into one of the deep temporal arteries. A very early arterial image demonstrates a single communication between the artery and an adjacent dilated vein. (Two other direct arteriovenous communications were present in this malformation). *E*, An image performed 2 seconds after *D* demonstrates the large tortuous venous component of the malformation. *F*, Postembolization external carotid arteriogram (frontal) demonstrates occlusion of the AVM with no residual opacification of the large venous component (compare with *C*).

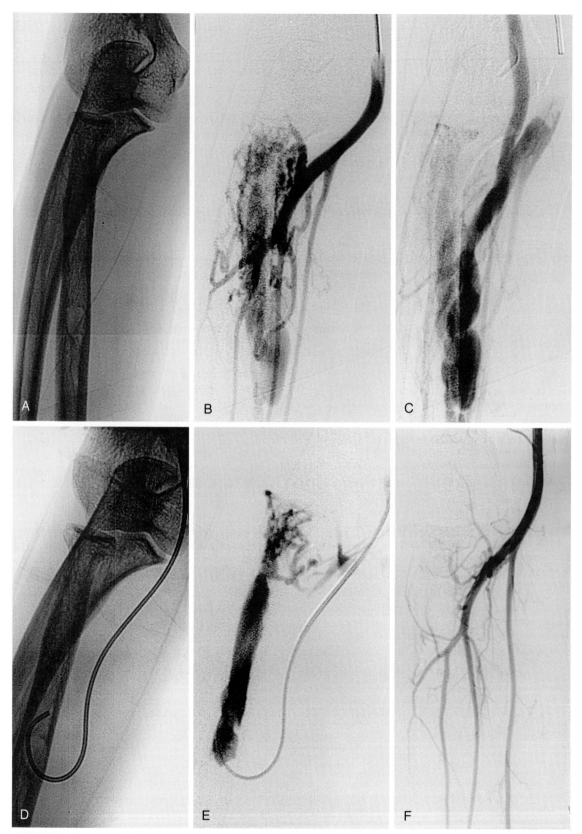

Figure 28–8. Right radial head arteriovenous malformation (AVM) with an arteriovenous anatomy treated by embolization via a retrograde venous approach. *A,* Control film of the right elbow demonstrates expansion of the medullary cavity of the proximal radial shaft with enlargement of the vascular foramen. *B,* Early arterial phase from a right brachial arteriogram demonstrates a high-flow AVM involving the radial head, which has numerous arterial feeding vessels. *C,* Later phase from same study demonstrates a large emissary vein from the radial shaft draining into a dilated forearm vein. *D,* The venous component of the malformation has been catheterized in a retrograde direction. *E,* Angiogram performed with a tourniquet inflated to a level higher than arterial pressure demonstrates almost complete stasis of contrast medium within the venous component of the malformation within the radial shaft. Embolization was performed with use of absolute alcohol. *F,* Right brachial arteriogram performed 6 months after embolization demonstrates an excellent result, with no residual arteriovenous shunting and with preservation of normal arterial branches.

ent. Whereas a retrograde venous approach has been used in the treatment of certain intracranial vascular malformations, it is a rare, and perhaps underused, technique in treatment of patients with peripheral high-flow vascular lesions.

Embolization with liquids via a direct puncture or retrograde venous approach is best performed with control of arterial inflow and venous outflow. This is relatively straightforward when the AVM involves the arm or leg because a tourniquet is all that is required. It is much more difficult, however, when the lesion involves, for example, the shoulder or pelvis, and in these circumstances, an arterial or venous occlusion balloon may be necessary.

The major potential complication of venous embolization when liquid agents are used is inadvertent occlusion of the normal venous drainage from surrounding tissues, with resultant venous hypertension and deep venous thrombosis. This is best avoided by performing test injections of contrast material to determine the amount of embolic agent that can be administered without causing spillover into normal veins and by injecting small, intermittent aliquots of the embolic agent rather than one large bolus. Absolute alcohol may be mixed with nonionic contrast material without precipitation. The present authors prefer, however, to use undiluted absolute alcohol to

preserve its maximal sclerosant activity. This makes it even more important to take great care not to instill too much alcohol during any one injection.

Absolute alcohol may cause a peripheral sensory or motor neuropathy, or both, if it leaks out into the adjacent soft tissues during embolization. This is a particular hazard if a direct puncture technique is being used, because leakage may occur along the needle track. There is less chance of this occurring, however, when a retrograde venous approach is being used, because the puncture site is often at some distance from the point of alcohol instillation, and this is perhaps a further advantage of using this route for embolization when the anatomy allows.

A further potential complication of this technique when both arterial inflow and venous outflow are being occluded is that of retrograde filling of the arterial feeding vessels and reflux of embolic material into the arterial side of the circulation. This is rarely seen, however, even when a tourniquet is inflated to above arterial pressure during contrast injection. The possibility of this occurrence, however, underscores the importance of performing test injections of contrast medium before the instillation of any liquid embolic agents.

Arteriolovenulous (Fig. 28–9) lesions are undoubtedly the most difficult to treat successfully by emboli-

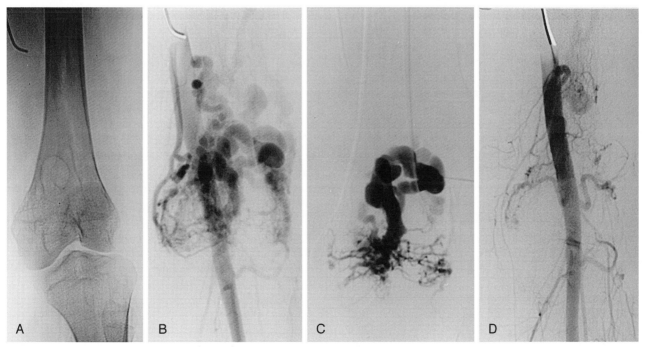

Figure 28–9. Extensive high-flow vascular malformation involving the whole of the left leg with an arteriolovenulous anatomy. The patient received treatment of the portion of the lesion around the knee via venous embolization with use of a flow-occlusion technique. *A,* Control film of left knee demonstrates areas of distal femoral bony erosion by a dilated venous component of the arteriovenous malformation (AVM). *B,* With the angiographic catheter in the distal superficial femoral artery, an angiogram demonstrates marked dilatation of the popliteal artery and of the geniculate branches that supply a high-flow lesion around the knee. *C,* A large draining vein has been punctured on the lateral aspect of the knee and a catheter has been introduced into this vessel. With a tourniquet inflated to a level higher than arterial pressure, a venogram demonstrates retrograde opacification of small venous tributaries that represent the venulous component of the AVM. Embolization was performed with use of absolute alcohol. *D,* Follow-up arteriogram performed 8 months after embolization demonstrates a considerable improvement with no residual arteriovenous shunting in the component of the malformation treated around the knee joint. The popliteal artery remains hypertrophied because of residual malformation involving the lower leg.

zation. The abnormal shunts are located between numerous small arterioles and venules, and as such, it is usually very difficult, if not impossible, to see where arteries end and veins begin. The first identifiable vein is, therefore, usually at some distance from the shunts. Embolization of these lesions has relied on the injection of particles, such as polyvinyl alcohol, and this procedure usually has to be repeated regularly, with the aim of reducing the rate of arteriovenous shunting and thereby relieving symptoms. This form of treatment is often surprisingly effective, although symptom recurrence is common.

The use of absolute alcohol from an arterial approach for this type of lesion has its proponents, but there is a significant serious complication rate with this technique related to necrosis of normal tissue, skin ulceration, and neural damage. A direct puncture technique is also difficult because of the small size of the shunts.

A retrograde venous approach has previously been regarded as being absolutely contraindicated in this anatomic type of AVM because of the risk of occluding venous outflow beyond the shunts and thereby worsening the venous hypertension within the lesion, with the potential of causing skin ulceration and hemorrhage. Such an approach may theoretically achieve a satisfactory result; however, this result would occur only if it were possible to fill retrogradely the small venules immediately beyond the shunts with a liquid embolic agent and thereby occlude the shunts themselves. However, there has been very little experience with use of this technique. The treatment of patients who have lesions involving the limbs might again be expected to be easier, because a tourniquet can easily be applied to occlude arterial inflow and venous outflow, thereby allowing satisfactory back-filling of the small venules (see Fig. 28–9).

Complications

The complications that are most commonly reported during embolization of vascular malformations are the inadvertent embolization of vessels other than those supplying the lesion, and the passage of emboli into the venous circulation. Provided the embolization is performed with meticulous care, these complications should be very uncommon.

The postembolization syndrome consists of a variable combination of pain at the site of the embolized arteriovenous malformation and includes pyrexia, leucocytosis, and a general feeling of malaise and is common after the procedure, particularly if the malformation is large. The condition generally lasts for only 24 to 48 hours but may persist for a week or more before it disappears. Symptomatic treatment is

usually all that is required. The more serious complication of infection at the site of embolization is exceedingly rare but could produce the same symptoms as the postembolization syndrome, and the possibility of this complication should always be considered. Blood cultures should be taken in any case featuring pyrexia and leucocytosis.

Embolization performed with absolute alcohol is associated with an increased number of complications, including tissue necrosis, neural damage, and death caused by acute pulmonary hypertension and cardiac arrest.

SURGICAL AND ADJUNCTIVE TREATMENT

Surgical Techniques

The surgical techniques used in the treatment of vascular malformations are excision, compartmentalization by suturing, and vascular reconstruction.

EXCISION

Patients who have small, superficial AVMs may occasionally be cured by surgical excision. Unfortunately, such AVMs represent by far the minority of lesions. Most are large and diffuse in nature and involve important normal adjacent structures and are, therefore, exceptionally difficult or impossible to excise. Patients who have high-flow lesions that are considered suitable for excision should undergo preoperative arterial embolization to reduce blood loss during surgery (see Fig. 28–6). Close collaboration between surgeon and radiologist is absolutely essential, and it is important that both parties recognize that the aim of embolization is to reduce only the vascularity of the malformation and not the extent of the resection. Satisfactory long-term palliation, or indeed cure, can only be achieved if the malformation is excised in its entirety. It is equally important that the surgeon be fully informed of the extent of the embolization that has been performed. Complete devascularization of a malformation is not always possible by embolization. For example, it is not uncommon for high-flow malformations involving the face to derive some supply via the ophthalmic artery. Embolization of this vessel is not recommended for obvious reasons, and if the contribution from this artery is significant, the surgeon must be forewarned.

Excision should be performed between 24 and 48 hours after the embolization because this is the time of maximal devascularization and the excision can usually be performed with use of small particles of polyvinyl alcohol. A particle size is chosen that can produce good peripheral occlusion within the malformation itself, without passing through to the venous side. Proximal arterial embolization with large particles, metallic coils, or glue should be avoided at all costs for two reasons: first, collaterals form almost immediately, and satisfactory devascularization cannot be achieved; and second, this form of embolization interferes with subsequent arterial access if the malformation recurs.

SUTURAL COMPARTMENTALIZATION

Popescu first described the technique of compartmentalization of vascular malformations of low-flow type (termed cavernous hemangiomas in his original paper),[12] and this may produce spectacular results in large lesions that are not amenable to surgical excision. In this technique, a large hand-held needle is used to under-run the malformation in a criss-cross fashion, and this induces thrombosis in all the compartmentalized segments of the lesion because of the obliteration of blood flow. Some skin necrosis between and underneath the sutures is not uncommon but usually heals with time.

VASCULAR RECONSTRUCTION

Because of the increased use of direct puncture techniques for the embolization of even high-flow malformations (see later discussion), the reconstruction of a suitable vascular access to a lesion for embolization is rarely required. This technique may occasionally be useful for patients, however, when an arterial embolization is deemed to be the best form of treatment and this procedure is denied because of previous proximal embolization or surgical ligation.

Laser Therapy

HEMANGIOMAS

As stated previously, the only true tumor within this group of lesions is hemangioma of infancy or strawberry mark. This is a unique tumor in that it is self-limiting, and eventually it involutes. The congenital hemangioma is not present at birth and is noted initially as a small red dot. Typically, there is remarkable growth that usually peaks when the infant is 3 months of age, although it can continue to grow until the patient is 1 year of age. The lesion then stabilizes in size and eventually begins to involute over a variable time frame. Most quoted figures are that 50% of these lesions are involuted in patients who are 5 years of age and 70% in patients who are 7 years of age. This means that if left untreated, approximately 50% of these children begin school with lesions still present. If these are large, deforming lesions of the face,

this can be a significant problem. Other problems that they can create are painful, ulcerated lesions in the perineal areas as well as pressure on the globe, with distortion of vision or blockage of vision and obstruction of the nose or mouth. Other classic problems involve Kasabach-Merritt syndrome (platelet trapping), and high-output cardiac failure and failure to thrive.

There is a great deal of literature on this subject but no general agreement on the desirability of treating patients with these lesions. Furthermore, there is no consensus about the types of lesions for which patients should be treated or how they should be treated. Lesions on the trunk that are not ulcerated or causing any functional problems are usually left to involute on their own. Ulcerated lesions in the region of the perineum have been treated very successfully with the argon or the potassium titanyl phosphate (KTP) laser. Initially, this may produce a more complicated wound, but in all the cases in our experience, the lesions involuted within a short period of time after laser treatment. Intralesional treatment is the most recent technique that the authors have used. A fiberoptic cable of a KTP:yttrium aluminum garnet (YAG) laser is placed in the center of the lesion via a catheter. The metal cannula is removed, and the plastic cannula is used as the port. The laser is turned on and its light can be seen via transillumination. Various quadrants of the lesion are heated with the laser. Almost always, there is resulting involution of the lesion. The treatment can be repeated as needed. It is a very simple treatment that takes only a few minutes, usually under general anaesthesia. Approximately one third of these patients develop ulceration as part of the involution process. Occasionally there is a nonresponding patient.[13] Other long-standing, well-recognized treatments that have been shown to be effective for hemangioma of infancy include intralesional steroid injections or systemic steroid therapy (2 mg/kg per day). Systemic therapy must be carried on for several weeks and gradually tapered. It can be a very significant treatment in many cases in which there are systemic problems. Gastrointestinal upset is common and usually treated prophylactically with cimetidine. Intralesional steroid injection is a very simple technique. In fact, this is often done in the doctor's office and does not involve systemic effects of steroids and can be repeated as needed. There are some reports of selective embolization of these lesions. There does not seem to be any consensus of opinion on the role of embolization, but it should be considered in complicated cases, such as Kasabach-Merritt syndrome or bleeding.

CAPILLARY MALFORMATIONS

The typical capillary malformation is also known as a portwine stain. It is a pink spot that is flat at birth.

However, it is not generally recognized that these are progressive lesions that become raised, nodular, and larger over passing decades. There are several lasers designed to treat these, one of which is the flashed pump dye laser that emits a yellow flash of light that is absorbed preferentially by hemoglobin and blood cells. It is recommended that these lesions be treated early so that they can be eliminated before the child reaches school age.

CONCLUSIONS

There can be little doubt that patients with *pulmonary arteriovenous malformations* are best treated by pulmonary artery catheterization and embolization rather than by thoracotomy and resection. As these lesions are relatively uncommon, however, their treatment by embolization probably qualifies as a procedure that is best performed in a few specialist referral centers. In such institutions, excellent results can be obtained.

Just as important as the treatment is the screening of family members, and this must be one of the areas to which the team involved with these individuals must turn their attention.

Systemic vascular malformations represent a diverse group of lesions whose treatment (when required) is difficult. New catheters and embolic agents have already greatly increased our ability to treat these lesions successfully, and direct puncture and retrograde venous approaches are proving to be very promising techniques. A thorough understanding of the nature of these lesions and their anatomy and response to treatment is essential. They are best assessed and treated by a multidisciplinary team, including a vascular radiologist, a vascular surgeon, a plastic surgeon, and an orthopedic surgeon. Treatment of patients who have these rare lesions should be limited to a small number of specialized centers.

REFERENCES

1. Mulliken JB: Classification of vascular birthmarks. *In* Mulliken JB, Young AE (eds): Vascular Birthmarks. Hemangiomas and Malformations. Philadelphia, WB Saunders, 1988, pp 24–37.
2. Woolard RH: The development of the principal arterial stems in the forelimb of the pig. Cont Embryol 14:139–154, 1922.
3. Young AE: Pathogenesis of vascular malformations. *In* Mulliken JB Young AE (eds): Vascular Birthmarks. Hemangiomas and Malformations. Philadelphia, WB Saunders 1988, pp 107–113.
4. Whyte MKB, Hughes JMB, Jackson JE, et al: Cardiopulmonary response to exercise in patients with intrapulmonary vascular shunts. J Appl Physiol 75:321–328, 1993.
5. Chilvers ER, Peters AM, George P, et al: Quantification of right to left shunt through pulmonary arteriovenous malformations using 99Tcm albumin microspheres. Clin Rad 39:611–614, 1988.
6. Coley S, Jackson JE: Endovascular occlusion with a new mechanical detachable coil. Am J Roentgenol 171:1075–1079, 1998.
7. Chilvers ER, Whyte MKB, Jackson JE, et al: Effect of percutaneous transcatheter embolization on pulmonary function, right-to-left shunt, and arterial oxygenation in patients with pulmonary arteriovenous malformations. Am Rev Respir Dis 142:420–425, 1990.
8. Dutton J, Jackson JE, Whyte MKB, et al: Pulmonary arteriovenous malformations: Results of coil embolization in 53 patients. Am J Roentgenol 165:1119–1125, 1995.
9. Szilagyi DE, Smith RF, Elliott JP, et al: Congenital arteriovenous anomalies of the limbs. Arch Surg 111:423–429, 1976.
10. Yakes WF, Haas DK, Parker SH, et al. Symptomatic vascular malformations: Ethanol embolotherapy. Radiology 170:1059–1066, 1989.
11. Houdart E, Gobin YP, Casasco A, et al: A proposed angiographic classification of intracranial arteriovenous fistulae and malformations. Neuroradiology 35:381–385, 1993.
12. Popescu V: Intratumoral ligation in the management of orofacial cavernous haemangiomas. J Maxillofac Surg 13:99–107, 1985.
13. Achauer BM, Celikz B, Vander Kam V: Intralesional bare fiber laser treatment of hemangioma of infancy. Plast Reconst Surg 101:1212–1217, 1998.

Chapter 29 Chemoembolization

David P. Brophy and Melvin E. Clouse

Quality of life and overall survival in patients with hepatocellular carcinoma (HCC) or metastatic liver disease depends on control of tumor growth and suppression of the secretory function of certain liver metastases. Various treatment modalities have evolved to improve quality of life and survival in these patients with cancer. Surgical resection remains the treatment of choice for hepatoma, although fewer than 15% of patients are considered suitable because of concomitant cirrhosis, diffuse tumor, or medical contraindications.[1] Similarly, only 10 to 15% of hepatic metastases from colon carcinoma may be considered suitable for hepatic resection.[2] Hepatic metastases from neuroendocrine tumors invariably are too diffuse to be considered for surgical resection.

Various intravenous chemotherapeutic regimens have shown response rates of 20 to 25% at best.[3] The most commonly used agents, adriamycin, 5-fluorouracil, mitomycin, and cisplatin, have not been proven to have any effect on survival either alone or in combination. Possible reasons for impaired response to systemic therapy include the ability of liver and tumor cells to express high levels of a multidrug-resistant gene product. Drug toxicity also is enhanced in patients with limited hepatic reserve, thus limiting dose.

Given the limited results with systemic chemotherapy, other routes of drug delivery have been explored; direct drug injection into tumor, intraperitoneal application, and intraportal or intra-arterial infusion all have been attempted to increase intratumoral drug concentration. The intra-arterial method is most appealing because the hepatic artery primarily supplies hepatic tumors, especially in the early stages, whereas the healthy liver has a dual blood supply, with oxygen requirements distributed between the hepatic artery and the portal vein. Because of this unique blood supply, experience gained from blind embolization and surgical devascularization of the hepatic artery, added to the theoretical advantages of local drug administration, has resulted in the investigation of arterial-directed treatment for hepatic neoplasms.

Chemoembolization (CE) refers to the intra-arterial or intraportal administration of both chemotherapeutic agent(s) and embolic material for the treatment of hepatic malignancy, usually HCC, neuroendocrine tumors, or hepatic metastases from colon carcinoma (Fig. 29–1). The embolization component causes ischemia and paralyzes tumor cell excretion of the chemotherapeutic agent. Also, by causing vascular occlusion, CE delays the transit of chemotherapeutic agents through the tumor vascular bed, thus increasing the length of exposure.

INDICATIONS FOR CHEMOEMBOLIZATION

CE is a palliative procedure. Operative removal, ranging from tumor enucleation to liver transplantation, offers the only potentially curative treatment for hepatic malignancy. CE should be administered to patients who have symptomatic hepatic malignancy or who are expected to die of extensive malignant hepatic disease.

Hepatocellular Carcinoma

HCC is a common cause of cancer-related death worldwide, responsible for more than 1 million deaths each year. Although common in the Far East because of the high prevalence of hepatitis B, it remains relatively uncommon in Europe and the United States. The prognosis is universally poor, with typical survival being 4 to 6 months depending on extent of disease, portal vein patency, alpha-fetoprotein, and liver synthetic function. Median survival is only 4 to 6 weeks with concomitant cirrhosis.[4]

Although surgery offers the only chance of cure, this is often either contraindicated because of multifocal disease or limited hepatic reserve or impossible because of the lack of donor livers. Because response rates to intravenous chemotherapy are only between 20 to 25%,[3] CE is preferred in this nonresectable HCC patient population (Fig. 29–2).

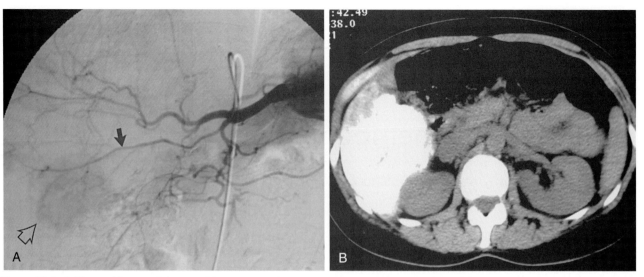

Figure 29–1. A 57-year-old man with hepatocellular carcinoma. *A,* celiac axis arteriogram shows a hypervascular lesion *(hollow arrow)* being supplied by an accessory right hepatic artery *(black arrow)*. *B,* Computed tomography (CT) scan post-chemoembolization (CE) of this vessel, confirms localization of oil contrast to the right posterior hepatic territory.

Even when HCC is amenable to surgery, recurrence rates are high and overall survival poor. Because HCC usually recurs in the remaining liver tissue, postoperative adjuvant CE has been performed and shows a potential for treating new small lesions, which are fed almost exclusively by the hepatic artery. In HCC cases, CE has been performed extensively before surgery. Neoadjuvant CE has made resection technically easier by causing tumor necrosis and by

making borderline lesions resectable. It also is argued that tumor seeding during resection is reduced and that microscopic unresected lesions are treated, thus reducing the rate of recurrence.[5]

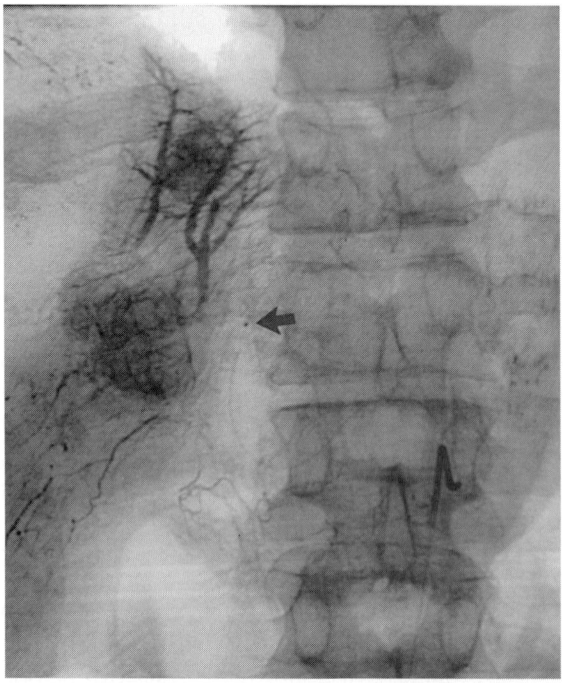

Colorectal Carcinoma

Of patients diagnosed with colorectal carcinoma (150,000/year in North America), 15 to 25% have metastatic liver disease at the time of diagnosis, with hepatic metastases developing in an additional 25% later in the disease. Most of the 70,000 people in the United States who die of colorectal carcinoma die of liver failure related to metastases. A median survival of 6 months from time of metastatic disease diagnosis can be expected. Hepatic resection is the treatment of choice and is the only potential for cure. After resection, a 25% 5-year survival rate can be expected. However, only 10 to 15% of patients with metastatic colorectal liver disease are considered suitable for liver resection. For the remaining patients, palliative treatment modalities include systemic intravenous therapy, CE, direct drug injection into the tumor, and laser or radiofrequency ablation. Unfortunately, the average response rate for intravenous chemotherapy is less than 25%, with a median survival of 11 to 12 months.[2]

CE is indicated either in patients with liver metastatic colorectal disease in whom surgery is not considered feasible because of tumor size or multiple liver foci or in patients refractory to other treatments for colorectal liver metastases. CE should only be performed if the metastatic disease is liver dominant because CE is a predominantly local treatment. When symptoms can be attributed to hepatomegaly because

Figure 29–2. A 45-year-old man with hepatocellular carcinoma. This completion film shows a microcatheter tip *(arrow)* in the left hepatic artery positioned through a 5-French Sos catheter. Opacification of the portal vein correlates with improved response to CE.

of tumor bulk, these lesions may be uniquely suited to local therapy.

Other Metastases

Patients with hepatic metastases from primary neuroendocrine tumors represent a large number of patients treated by chemoembolization. Although the growth of these tumors is typically indolent, peptide secretion from functioning metastatic islet cells or carcinoid tumors can result in compromising symptoms. Mass effect within the liver also may be a cause of debilitating symptoms. Only 7% of patients with metastatic neuroendocrine tumors are considered suitable for hepatic resection, and then 90% of the liver may need to be resected for this treatment to be effective. With various intravenous chemotherapy regimens, islet cell tumors have response rates of up to 69%, whereas carcinoid metastases show only a 20% response rate. CE is indicated in patients with symptomatic metastatic neuroendocrine tumors (Fig.

29–3), and because the liver component of neuroendocrine tumors is invariably responsible for symptoms, these tumors are suited ideally to local therapy.[6] CE also has been reported in the treatment of liver metastases from ocular melanoma, renal carcinoma, breast carcinoma, leiomyosarcoma, and a few other rare tumors. For these tumors, CE data are mainly anecdotal.

TECHNIQUE

Patient Selection

As with all cytotoxic treatments, tissue biopsy should be obtained before commencement of therapy. An exception is a cirrhotic patient with a mass on cross-sectional imaging and an alpha-fetoprotein of greater than 500, where a presumptive diagnosis of HCC can be made and treatment considered without biopsy.

Poor liver function and advanced cirrhosis can make CE not only less effective, but also excessively risky. Patients scoring 2 or higher on the Eastern

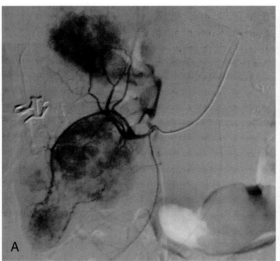

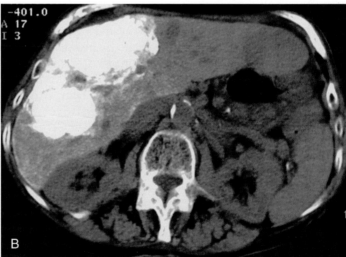

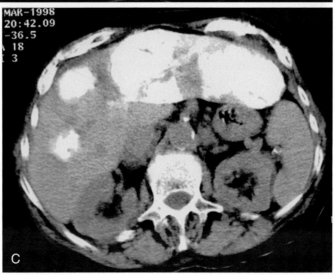

Figure 29–3. A 60-year-old woman with metastatic carcinoid. *A,* Initial selective right hepatic arteriogram with a 5-French C2 catheter shows multiple hypervascular right lobe lesions. *B,* CT scan 24 hours after right hepatic artery treatment shows preferential uptake of iodinated oil contrast within the lesions with relative washout from the surrounding right hepatic parenchyma. *C,* Twelve months later, a chemoembolization of the left hepatic artery was performed because of abdominal pain, enlarging left hepatic lesions and elevated 5-hydroxyindoleacetate. CT scan at that time, although showing localization of iodinated oil to the left sided lesions, also confirms response of the right-sided lesions to treatment 12 months previously.

Cooperative Oncology Group or World Health Organization performance scales probably should be excluded from CE.

Before considering CE, a multidisciplinary approach (including medical and surgical oncologists and radiologists) and appropriate workup are necessary to confirm that the patient is unsuitable for a potentially curative surgical procedure and that CE is a reasonable treatment because of previous therapy failure or doubtful efficacy of other therapy.

Currently, the primary liver imaging modality is a triple-phase (noncontrast, arterial, and portal) spiral or helical computed tomography (CT) because CT provides the best anatomic overview for the interventionist. Hypervascular lesions, which respond best to CE, typically are detected during the arterial phase. Regenerative nodules, fat or fibrous tissue infiltration, and vascular shunting often make determination of the extent of malignancy in cirrhotic patients difficult. Imaging should evaluate the exact segmental location, size, and number of lesions, with reference also made to the apparent vascularity, or lack thereof. The predominant location by vascular territory should be estimated and note made of unusual anatomy or postsurgical changes (atrophy–hypertrophy complex, exophytic tumor). The presence of associated pathology such as biliary obstruction, vascular compromise (portal vein occlusion, hepatic infarction), and extrahepatic disease should be determined. If extrahepatic disease is considered to be the main source of symptoms or life-threatening disease, then an alternative treatment to CE should be contemplated because CE treats only hepatic disease. On rare occasions on which the extrahepatic disease is indolent or responding to other treatments while the intrahepatic disease tumor is progressing, patients with extrahepatic disease are treated with CE. With good arterial phase imaging, it may be possible to identify aberrant arterial supply to the liver, such as hepatic artery arising from the superior mesenteric artery or the left gastric artery. CT also is used for patient follow-up post-CE.

Determining the patency of the superior mesenteric, splenic, main portal, and right and left portal veins is crucial if complications of CE are to be avoided. Because CE results in cessation of hepatic arterial supply to the hepatic lobe or segment being treated, that portion of liver temporarily becomes dependent on the portal system for its blood supply. If portal supply is compromised, subsegmental or segmental rather than lobar CE with a smaller volume of embolic agent is advised, particularly if hepatopetal collateral branches cannot be demonstrated by either color Doppler ultrasound, magnetic resonance venography, or delayed phase splenic/mesenteric angiography. Although CE has been performed in cases of complete portal vein occlusion, morbidity is increased. It is our experience that marked hepatofugal flow also is associated with morbidity because of liver infarction and the passage of embolic material into the systemic circulation via arterioportal and then spontaneous portosystemic shunts.

CE is contraindicated in biliary obstruction unless biliary drainage keeps the bilirubin below 3 mg/dl (52 µmol/L). Even when bilirubin is below this level, segmental biliary dilation precludes treatment of that segment because of the risk of infarction. The presumed mechanism is that the resistance to biliary outflow increases the pressure in the sinusoids, which in turn compromises portal inflow, making the involved liver more dependent on hepatic arterial flow and therefore susceptible to infarction after CE.[7]

Limited liver function reserve is a contraindication to CE. Ascites refractive to dietary control, diuretics and fluid restriction, encephalopathy that cannot be easily controlled medically, and poor synthetic hepatic function all are indicators for severe liver dysfunction. CE is less effective and is associated with higher morbidity in patients who are classified with Child's class C liver disease. In patients with borderline dysfunction, CE can cause hepatic decompensation and worsen hepatic failure, precipitating encephalopathy and ascites. Generally, patients being considered for CE should have reasonably maintained liver function, that is, albumin greater than 2.8 g/dl and international normalized ratio (INR) of less than 2. A subgroup of patients with a combination of greater than 50% of liver volume replaced by tumor, aspartate transaminase greater than 100 IU/L, lactate dehydrogenase greater than 425 IU/L, and a total bilirubin greater than 2 mg/dl (34.5 µmol/L)[8] are at increased risk of acute hepatic failure after CE. If these patients are to be treated, segmental or subsegmental CE with less embolic material is advised.

Other important laboratory parameters include renal function, in which a creatinine level of less than 2 mg/dl (180 µmol/L) is preferred because the renal excretion of both iodinated contrast and tumor necrosis products can cause renal function deterioration. Blood counts are rarely abnormal in patients being considered for CE, unless the patient has HCC with cirrhosis and hypersplenism. White cell counts greater than 2000/mm³ and platelet counts greater than 50,000/mm³ are preferred in this scenario.

Patient Preparation and Preprocedural Care

Once the patient is considered suitable for CE, there should be an in-depth discussion not only with the patient but also with the family. Alternative treatments and the option of no treatment should be addressed. The patient and family should have a clear understanding of the aims and expectations of the treatment: CE should be presented as a palliative rather than curative procedure. Up to 90% of patients have some degree of "postembolization syndrome," characterized by epigastric/right upper quadrant pain, fever, nausea, and vomiting. The severity of these symptoms varies enormously between patients and lasts anywhere from hours to several days. Narcotics and antiemetics are given prophylactically, which should abate these symptoms. More serious complications occur in less than 4% of cases, some of which can result in death. In uncomplicated cases, average length of hospital stay is between 2 and 3 days. It should be pointed out that depending on arterial anatomy, two to four separate sessions of CE are required to treat the entire liver, after which response is assessed by repeat imaging and tumor markers. If regrowth or new tumors are detected, additional CE may be indicated.

Although oral intake is restricted from midnight the night before the procedure, clear fluids are allowed up to 2 hours before the procedure begins. Because good hydration at the time of the procedure is the key to preventing contrast related renal insufficiency,[9] aggressive intravenous fluids (e.g., normal saline or dextrose 5%/½ normal saline at 150–300 ml/hr) are begun as soon as the patient arrives at the hospital.

Patients are admitted the day of CE at our institution. One to 2 days before CE, oral allopurinol 300 mg twice daily is administered. This xanthine oxidase inhibitor decreases the incidence of hyperuricemia and related renal insufficiency that can be associated with tumor lysis. Before treatment of metastatic neuroendocrine tumors, patients are started on a long-acting somatostatin analogue, octreotide 100 to 200 mg subcutaneously twice daily. This can be started the morning of the procedure.

Although not all investigators agree with prophylactic antibiotics, it has been shown that broad spectrum antibiotics can decrease infectious complication rates (0% vs. 6.6%).[10] Intravenous cefotetan (1 g) or cephazolin (1 g) with metronidazole (500 mg) is effective.

Patients are premedicated with hydromorphone 1 to 3 mg subcutaneously and hydroxycine 25 to 50 mg orally, with additional midazolam and fentanyl administered during the procedure. Prochlorperazine can be given orally before the procedure as a prophylactic antiemetic. Ondansetron is a very effective antiemetic alternative that also can be given orally 1 hour before the procedure. Intravenous steroids (dexamethasone) also are administered by some institutions as a premedication.

Some institutions routinely place urinary bladder catheters and order full bowel preparation before the procedure. However, this is probably unnecessary.

Portal or Arterial Chemoembolization

CE has been administered into the hepatic artery and/or the portal vein. Separate intra-arterial and intraportal injections do not result in different patterns of oil droplet accumulation in or around even hypovascular tumors. This may be attributed to arterioportal shunts that allow oil droplets to pass from the arterial to the portal system.[11] Therefore, there is no advantage in intraportal CE alone or in combination with the intra-arterial CE, and given the associated additional morbidity, intraportal CE is not justified.

Choice of Chemotherapeutic Agents

Despite claims that the CE technique has been established and that CE currently is a "standard procedure," there is no consensus on which chemotherapeutic or embolic agents should be used.

Many agents or combinations of chemotherapeutic agents have been used for CE. Doxorubicin, mitomycin C, and cisplatin are the most commonly reported. In Europe and the Far East, doxorubicin, either alone or in combination with mitomycin C, is used most commonly. In the United States, doxorubicin or cisplatin alone or a combination of cisplatin, mitomycin C, and doxorubicin are used most often. Typical doses are 40 to 60 mg doxorubicin, 100 to 150 mg cisplatin, and 10 to 20 mg mitomycin C. All these agents are broad spectrum antibiotics and, more importantly for angiographic purposes, can be administered in effective small-volume doses. No convincing comparative studies have shown any significant advantage of one regimen over another. Although systemic toxicity of these drugs always must be considered, most toxicity can be attributed to local hepatic ischemia or nontarget CE.[12]

Embolization Materials

Various techniques of embolization and types of embolization materials have been used for CE. Hepatic embolization alone, without administration of a chemotherapeutic agent, may be performed. This gives response rates of between 80 and 90% for palliation of carcinoid and islet cell hypervascular tumors. Response rates for hepatoma are more modest, at 50 to 60%, with slight increase in survival.[13] However, hepatic artery embolization alone is limited by the ability of the liver to form collateral vessels, and therefore, any benefit tends to be transient. Embolization alone does not extend survival for patients with colorectal metastases.[12]

For CE, the chemotherapeutic agent is dissolved

in 10 to 15 ml of water-soluble nonionic contrast material, which in turn is mixed with an embolic agent. In the treatment of HCC in particular, this embolic agent usually is iodinated poppy seed oil. Because this oil selectively accumulates in HCC, it has been used to improve the efficacy of HCC diagnosis. In CE, its use has resulted in improved targeting of chemotherapeutic drugs to tumor when incorporated into a chemotherapy regimen. Various techniques of combining chemotherapy drugs and oil have been used. These include suspending the drug in oil or using lipophilic chemotherapeutic agents. An emulsion of iodinated oil with aqueous solution of drug and nonionic contrast material, however, is used most commonly. The oil-based contrast material, an essential component of the treatment, acts as a transport medium for the chemotoxic agent and also, because of its high viscosity, results in a degree of vascular embolization. It has an affinity for tumor vasculature that has made it useful in the identification of liver tumors. As it traps the chemotherapeutic agent with it, the iodinated oil contrast prolongs the transit time of the chemotoxic agent at the site where it is needed most. Because hepatic tumors do not have Kupffer cells and normal lymphatic vessels to clear the chemotherapeutic agent, vascular inflow and outflow are the main means of drug removal. It is suggested that if iodinated oil traverses the sinusoids and is seen in the portal vein, then more effective tumor necrosis can be expected (Fig. 29–2).

When CE with iodinated oil and a chemotherapeutic agent is followed by embolization with particulate agents, improved results have been obtained.[12] The combination of oil and particles occludes both the portal venules and the terminal arterioles, therefore sandwiching the drug while maintaining ischemia and increasing dwell time of chemotherapy agent. Such particulate agents include gelatin powder, polyvinyl alcohol particles, starch microspheres, and collagen particles. These particulate embolic agents have been given in a mixture with, or separately after, the emulsion of chemotherapy drugs, iodinated oil, and water-soluble contrast.

No compelling clinical evidence suggests a benefit of one embolic agent over another, although the effects of different particle sizes, different emulsion preparations, and the duration of vascular occlusion are being investigated.

Embolization Technique and Anatomic Considerations

The patient is prepared and draped in a sterile fashion, with angiographers wearing full sterile outfit, including gloves, hat, and gown. All personnel in the angiography room should be wearing protective eyewear or glasses. Conscious sedation is routine. Rarely, particularly in nervous younger patients, heavier sedation using propathol with monitored anesthesia care may be needed. Initial diagnostic visceral angiography is performed, usually via the right common femoral artery. After local anesthesia is infiltrated around the artery, a modified Seldinger technique with a single-wall needle is used to acquire arterial access. A 5-French sheath is positioned routinely through which a 5-French Cobra or Simmons catheter invariably achieves selective cannulation of the proximal superior mesenteric artery and celiac axis. Mesenteric and hepatic arteriography are performed to map out vascular anatomy and areas of tumor vascularity and to assess all sources of hepatic arterial supply and portal vein patency.

The superior mesenteric artery (SMA) usually is selected first, particularly in cirrhotic patients with splenomegaly when injection into the celiac axis or even splenic artery may not give optimal opacification of the portal vein. Injection into the proximal SMA may show a replaced or accessory right hepatic artery. Delayed-phase SMA angiography invariably allows adequate portal vein opacification if the portal venous system has not been imaged recently by cross-sectional techniques. Patency of the portal vein has been considered necessary for safe CE of the hepatic artery. However, CE can be performed in the presence of complete portal vein occlusion, provided that there is satisfactory collateral portal flow. If the portal vein is occluded, particulate embolization to produce stagnant flow probably should be omitted. If there is any doubt, however, a segmental or subsegmental CE can be undertaken to reduce the risk of liver infarction and liver failure.

The celiac axis then is cannulated, followed by selective arteriography of the common, proper, right, and left hepatic arteries, as necessary.

Variant hepatic arterial anatomy is present in almost half the population. Complete celiac and mesenteric arteriography is mandatory during the first CE to map out the arterial supply to the liver and to map out any replaced or accessory hepatic branches. Procedure-related complications, such as gastric and duodenal ulcers, can be averted by careful angiography and avoidance of intestinal branches. Knowledge of the normal and variant visceral arterial anatomy is invaluable in preventing nontarget CE and complications. The entire purpose of the CE procedure is defeated if complications keep patients in the hospital for prolonged periods of time.

1. The most common anatomic variant is a right hepatic artery branching off the proximal SMA (15% of population) to supply posterior segments of the right lobe or indeed, the complete right lobe. If this vessel is challenging to cannulate, either a Rosch

hepatic catheter or formation of a Waltman loop with a Cobra catheter can be helpful. A coaxial 3-French microcatheter is another option for selecting replaced or accessory right hepatic arteries.

2. Failure to identify the supply to the left lobe suggests the left hepatic artery arising from the left gastric artery. The entire left hepatic artery or lateral segmental branch can be replaced by the left gastric artery. This variant occurs in 11% of the population. Careful attention should be paid to the initial celiac axis arteriogram to ensure that the left gastric artery is seen to fill. If the catheter is too far into the celiac trunk and no contrast refluxes at the time of injection, the left gastric and therefore a left hepatic artery arising from it can be missed. Cannulation of the left gastric artery can require the use of a Waltman loop, and a coaxial catheter may be needed to manipulate beyond all gastric branches. The Waltman loop technique frequently facilitates not only easy cannulation of the left gastric artery but also both phrenic arteries (Fig. 29–4).

3. There are a wide range of less frequent hepatic arterial variants: right hepatic artery originating from the aorta, the common hepatic artery being replaced arising from the SMA, the common hepatic artery originating directly from the aorta, and the entire celiac and SMA distribution arising from a single trunk. Rarely, the left gesture-hepatic trunk or the right hepatic artery can have their own separate origin off the abdominal aorta. Because of this variability, the entire hepatic arterial supply should be well visualized before a patient undergoes chemoembolization.

In addition to the hepatic arterial supply, there are a few intestinal branches that are important to identify. The right gastric artery runs along the lesser curvature of the stomach and anastomoses with the left gastric artery. Although this vessel can arise from the proper (40%), left (40%), or right (10%) hepatic artery or the gastroduodenal artery (8%), it may not be angiographically visible. CE of this branch can cause severe antral ulceration with extended hospital stay and recovery. If there is a concern that chemoembolic material may enter this vessel, it can be embolized selectively with coils to protect the gastric mucosa from reflux of chemoembolic material. Left gastric collateral vessels perfuse the territory supplied by the right gastric artery.

Sometimes the gastroduodenal artery may arise uncomfortably close to the origin of the middle and/or left hepatic artery and can require coil embolization to prevent reflux. Collateral branches from the pancreaticoduodenal arcade perfuse territory supplied by the gastroduodenal artery.

Very rarely, a large falciform artery originating from the left hepatic artery also may have to be embolized before CE of the left hepatic artery.

Another branch that may cause problems is the supraduodenal artery. This vessel may arise from either the proper hepatic, right hepatic, left hepatic, gastroduodenal artery or pancreaticoduodenal arteries.

Initially, there was much concern over allowing chemoembolic material into the cystic artery, but treatment of the right hepatic artery, when given from a position proximal to the cystic artery, surprisingly rarely caused significant cholecystitis. This may be related to early stagnation of flow in the small cystic artery, preventing passage of smaller embolic material toward the end of the CE treatment. Patients can remain asymptomatic despite follow-up noncontrast CT scans clearly showing uptake of chemoembolic material in the gallbladder wall. It may be that symptoms of cholecystitis are mistaken for postembolization syndrome for which the patient already is receiving prophylactic antibiotics for potential liver infection and prophylactic pain medications.

Vascular defects also may be caused by tumor-related arterial compromise. Correlation with preprocedural CT can be very useful when there is gross architectural distortion by large tumors. Peripheral hepatic tumors may have alternative arterial supply from adjacent parietal arteries, such as the internal mammary and phrenic arteries.

Some patients may present for CE after postoperative recurrence or after hepatic arterial infusion has failed. These patients pose a challenge because their

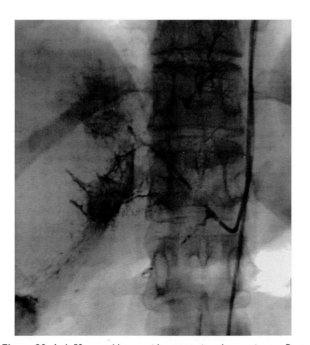

Figure 29–4. A 53-year-old man with metastatic colon carcinoma. Post-treatment film shows the results of an uncomplicated CE of the right phrenic artery, which was supplying left hepatic lesions. This treatment was facilitated by formation of a Waltman loop, allowing stable cannulation.

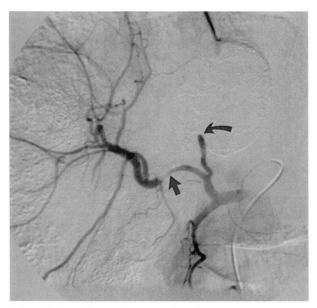

Figure 29–5. A 35-year-old woman with metastatic islet cell carcinoma. Common hepatic arteriogram post-right hepatic artery CE shows dissection of the right hepatic artery *(straight arrow)*, a catheter-related complication of right hepatic artery CE. Also seen is arterial occlusion related to treatment deposition in the vasa vasorum from prior CE of the left hepatic artery *(curved arrow)*.

anatomy may be altered severely. If the celiac axis or common hepatic artery is occluded, collateral branches are likely to have formed from the SMA circulation. A 3-French microcatheter usually is required to negotiate these tortuous collaterals.

Inevitably with each CE, some of the drug is deposited in the vasa vasorum of the hepatic artery, which then can occlude (Fig. 29–5). In the face of hepatic artery occlusion, the hepatic tumor can parasitize arterial supply from neighboring vessels, such as the inferior phrenic, internal mammary, pancreaticoduodenal, adrenal, and intercostal arteries (Figs. 29–6 and 29–7). These vessels can be embolized safely but can require superselection to avoid extrahepatic sites.

Opacification of the portal vein in the late phase of a proper hepatic arterial injection indicates arterioportal shunting that, if gross, likely is associated with hepatofugal portal venous flow, and we would caution against CE because of the risk of hepatic infarction and passage of chemoembolic agent into the systemic circulation via spontaneous portosystemic shunts. Occasionally in patients with HCC, smaller arterioportal shunts only can be appreciated when the portal vein becomes opacified with chemoembolic mixture after CE. In our experience, this has occurred without complication.

Again, one of the most important factors in preventing complications from CE is a thorough knowledge of the normal and variant anatomy. Identification of replaced and accessory arteries prevents unnecessary treatment failures. Recognition of intestinal branches that commonly arise from hepatic arteries prevents potentially serious complications. Meticulous technique is required for a successful chemoembolization program.

A diagnostic arteriogram always is performed with the drug delivery catheter in its final position. Again, this is to confirm that the territory to be treated will not result in chemoembolic agent being delivered to nontarget locations. Once hepatic arterial access to the desired liver segment or lobe is secured, preparation of both the chemotherapeutic agent and embolic material can begin. We presently are using doxorubicin to treat HCC and neuroendocrine tumors, whereas a combination of 5-fluorouracil and mitomycin C is administered for metastatic colorectal carcinoma. All chemotherapy preparation should be performed in the pharmacy. The usual dose of doxorubicin is between 30 and 60 mg, depending on the size of the territory to be embolized. Doxorubicin is emulsified with iodinated oil and water-soluble contrast. For metastatic colorectal carcinoma, usually 1g 5-fluorouracil and 10 mg mitomycin C are mixed and emulsified with both iodinated oil and water-soluble contrast in a fashion similar to doxorubicin. For both regimens, there may be occasion to alter the composition of the emulsion according to angiographic findings: such as decreasing iodinated oil when there is portal vein compromise, which also may require segmental rather than lobar artery treatment and increasing iodinated oil when treating a particularly hypervascular tumor.

Once mixed and emulsified, this emulsion should be kept agitated until injection. The iodinated oil and chemoembolic mixture is held in suspension, and

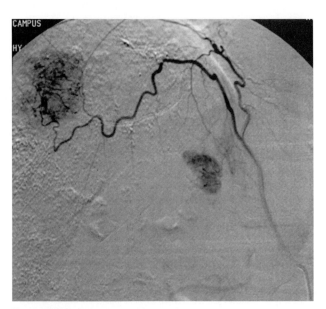

Figure 29–6. Arteriogram shows right phrenic artery supplying liver dome lesions in a patient with hepatocellular carcinoma previously treated by chemoembolization.

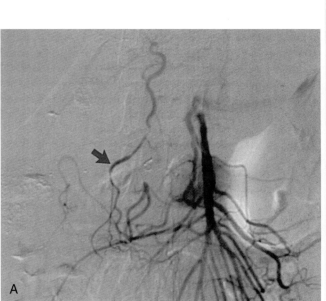
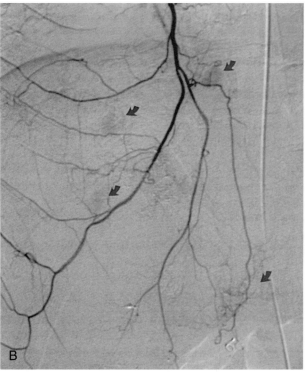

Figure 29–7. A 49-year-old woman with metastatic colon carcinoma who previously had CE via both right and left hepatic arteries. *A,* superior mesenteric arteriogram shows reconstitution of the left hepatic artery via the posterior pancreaticoduodenal arcade *(straight arrow).* The splenic artery fills via the artery of Bühler with the common hepatic artery not opacifying. *B,* Right internal mammary arteriogram shows focal areas of tumor blush *(curved arrows),* which corresponded with recurrent disease on CT scan.

therefore, continuous shaking is required up to the time of administration. Also, premature aspiration of chemotoxic emulsion should be avoided because prolonged contact between the plastic syringe and chemotoxic agent can result in a caustic reaction. For this reason also, the same delivery syringe should not be used for more than one aspiration and injection.

Just before administering the chemotherapeutic emulsion, additional pretreatment with narcotics and sedation can be given intravenously. In addition, 10- to 30-mg boluses (up to a total of 100 mg) of intra-arterial lidocaine can be given before and between the injections of chemoembolic emulsion. The chemotherapeutic emulsion is given in 1- to 10-ml aliquots, depending on the dynamics of flow and size of catheter, under intermittent fluoroscopic control. The contrast provided by the iodinated oil, and the water-soluble contrast ensures visualization of the injection for accurate delivery. Care must be taken during injection; unwanted reflux into other visceral branches can result from too vigorous injection. The injection of this emulsion through microcatheters can be facilitated by the use of small 1- to 5-ml syringes.

Immediately after administration of the chemoembolic emulsion, particulate embolization is performed. Most commonly, gelatin in either a pledget or powder form is used. The angiographer dissolves 1 of gelatin powder in a mixture of 15 to 25 ml of nonionic contrast (300 mg/ml organically bound iodine) with 2 to 4 ml of absolute alcohol until a "thin apple sauce" consistency is achieved. This small amount of alcohol facilitates mixing of the dry gelatin with the contrast and is not meant to cause undesirable thrombotic arterial occlusion. Up to 10 ml of this paste can be administered under fluoroscopic control at a rate that avoids reflux and to a point at which there is stagnant or almost stagnant antegrade flow.

Lesser volumes are recommended if less dynamic flow is present and in the event of portal vein compromise or borderline liver function reserve. While the catheter is still in the embolized artery, the catheter should be flushed with saline under fluoroscopic control to prevent nontarget embolization during removal of catheter.

Posttreatment Care

After removal of the catheter, the patient is kept on bedrest for 5 to 6 hours. Vigorous hydration is maintained with intravenous fluids (3 L of normal saline or dextrose/saline, 150 ml/hr). Clear fluids are allowed to advance to regular diet as tolerated. Routine postprocedural vital signs are obtained with checks on the catheter entry limb for pulses and possible hematoma.

Immediate postprocedure time is usually the most difficult for the patient. Narcotics, prochlorperazine, and acetaminophen are supplied liberally for control of pain, nausea, and fever. Location of pain can correspond roughly to the liver segment embolized: right lobe treatment causes right upper quadrant and loin pain whereas left lobe treatment is associated with anterior chest and epigastric pain. However, some patients relate a diffuse, poorly localized abdominal discomfort. Substantial improvement in pain level can be expected in the first 12 hours. Spirometry must be encouraged actively to maintain effective pulmonary toilet during this time. Once initial pain subsides, worsening or recurrent pain is not expected, and if it occurs, it should alert the attending physician to complications, such as cholecystitis, gastrointestinal erosions, hepatic infarction, or tumor rupture.

In rare cases, ondansetron may be required for nausea. Vomiting unresponsive to medications, occurring in association with hepatic encephalopathy, may necessitate placement of a nasogastric tube to prevent aspiration and possible pneumonia. Fever can be expected in the first week posttreatment and does not require cultures. Symptomatic treatment with acetaminophen or another antipyretic agent is usually effective. High-spiking fevers, significant leukocytosis, and a second rise in C-reactive protein after initial fall, particularly 72 hours post-CE, should be evaluated further as evidence of complications such as cholecystitis, liver abscess, bowel infarction, pancreatitis, or pneumonia.

While in the hospital, the patient's complete blood count, creatinine, and liver function tests are checked daily. Increases in transaminases peak on the second day post-CE and are expected to return to pre-CE levels within 5 to 14 days. Bilirubin increases also, usually peaking on day 3 post-CE, returning to pre-CE levels within 1 to 4 weeks.[14]

The patients are discharged as soon as oral intake is established and parenteral narcotics are not required for pain control. The average length of hospital stay currently is between 1.5 and 2 days. Intravenous antibiotics (cephazolin 500 mg/8 hr and metronidazole 500 mg/12 hr) are converted to oral antibiotics (ciprofloxacin or augmentin) and continued for 5 days. Antiemetics and narcotics are prescribed as needed. Cirrhotic patients are prescribed lactulose for 7 days to decrease the incidence and severity of hepatic encephalopathy.

Before discharge, a noncontrast CT scan is performed to confirm quality and location of CE, to identify nontarget CE, to plan the next treatment, and to act as a baseline for future CT scan interpretation (Fig. 29–8). The patient returns for treatment of the remaining lobe 1 month later. Depending on arterial anatomy, two to four treatments are required to treat the whole liver, after which response is determined by repeat imaging and tumor markers.

RESULTS

Hepatocellular Carcinoma

Evaluation of the literature with regard to the transcatheter treatment of HCC is difficult. Although treatment outcomes are related to extent of disease and degree of liver dysfunction, tumor size and Child/Okuda classifications are not reported consistently by many authors. CE results have been reported extensively in patients with HCC, with the largest experience coming from the Far East. CE with oil and Gelfoam have been shown histologically to be far more effective at tumor necrosis than CE with oil or oil alone. Combining results from series treating unresectable HCC, biologic and morphologic response rates in 800 patients have been between 60% and 83%. Most favorable results were found using combinations of iodinated oil, Gelfoam, and a chemotherapeutic agent. Cumulative probability of survival was 50 to 88% at 1 year, 33 to 64% at 2 years, and 18 to 51% at 3 years. Improved survival can be expected in patients with tumor involving less than 40% of liver volume and better classification of cirrhosis (Child, Okuda) and where there is retained iodinated oil within tumor post CE.[12, 13]

Despite the large number of single-regimen studies, very few comparative studies have compared CE with alternative therapies. A multicenter prospective randomized study comparing CE and supportive treatment was terminated because it showed only a 20% difference in survival at 8 months.[15] Because of the high exclusion rate in this study and the limited focus on short-term survival among patients with minimal disease, the conclusion of this study cannot be applied to most patients with HCC presenting for CE. In a further multicenter study, which incorporated far more patients with Child's B and Child's C cirrhosis, there was a significant increase in survival at 1 to 4 years in their CE group (64%, 38%, 27%, and 27%) compared with the supportive care group (18%, 6%, 5%, and 0%).[13]

Colorectal Carcinoma

Trials evaluating the results of CE in metastatic colorectal carcinoma are limited to less than 400 patients. These studies used iodinated oil, gelatin, or collagen in combination with multiple chemotherapy regimens. Radiologic and biologic (CEA) criteria were used to determine response. Most patients already had failed systemic and/or intra-arterial infusion chemotherapy. Response rates have ranged between 25%

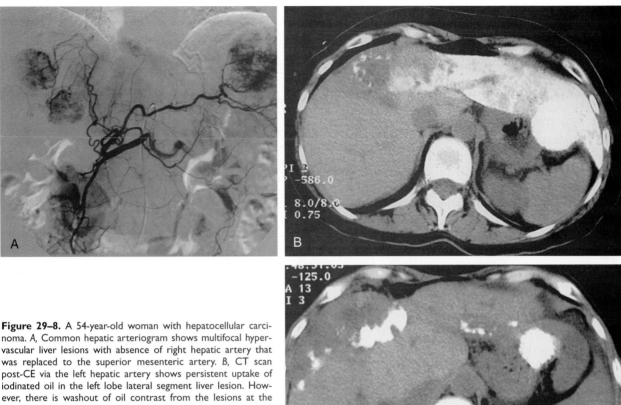

Figure 29–8. A 54-year-old woman with hepatocellular carcinoma. *A,* Common hepatic arteriogram shows multifocal hypervascular liver lesions with absence of right hepatic artery that was replaced to the superior mesenteric artery. *B,* CT scan post-CE via the left hepatic artery shows persistent uptake of iodinated oil in the left lobe lateral segment liver lesion. However, there is washout of oil contrast from the lesions at the interlobar region suggesting that there is dual (right and left) supply to these lesions. *C,* The right hepatic artery was treated 6 weeks later. Follow-up CT scan 13 months later confirms a reduction in size of the left-sided lesion. However, there is recurrent disease evident at the periphery of the treated lesions.

and 100% depending on the criteria used for measurement. Median survival was between 7 and 23 months. Good performance status at onset of treatment, reduction in size of lesion, homogenous distribution of iodinated oil, and subsequent central necrosis, increased tumor vascularity, and the use of multiple chemotherapeutic agents all have been suggested to be associated with an improved response.[16]

Other Metastases

Devascularization has been established as a treatment for hypervascular tumors such as neuroendocrine tumors. The results of CE for the treatment of neuroendocrine tumors compare favorably with those of embolization alone, with CE having a mean symptom-free interval of 22 to 29 months compared with 5 to 10 months with embolization alone.[17] Symptomatic and biologic response can be expected in greater than 87% of cases with both techniques. No

differences in response rates or survival have been shown between CE and embolization. Symptomatic responses may be difficult to evaluate because symptoms may be partly controlled by octreotide. A prospective study is necessary to determine the relative benefits and roles of embolotherapy, CE, and octreotide either alone or in combination.

Hepatic metastases from ocular melanoma are frequently aggressive, with median survival of 2 to 6 months. In the largest studies using CE, the median survival rates were 11 months in 30 patients.[18]

Hepatic metastases from lung, breast, kidney, pancreas, small bowel, cholangiocarcinoma, ovary, bladder, thymus, and adenocarcinoma of unknown origin have been grouped together in CE reports claiming 60 to 75% response rates and median survival of 8 to 11 months.[12] Hepatic metastases from sarcomas, because they respond poorly to both systemic chemotherapy and radiotherapy, have been treated with CE. Anecdotal reports have suggested durable responses.

FOLLOW-UP AND REINTERVENTION

Tumor markers, liver function tests, and CT scans are performed at 1 month, 2 to 3 months and 4 to 6 months post-CE, and at 3-month intervals thereafter. The decision to re-embolize a lobe or segment of the liver in an individual patient is based on a combination of clinical symptoms, serum tumor markers, response to initial treatment, and findings on CT. Interpretation of CT findings can be difficult because tumor recurrence and tumor necrosis can have similar appearances. Focal enhancement on contrast-enhanced CT scans can suggest recurrence, particularly when the tumor is known to be hypervascular. Recurrence, however, commonly manifests as new lesions rather than recurrence of treated lesions. Additional treatment requires that liver function tests have returned to baseline or at least show a downward trend, indicating recovery of normal liver parenchyma from previous treatment. Given the palliative nature of CE, asymptomatic recurrence sometimes is left untreated in our institution, although many investigators take a more aggressive approach to re-embolization. Before *any* CE treatment, risk factors for complications must be assessed and CE either modified or not given at all if significant risk exists.

COMPLICATIONS AND HOW TO AVOID THEM

The widespread acceptance of CE for liver tumors is related at least in part to the relative safety of performing devascularization in this territory and to the treatment being well tolerated in most cases. However, CE can cause serious complications and even death. Major complications of CE include hepatic failure or infarction, biliary necrosis, hepatic abscess, tumor rupture, surgical cholecystitis, and nontarget embolization of the gastrointestinal tract. With proper patient selection and careful attention to technique, the incidence of these serious complications is 3 to 5% with 30-day mortality rates between 1% and 4%.[14]

Postembolization Syndrome

The most common consequence of CE is postembolization syndrome (PES). This refers to a constellation of symptoms, such as pain, nausea, fever, and malaise, which can occur after either bland or chemotherapeutic visceral embolization. Although it occurs in 85 to 90% of patients, it is severe in only 15%, requiring prolonged hospital admission.[19] Administration of intra-arterial lidocaine during CE is thought by some to significantly reduce the severity and duration of pain after the procedure. Treatment is symptomatic, with a combination of analgesics, antiemetics, and antipyretic agents. When PES is severe, other complications, such as sepsis, should be considered. Severe PES is thought to be closely related to the degree of tumor necrosis. Patients should be at bedrest for a time after CE because portal venous flow is increased by 30% in the supine compared with the erect position. Larger tumors and the use of larger quantities of particulate embolic material correlate with the severity of PES and the increased likelihood of septic complications. Malaise after treatment may persist for a few weeks.

Hepatic Complications

Hepatic failure can occur if there is limited hepatic reserve, for example, in patients with Child's C cirrhosis, tumor taking up greater than 70% of the liver parenchyma, portal venous compromise, biliary obstruction, and an excessive amount of iodinated oil embolization. Usually liver failure is transient, but irreversible hepatic failure can occur in 3.1% of cases. Disseminated intravascular coagulopathy can further complicate hepatic infarction.[14]

Portal vein occlusion is a well-known risk factor for liver infarction. In such patients, superselective treatment with less aggressive administration of embolic material can be performed if the tumor is limited and there is adequate liver function. When the parenchymal tumor is extensive, CE is contraindicated because of the risk of hepatic failure.

Liver infarction also can occur without portal vein occlusion. Hepatic arterioportal shunts can be demonstrated angiographically in 28.8% of patients presenting with HCC. With CE, arterioportal shunts predispose to liver infarction as the CE mixture injected into the hepatic artery accumulates in the peripheral portal vein through the arterioportal communication. This results in tumor necrosis as well as infarction, with subsequent atrophy of the surrounding parenchyma. If an arterioportal shunt is seen pre-CE, a more selective treatment with less embolic material can be performed safely. If liver infarction is suspected, prophylactic antibiotics should be administered.

Intrahepatic biloma is a consequence of bile duct stricture secondary to peripheral duct necrosis caused by microvascular damage of the peribiliary capillary plexus. Its clinical course is usually spontaneous regression, but it can be fatal if infected.

Liver abscess is associated with CE of larger tumors, biliary obstruction, and intrahepatic biloma formation. Because the presence of gas within a lesion is not unusual and can occur with necrosis alone, it does not necessarily imply infection (Fig. 29–9). Correlation

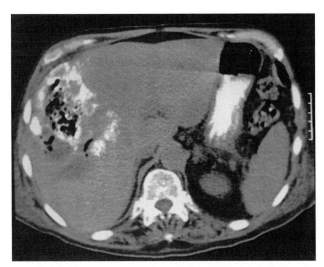

Figure 29–9. A 64-year-old man with hepatocellular carcinoma. Gas collections within a large tumor 2 months post-CE. These gaseous areas commonly are seen post-CE most frequently are not associated with clinical infection.

with clinical and laboratory findings is warranted. Diagnostic aspiration may be indicated, particularly if symptoms do not improve within 5 to 6 days post-CE.

Although tumor rupture and hemorrhage usually can be controlled with conservative measures, this complication is potentially fatal. The tumor in these cases is usually very large, with the corresponding portal venous trunk occluded. Another predisposing factor is recent percutaneous biopsy. CE should be deferred when there has been a recent biopsy.

Multiple intrahepatic aneurysms can be seen after CE. These are rare findings that can spontaneously disappear during follow-up. The risk of rupture is not known.

Life-threatening carcinoid crisis and other humoral effects related to release of serotonin and vasoactive intestinal polypeptide should be anticipated when treating neuroendocrine tumors such as carcinoid and islet cell tumors. Treatment with octreotide periprocedurally is recommended.[11]

Extrahepatic Complications

Nontarget CE can be prevented with attention to variant anatomy, stable catheter positioning, regular flushing, awareness of gross vascular shunts, and careful delivery of the chemoembolic agent. Cholecystitis requiring specific treatment is a rare complication of CE.[14] The real incidence of cholecystitis is probably higher because its clinical manifestations can be masked by symptoms of PES, altered liver function tests post-CE, and the administration of analgesics and prophylactic antibiotics. Most investigators do not specifically consider the cystic artery when treating the right hepatic artery, so that the cystic artery

commonly receives the cytotoxic agent and some iodinated oil. However, there is a very low incidence of cholecystitis requiring specific treatment, even when oil is identified in the gallbladder wall on follow-up CT (Fig. 29–10). Nevertheless, CE of the cystic artery can cause gangrenous cholecystitis, gallbladder perforation, and emphysematous cholecystitis requiring either surgical cholecystectomy or percutaneous cholecystostomy. CE of the cystic artery should be avoided by advancing the catheter beyond the identified cystic artery origin and by avoiding reflux during injection of chemoembolic agent, particularly if the cystic artery is enlarged (Fig. 29–11). Reflux of CE material into the gastroduodenal artery (GDA) is the most likely mechanism of hyperamylasemia and acute pancreatitis post-CE. More selective catheterization and avoidance of reflux can prevent this. In patients in whom this may not be possible, the GDA territory can be protected from small-particle embolization by occluding the GDA origin with coils.

Gastroduodenal intestinal erosions and ulceration can result from inadvertent CE of gastrointestinal branches. Because of collateral circuits in the gastroduodenal region, coil embolization of the GDA, right gastric artery, and left gastric artery from a left gastrohepatic trunk can protect these vessels from reflux of chemoembolic material. Reflux into the SMA from an accessory or replaced right hepatic artery can be prevented by coil embolizing the right accessory or replaced hepatic artery, which allows the use of the proper hepatic artery from the celiac artery to embolize the right lobe.

Rarely, splenic artery CE can occur. The mechanism for this can be either severe celiac axis stenosis with retrograde flow in the common hepatic artery, increased splenic artery flow in cirrhotic patients with splenomegaly, or catheter-induced spasm in the proper hepatic artery.

Alternatively, larger quantities can exit the liver through hepatic artery to hepatic vein shunts that can be seen angiographically in 2.4% of patients presenting with HCC.[20] The amount of oil injected and the presence of these arteriovenous shunts are factors that determine the occurrence of symptomatic pulmonary embolism and pulmonary infarction. Injection of more than 20 ml of iodinated oil increases the risk of clinical pulmonary embolism in patients with HCC.[14] Pneumothorax can complicate pulmonary infarction.

After CE, liver tumors often parasitize arterial supply from neighboring arteries, such as the inferior phrenic artery, the internal mammary artery, the adrenal artery, and the intercostal artery. If further treatment is indicated, care must be taken to outline branches from these vessels. Pulmonary, cutaneous, renal, and spinal cord embolizations all have been

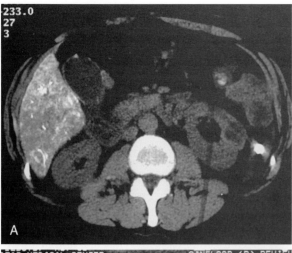
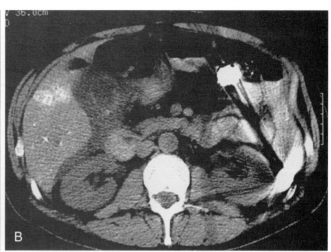
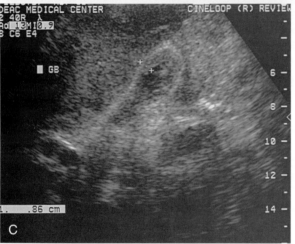

Figure 29–10. A 57-year-old man with colon carcinoma treated by right hepatic artery CE complicated by cholecystitis. *A,* CT scan 24 hours post-CE shows localization of iodinated oil in the gallbladder wall. The patient had worsening abdominal pain after CE. *B,* Further CT scan 10 days later shows gallbladder wall thickening with free fluid in the gallbladder fossa and Morison's pouch. *C,* With conservative management, which included antibiotics, the patient made a full symptomatic recovery with an ultrasonogram 1 month later, showing slight residual gall bladder wall thickening.

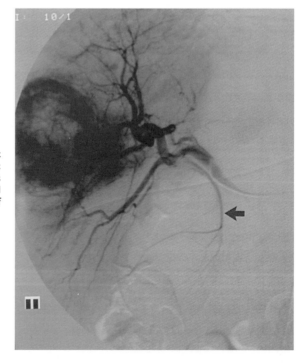

Figure 29–11. A 65-year-old man with hepatocellular carcinoma. Selective right hepatic arteriogram shows large hypervascular right hepatic lobe lesion. The cystic artery is opacified *(arrow).* To prevent complications, CE of nontarget arteries is avoided: the catheter is advanced distal to the nontarget artery before CE, and care is taken not to allow reflux into nontarget arteries during injection of CE material.

recorded as complications of treating these vessels when they supply hepatic tumor.

Passage of chemoembolic material to the cerebral circulation can occur. The mechanism involved could be either an arteriovenous shunt in the liver with transient elevated right-sided cardiac pressures in the presence of an atrial septal defect or an arteriovenous shunt in both the liver and the lung, both of which are associated with cirrhosis.

Renal Failure

Acute renal failure or diminished renal function is a well-known complication of iodinated contrast, particularly in those patients with already compromised renal function. With CE, the risk is increased because cell necrosis products are released into the circulation, further burdening renal tubules. The risk of renal compromise is decreased by prescribing allopurinol and ensuring adequate hydration by the time contrast is administered and during the postprocedure period.

FUTURE DEVELOPMENTS

Experience with CE and advances in catheterization techniques have made CE a safe and well-tolerated procedure. Recent reports have commented on other roles for CE.[21] However, more randomized, controlled studies are needed to determine the best CE regimens for different tumors and to identify patient populations most likely to benefit from such treatment. The efficacy of adjuvant and neoadjuvant CE for increasing resectability and preventing recurrent disease also needs to be outlined. Future studies need to define the relative roles of CE and emerging treatments, such as percutaneous ethanol ablation of tumors, cryoablation, and radiofrequency ablation.

REFERENCES

1. MacIntosh EL, Minuk GY: Hepatic resection in patients with cirrhosis and hepatocellular carcinoma. Surg Gynecol Obstet 174:245, 1992.
2. Scheele J, Stangi R, Altendorf-Hofmann A: Hepatic metastasis from colorectal carcinoma: Impact of surgical resection on the natural history. Br J Surg 77:1241, 1990.
3. Lehnert T, Herfarth C: Chemoembolization for hepatocellular carcinoma: What, when, and for whom? Ann Surg 224:1, 1996.
4. Di Bisceglie AM, Rustgi VK, Hoffnagle JH, et al: Hepatocellular carcinoma. Ann Int Med 108:390, 1988.
5. Harada T, Matsuo K, Inoue T, et al: Is preoperative hepatic arterial chemoembolization safe and effective for hepatocellular carcinoma? Ann Surg 224:4, 1996.
6. Moertel CG, Lefkopoulo M, Lipsitz S, et al: Streptozocin-doxorubicin, streptozocin-fluorouracil, or chlorozotocin in the treatment of advanced islet-cell carcinoma. N Engl J Med 326:519, 1992.
7. Doppman JL, Girton M, Vermess M: The risk of hepatic artery embolization in the presence of obstructive jaundice. Radiology 143:37, 1982.
8. Soulen MC: Chemoembolization of hepatic malignancies. Oncology (Huntingt) 8:77, 1994.
9. Solomon R, Werner C, Mann D, et al: Effects of saline, mannitol and furosemide on acute decreases in renal function induced by radiocontrast agents. N Engl J Med 331:1416, 1994.
10. Berger DH, Carrasco CH, Hohn DC, et al: Hepatic artery chemoembolization or embolization of primary hepatic tumors: Post treatment management and complications. J Surg Oncol 60:116, 1995.
11. Cay O, Kruskal J, Thomas P, et al: Targeting of different ethiodized oil-doxorubicin mixtures to hypovascular hepatic metastases with intra-arterial and intraportal injections. J Vasc Intervent Radiol 7:409, 1996.
12. Soulen MC: Chemoembolization of hepatic malignancies. Semin Intervent Radiol 14:305, 1997.
13. Bronowicki JP, Vetter D, Dumas F, et al: Transcatheter oily chemoembolization for hepatocellular carcinoma. Cancer 74:16, 1994.
14. Chung JW, Park JH, Han JK, et al: Hepatic tumors: Predisposing factors for complications of transcatheter oily chemoembolization. Radiology 198:33, 1996.
15. Group d'Equipe et de traitment du carcinome hepatocellulaire: A comparison of Lipiodol chemoembolization and conservative treatment for unresectable hepatocellular carcinoma. N Engl J Med 332:1256, 1995.
16. Inoue H, Kobayashi H, Itoh Y, et al: Treatment of liver metastases by arterial injection of adriamycin/mitomycin C Lipiodol suspension. Acta Radiol 30:603, 1989.
17. Therasse E, Breittmayer F, Roche A, et al: Transcatheter chemoembolization of progressive carcinoid liver metastasis. Radiology 189:541, 1993.
18. Mavligit GM, Charnsangavej C, Carrasco CH, et al: Regression of ocular melanoma metastatic to the liver after hepatic arterial chemoembolization with cisplatin and polyvinyl sponge. JAMA 260:974, 1988.
19. Cockburn JF, Jackson JE, Allison DJ: Complications of embolization. *In* Ansell G, Bettman MA, Kaufman JA, et al (eds): Complications in Diagnostic Imaging and Interventional Radiology, 3rd ed. Boston, Blackwell Science Inc, 1996, pp 392–407.
20. Ngan H, Peh WC: Arteriovenous shunting in carcinoma: Its prevalence and clinical significance. Clin Radiol 52:36, 1997.
21. Wu CC, Ho YZ, Ho WL, et al: Preoperative transcatheter arterial embolization for the treatment of primary hepatocellular carcinoma: A reappraisal. Br J Surg 82:122, 1995.

Covered Stents and Endovascular Grafts

Chapter 30 Endovascular Grafting for Occlusive Aortoiliac Disease

Surgical Contributors: *Luis A. Sanchez, Takao Ohki, Reese A. Wain, and Frank J. Veith*

Aortoiliac occlusive disease is a significant cause of lower extremity ischemic symptoms, alone or in combination with infrainguinal occlusive disease. The appropriate treatment of patients with lesions in the aortoiliac segment depends on the extent of the lesion, the presence of bilateral and infrainguinal disease, the symptoms at presentation, and the patient's medical condition at the time of treatment. Over the past four decades, the treatment of patients with aortoiliac occlusive disease has significantly improved as a result of advances in surgical techniques, perioperative patient care, and available endovascular instrumentation. The first procedure to enjoy widespread use was arterial endarterectomy, which was described in 1947 by dos Santos[1] and later, in the United States, by Wylie.[2] Endarterectomy was the most frequently performed procedure for treatment of patients with aortoiliac occlusive disease from the 1950s through the 1960s. Concurrently, new prosthetic grafting techniques were developed for the treatment of patients with aneurysmal and occlusive disease.[3–5] During the 1970s and 1980s, aortofemoral grafting was the most frequently performed intervention for patients with aortoiliac occlusive disease because of its broad applicability and perceived improvements in long-term results.[6, 7] Extra-anatomic prosthetic bypasses were important for the treatment of patients with intracavitary arterial infections, and were increasingly used for patients with significant medical contraindications for aortic surgery.[5]

Endovascular techniques for the treatment of patients with atherosclerotic lesions were initially reported by Dotter and Judkins[8] in 1964, but it was not until Gruntzig and Hoppff[9] described the double-lumen balloon catheter in the 1970s that balloon angioplasty became a popular technique. Balloon angioplasty has proved to be extremely successful in the treatment of patients with localized aortoiliac lesions.[10, 11] Angioplasty results have improved with use of intraluminal stents, serving to increase the acceptance, and expand the indications for, the use of this less invasive technique.[12, 13] In the mid-1980s and early 1990s, angioplasty and stenting became the procedures of choice for the treatment of patients with short segment aortoiliac stenoses and occlusions. These techniques have increased the applicability of femorofemoral bypasses for moderate- to high-risk patients who have severe bilateral aortoiliac occlusive disease, and they are very helpful adjuncts for the treatment of patients who have complex multilevel arterial occlusive disease.[14, 15]

Unfortunately, the results of angioplasty in patients with aortoiliac occlusive disease and of stenting in patients with extensive occlusive lesions are less favorable than those obtained for patients with localized lesions.[11, 16] Endovascular grafts, which were initially used for the treatment of aortic aneurysms,[17] have been successfully adapted to the treatment of aortoiliac occlusive disease.[18–23] By combining the durability of prosthetic grafts and the minimally invasive techniques used for angioplasty and stenting, endovascular grafts may have significant advantages over existing methods for treating complex aortoiliac occlusive disease. The advantages of endovascular grafts may be most useful for patients who are poor candidates for standard surgical techniques or existing interventional approaches. In such patients, such interventions are difficult, unsafe, or associated with poor long-term results.

ENDOVASCULAR GRAFTING

Technique

In the developmental stages, two different techniques have been clinically applied. One involves the percutaneous insertion of a ready-made, Dacron-covered, self-expanding nitinol stent (Cragg Endopro System I),[24, 25] which can be inserted through a sheath and then released by pulling back the sheath against a pusher. These grafts have been used for patients with residual stenoses or dissections after angioplasty, restenoses, ulcerated lesions, and long (>6 cm) iliac artery lesions as well as aneurysms. There are encouraging early results with technical success in all cases and patency rates of 80 to 100% at 8 months of follow-up in patients with intermittent claudication.[24, 25] Several other systems are now available, including the JoMed and the Corvita stent graft.

In our experience with endovascular grafts at Montefiore Medical Center, we have relied on an operative rather than a percutaneous approach. The patients whom we treated have had extensive aortoiliac occlusive disease in combination with infrainguinal disease, which has led to limb-threatening ischemic symptoms in all cases. Our endovascular devices are constructed from 6-mm polytetrafluoroethylene (PTFE) thin-wall grafts and Palmaz balloon-expanable stents (P 294, P 308). The stents are sutured to the proximal end of the prosthetic graft with four sutures so that the prosthetic graft overlaps 50% of the stent. The endovascular grafts are mounted on 6 to 8 mm × 4 cm angioplasty balloons and placed within a delivery sheath along a second angioplasty tip balloon that provides a tapered tip to the introducer sheath (Fig. 30–1).

Access vessels are exposed through limited femoral incisions under local, regional, or general anesthesia, depending on the patient's medical condition. Arterial recanalization is usually undertaken by an up-and-over approach from a contralateral percutaneous femoral puncture. This approach leads to safer and often easier arterial recanalization from the patent proximal lumen in occluded vessels. If the contralateral iliac artery is similarly occluded or severely diseased, a retrograde approach is used. Recanalization

of the aortoiliac segment can be more troublesome with this approach because of the difficulty in re-entering the true lumen of the aorta or the proximal iliac artery from a dissection plane.

After successful recanalization of the diseased aortoiliac segment, the entire segment is dilated with an 8-mm angioplasty balloon to create a channel in which the endovascular graft will be placed. The delivery system is then introduced over the guide wire and advanced to the planned deployment site. The tip balloon is deflated and withdrawn. The introducer sheath is withdrawn, and the stent portion of the endovascular graft is deployed with use of the angioplasty balloon. The sheath is completely removed, the distal end of the graft is retrieved from the femoral arteriotomy, and the entire graft is sequentially dilated with the angioplasty balloon. Management of the distal anastomosis is dependent on the individual patient's pattern of disease.[26] Endovascular grafts can be terminated in the common femoral artery with creation of an endoluminal anastomosis. The femoral artery is then closed with a patch or the hood of a second bypass graft. Other patients can have the distal end of the endovascular graft anastomosed in standard fashion to the best outflow vessel or a separate bypass graft.

Results

Over a 5-year period, 52 patients at our institution underwent 58 endovascular grafts for severe limb-threatening ischemia (Fig. 30–2). Fifty-two percent of

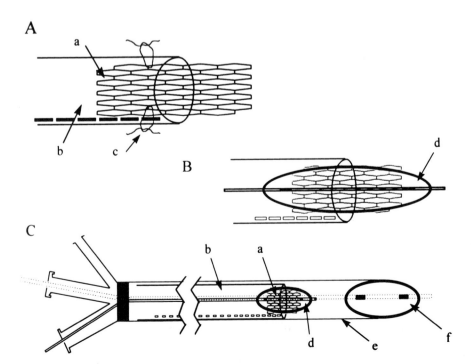

Figure 30–1. Endovascular graft assembly. *A,* A 30-mm Palmaz balloon expandable stent (a) is sutured to a 6-mm, thin-walled polytetrafluoroethylene (PTFE) graft (b) with interrupted sutures (c). *B,* The endovascular graft is mounted on an 8-mm × 3 cm angioplasty balloon (d). *C,* Before insertion, the device is loaded into a 20 French delivery sheath (e). A separate tip balloon (f) extends from the proximal portion of the sheath and provides a smooth, tapered profile to the delivery system, which facilitates its insertion.

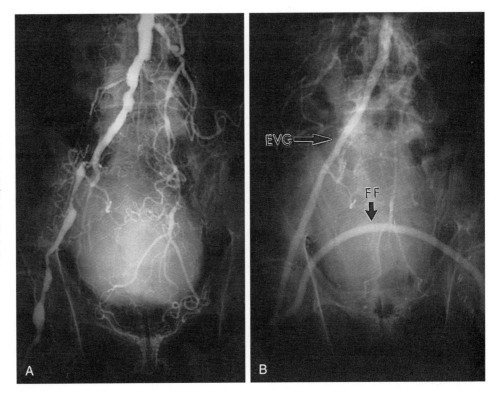

Figure 30–2. Seventy-year-old patient who presented with bilateral lower extremity ischemia. *A,* The preoperative arteriogram shows a diffusely diseased right iliac artery system with complete occlusion of the left iliac system. *B,* An endovascular graft (EVG) was placed through the right iliac system and secured proximally at the distal aorta. A femorofemoral (FF) bypass was used to reperfuse the contralateral lower extremity.

these patients required synchronous conventional lower extremity bypasses in addition to the endovascular grafts to resolve the advanced ischemic symptoms. The 5-year primary patency rate in this difficult group of patients was 66%, with a secondary patency rate of 72%. The 5-year limb salvage rate was 89%.[27]

Endovascular grafts are ideally suited for treatment of high-risk patients and those in whom conventional surgery or other interventional procedures are contraindicated or technically impossible. This technique has many of the advantages of minimally invasive endovascular procedures. The procedure can be performed with minimal use of anesthesia, which thereby avoids the cardiac and pulmonary stresses of general anesthesia. It prevents transperitoneal or retroperitoneal access to the aortoiliac system, which is often associated with cardiac, pulmonary, and other local complications. A patient who has an entire length of diseased artery, even if it is heavily calcified, can be treated. In addition, this technique allows the treatment of concurrent femoral artery disease and sequential treatment of infrainguinal disease if necessary. Disadvantages include the occasional sacrifice of collateral vessels and the large introducer systems currently used.

We are encouraged by the high technical success rate, the low morbidity and mortality rates, and the superior 5-year primary (66%) and secondary (72%) patency rates in this difficult group of patients who have multilevel arterial occlusive disease, threatened limbs, and severe medical comorbidities. The results

of the first generation of endovascular grafts approach the 75 to 90% 5-year patency rates[25, 29] associated with aortofemoral bypasses for extensive aortoiliac occlusive disease. These endovascular grafts share many of the advantages of aortofemoral reconstructions. These include direct aortic inflow, ability to treat bilateral disease, and opportunity to correct outflow femoral disease at the time of the reconstruction. In addition, endovascular grafts can be performed in patients who have medical or surgical contraindications for direct aortoiliac reconstructions and can be combined with infrainguinal reconstructions in patients who require a single sitting to under complete revascularizations for limb salvage. On the other hand, end-to-side aortofemoral reconstructions preserve important collateral branches that have developed over the years, and aortofemoral bypasses can be used to treat patients with pararenal aortic occlusions.

The short- and long-term results of endovascular grafts to treat patients with severe aortoiliac occlusive disease also compare favorably with those published for treatment of patients who have extra-anatomic bypasses (5-year primary patency rates of 45 to 85%).[30, 31] Endovascular grafts share many of the advantages of axillofemoral reconstructions. These include the use of local or regional anesthesia to limit perioperative complications, the ability to treat patients with significant medical comorbidities, and the potential to treat patients with failed aortofemoral reconstructions. In addition, endovascular grafts obtain in-line inflow from the aorta or the proximal iliac artery, thus avoiding the risk of potential injury to uninvolved donor arteries. On the other hand, extra-anatomic reconstructions are often the only alternative for the treatment of patients who have infected aortic grafts and other aortoiliac arterial infections.

Angioplasty, with or without stents, has become the procedure of choice for patients who have short aortoiliac lesions, with primary patency rates between 80 and 95% after 2 years.[10-13] More recently, primary stenting has been performed after recanalization of occluded iliac arteries, with primary patency rates of 78% and secondary patency rates of 86% after 1 year.[32] Endovascular grafts have patency rates comparable with those of aortoiliac stenting and share the advantageous, minimally invasive nature of the procedure compared with that of open surgical options. In addition, endovascular grafts can successfully treat extensive aortoiliac occlusive disease, allow treatment of concurrent femoral and distal arterial occlusive disease, and limit the development of intimal hyperplastic lesions to the ends of the endovascular graft.

These first-generation endovascular grafts will likely continue to improve and have an important role in the treatment of extensive aortoiliac and femoropopliteal occlusive disease. Introducer systems are becoming streamlined for easier and safer introduction, and new endovascular grafts are fully supported to diminish problems of extrinsic compression and kinking within tortuous vessels. Currently, a variety of devices are in the process of being evaluated for the endovascular treatment of arterial occlusive lesions, including: the Corvita Endoluminal Graft, the Hemobahn, the Passager, and the Wallgraft.

CONCLUSION

Endovascular grafts can be extremely useful for the treatment of a high-risk subset of patients with severe aortoiliac occlusive disease. Further improvements in endovascular graft design and deployment techniques will support the continued growth of this evolving field. New endovascular procedures will likely change the indications for which arterial angioplasty and stenting, aortofemoral bypasses, and extra-anatomical procedures have traditionally been performed. The indications for the use of endovascular grafts are likely to grow as new devices are evaluated and long-term results become available.

REFERENCES

1. dos Santos JC: Sur la Désobstruction des Thromboses Artrievelles Anciennes. Memoires de L'Académie de Chirurgie 73:409–411, 1947.
2. Wylie EJ: Thromboendarterectomy for arteriosclerotic thrombosis of major arteries. Surgery 32:275–285, 1952.
3. DeBakey ME, Creech O Jr, Cooley DA: Occlusive disease of the aorta and its treatment by resection and homograft replacement. Ann Surg 140:290–310, 1954.
4. Julian OC, Dye WS, Lowin JH, et al: Direct surgery of arteriosclerosis. Ann Surg 136:459–474, 1952.
5. Blaisdell WF, Hall AD: Axillary-femoral artery bypass for lower extremity ischemia. Surgery 54:563–568, 1963.
6. Brewster DC, Darling RC: Optimal methods of aortoiliac reconstruction. Surgery 84:739–748, 1978.
7. Crawford ES, Bomberger RA, Glaeser DH, et al: Aortoiliac occlusive disease: Factors influencing survival and function following reconstructive operation over a twenty-five-year period. Surgery 90:1055–1067, 1981.
8. Dotter CT, Judkins MP: Transluminal treatment of arteriosclerotic obstruction: Description of a new technique and a preliminary report of its application. Circulation 30:654–670, 1964.
9. Gruntzig A, Hopff H: Perkutane rekanalisation chronischer arterieller verschlusse mit einem neuen dilatationskatheter: Modifikation der dotter technik. Dtsch Med Wochenschr 99:2502–2511, 1974.
10. Johnson KW: Factors that influence the outcome of aortoiliac and femoropopliteal percutaneous transluminal angioplasty. Surg Clin North Am 72:843–850, 1992.
11. Johnson KW: Iliac arteries: Reanalysis of results of balloon angioplasty. Radiology 186:207–212, 1993.
12. Sigwart U, Puel J, Mirkovitch V, el al: Intravascular stents to prevent occlusion and restenosis after transluminal angioplasty. N Engl J Med 316:701–706, 1987.
13. Palmaz JC, Laborde JC, Rivera FJ, et al: Stenting of the iliac arteries with the Palmaz stent: Experience from a multicenter trial. Cardiovasc Intervent Radiol 15:291–297, 1992.
14. Brewster DC, Cambria RP, Darling RC, et al: Long-term results of combined balloon angioplasty and distal surgical revascularization. Ann Surg 210:324–331, 1989.
15. Schneider PA: Balloon angioplasty and stent placement during operative vascular reconstruction for lower extremity ischemia. Ann Vasc Surg 10:589–598, 1996.
16. Sapoval MR, Chatellier G, Long AL, et al: Self-expandable stents for the treatment of iliac artery obstructive lesions: Long-term success and prognostic factors. Am J Roentgenol 166:1173–1179, 1996.
17. Parodi JC, Palmaz JC, et al: Transfemoral intraluminal graft implantation for abdominal aortic aneurysms. Ann Vasc Surg 5:491–499, 1991.
18. Marin ML, Veith FJ, Cynamon J, et al: Initial experience with transluminally placed endovascular grafts for the treatment of complex vascular lesions. Ann Surg 222:449–469, 1995.
19. Parodi JC: Endovascular repair of abdominal aortic aneurysms and other arterial lesions. J Vasc Surg 21:549–557, 1995.
20. Marin ML, Veith FJ: The role of stented grafts in the management of failed arterial reconstructions. Semin Vasc Surg 7:188–194, 1994.
21. Marin ML, Veith FJ: Clinical application of endovascular grafts in aortoiliac occlusive disease and vascular trauma. Cardiovasc Surg 3:115–120, 1995.
22. Sanchez LA, Marin ML, et al: Placement of endovascular stented grafts via remote access sites: A new approach for the treatment of failed aorto-ilio-femoral reconstructions. Ann Vasc Surg 9:1–8, 1995.
23. Marin ML, Veith FJ, Sanchez LA, et al: Endovascular aortoiliac grafts in combination with standard infrainguinal arterial bypasses in the management of limb-threatening ischemia: Preliminary report. J Vasc Surg 22:316–325, 1995.
24. Henry M, Amor M, Ethevenot G, et al: Initial experience with the Cragg Endopro system 1 for intraluminal treatment of peripheral vascular disease. J Endovasc Surg 1:31–43, 1994.
25. Pernes JM, August MA, Hovasse D, et al: Long iliac stenosis: Initial clinical experience with the Cragg endoluminal graft. Radiology 196:67–71, 1995.
26. Lyon RT, Veith FJ, Marin ML, et al: Alternative techniques for management of distal anastomoses of aortofemoral and iliofemoral endovascular grafts. J Vasc Surg (in press).
27. Wain RA, Marin ML, Veith FJ, et al: Analysis of endovascular

graft treatment for aortoiliac occlusive disease: What is its role based on 5-year results. (Unpublished data).

28. Szilagyi DE, Elliot JP, Smith RF, et al: A thirty-year survey of the reconstructive surgical treatment of aortoiliac occlusive disease. J Vasc Surg 3:421–436, 1986.

29. Brewster DC: Clinical and anatomical considerations for surgery in aortoiliac disease and results of surgical treatment. Circulation 83[suppl]:I-42–I-52, 1991.

30. Rutherford RB, Patt A, Pearce WH: Extra-anatomic bypass: A closer view. J Vasc Surg 5:437–446, 1987.

31. Taylor LM, Moneta GL, McConnell D, et al: Axillofemoral grafting with externally supported polytetrafluoroethylene. Arch Surg 588–95, 1994.

32. Vorwerk D, Guenther RW, Schumann K, et al: Primary stent placement for chronic iliac artery occlusions: Follow-up results in 103 patients. Radiology 194:745–749, 1995.

Chapter 31 — Endovascular Repair of Abdominal Aortic Aneurysms

Endovascular Contributors: Ulrich Blum, Peter McCollum, Brian R. Hopkinson, Geoffrey White, Martin Hauer, James Gunn, S.W. Yusuf, James May, Götz Voshage, Peter Harris, J. Macierewicz, and Paul Petrosek

Abdominal aortic aneurysm (AAA) is a disease entity that is associated with significant comorbidity in most patients, particularly in relation to cardiovascular disease. This fact might be expected to influence the perioperative mortality of surgical repair more so than any other feature. Despite this, there remains a disturbingly large variation in reported elective surgical mortality in all types of patients with AAA that appears to be independent of perceived preoperative surgical risk. This simple stark fact suggests that some centers have a much better team approach to the management of these patients than have others. Most importantly, it highlights the critical operative influence that the individual surgeon has on his or her long-term outcome figures.

Any operation that is performed in an effort to save lives must be seen to significantly improve on the natural history of the underlying disease and its comorbid factors. Thus, although it is attractive to suggest that small aneurysms should be repaired at the first opportunity, there is no evidence to substantiate this viewpoint and there is abundant evidence to suggest that only large aneurysms require intervention (either surgical or endovascular repair [EVAR]). Recent data from the U.K. small aneurysm study have shown no benefit for conventional surgery on aneurysms that are between 4 cm and 5.5 cm in diameter after a 5-year follow-up period.[1] There are several reasons why this may be the case. First, there was a 5.8% perioperative mortality in this multicenter study, which some may believe is high but which nevertheless reflects actual practice. Second, there was a relatively small rate of AAA expansion in these patients and a very small rupture rate in aneurysms less than 5.5 cm (7 patients). Patients whose AAA eventually exceeded this figure were later offered surgery. Lastly, many patients in this study died of other causes (133 of 150 deaths). This finding also was reported by Galland and associates in a series of 267 patients.[2]

These data have enormous implications for the surgical management of AAA patients who are usually otherwise asymptomatic. It is clear that guidelines will come into force that only mandate intervention in large aneurysms (> 5.5 cm) unless there are relevant symptoms. On the basis of the small aneurysm study, it is very unlikely that even a significant reduction in perioperative mortality (such as may potentially be offered by EVAR) ever would justify intervention on asymptomatic small aneurysms.

DEFINITION AND CLASSIFICATION

The abdominal aorta has a normal size range of approximately 1.2 to 2 cm at the infrarenal segment depending on the age, sex, and size of the patient. The Society for Cardiovascular Surgery has defined an aneurysm as a 50% dilation of a normal sized artery.[3] Thus, aortas with a size of greater than 3 cm can be regarded as aneurysmal, and aneurysmal disease is found most frequently in the infrarenal aorta. Aortic aneurysms are generally fusiform with underlying atherosclerosis as the predominant etiology. Type B dissections or true infrarenal aortic dissections are a rarer cause of abdominal aortic dilatation. Likewise, aortic pseudoaneurysms are occasional findings in patients with previously placed abdominal grafts. Most AAAs (> 95%) lie below or just at the level of the renal arteries. When the renal vessels genuinely are involved, the aneurysm is generally a type IV "thoracoabdominal" aneurysm. The lower extent of the usual AAA may either lie at the aortic bifurcation or extend into the common or sometimes the internal iliac arteries. Often, there may be associated anneurysms in other sites, with the popliteal and femoral arteries being the most frequently involved. In some patients, the aneurysm appears to be encased in a pearly white icing that is densely adherent to surrounding structures. These "inflammatory" aneurysms are more challenging surgically but still have the propensity to enlarge and rupture.

OVERVIEW OF ENDOVASCULAR REPAIR OF ABDOMINAL AORTIC ANEURYSMS

When Parodi undertook the first transluminal operation to repair an AAA in 1990, the potential of this approach was recognized immediately and a whole new area of technology was initiated that currently is evolving so rapidly that it is hard even for vascular specialists to keep pace with it.[4] As with the new therapies throughout the history of medicine, endovascular aneurysm repair first generated optimism about its potential that was perhaps excessive but recently been viewed rather pessimistically as previously unsuspected hazards and drawbacks have become more apparent. Initially, the only information on which to base any judgment about the efficacy of endovascular aneurysm repair was anecdotal and therefore completely unreliable, but large-scale registries that were established in the mid 1990s have provided reliable information on the outcome of endovascular aneurysm repair in large populations of patients observed for follow up for several years.[5–7] Based on this information, it is now possible to make a realistic appraisal of the efficacy of this new approach in its present state of technology and, just as importantly, to point the way for further research and development.

It took only one patient to establish the feasibility of deploying a stent graft within an AAA; however, it is now confirmed that successful deployment of aortic endografts can be achieved with a remarkable degree of consistency and with a very low risk of complications. In 1138 consecutive patients registered on the Eurostar Database, the procedure was completed successfully in 98%. Minor technical problems were encountered during deployment in 17%, but these were resolved by appropriate endovascular manipulations in the majority. Only one patient died during the course of the operative procedure, but another 25 patients died within 30 days, giving an in-hospital mortality rate of 2.5%. Nearly all the patients who died had severe comorbidity. Other benefits predicted for the endovascular approach to aneurysms, based on the fact that it is relatively noninvasive, also have been realized with more rapid recovery times, considerably reduced requirement for intensive care facilities, and shorter hospital stay in comparison to conventional open surgery. It is assumed that this greater efficiency will yield benefits in terms of cost reduction in due course, although currently the cost benefits are balanced to some degree by the high price of the endovascular devices themselves and the need for regular objective postoperative surveillance of the new technology. A unique phenomenon associated with endovascular repair of aneurysms that justifiably has attracted a great deal of attention is that of endo-

leak. This has been defined by White and colleagues as "a condition associated with endoluminal vascular grafts, defined by the presence of blood flow outside the lumen of the endoluminal graft, but within an aneurysm sac or adjacent vascular segment being treated by the graft."[7] If the aneurysm sac has not been excluded completely from the circulation, there is an assumption that the aneurysm has not been cured and that the patient is, therefore, still at risk from rupture. The source of the endoleak may be one or more of the anastomoses or the body of the graft itself through defects in the fabric or disjunction of the modular parts or there may be back bleeding in the sac from aortic side branches. An endoleak may be present from the time of operation—early or primary endoleak—or may develop later secondary endoleak. The reported incidence of primary endoleaks has ranged widely from 5 to 44%.[8–11] Although it is accepted that the prevalence of endoleak may depend on factors such as patient selection and operative skill, the observed incidence of this phenomenon depends on the care taken and the method used to detect it. The protocol for the Eurostar Registry requires patients to be examined by contrast-enhanced computed tomography (CT) scanning on discharge and at 6 weeks, 3 months, 6 months and 1 year after surgery. In 895 patients, an endoleak was present on discharge in 14%, and this was roughly consistent with the incidence reported from the U.K. Reta Registry and the large aggregated series from Australia. Even more disturbing was the finding that in another 18% of patients, a new endoleak developed during the first year after operation. Early endoleaks are caused by failure to achieve a "seal" between the endograft or the vessel wall or relate to back filling of the sac from aortic side branches, and it was reasonably predictable that they would occur in a certain proportion of patients. However, new endoleaks developing some time after surgery must be related to ongoing pathologic processes or structural changes in the device itself, and it had been hoped initially, perhaps naively, that this would not occur. Mechanisms for the development of late endoleaks that had been anticipated were continued expansion of the neck of the aneurysm and stent migration. Although these mechanisms have occurred, a considerable number of late endoleaks were found to be arising from the body of the endograft, and this had not been anticipated. The mechanisms involved structural changes within the endografts over time, the most frequent and easily recognized consequence of which is disjunction of the modular parts. However, tears in the fabric of the graft occurring some time after the operation also have occurred, with serious consequences.

Images obtained on completion of endovascular repair of an AAA invariably show that the endograft lies either straight within the aneurysm sac or is gently curved. Occasionally, there may be slight angulation in the body of the graft, reflecting angulation at the neck of the aneurysm itself. However, 1 year later, up to 70% of some types of endograft have become severely buckled or kinked, sometimes with associated clinical complications, such as dysjunction of the modular parts with a new endoleak or occlusion of one of the limbs.[12] Studies of this phenomenon have shown that the principal cause is reduction in the longitudinal dimension of the aneurysm as part of a general process of shrinkage of an aneurysm that has been effectively excluded from the circulation. Paradoxically, this means that successful exclusion of an aneurysm can itself be a cause of late complications and is a problem to be addressed by engineers involved in stent graft design. The most effective stent grafts are likely to be those that can accommodate changing vascular morphology over time while simultaneously preserving their structural integrity. Although it has been observed that the diameter of the neck of the aneurysm does increase after endovascular repair, this appears to be a short-term effect and simply may be the result of the radial force exerted by the proximal stent. Progressive dilatation of the neck leading to late proximal endoleaks so far has not been observed with any frequency. Migration of the stents from the proximal and distal anastomotic sites has been largely overcome by systematic oversizing of the device relative to the diameter of the arteries and by the application of hooks and barbs that appear to be very effective in securing the devices.

All endoleaks may not be equal importance. There is anecdotal evidence to indicate that large endoleaks originating from the proximal anastomosis are particularly dangerous. Virtually all these result from failure to achieve effective seal at the proximal anastomosis at the original operation and it currently is accepted that such endoleaks must not be left unresolved. If balloon dilatation or the deployment of an extender cuff is not effective, then conversion to open repair should be considered. An alternative approach that has been attempted is the application of an external band applied around the aorta at the level of the stent, but the efficacy of this approach is, as yet, unproven. Some proximal endoleaks apparently resolve spontaneously. The mechanism is sealing of the anastomotic defect by thrombosis. However, continued expansion of the aneurysm sac has occurred under these circumstances, and there is experimental evidence to show that although a plug of thrombus may arrest blood flow into the aneurysm, it does not necessarily isolate the sac from arterial pressure. Therefore, a wait-and-see policy with respect to proximal endoleaks in the hope that they may seal spontaneously is unsafe. Most endoleaks that develop at the distal anastomosis can be resolved by secondary endovascular interventions and are, therefore, less problematic. The clinical significance of endoleaks related to patent lumbar or inferior mesenteric arteries is as yet undetermined. When such endoleaks persist, it can be assumed that the aneurysm sac does remain pressurized. However, even if rupture should occur, the consequences perhaps would not be so dire as those normally associated with this event.

The primary objective of treatment for aortic aneurysms is to prevent death of the patient from rupture of the aneurysm; this should be kept in mind. Although the attributes associated with a less invasive procedure undoubtedly confer on endovascular grafting significant advantages over the conventional operation, this new approach may not be as effective in achieving the primary objective. Rupture of the aneurysm within 1 year after endovascular repair was reported in 6 of 895 patients entered on the Eurostar Registry, and there has been other anecdotal reports of late rupture.[13] However, a small risk of failure does not necessarily outweigh the benefits of endovascular repair, provided that those at risk can be identified and secondary intervention undertaken to eliminate or minimize this risk. Given the present state of the art, endovascular repair does not guarantee freedom from problems or elimination of the risk of rupture for every patient that is treated by this means. For this reason, careful postoperative surveillance is mandatory.

The optimum technique for postoperative surveillance has yet to be determined. Thus far, reliance has been placed primarily on contrast-enhanced CT scanning to detect endoleaks, although evidence is accumulating that duplex ultrasound scanning with enhancement may be equally effective at lower cost. However, to focus on the detection of endoleaks alone as defined by White may be inappropriate and unsafe. It now is known that blood flow into the sac at a rate of 1 ml/min or less is capable of sustaining high pressure, and flow rates of this magnitude cannot be detected by any currently available system of imaging.[14, 15] Furthermore, thrombus may transmit pressure without any movement of blood. Although it is appropriate to look for and treat potentially dangerous endoleaks, continued expansion of the aneurysm sac is probably the most reliable indicator of a failed procedure. Even in the absence of a detectable endoleak, this should be regarded as an indication for secondary intervention, which in the absence of an identifiable and correctable cause, is likely to mean conversion to open repair. In the future, it may be possible to measure pressure or "endotension" within the sac safely over time, and, in theory at least, this would have major advantages over methods based on visualization of flow.

Despite the apparent drawbacks, there can be little doubt that endovascular grafting will have an important role in the treatment of patients with AAAs in the future. As technology evolves, solutions to the mechanical problems that have surfaced in relation to early endovascular devices undoubtedly will be found. We also can expect to see simpler and more efficient introducer systems and clearer definition of the requirements for follow-up assessment. At the time of writing, there is still some way to go both in terms of refining the new technology of endovascular aneurysm repair and, just as importantly, in evaluating the clinical results over time. Large-scale randomized trials are planned that to help establish its proper role alongside established options for the management of patients with AAAs. Until these processes are completed, endovascular repair is not yet ready for adoption as the standard treatment for most patients with this condition.

ENDOVASCULAR ABDOMINAL AORTIC ANEURYSM REPAIR USING THE AORTO UNI-ILIAC APPROACH

Over the past few years, several devices for endovascular aortic aneurysm repair have been developed and used in clinical trials.[16] Our initial experience with the Chuter-Gianturco bifurcated device showed that only a small proportion of patients were found to have a suitable anatomy for this system.[17] Further analysis of the measurements of the aortoiliac segment obtained with spiral CT scan in our unit confirmed that the available aorto aortic and bifurcated devices were suitable for approximately 10% of patients.[18] This necessitated the use of an aorto uni-iliac approach,[19] which enabled us to treat most aneurysms with endovascular techniques, and the bulk of our experience is with this type of repair. Recently, the Zenith™ modular bifurcated system developed by Hartley & Lawrence-Brown has become available in a wide range of sizes and has been found to be suitable for many patients who previously would have been unsuitable for many patients who previously would have been unsuitable for bifurcated repair. The details of Zenith system can be found elsewhere.[20] In this section, the indications for endovascular aneurysm repair and the technique of aorto uni-iliac repair using the Malmo-Nottingham system is presented.

Indications

Because the long-term results of endovascular aortic aneurysm repair currently are not known, open repair remains the preferred method for patients younger than 65 years of age who are fit for open repair. With regard to the size of aneurysm, the indications for the use of endovascular technique should be the same as

that for open repair and should be based on the available evidence.[1] Moreover, there is some evidence[21] that small aneurysms (4.5–5.5 cm) are no more suitable for endovascular repair than intermediate-sized (5.5–6.9 cm) aneurysms. A policy of surveillance for small aneurysms therefore does not seem to have a disadvantage of aneurysms becoming less suitable for endovascular repair as they grow in size within this range.

Endovascular techniques have evolved to provide a less invasive alternative to aortic aneurysm repair, and physiologic studies on patients undergoing uncomplicated endovascular repair confirm that less hemodynamic change,[22] renal damage,[23] colonic ischemia,[24] and ischemia–reperfusion injury[25] occur with endovascular repair compared with open repair. However, it remains to be seen whether endovascular repair is safe and effective in patients who are considered to be at high risk or unfit for open surgery. Data available so far from uncontrolled observational studies suggest that outcome of endovascular repair in these patients depends not only on the severity of organ dysfunction but also on the system involved and the anatomy of the aortoiliac segment. Controlled trials are required to determine the role of endovascular repair in high-risk surgical patients. In the meantime, the decision to use endovascular repair in such patients must be made in the light of the fact that many patients in this group may die of their medical problems with an intact aneurysm.[26]

Aortic aneurysms may become symptomatic because of rapid enlargement or development of periaortic inflammation. The outcome of open surgery in symptomatic patients has been reported to be worse compared with that of patients with totally asymptomatic aneurysms.[27] Provided that the anatomy is favorable and the procedure can be undertaken without a significant delay, then endovascular repair may be a better option for these individuals. The effect of endovascular exclusion on periaortic inflammation is not well understood at present, but relief of ureteric obstruction has been seen after endovascular repair of an inflammatory aneurysm.

The morbidity and mortality rates of open surgery for ruptured aneurysm have remained high, and endovascular repair has the potential for improving the outcome for these patients. The logistics of emergency endovascular repair are complex, and although the first endovascular repair of a ruptured aneurysm[28] was performed in 1994, only a small number of patients with ruptured aneurysms have been treated thus far with endovascular techniques. Effective exclusion of a ruptured aneursysm is possible with an endoprosthesis, and these aneurysms remain excluded and undergo a reduction in size.[29] As the experience with elective endovascular repair increases and the devices become more readily available, contained rupture in stable patients will become an important indication.

Endovascular repair using a bifurcated endoprosthesis provides a more anatomic repair and avoids the use of a femorofemoral bypass. It is our preference is to use a bifurcated endoprosthesis in patients who have a suitable anatomy for such a repair. However, there are many patients who are unsuitable for a bifurcated repair mainly because of the iliac anatomy. The aorto uni-iliac approach allows endovascular repair in such patients. Several methods of aorto uni-iliac repair have been described. Some involve routine exposure of the iliac arteries, sacrifice of the internal iliac artery, and anastomosis of the distal end of the graft to the common femoral artery. The technique used in our unit does not require any of these maneuvers. The common femoral arteries are used for the introduction of the endoprosthesis, and the internal iliac arteries are not sacrificed routinely. Following is a description of the method used in our unit.

Technique of Aorto Uni-Iliac Repair

PREOPERATIVE ASSESSMENT

Spiral CT angiography is the preferred method of preoperative assessment in our unit.[30] The data obtained are processed, and images of the aortoiliac segment are reconstructed in multiple planes to obtain measurements of the neck diameter, neck length, common and external iliac diameters, and the distance from the renal artery to the aortic and iliac bifurcations. Other important features documented include tortuosity and calcification of the iliac arteries, shape and lining of the neck, angle between the aortic neck and the suprarenal aorta, angle between the neck and the aneurysm, and the angle between the aneurysm and the common iliac arteries. Software that allows three-dimensional reconstruction of the aortoiliac segment and a model of the endoprosthesis to be superimposed to determine the size of the endoprosthesis are being developed and may allow a more accurate selection of endoprosthesis.[31]

An endoprosthesis of appropriate size is constructed for each patient from the components mentioned in the following paragraphs. Although technically it is possible to implant wider grafts, patients with neck diameters up to 30 mm and common iliac diameters up to 24 mm are considered suitable. If the iliac artery is wide, then it must be free of thrombus. Similarly, there must be no significant filling defects in the neck, suggesting the presence of atheroma or thrombus because these features prevent a satisfactory seal around the stent graft. The other adverse features that are likely to result in technical difficulties

or failures are an angle greater than 45 degrees between the long axis of the neck and the long axis of the aneurysm, and an angle greater than 60 degrees between the long axis of the aneurysm and the common iliac artery. Tortuous and heavily calcified iliac arteries also can make the procedure difficult.

ENDOPROSTHESIS

The endoprosthesis consists of a Gianturco Z stent skeleton and Twill weave uncrimped Dacron graft. Two segments of graft are sutured obliquely to create a tapered graft (Fig. 31–1). The graft diameter is approximately 10% greater than the diameter of the aortic neck and the iliac artery. For a wide neck, greater oversizing may be used, that is, a 32-mm graft for a 28-mm neck and a 34-mm graft for a 30-mm neck diameter. The length of the graft can be more difficult to determine, particularly in large aneurysms with a large cavity. In these cases, measurements should be obtained by CT scan and calibrated angiogram, and contingency plans should be made to extend the graft with an iliac extension piece should this become necessary. The proximal most stent for attachment to the aneurysm neck has four caudally pointing barbs and four cranially pointing hooks, and the rest of the stents are without any hooks or barbs (Fig. 31–2). The height of the proximal stent is 25 mm,

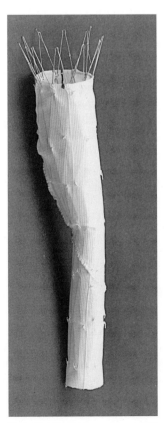

Figure 31–1. The Nottingham aorto uni-iliac device.

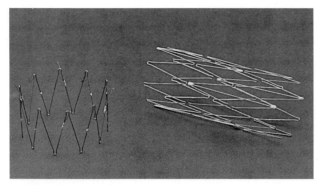

Figure 31–2. The barbs and hooks on the Nottingham device.

and the resting or unrestrained diameter is 45 mm. The stents are sutured to the graft with 5/0 Goretex suture. Depending on the neck length, diameter, and shape, an uncovered suprarenal stent may be used. If the neck is parallel and long enough to accommodate a complete stent that is 25 mm long, then a suprarenal stent is not necessary. Otherwise, an uncovered suprarenal stent is required, and if the renal artery origin is not diseased, then routine use of an uncovered suprarenal stent may make the proximal attachment more secure. The decision to use a suprarenal stent therefore has to be made for each individual case based on the measurements and the quality of the infrarenal aortic neck and the state of the renal artery ostia. The autoclaved endoprosthesis is mounted on a graft carrier and inserted into a 21-F loading sheath (Fig. 31–3) at the time of the procedure. A long thread is passed through the opposite bends of the top Gianturco stents and then through the central lumen of the graft carrier and secured at the caudal end of the carrier with rubber-covered forceps. This provides cranial traction to the endoprosthesis as it is introduced through the sheath and in effect allows the endoprosthesis to be pulled rather than pushed up. The advantage of this mechanism is that the endoprosthesis is not at a risk of being displaced downstream during deployment and therefore no manipulation of blood pressure is required. It also keeps the proximal stent partially restrained even when the

entire endoprosthesis has been released and allows fine adjustment even at the last stage of deployment.

In our unit, the procedure is performed in the operating room under general anaesthesia with preparation for conversion to an open procedure, should that become necessary. Interventional radiology suites usually are better equipped with regard to imaging equipment, and if a similar level of sterility, nursing support, and access to instruments as a vascular operating room can be achieved, then the procedure can be performed in such a location. We use a mobile image intensifier with facilities for digital subtraction imaging, playback, and hard copy output for intraoperative imaging. A small range of equipment is required routinely, as follows:

19-gauge needle

0.035-inch J-tipped guide wire

7-F sheaths

Superstiff Amplatz 0.35-inch guide wires 180 cm/ 260 cm

7-F marker angiography catheter

5-F Cobra catheter

Delivery system consisting of the 21-F delivery sheath, a preloading sheath, and the graft carrier.

Both common femoral arteries are exposed. Tapes are passed around the common femoral artery and converted into a snare by feeding them through a plastic tube (Kwill). This enables hemostasis during the introduction of sheath through an arteriotomy. A guide wire is introduced via an anterior wall femoral puncture on the side chosen for the deployment of the iliac end of the endoprosthesis. If the arteries are particularly tortuous, then a Cobra catheter and sometimes a Terumo guide wire is used for negotiating the aortoiliac segment. A 7-F pigtail angiographic catheter with radiopaque marks at 1-cm intervals over 15 cm is introduced over the guide wire via a 7-F sheath and positioned at the level of the renal artery. With a 7-F catheter, a hand injection is usually adequate for obtaining an aortogram to identify the origins of the renal arteries and to measure the distance from the renal artery to aortic and iliac bifurcation. In patients with impaired renal function, we use a combination of carbon dioxide (CO_2) and iodinated contrast to minimize the total dose of iodinated contrast. The angiography catheter then is removed and reintroduced over a guide wire via a 7-F sheath placed in the contralateral femoral artery.

A 21-F sheath is introduced over the guide wire through a longitudinal arteriotomy and hemostasis is maintained by tightening the tapes around the artery. If difficulty is anticipated because of aortoiliac tortuosity, then a 260-cm stiff brachial-to-femoral guide wire is used. This, however, is required infrequently,

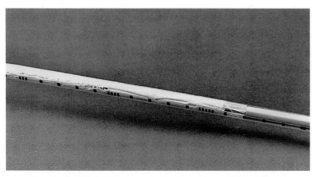

Figure 31–3. The loading sheath for the Nottingham device.

and because we have encountered embolic complications with this technique, we therefore recommend selective use only. The end of the sheath is positioned in the lower thoracic aorta wall above the origins of the renal arteries. The dilator is slowly withdrawn, and the sheath is clamped with a pair of rubber-covered clamps to achieve hemostasis. The preloading sheath containing the endoprosthesis is locked to the introducing sheath, and the endoprosthesis is advanced to the level of the renal artery. The position of the renal artery is confirmed again with an angiogram and the process of deployment commenced. The position of the endoprosthesis and its relationship to the origin of the renal artery is kept under constant check with frequent injection of small volume of contrast through the angiography catheter. The first covered stent is deployed immediately below the renal artery origin without compromising its origin. Once the entire endoprosthesis has been released by completely withdrawing the sheath, the suture line used for mounting the endoprosthesis on the carrier is removed, allowing the proximal stent to fully expand. The attachment of the proximal stent to the delivery system with the suture line keeps the proximal stent stable and prevents any displacement by the blood flow during deployment.

A guide wire is introduced through the central lumen of the carrier to maintain access through the endoprosthesis before removal of the carrier. The angiography catheter, which at this stage is lying between the endoprosthesis and the aortic wall, is withdrawn gently over a guide wire. This catheter then is introduced over the guide wire through the endoprosthesis into the suprarenal aorta. An angiogram can be performed at this stage to confirm that the renal arteries are patent and that there is no paragraft perfusion along the proximal end of the prosthesis. A 21-F sheath then is introduced via a longitudinal arteriotomy in the contralateral femoral artery over a guide wire into the aneurysm sac.

The guide wire is removed, and an aneurysmogram is performed by injecting through the lumen of the dilator. This is done to detect any patent lumbar artery or inferior mesenteric artery. If any patent branch is found arising from the aneurysm sac, then large embolilzation particles made of Gelfoam are introduced into the sac. After this, a Gianturco stent covered with Dacron graft is deployed inside the common iliac artery to act as an occlusion device. The procedure is completed with a traditional femorofemoral bypass (Fig. 31–4A, B,) and a final angiogram to ensure that:

1. The renal arteries are patent.
2. There is no paragraft perfusion on the aneurysm sac.
3. There is no perfusion of the sac along the occluding device in the iliac artery.

4. The internal iliac arteries are patent.
5. The femorofemoral crossover graft and the distal superficial femoral and profunda arteries are patent (Fig. 31–5).

Postoperative surveillance is carried out with contrast-enhanced CT scan, performed within the first week of the procedure and subsequently at 3 months, 6 months, and annually.

Results

Between March 1994 and January 1998, a total of 134 aortic aneurysms were repaired in our unit using the aorto uni-iliac method. Of these 134, 7 procedures were performed for ruptured AAA, 4 for aortocaval fistulas, 9 for urgent repair for symptomatic AAA, and 114 for elective repair of asymptomatic AAA. Of these 114 patients, 70 (61.4%) were considered to be high risk for open surgery and most had been referred by other centers. The mean age of the entire group was 72 years (range 51–86 years).

A breakdown of the perioperative mortality for each subgroup is shown in Table 31–1 and a breakdown of the cause of death shown in Table 31–2.

There are several questions regarding the long-term outcome of endovascular repair, such as late migration, distortion of prosthesis, dilatation of the aneurysm neck, and the fate of side branch endoleaks, that need to be answered before the long-term safety and efficacy of endovascular repair becomes clear. Careful follow-up and documentation therefore remains an important responsibility of any clinician embarking on the use of this technique, and this preferably should be within a multicenter clinical trial.

ENDOVASCULAR ABDOMINAL AORTIC ANEURYSM REPAIR USING BIFURCATED DEVICES

The development of fabric-covered stents opened a new dimension for non-surgical therapy of aneurysmal disease.[32] Successful endoluminal grafting for abdominal and thoracic aortic aneurysms has been demonstrated by many centers. There are a growing number of communications reporting on different endovascular stent-graft devices documenting clinical effectiveness associated with relatively low morbidity and mortality rates and quick patient recovery.[33–43] With respect to reliability of endovascular techniques compared with standard surgical repair, there are three issues still remaining unknown:

1. Will endovascular therapy prevent expansion of the aneurysm and delayed aneurysm rupture?

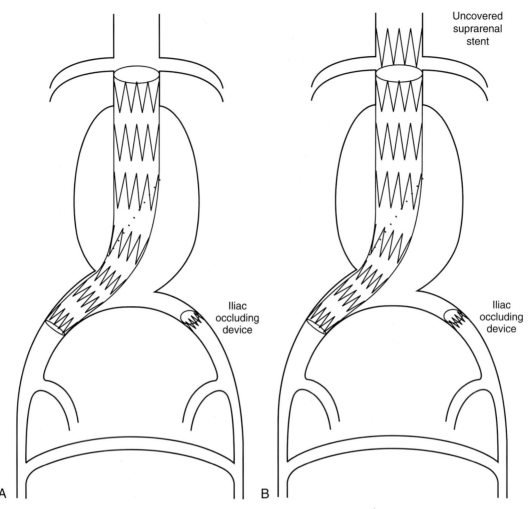

Figure 31–4. *A,* The endoprosthesis extends from just below the renal artery to the more favorable common iliac artery. An occluding device is placed in the contralateral common iliac artery, and a traditional femorofemoral bypass is performed. *B,* In the absence of a long (>25 mm length) and good quality neck an uncovered stent is placed across the origins of the renal artery to provide secure attachment to the suprarenal aorta.

2. Will graft and stent material remain durable and retain its structural integrity?
3. Will the dilating process be retarded by successful aneurysm exclusion?

To examine these issues and to define the clinical utility of this new interventional technique, a large three-center study was undertaken to prospectively study initially polyester-covered nitinol stents and then endoprostheses based on a nitinol framework incorporating a polytetrafluoroethylene (PTFE) fabric cover for the treatment of infrarenal AAAs. Detailed outcome analysis and results are discussed subsequently.

Types of Endoprosthesis

The present generation of modular bifurcated endoprostheses are based on the original Miahle Stentor device (Fig. 31–6). These consist of a main body, including an ipsilateral iliac limb and a separate plug-in contralateral limb. The devices are constructed from an endo- or exoskeleton of self-expanding nitinol stent with an ultra thin Dacron graft covering. When an endoskeleton has been used, hooks may be incorporated in the uppermost stent to provide secure fixation. The endoprostheses using an exoskeleton generally rely on radial force for upper fixation alone and the incorporation of the stent struts into the normal vessel wall over time (see Chapter 2). The plug-in contralateral limbs all are self-expanding and rely on radial strength to obtain a seal in the iliac arteries.

Variations on these standard devices have been evolved to allow the use of the endoprosthesis when there is a short proximal neck. Such an example is the Cook Zenith device, which uses an uncovered Gianturco suprarenal stent similar to the Nottingham uni-iliac device (see Fig. 31–1).

Deployment Technique

The technique described relates to the basic implantation procedure suitable for most modular bifurcated

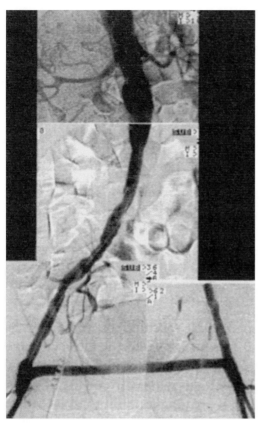

Figure 31–5. A completed aorto uni-iliac procedure with femorofemoral crossover.

endoprostheses. The technique is the editors' overview, and the reader should note that there are many possible individual variations of technique.

At commencement of the procedure, once the patient is anesthetized and has a bladder catheter inserted, he or she is placed supine on the angiographic or operating table with a radiopaque ruler or other marker system positioned under the patient. Although in many centers, endovascular repair is performed under general anaesthesia, the use of spinal anesthesia is becoming more frequent.

A 4-F pigtail catheter is inserted into the left brachial artery percutaneously and advanced under fluoroscopic control into the descending aorta to lie above the renal arteries and allow control angiography. Heparin is administered in a dose of 5000 to 10,000 units, and antibiotic prophylaxis is given.

Table 31–1. Perioperative Mortality Breakdown

Ruptured AAA	3/7 (43%)
Aortocaval fistulas	1/4 (25%)
Urgent for symptomatic	0
Elective for nonruptured	11/114 (9.6%)
Elective in high-risk group	9/70 (12.9%)
Elective in acceptable risk group	2/44 (4.5%)

AAA = abdominal aortic aneurysm.

Table 31–2. Causes of Postoperative Deaths

Ruptured AAA

Two patients died after open conversion. It was not possible to introduce the delivery system into the aorta because of tortuous and calcified iliac arteries. One patient died of PE after successful EVR.

Aortocaval Fistula

One patient died after conversion to open procedure because of a top endoleak.

Elective High-Risk Group

Myocardial infarction	3
Stroke	1
Renal failure	1
Multisystem organ failure after conversion	2
Ruptured AAA secondary to persistent top endoleak	1
Pneumonia after laparotomy for periaortic ligatures	1

Elective Acceptable Risk Group

Myocardial infarction	1
Septicemia from MRSA infection of femorofemoral crossover graft	1

AAA = Abdominal aortic aneurysm; EVR = endovascular repair; MRSA = methicillin-resistant *Staphylococcus aureus*; PE = pleural effusion.

Bilateral groin incisions are made (or unilateral if a percutaneous contralateral iliac limb is to be used). The ipsilateral artery has a small arteriotomy made, and a steerable wire and catheter are advanced into the descending aorta. The steerable wire then is replaced with a stiff wire such as the Amplatz super

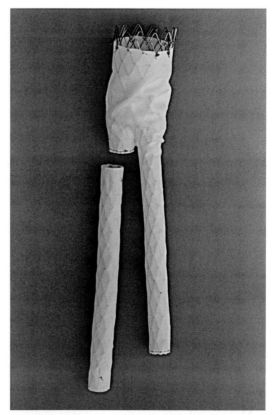

Figure 31–6. The Miahle Stentor device.

stiff. A digital subtraction angiogram then is performed via the brachial catheter, and the level of the renal arteries relative to the opaque ruler is noted (Fig. 31–7A).

After extension of the arteriotomy, the delivery system of the endoprosthesis then is advanced over the stiff wire until the markers for the top of the stent graft lie above the level of the renal arteries. At this time, the delivery system also is rotated to ensure that the long iliac limb is on the correct side. Radiopaque markers built in to the stent graft are used to ensure its correct orientation within the aorta.

The image intensifier is centered over the renal arteries and a further angiogram performed via the brachial catheter using a more magnified field of the image intensifier. The exact relationship of the renal arteries to the ruler is noted, and from this time, no further movement of the image intensifier or table is

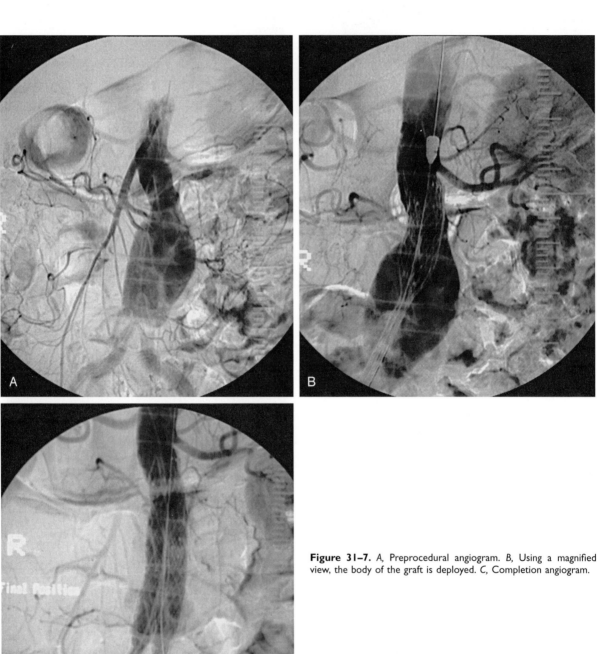

Figure 31–7. *A,* Preprocedural angiogram. *B,* Using a magnified view, the body of the graft is deployed. *C,* Completion angiogram.

allowed until the body of the graft is deployed (see Fig. 31–7B). Although in many patients, conventional contrast angiography is appropriate, when there is impairment of renal function, CO_2 angiography may be of great value in reducing the overall contrast burden.

Graft deployment is commenced above the renal arteries. Once the first few centimeters have been deployed, the whole assembly gradually is pulled caudally until the markers indicating the top of the fabric lie just below the renal arteries (see Fig. 31–7B). After this maneuver, the remainder of the graft is deployed into the ipsilateral iliac artery.

A 10-F sheath then is inserted into the contralateral femoral artery, and a guide wire is passed into the open gate of the stent graft before insertion of the iliac limb. The editors favor passage of a long steerable wire via the brachial catheter to negotiate the open limb of the device and into the aneurysm sac, where it is snared via the contralateral femoral sheath. Some operators favor a direct approach from the contralateral femoral artery with a steerable wire and shaped catheter, whereas others attempt to cross over from the already deployed ipsilateral iliac limb. Whichever method is used, prolonged manipulation inside the aneurysm sac should be avoided to lessen the chance of embolization. In addition, the contralateral femoral artery should be clamped below the sheath to prevent distal embolization. Once the open limb of the stent graft has been catheterized, the contralateral limb is deployed.

Thus, detailed angiography via the brachial catheter is obtained to check for endoleaks (see Fig. 31–7C). Figure 31–8A to D illustrates in diagramatic form the technique of implantation. A further CT examination is performed before discharge from hospital to confirm successful exclusion of the aneurysms (Fig. 31–9).

Complications

The complications of endovascular repair of AAAs can be divided into early and late events.

EARLY COMPLICATIONS

These may be related to technical failures of the device or to procedural problems. The technical failures are:

1. Failure to deliver the device because of tortuosity of vessels, misplacement, or primary failure of the delivery system. In all these instances, conversion to surgical repair is the most likely consequence.
2. Delivery of the device in an apparently correct position but with the presence of persistent primary endoleaks (Fig. 31–10A, B).
3. Delivery of the device with exclusion of potentially important branches. The most important of these are the renal and internal iliac arteries. If both internal iliac arteries are patent, then one may be excluded safely. However, if either both or a single

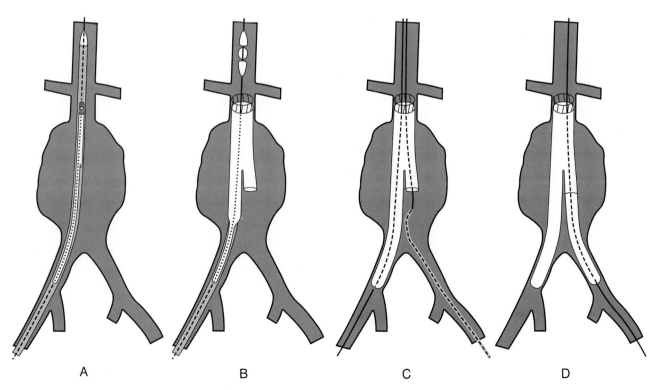

Figure 31–8. A–D, The technique of implantation.

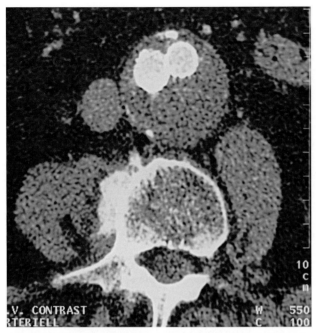

Figure 31–9. Postprocedural computed tomography (CT) at level of iliac limbs showing no evidence of an endoleak.

internal iliac artery is covered by the graft, then the possibility of buttock claudication or even colonic ischemia is likely. Colonic ischemia occurs particularly when the inferior mesenteric artery is not patent and the blood supply to the distal colon occurs via the internal iliac arteries.

Figure 31–11*A* to *C* shows a thoracoabdominal

aortic aneurysm repaired by a tube graft in which the celiac trunk inadvertantly has been excluded.

Procedural Problems

Procedural problems include the following:

1. Damage to access vessels or the aorta. In such instances, either immediate endovascular or surgical repair is required. Perforation of the aorta may require immediate surgical conversion, whereas iliac and femoral artery damage may be repaired locally.
2. Distal athero- or thromboemolization. This is always a potential problem, particularly when prolonged manipulations are performed within the aneurysm sac. Clamping of the femoral arteries before such manipulations should minimize this complication.

LATE COMPLICATIONS

Most late complications relate to late endoleaks or graft thrombosis.

Late endoleaks. These can be caused by

1. Slippage of the top stent due to either undersizing or continued expansion of the aneurysm neck.
2. After successful exclusion, longitudinal shrinkage of the aneurysm leading to buckling of the device and limb dislocation (Fig. 31–12).

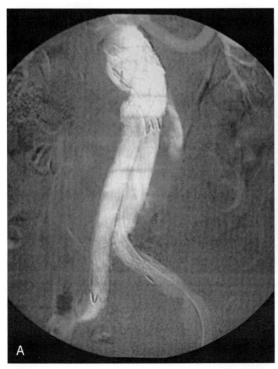

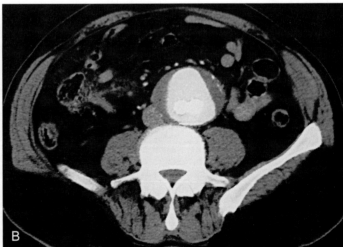

Figure 31–10. *A*, Postprocedural angiogram showing proximal endoleak. *B*, CT of same patient confirming persisting endoleak.

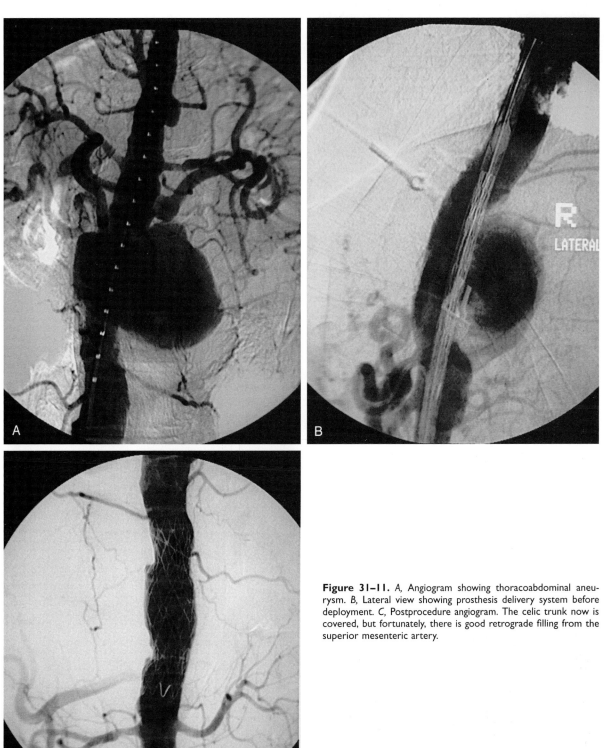

Figure 31–11. *A,* Angiogram showing thoracoabdominal aneurysm. *B,* Lateral view showing prosthesis delivery system before deployment. *C,* Postprocedure angiogram. The celic trunk now is covered, but fortunately, there is good retrograde filling from the superior mesenteric artery.

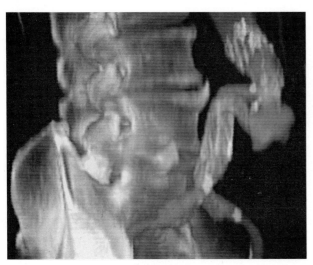

Figure 31–12. After initial successful occlusion, the aneurysm has shrunk longitudinally, leading to buckling of the device and dislocation of the plug-in limb.

3. Mechanical failure and disintegration of the implanted device. Figure 31–13 shows the radiograph of an explanted device. The sutures between the second and third stents have broken. Figure 31–14A to C shows an explanted device with a tear in the fabric at the junction between the fixed limb and the body of the graft.
4. Endoleak at the distal insertion site into the iliac artery caused by either continued expansion of an already dilated iliac artery or by displacement of the iliac limb.
5. Persistent filling of the sac from retrograde flow via the inferior mesenteric artery or patent lumbar vessels. When the graft is intact, it may be possible to seal the endoleak by placement of an additional covered stent. Lumbar and inferior mesenteric artery endoleaks may be treated by embolization. Otherwise, persistent endoleaks are an indication for conversion to conventional repair as rupture is a distinct reality.

Graft Thrombosis. If one or the other iliac becomes occluded, then angiography should be performed to determine the cause. If the limb is kinked, it may be possible to perform thrombolysis and then straighten the kink by insertion of an additional endovascular stent. If this is not possible, then a femoro-femoral crossover may be performed.

The German-Swiss Three-Center Experience

Since 1994, bifurcated stent grafts for the endovascular repair of infrarenal AAA have been implanted in a total of 296 patients with a mean age of 70 (range 49–90) years. For analysis of the initial and follow-up results, the patients were divided into three subgroups: group 1 included patients treated between August 1994 and April 1996 with use of the original stent graft device (Miahle Stentor), group 2 included patients treated between May 1996 and December 1997 with a refined prosthesis (Vanguard), and group 3 patients were treated between September 1997 and December 1998 with a newly designed bifurcated stent graft (Excluder).

The patients were selected based on anatomic suitability.[41] Inclusion criteria were aneurysms classified as type A, B, or C (see Fig. 31–6). Type A aneurysms had a proximal and distal aortic neck of greater than 15 mm in length without iliac involvement. Type B aneurysms had involvement of the aortic bifurcation and a proximal aortic neck of greater than 15 mm in length, and a diameter less than 12 mm of the common iliac artery. Type C aneurysms had a proximal aortic neck greater than 15 mm in length and involvement of the common iliac arteries without involving the iliac bifurcation.

Patient exclusion criteria were aortic aneurysms with both internal iliac arteries involved in the aneurysm (type D aneurysm), patients whose proximal aortic neck was less than 15 mm in length (type E aneurysm) (Fig. 31–15), patients with a diameter less than 7 mm of the iliac arteries, patients with stenosis or occlusion of the superior mesenteric artery, and patients who could not be observed for follow-up. In

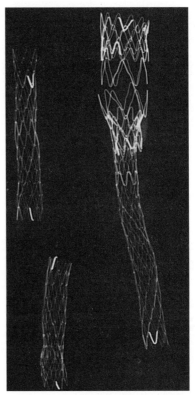

Figure 31–13. Radiograph of explanted device showing suture breakage between the second and third stents of the body of the graft.

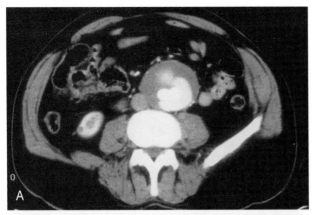

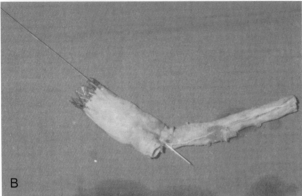

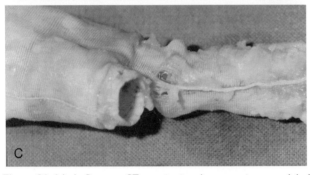

Figure 31–14. A, Contrast CT examination demonstrating an endoleak at 18 months postimplantation. B, The explanted device showing a tear in the fabric at the junction of the body and fixed limb. C, Magnified view of part B.

addition, patients with marked tortuosity of the iliac arteries (< 90 degrees) or angulation of the proximal neck (> 60 degrees) were excluded from the study.

To define the anatomy of the aortic aneurysm, multiplane conventional angiography with use of a calibrated catheter, spiral CT, and magnetic resonance angiography were performed. Measurements included the distance between the renal arteries to the aneurysm and the aortic bifurcation, the length and the diameter of the proximal and distal neck of the aneurysm, and the diameter of the proximal and distal common iliac arteries.

The stent grafts implanted in patient groups 1 and 2 were self-expanding endoprostheses based on a nitinol alloy framework annealed into a tubular zig-

zag configuration by a 7-0 polypropylene thread and incorporating a thin woven polyester fabric graft over a nitinol wire stent frame[41] (see Fig. 31–6). The endoprosthesis currently under evaluation (patient group 3) is based on a nitinol framework covered with a thin PTFE-graft on the inside (Fig. 31–16). Both types of bifurcated endoprostheses are modular systems and have two components. The primary component consists of an aortic section with a fixed ipsilateral iliac limb with an attachment site for the second iliac limb section.

Endoluminal treatment was performed under general (n = 239) or local anesthesia combined with analgosedation (n = 57) in the angiography suite (in the German hospitals) or operating room (in the Swiss hospital) as teamwork between interventional radiologists and vascular surgeons. The vascular surgeon performed the arteriotomy, and the radiologist placed the endoprosthesis. All patients were prepared for surgical repair in case of failed endoluminal technique.

FOLLOW-UP

The follow-up protocol included spiral CT and plain abdominal radiographs. CT control studies were performed before discharge, at 6 and 12 months, and then every year on an outpatient basis. Plain radiographs were taken at 12 months and then annually.

CT measurements were performed with use of the caliper method at the level of the most caudal renal artery, 30 mm further caudally, at the level of the maximum aneurysm diameter, 10 mm above the iliac bifurcation, and, to assess the diameter of both proximal iliac arteries, 10 mm below the iliac bifurcation. All postinterventional CT measurements were taken in comparison with the preinterventional CT.

Plain radiographs were taken to assess the position of the stent graft device related to anatomic landmarks and to evaluate the structural integrity of the endoprostheses. The upper, middle, and lower rings of the aortic section of the polyester covered nitinol stents (group 1 and 2) were analyzed and the number of suture breaks of the nitinol framework counted.

DEFINITION OF RESULTS

Primary technical success was defined as complete if the AAA was excluded from the circulation with restoration of normal blood flow without evidence of an endoleak and lack of increase in aneurysm size. Failure was defined as demonstration of an endoleak or increase in aneurysm size during follow-up. Secondary technical success was achieved if a second endoluminal procedure was required to completely exclude the AAA from the blood circulation.

Endoluminal

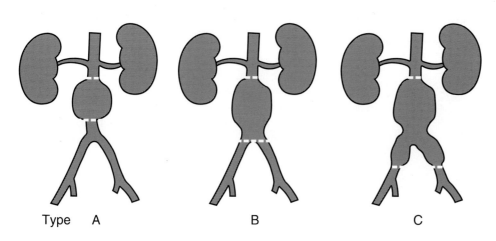

Type   A   B   C

Figure 31–15. Morphology of abdominal aortic aneurysms.

Surgical

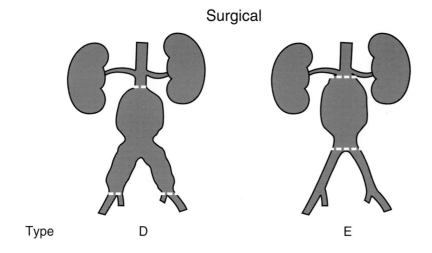

Type   D   E

RESULTS

Endoleaks have been reported by all the authors using different devices ranging between 9% and 47%.[33–35, 37–44] In this prospective study, we implanted in 296 patients bifurcated stent grafts based on a self-expandable Nitinol framework covered with a polyester (study group 1 and 2) or PTFE fabric graft for the endovascular repair of AAA (group 3). Technical results are given in Table 31–3. Incomplete sealing between the stent graft and the aorta, defined as technical failure, was a major problem in study group 1. Primary failure (18%) was the result of problems with access, proximal or distal endoleaks, or reperfusion via lumbar collateral vessels. In a second series including 159 patients (group 2), the refined version of the stent graft was implanted. With increasing experience and strict application of the inclusion and exclusion criteria, particularly excluding patients with pronounced tortuosity of iliac arteries and marked angulation of the proximal aneurysmal neck, an initial technical success rate of 95% was achieved. Perigraft

flow due to reperfusion via lumbar arteries was the main problem in this study group.

In a small series of 31 patients (group 3) treated with a new stent graft combination, the initial technical success was promising. A 10% rate of endoleaks was the result of backbleeding into the aneurysm sac via lumbar/hypogastric arteries. Table 31–4 lists the early complications and Table 31–5 lists the long-term follow-up.

During follow-up, CT and plain radiographs demonstrated de novo endoleaks 6 to 43 months after stent graft implantation in 16 patients (group 1) and 18 patients (group 2), respectively, that were caused by distal migration of the endoprosthesis, dislodgement of the iliac limbs from the distal attachment site, disconnection of the contralateral limb from the attachment site, polyester tears, or lumbar reperfusion. Some important lessons emerge from these patients: there was significant increase in aneurysm size requiring explantation of the implant in 7 and reintervention to seal the endoleak in 18 additional

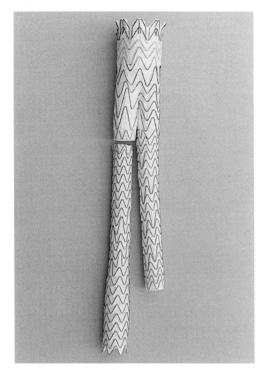

Figure 31–16. The Excludor Prograft.

Table 31–4. Complications in 296 Patients Treated With Stent Grafts for Infrarenal Abdominal Aortic Aneurysm

Group	No. Patients	(%)
Group 1 (N = 107)		
Local		
Femoral artery damage	2	
Arteriovenous fistula	1	
Groin hematoma requiring surgery	1	
Lymph fistula	1	
Groin infection after arteriotomy	1	
Limb occlusion*	1	
Remote		
Peripheral macroembolization	3	
Peripheral microembolization	1	
Systemic		
Rupture of iliac artery†	1	
Embolic graft occlusion‡	1	
Acute hepatic failure§	1	
Total	14	13
Group 2 (N = 158)		
Local		
Femoral artery damage	1	
Groin infection after arteriotomy	3	
Lymph fistula	1	
Remote		
Peripheral microembolization	2	
Total	7	4
Group 3 (N = 31)		
Local		
Femoral artery damage	1	
Systemic		
Acute aortic rupture‖	1	
Total	2	7

*Requiring local thrombolysis.
†Requiring emergency surgery.
‡Resulting in foot amputation.
§Resulting in death 8 d after the procedure.
‖Resulting in death 4 h after the procedure.

patients. Delayed aortic rupture occurred in two patients who underwent enlargement of the aneurysm without any evidence of an endoleak as shown by CT, and in one additional patient who developed a de novo leak 12 months after stent graft implantation. Expansion of the aneurysm sac, most likely caused by continued pressure on the aortic wall, demonstrates the potential clinical significance of persistent

Table 31–3. Initial Technical Results in 301 Patients Treated or Attempted to Be Treated with Stent Grafts for Infrarenal Abdominal Aortic Aneurysm

Group 1 (n = 111)		
Initial success*	No. Patients	82%
Endoleak (no.)		16
Proximal attachment site	5	
Distal attachment site	3	
Polyester tear	6	
Lumbar refilling	4	
Conversion to surgery		4
Group 2 (n = 159)		
Initial success*	N	95%
Endoleak (no.)		7
Attachment site second iliac limb	1	
Lumbar refilling	6	
Conversion to surgery		1
Group 3 (n = 31)		
Initial success*	N	90%
Endoleak (no.)		3
Lumbar refilling	3	

Values are number of patients.
*Initial complete exclusion of abdominal aortic aneurysm from circulation with restoration of normal blood flow.

or untreated leaks associated with an increase of the aortic diameter over time, which has been communicated in several reports.[13, 37, 38, 45–47] Conversely, patients with sealed endoleaks and those free of endoleaks underwent significant shrinkage of their aneurysms, confirming the observation of other authors.[37, 39, 48]

The finding that "successful" coil embolization of lumbar collateral vessels with reperfusion of the aneurysm failed to interrupt pressure transmission to the aneurysmal wall in four patients confirmed the experimental work of Marty and associates.[49] These authors investigated the efficacy of coil embolization in the management of endoleaks and concluded that this technique failed to reduce intra-aneurysmal pressure and may not be a reliable therapeutic option for this type of endoleak. Thus, patients with persistent lumbar reperfusion or sealed lumbar refilling associated with expansion of aneurysm size may be at

Table 31–5. Follow-Up and Secondary Technical Success in 230 Patients Treated with Bifurcated Stent Grafts for Infrarenal Abdominal Aortic Aneurysm

Group		No. Patients	(%)
*Group 1**		67	69
De novo endoleak†		24	
Proximal attachment site	5		
Attachment site second iliac limb‡	5		
Distal attachment site	7		
Polyester tear	5		
Lumbar refilling	2		
Late aortic rupture§		3	
Aneurysm growth‖		5	
Graft infection¶		1	
Limb thrombosis**		1	
Group 2††		117	88
De novo endoleak‡‡		18	
Proximal attachment site	4		
Attachment site second iliac limb‡	5		
Distal attachment site	5		
Lumbar refilling	4		
Aneurysm growth§§		7	
Group 3 (n = 28)‖‖		31	90
Endoleak		2	
Lumbar refilling	2		
Graft infection¶¶		1	

*Mean follow-up 35 months.

†Nine of 24 endoleaks treated endoluminally; spontaneous seal in 2 patients.

‡Successfully treated with use of an additional overlapping endograft.

§Two of 3 patients successfully treated by means of surgery. Third patient died from late aortic rupture after 12 months.

‖Explantation of stent graft in 3; 2 patients considered for surgical repair.

¶Twelve months after endoluminal treatment clinical evidence of aortointestinal fistula resulting in explantation of endograft.

**Recurrent occlusion of left iliac limb, finally explantation of stent graft.

††Mean follow-up 17 months.

‡‡Nine of 18 de novo endoleaks treated by means of endoluminal technique.

§§Stent graft in 2 patients explanted; explantation in 5 additional patients considered.

‖‖Mean follow-up 7 months.

¶¶Explantation of stent graft after 6 months.

continued risk for rupture and should be considered for surgical repair.

Long-term fixation of endografts depends on the integrity and structural stability of the aorta, especially at the proximal aortic "anastomotic" site. Careful CT evaluation in study groups 1 and 2 demonstrated a slight increase in diameter (2–5 mm) at the proximal aortic cuff over 4 years in four patients. This observation has been reported by other groups following patients after endovascular repair of AAA[48, 49]; however, it was not found by Matsumara and colleagues.[44] Two retrospective studies evaluating the proximal aortic cuff by angiography and CT, respectively, in patients who had undergone conventional surgical repair for AAA demonstrated a significant increase of the diameter (4–5 mm) of the proximal aortic cuff in 8 to 25%.[50, 51] These data, based on follow-up of patients treated endoluminally or

conventionally, suggest that the indication for endoluminal treatment of infrarenal AAA with stent grafts in patients with long life expectancy may be reconsidered.[43]

Based on our initial and long-term follow-up results, endoluminal repair of infrarenal AAAs with use of bifurcated endografts associated with quick hospital recovery and low morbidity and mortality may be a feasible alternative to conventional surgery, especially for patients at high surgical risks. However, currently there are no long-term data available with respect to the fate of the proximal aortic cuff, possibly resulting in the late aortic rupture, which remains a serious concern.

SUMMARY

In a prospective study involving three centers, bifurcated stent grafts for the endovascular repair of infrarenal AAAs were implanted in a total of 296 patients. The purpose of the study was to define the clinical utility of stent grafts for the endoluminal treatment of infrarenal AAAs. Patient selection was based on anatomic suitability. For the analysis of the initial and follow-up results, the patients were divided into three subgroups: group 1 included patients treated with use of the original polyester-covered nitinol stent; group 2 included patients treated with the refined version of the endoprosthesis; and group 3 patients were treated with a newly designed bifurcated stent graft device.

In group 1 (n = 111), primary technical success was achieved in 82% of the patients. The initial technical success in subgroup 2 (n = 159) was 94% and in subgroup 3 (n = 31) was 90%. Minor and major complications related to the intervention, including two perioperative mortalities, were observed in 25 patients (8%).

During follow-up, serious problems, such as distal migration of the stent graft, dislodgement from the distal attachment site, or disconnection of the second iliac limb, were seen in 17 patients (group 1). Delayed aortic rupture occurred in three additional patients, 2 of whom survived after successful surgical repair. Secondary technical success was achieved in 69% in group 1, in 88% in group 2, and in 90% in group 3.

Based on initial and long-term follow-up results, endoluminal repair of infrarenal AAA with use of bifurcated endografts may be a feasible alternative to conventional surgery, especially for patients at high surgical risks. However, currently there are major concerns with respect to the structural integrity of stent graft material and the fate of the proximal aortic cuff in the long-term.

FURTHER CONSIDERATIONS IN ENDOVASCULAR AORTIC ANEURYSM REPAIR

Anatomy

The anatomic criteria required for endovascular repair are given in Table 31–6. The principal criterion limiting suitability is the need for an adequate length of normal artery proximal and distal to an aneurysm for graft attachment. Because most of abdominal aneurysms extend almost to the aortic bifurcation, most patients brought to endoluminal repair require a bifurcated (aorto bi-iliac) device. This contrasts with conventional repair, in which most patients receive a tube graft because it is usually possible to suture directly to the orifices of the common iliac arteries.

Access to an infrarenal aneurysm for current devices is most commonly transfemoral. Sheath diameters are typically 21 F (outside diameter) for aortic graft components and 18 F for iliac graft limbs or graft extensions, thus open arteriotomy is required. These large sheaths necessitate minimum insertion pathway diameters of 7 mm and 6 mm, respectively. External iliac artery tortuosity has not been a significant impediment in our experience because the vessel can be mobilized at the inguinal ligament and manually straightened, in a "pull-down" maneuver. Common iliac tortuosity with calcification poses greater difficulty to sheath passage because this artery is less affected by pull-down straightening. The most difficult scenario for sheath passage is a combination of heavily calcified common iliacs with at least one angulation greater than 90 degrees. Extreme tortuosity without calcification often can be easy to negotiate because these vessels tend to be elastic and can be straightened by a combination of iliac pull-down and application of tension on a super-stiff guidewire.

Aneurysm proximal neck shape is an important determinant of graft attachment. A neck with cone-shaped, divergent walls (from proximal to distal) may be less favorable for lasting graft attachment than a funnel-shaped neck (convergent walls) or a neck with parallel walls.[52] At the proximal neck, it is essential to obtain good apposition of the endovascular prosthesis to its attachment zone to prevent endoleak.

Table 31–6. Anatomic Criteria

I	Infrarenal segment of thrombus-free normal aorta of length ≥15 mm and diameter of ≥26 mm
II	Minimal iliac artery diameter of ≥7 mm
III	Angulation of proximal aortic neck of 60 degrees
IV	Angulation of iliac arteries of <90 degrees*

*As defined by Ad Hoc Committee for Standardized Reporting Practices in Vascular Surgery.

Heavy calcification (>⅓ circumferential) or the presence of thrombus at the neck may preclude graft attachment, particularly for devices that rely on wire-form barbs or times for fixation.

Severe angulation along a relatively short proximal neck (15–20 mm) makes graft attachment along the entire length of neck difficult because the outer (concave) aortic wall is longer than the inner (convex) wall. In such cases, if the delivery sheath does not closely follow the aortic centerline, a graft attaches higher on the nearest wall of aorta, potentially causing graft kinking within the neck and leaving a segment of the opposite wall uncovered.

Aneurysm Size

The probability of aneurysm rupture correlates with maximum transverse diameter and rate of expansion. The risk of rupture for small AAAs (< 5 cm in diameter) is extremely low—less than 1% per year.[1] This is increased for rapidly expanding aneurysms (i.e., those enlarging more than 5 mm in 6 months), which consistently demonstrate a greater propensity to rupture.[53] For any aneurysm patient, surgical repair is prudent if procedural mortality is less than the risk of spontaneous aneurysm rupture, at a given size. With conventional (open) repair, this compromise of risk is reached at an aneurysm diameter of 5 cm in experienced centers, where the mortality rate is less than 5%.

Endovascular repair poses a dilemma because there is a procedural advantage in repairing small aneurysms, which tend to have longer proximal necks but are at low risk of rupture. Early in our experience, we prospectively compared endovascular repair versus no treatment for aneurysms less than 5 cm in diameter.[54] There was no difference in mortality between treated and untreated groups at a mean follow-up interval of 21 months. Of 38 endovascularly treated patients, 1 died as a result of surgery, and 1 of 58 patients in the no treatment group experienced aneurysm rupture. However, those patients brought to aneurysm repair suffered significant morbidity, including a 14% rate of conversion to open repair and a 14% incidence of major vascular complications. These results did not justify endovascular repair of small aneurysms at this time. Our current practice limits the procedure to aneurysms which are (1) greater than 5 cm, or more than twice normal aortic diameter in a person of small body mass, or (2) less than 5 cm and symptomatic or enlarging 5 mm or more over a 6-month period.

Endovascular Repair in the Surgically Unfit Patient

The minimally invasive nature of endovascular repair lends itself to unique indications. These include surgically high-risk patients in whom conventional repair would cause prohibitive morbidity and patients with anatomy that is either inaccessible or cannot be treated effectively by exogenous access to the aorta (e.g., multiple previous operations, radiation damage, etc).

Repair of aortic aneurysms in these high-risk patients is contentious because their risk of death from the natural history of medical comorbidity may be greater than the risk of aneurysm rupture. However, for all AAA patients, the survival rate at 6 years postoperatively averages only 60%, one third less than age-matched nonaneurysmal populations.[55] The leading cause of late death after surgical repair is pre-existent cardiac disease, accounting for twice as many deaths in aneurysm patients vs. the general (nonaneurysmal) population.[55] Thus, aneurysm repair may be as much as a palliative procedure as it is prophylactic. Considered in this light, the endovascular technique is less morbid than conventional surgery in groups matched for medical risk. The U.S. AneuRx Multicenter Clinical Trial demonstrated that the major morbidity rate was reduced from 23% after conventional surgery group to 12% after stent graft treatment.[56] The latter group demonstrated significant reductions in operative blood loss, time to extubation, intensive care unit (ICU) stay, and total hospital stay. These findings suggest that endovascular aneurysm repair may be an ideal treatment for patients with significant medical morbidity who are expected to live indefinitely but would not be able to survive aneurysm rupture or conventional repair.

Endovascular repair also may be an ideal form of treatment when access to the aorta is difficult, as with extreme obesity, previous laparotomy or thoracotomy, or in situations of scarring, inflammation, or infection around the aorta itself. Such unusual cases merit independent review because all are unique. As an example, we recently performed endovascular repair on one patient who had undergone sternotomy and aortic arch replacement for aneurysmal transformation of a DeBakey type I dissection. The proximal descending aorta had been sutured over an elephant trunk of the arch graft, for future staged repair. Two weeks postoperatively, a left empyema and severe back pain developed, suggesting that the descending thoracic aneurysm had become symptomatic. This large aneurysm underwent successful endovascular repair, avoiding a second invasive surgery through a different incision (left thoracotomy), which would have transversed an infected field. This case illustrates three points: (1) endovascular repair may be used as an adjunct to open surgical repair; (2) the remote access point used for endovascular repair is not affected by processes that would preclude open repair (empyema); and (3) an endovascular prosthesis may be preferable in situations in which an artery can be difficult to suture, as with aortic dissection or in trauma.

Complications of Endovascular Repair

MORTALITY

Most published reports have shown that perioperative mortality after endoluminal aneurysm repair is similar to that reported for open repair.[1, 41, 57] In our experience, overall mortality after endoluminal repair averages approximately 4%, comparing favorably to large studies of elective conventional repair, including the U.K. Small Aneurysm Trial (5.8%), the Canadian Aneurysm Study (4.7%), and Michigan statewide mortality (5.6% in 1990).[1, 55, 57, 58] The minimally invasive nature of endoluminal surgery suggests that mortality should be less than with open surgery, however, the experimental nature of the technique probably has caused a selection bias for high-risk patients who have been offered the procedure on a compassionate basis. At times, our own cohort has included up to 44% of patients referred for endoluminal repair by outside vascular surgeons who had deemed them at excessive risk for conventional repair.[59] The impact of comorbidity in this group is best illustrated by our finding that among our first 113 endoluminal repairs, all deaths after intraoperative conversion (to open repair) occurred in high-risk patients.[60] There was a 43% mortality rate among "unfit" patients requiring conversion vs. no mortality among fit patients requiring conversion. Similarly, early in the experience of the U.K. Registry for Endovascular Treatment of Aneurysms, it was reported that 35% of all patients were "unfit" for open surgery.[6]

Among the "unfit" group, mortality after endovascular repair was more than twice that of average-risk, "fit" patients (14.6 vs. 6.6%). In contrast to these results, more recent results from the U.S. AneuRx Multicenter Trial have demonstrated low mortality (2.6%), despite 26% of patients being classified as American Society of Anesthesiologists (ASA) Class IV.[56] These substantially better results may reflect current improvements in endovascular technique and graft design, which are not represented fully by our cumulative experience (1992–present) or the early U.K. experience.

TECHNICAL COMPLICATIONS

There are a number of technical complications that are related specifically to the endoluminal method of repair. Although we have observed a greater incidence of local and systemic morbidity in endovascularly treated patients compared with those undergoing conventional repairs, other large series have reported reductions (Table 31–7). Initially it was thought that technical complications were part of the learning curve for a new technique, but it may well be that these are inherent risks of passing firm sheaths through tortuous and diseased arteries. The obligatory use of large-diameter delivery systems (for all current aortic prostheses, sheath diameters are > 20 Fr) can result in femoral and iliac artery injury. Wound complication rates reflect the requirement for surgical exposure of these vessels. When our collective endovascular experience was analyzed according to date of implant (initial 3 years vs. past 2.5 years), we found no significant difference in incidence of adverse events between early and late time periods (49% vs. 44% "device adverse events," as defined by the U.S. Food and Drug Administration [FDA]).[58] This was despite the fact that our late experience was heavily weighted with second-generation, purpose-designed prostheses, whereas most early cases used first-generation or "homemade" devices, custom fabricated from conventional angiography components and off-the-shelf grafts. The contribution of a learning curve to results was substantially discounted in our experience by our finding that adverse events were not reduced during our later experience, despite the fact that the need for emergent conversion was lowered significantly in this group.

Renal failure after endoluminal AAA repair is a serious systemic complication. Patients requiring postoperative dialysis in our series experienced a 43% mortality rate.[58] This finding mirrors the experience reported for conventional repair, in which persistent postoperative renal failure has been associated with ninefold greater mortality.[13] Although most endovascular series report a low incidence of this complication (our rate of 3.6% was the highest of the 3 largest series), the incidence remains greater than that reported for open repair.[58, 61] Renal failure after endovascular grafting may be secondary to the administration of large quantities of intravenous contrast, embolization of thrombus or atheroma during instrumentation, or inadvertent covering of the renal ostia by endograft. Although renal embolization is usually occult, manifest by a transient rise in creatinine or segmental infarct on postoperative CT, renal artery coverage by graft causes greater morbidity. In our experience, this has occurred twice in 199 cases; both cases required conversion to open repair and subsequent hemodialysis.[58, 59]

The occurrence of a postimplantation syndrome, manifest by spontaneously resolving pyrexia of unknown origin, is reported sporadically after endoluminal repair in up to 56% of cases.[41] It has been suggested that the mechanism of this event is immune system activation by prosthesis components, disturbed aneurysm thrombus, or transient visceral ischemia. Although one author has shown that endoluminal repair increases circulating tumor necrosis factor compared with conventional repair, others have reported lesser immune activation after endoluminal repair.[61, 62] Visceral ischemia is not more prevalent in any endoluminal series, and at least one group has shown that rectal mucosa is rendered less ischemic by endovascular vs. open aneurysm repair.[62]

Repeated instrumentation of the iliac arteries and aneurysm sac may increase the risk of peripheral embolization during endovascular repair; however, this also has not been proven by experience. Embolic events requiring reoperation are reported by the three largest endovascular series report to be nearly equal to the 3.3% incidence noted in the Canadian Aneurysm Study of 666 conventional repairs.[61] It is unclear whether iatrogenic femoral or iliac artery injury or acute distal limb ischemia are significantly increased by endovascular repair. In our experience, up to 12% of endovascular patients have required immediate or delayed intervention for ischemia or vessel injury, although others have reported this incidence to be as low as 2.6%, roughly equivalent to open repair.[41, 58, 61]

ENDOLEAK

Endoleak is defined as persistent blood flow outside an endovascular graft but within an aneurysm sac. This commonly is described as *primary*, if it arises at the time of graft implant, or *secondary* when arising

Table 31–7. Endovascular vs. Open Abdominal Aortic Aneurysm (AAA) Repair: Large Series Results

	Endovascular			Open
	Sydney[58] (n = 190)	AneuRx[56] (n = 190)	Blum[41] (n = 154)	Canadian Aneurysm Study[61] (n = 666)
30-day mortality	8 (4.2%)	5 (2.6%)	1 (0.6%)	5.4%
Renal failure*	7 (3.6%)	0	2 (1.3%)	0.6%
Wound complication†	1 (0.5%)	1 (0.5%)	3 (2%)	2%
Embolization†	—	0	4 (2.6%)	3.5%
Femoral/iliac injury/distal ischemia†	24 (12.6%)	10 (5.2%)	4 (2.6%)	3.5%

Blanks indicate complication(s) not specifically reported.
*Requiring temporary or permanent dialysis.
†Requiring concurrent or subsequent operative intervention.

in a delayed fashion. Primary or early endoleak results from errors of judgment in case or device selection or errors of technique. Secondary or late endoleak results from device failure or a loss of attachment to a dilating proximal or distal neck.

We have suggested a classification system for endoleak that is based on the source of leakage but also has prognostic significance[63, 64] (Table 31–8).

Type I Endoleak: Perigraft Endoleak or Graft-Related Endoleak

This occurs when a persistent perigraft channel of blood flow develops because of inadequate or ineffective seal at the graft ends (at the proximal or distal graft aspects) or "attachment zones."

Type II Endoleak: Retrograde Endoleak or Nongraft-Related Endoleak

This occurs when there is persistent collateral blood flow into the aneurysm sac flowing retrogradely from patent lumbar arteries, the inferior mesenteric artery, or other collateral vessels. In this case, there is a complete seal around the graft attachment zones so that the complication is not related directly to the graft itself.

Type III Endoleak: Fabric Tear or Modular Disconnection

Endoleak at the midgraft region may be the result of leakage through a defect in the graft fabric or between the segments of a modular, multisegment graft. This subgroup of endoleak essentially is caused by mechanical failure of the graft, secondary to early component defect or late material fatigue. Some cases may be associated with the effects of hemodynamic forces or changes in aneurysm morphology with shrinkage.

Type IV Endoleak: Graft Porosity

Type IV endoleak is any minor blush of contrast on completion angiogram or subsequent contrast studies, which is presumed to be emanating from blood diffusion across the pores of a highly porous graft fabric or perhaps through the small holes in the graft fabric caused by sutures, stent struts, and so forth. This is usually an intentional design feature rather than a form of device failure. In practice, differentiation of type IV endoleak from type III often proves very difficult and may require postoperative, directed angiography. As yet, the long-term effects of type IV endoleak are unknown.

Endoleaks: Undefined Origin

In many cases, the precise source of endoleak is not be clear from routine follow-up imaging studies, and further investigation may be required. In this situation, it may be appropriate to classify the condition as "endoleak, undefined origin" until the type of endoleak is defined by further studies.

Non-Endoleak Aneurysm Sac Pressurization: Endotension

In these cases, no endoleak is demonstrated on imaging studies, but pressure within the aneurysm sac is elevated and may be very close to systemic pressure.[64] The seal is formed by semiliquid thrombus, and the pressure in the sac is similar to pressures measured in endoleak. The aneurysm often is clinically pulsatile, and wall pulsatility also may be detected and monitored by specialized ultrasound techniques.[65]

In clinical practice, we have learned that high pressure may be maintained within the AAA sac with no evidence of "leak" or blood flow outside the graft in cases in which a rim of thrombus is interposed between the sac contents and the aortic lumen. We have observed this in three patients in whom the proximal stent slipped distally within the proximal aneurysm neck; the aneurysm became pulsatile once more and was enlarging on progress CT scans, but no contrast media was detected outside of the graft (unpublished data, 1998). This condition, which some have referred to as "endopressure," "pressure leak," or "endotension," does not fit conveniently into the definition of endoleak but obviously is closely associated and probably represents an intermediate state. We believe, therefore, that this condition should be recognized as a related group ("non-endoleak aneurysm sac pressurization").

Although all endoleaks can be associated with aneurysm enlargement (and eventual rupture), this has been encountered most frequently with those that are communicating directly with aortic lumen (types I and III).[37, 63–65] "Noncommunicating" endoleaks also

Table 31–8. Endoleak Classification and Causes[62, 63]

Type I	Graft dislodgment or ineffective seal to normal artery above and below an aneurysm
Type II	Retrograde perfusion of branch vessels of an aneurysm sac
Type III	Perfusion through porous graft fabric
Type IV	Graft fabric degeneration or tear during implant

can occur, arising through retrograde perfusion of lumbar arteries or a patent inferior mesenteric artery. Lumbar endoleaks frequently are fed through collateral branches of either hypogastric artery. In these cases, selective coil embolization of the feeding branch can obliterate aneurysm sac flow and prevent aneurysm expansion.

Persistence of any endoleak beyond 3 to 6 months mandates selective aortic and iliac angiography to localize its source. Secondary treatment is required for any endoleak that is accompanied by aneurysm enlargement. For communicating endoleaks, this may require placement of additional endovascular graft(s) or conversion to open repair. In contrast to noncommunicating leaks, coil embolization of communicating endoleaks may not prevent further aneurysm growth. Experimental evidence demonstrates that aneurysm sac pressure remains high with this type of endoleak, despite apparent radiologic sealing.[49] Somewhat similarly, any patient who experiences aneurysm enlargement without evidence of endoleak should be considered to have endotension or an occult leak because this situation has been associated with aneurysm rupture.[47]

DEVICE FAILURE

The endoluminal method of AAA repair has drawn attention to the changes in morphology of the aorta and iliac arteries that accompany increasing size of the aneurysm. Aneurysms increase in size longitudinally in addition to transverse expansion. This increase in longitudinal expansion is accommodated by a corresponding increase in tortuosity of the aorta and iliac arteries. It has long been recognized that iliac tortuosity has important implications for gaining access to the aorta for an endograft. Tortuosity in the proximal neck of the aneurysm may lead to migration and endoleak if the neck is short as well as tortuous.

The changes in morphology that accompany successful endoluminal repair have been recognized since 1995 and reported by a number of groups.[44, 45, 66–68] These include a reduction in the maximum transverse diameter of the aneurysm and an increase in diameter of the proximal neck of approximately 10%. In addition to contrast-enhanced CT demonstrating exclusion of the aneurysm sac from the general circulation, one important criterion of successful endoluminal repair is a reduction in maximum transverse diameter of the aneurysm.

A phenomenon that has been recognized only in the past 2 years is distortion in prostheses after endoluminal AAA repair. This may involve changes in shape and position and occurs most commonly in the form of kinking in the limbs of bifurcated prostheses at their junction with the trunk, but it also may occur in tube endografts. These structural changes

may lead to thrombosis of graft limbs or result in either dislocation of component parts of a modular prosthesis or dislocation of the limbs of an endograft from the native common iliac arteries. Both forms of dislocation result inevitably in endoleak.

The possible causes of kinking distortion are:

1. Increase in length of the prosthesis after deployment;
2. Reduction in the length of the aneurysm sac; and
3. Migration of the prosthesis from the proximal or distal anchoring sites in the native arteries.

In a recent study, we demonstrated that two commonly used self-expanding prostheses frequently lose up to 15% of their length during deployment.[69] This may be an inherent property of the self-expanding stent framework of the devices, exacerbated by longitudinal pushing forces applied to the graft during deployment, resulting in an "accordion" effect. Harris and colleagues[12] noted a similar shortening from the listed length in 15 of 16 patients (21.5 mm mean). Such foreshortening of prostheses during deployment raises the question of subsequent re-expansion to the original length, resulting in graft kinking. Direct evidence for this, however, is lacking, but three explants with severe deformity reported by Umscheid and Stelter[70] were found to be the same length as the packaged specifications. They concluded that increase in length of the prostheses could not, therefore, be responsible for kinking. It could be argued, however, that because many prostheses deploy in a foreshortened state, the observations of Umscheid and Stelter may have represented re-expansion back to the original length with resulting distortion.

Harris and colleagues present convincing data on the relationship between longitudinal shortening of AAA and kinking.[12] Migration of the prosthesis from the proximal or distal anchoring sites in the native arteries is the third possibility in explaining the etiology of kinking distortion. Such dislocation, however, might be the result of kinking rather than the cause of it. At this stage of our knowledge concerning the late effects of endografting, it would appear that all three possible causes of kinking may contribute to this problem, but that longitudinal foreshortening of the aneurysm sac is probably the major factor.

In addition to distortion, endoluminal prostheses are at risk of structural deterioration. This may involve fatigue fracture in the metal frame, disintegration of sutures holding the metal frame together or attaching the stents to the fabric, and fabric deterioration ranging from small defects to disintegration of the graft. These forms of structural deterioration may lead to graft distortion and failure. It seems very likely that the incidence of such material fatigue increases with time.

Management of Failures

Accumulating experience shows that secondary interventions are required to achieve successful outcome for a significant proportion of endovascular aneurysm repair cases. These secondary interventions may be required either in the perioperative 30-day interval or at any time during long-term follow-up. We evaluated the incidence and type of interventions required for the management of late complications in a series of consecutive patients undergoing endoluminal grafting of AAA with a range of devices.[71]

Data regarding the occurrence of late complications requiring reintervention were recorded prospectively for the initial 230 consecutive AAA cases done over a 6-year period, including balloon-expanded (BE; n = 97) and self-expanding (SE; n = 133) endovascular graft devices. Complications or cases of device failure that required radiologic, endovascular, or open surgical revision were documented.

Delayed endoleak has occurred to date in 27 of the 230 cases (12%), and other complications requiring intervention have occurred in 14 patients (6%).[71] The etiology of late endoleak was type I in 15, type II in 4, type III in 5, endotension in 2, and endoleak of unknown etiology in 1. Interventions were percutaneous (coil embolization; n = 4), repeat or supplementary transluminal graft procedure (n = 14), or conversion to open repair (n = 10, including 4 patients who had ruptured AAAs that resulted from untreated late endoleak). Late endoleak (predominantly type I) occurred more frequently in tube graft cases vs. other graft configurations. With bifurcated grafts, modular device limb disconnection (type III) was the most frequent cause of late endoleak. Embolization was used only for type II endoleak and was successful in all four cases. Repeat endografts were successful in 12 of 14 cases (86%). There were no perioperative deaths associated with reinterventions for late endoleak. The other reasons for late interventions were: graft limb occlusion (n = 6), graft limb stenosis (n=5), and non-endoleak pressurization of the sac (endotension n = 3). Late femorofemoral crossover grafts had a high incidence of wound complications.

This study has shown a relatively high incidence (18%) of late complications requiring reintervention within a few years after endovascular repair with first- and second-generation designs of endoluminal grafts. Most were corrected by endovascular transluminal techniques. These findings have important implications for patient follow-up and case selection. Patients undergoing successful endovascular repair should be informed that late secondary procedures may be required.

There also has been concern about late device failure. Continuing successful exclusion of the aneurysm sac from the circulation is dependent on the availability of permanent radial force in the prosthesis to maintain a seal between the prosthesis and the normal aortic wall or between component parts of a modular prosthesis. The evidence to date demonstrates a small but steady attrition rate because of this problem. Rapid changes have taken place over the past 6 years since the first report of the technique being used in the clinical setting. First-generation unsupported balloon-expandable devices requiring large-caliber introducing sheaths have been replaced with second-generation self-expanding devices with metallic support throughout, which can be delivered through small-caliber sheaths. These changes need to be taken into account when interpreting the data. It also should be noted that although concurrent trials with endoluminal and open repair of AAA have been carried out, no randomized trials have been reported.

Currently, endoluminal repair may be summarized as being as safe as open repair but having a higher early and late failure rate, which is compensated for by decreased blood loss, requirement for intensive care, and reduced length of hospital stay.

SURGICAL REPAIR OF ABDOMINAL AORTIC ANEURYSMS

Patients who have aneurysms deemed suitable for elective conventional surgical repair require careful workup before surgery. Almost all patients will have had ultrasound evaluation and most will have had CT scanning, with or without angiography, to evaluate the possibility of endovascular repair (Fig. 31–17). The predominant cause of perioperative morbidity and mortality in elective aneurysm repair is cardiovascular; the incidence of overt and covert myocardial infarct has been stated to be as high as 15%. Every effort therefore should be made to ensure that the patient is reasonably fit for major surgery. Cardiac assessment may be performed by echocardiogram and radioisotope studies to assess ventricular function and ejection fraction. Unfortunately, a good ejection fraction does not always mean that the cardiac status is satisfactory; patients with main stem stenosis may not be recognized. Alternative strategies such as routine coronary angiography are excessively invasive, expensive, and can pick up clinical insignificant disease. Hence, there is always some cardiac risk with aneurysm repair. When extensive cardiac disease is found, a careful decision is required about the merits of performing surgery at all, doing preliminary cardiac revascularization (as often is carried out in North America) or proceeding with AAA repair.

Formal routine respiratory assessment other than chest radiograph is not necessary unless there is a history of dyspnea or there are clear physical signs. A mild degree of pulmonary dysfunction is common

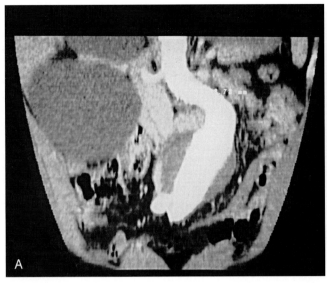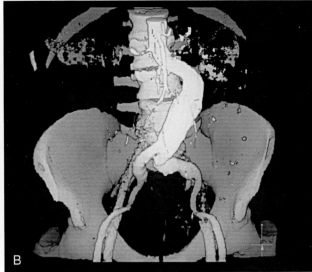

Figure 31–17. *A,* Oblique multiplanar reconstruction (MPR) from spiral CT examination. Accurate measurements can be made in multiple planes for sizing of the device. *B,* Three-dimensional (3-D) CT reconstruction allows appreciation of the topography of the aneurysms and iliac vessels before repair.

in this age group, who often have a significant smoking history. Renal dysfunction generally is reflected only by routine serum urea and creatinine levels, which are insensitive indices of early renal failure. Because there is a much higher morbidity with renal compromise, any doubt about the status should be evaluated carefully with 24-hour clearance and renal isotope scans and arteriography where relevant.

Anesthesia

Most patients are managed best with a general anesthetic, although there is an increasing trend to use adjuvant epidural blockade, which may potentially modulate the major pressure and fluid changes seen at clamping and declamping as well as protect bowel function and provide postoperative pain relief. Hard evidence for the efficacy of this approach still is lacking, although epidural blockade also may reduce the incidence of myocardial events. The use of beta blockade also has been shown to be of benefit in aortic surgery in terms of reduced cardiac morbidity and probably should be employed routinely if there are no contraindications.

Current opinion appears to favor the use of preoperative hemodilution, principally normovolemic. This requires that blood is removed and replaced with a plasma expander until the hematocrit is less than 30. This blood is then available for retransfusion at the end of the procedure and in most cases may obviate the need for autologous transfusion. Increased awareness of patients concerning hepatitis, human immunodeficiency virus (HIV), and Jakob-Creutzfeldt disease has highlighted the need to avoid transfusion when at all possible. Adjuvant methodologies to pre-serve blood loss, such as intraoperative cell savers, also help to reduce transfusion requirements.

The operative procedure for elective and emergency repair are covered in standard texts.[50, 51]

Postoperative Recovery

There is considerable evidence that most elective aneurysm patients may be managed optimally in a high dependancy unit (HDU) for 48 hours without the need for using expensive ICU resources. Predominantly, patients require monitoring of their blood pressure, urine output, pulse, electrocardiogram (ECG), oxygen (O_2) saturation, and fluid balance as well as management of any epidural analgesia. All these are performed easily in the HDU. This implies that patients are extubated immediately postoperatively, and again, there is good evidence that this is the optimal management for uncomplicated aortic surgery.

One of the main difficulties with any major surgery is the onset of hypothermia, but this is now well recognized and patients are kept warm in the operating room and postoperatively by means of heated blankets and warmed intravenous fluids. All patients require postoperative serum urea and electrolytes and a full blood count to be performed on the day of surgery, and blood transfusion should be started if the patients hemoglobin falls below the agreed trigger point (usually 9–10 g per 100 ml). Most patients may begin sitting on the first postoperative day and will be able to take a few steps around their bed, especially if adequate analgesia is provided. More aggressive mobilization is continued on the second and subsequent postoperative days.

Chest physiotherapy should be routinely performed postoperatively to ensure good ventilation and reduce the risk of infection. Subcutaneous heparin is continued throughout the postoperative period to reduce the risk of deep vein thrombosis (DVT). Epidural catheters usually are removed after 48 or 72 hours and replaced by oral analgesia or patient-controlled analgesia (PCA). Oral fluids usually can be started slowly after 24 hours and gradually increased with a corresponding reduction in intravenous fluids. Oral food can be started as soon as there is evidence of returning bowel function because this appears to improve the integrity of the intestinal mucosa and reduce bacterial translocation.

Transfer to the regular ward is possible in most cases by day 2 or 3, and patients are returned to full mobilization according to their ability. Discharge is usually possible between 7 and 12 days postoperatively. Patients are rarely back to their full health and ability before 3 months and should be warned of this in advance so they do not become too depressed.

Complications

The complications of open abdominal aortic surgery may be divided into those complications that may occur after any major surgery and those complications that are peculiar to aortic surgery. By far the most important complications relate to the heart because up to 10% of patients undergoing aortic surgery may suffer a myocardial infarct either overtly or subclinically. In addition, there can be further morbidity from arrhythmias. Cardiac complications may be reduced, but not eliminated, by careful attention to preoperative assessment and perioperative monitoring, keeping blood loss to a minimum and the use of beta blockade and epidural analgesia. The judicious use of postoperative fluids is also critical; hypotension may occur with underhydration, especially with sympathetic blockade secondary to epidural anesthesia. Overenthusiastic hydration conversely may push the patient into cardiac strain and later failure. Hence, careful balancing of fluid and electrolyte requirements is essential in the first 48 hours.

Respiratory complications are also common partly because these patients invariably are smokers and partly because open aortic surgery involves a major abdominal incision and prolonged general anesthesia with subsequent reduction in ventilation. These complications are clearly more likely in patients who have underlying pre-existing respiratory disease.

Outcome

The overall mortality for conventional, open aortic surgery varies widely according to known concurrent disease and associated factors. The mortality rate range for elective surgery may be anything from 1% to as much as 20%, although generally it is in the range of 2% to 10%. Perioperative mortality also varies according to what is classified as "elective" surgery. It is clear that there is a major difference between the results of surgery for patients coming off a waiting list (who are presumably well evaluated) and patients who are admitted acutely with nonruptured aneurysms. These patients have an increased risk of perhaps three to five times that of a pure elective case. Ruptured aneurysms have an in-hospital mortality rate of between 30% and 90%, depending largely on the availability of a vascular specialty service. Among the most important adverse factors are age, underlying ischemic heart disease, renal disease, and respiratory compromise, and it is no coincidence that these entities are also the most common complications of aortic surgery.

The selection of poor candidates for surgery probably has more influence on perioperative results than difficulties with the actual surgery undertaken, although the experience of the individual unit and the caseload also play a major part. Hence, the most benefit to be gained is in the perioperative assessment and selection of patients. Clearly, it is equally important not to deny surgery to someone who manifestly requires intervention, if at all possible; however, in some instances, there is every likelihood that the patient could be regarded as too high a risk for elective surgery. This should not necessarily prevent the unfit patient from undergoing emergency repair for aortic rupture at some future point because without surgery at this point he or she will certainly die, in contrast to the elective scenario. At present, the role of EVAR also should be judged against the fitness of the patient. Otherwise, many unfit patients may undergo EVAR who subsequently would have died of causes other than their aneurysm.

Despite this, in appropriate patients, open surgery conveys a major survival benefit coupled with a demonstrable improvement in the quality of life. In addition, there is evidence that survivors of aortic aneurysm surgery have a life expectancy equivalent to a healthy age-matched population. The cost of open repair compares very favorably with EVAR at present. The U.K. small aneurysm trial[1] estimated the average cost to be $7500 per case. This was considerably more than surveillance in the trial ($6000, which included those cases that later required surgery). The cost of EVAR is considerable at present and the need for regular CT scanning postoperatively adds a significant extra charge. Hence, it is extremely important to demonstrate that EVAR has long-term robustness and that it will be cost-effective, or at least cost-neutral, in the future.

Conclusions

Conventional aortic aneurysm surgery is a major procedure that carries a significant operative mortality and morbidity. Despite this, excellent results can be obtained in major centers with a team approach. Importantly, it is a procedure that will last the patient's remaining lifetime in most cases. As elective aortic aneurysm repair is a procedure that is performed primarily to improve long-term survival, any intervention must satisfy the test of durability. Therefore, the gold standard for the management of aortic aneurysms greater than 5.5 cm in diameter currently is still open, conventional repair. The success or otherwise of alternative intervention strategies such as endovascular aneurysm repair must be judged against this standard. Critically, the U.K. small aneurysm study[1] has demonstrated the relative uselessness of performing open surgery in asymptomatic aneurysms smaller than 5.5 cm, and the same most likely can be held true for endovascular repair of these smaller aneurysms.

The future may well see improvements in the applicability and durability of endovascular repair for aortic aneurysms; however, it is likely that pharmaceutical manipulation of patients at risk will become increasingly important in conjunction with adequate screening programs to pick up early aneurysms. Such therapies may include the inhibition of matrix metalloproteinases (MMPs) or alternative methods for the preservation of the collagen infrastructure in the aorta. For the present, many elective and most ruptured aneurysms will continue to be treated by conventional, open surgery. It nonetheless will become increasingly important to document an individual unit's results for surgery and to fall within acceptable ranges for operative mortality in these cases. It is becoming increasingly unacceptable for surgeons to do the "occasional" elective aortic aneurysm, and this may mean that aortic surgery will become limited to major vascular centers with adequate resources and expertise.

REFERENCES

1. The UK Small Aneurysm Trial Participants: Mortality results for randomized controlled trial of early elective surgery or ultrasonographic surveillance for small abdominal aneurysms. Lancet 352:1649–1655, 1998.
2. Galland RB, Whitely MS, Magee TR: Fate of patients undergoing surveillance of small abdominal aortic aneurysms. Eur J Vasc Endovasc Surg 16:104–109, 1998.
3. Johnstone KW, Rutherford RB, Tilson MD, et al: Suggested standards for reporting on arterial aneurysms. J Vasc Surg 13:444–450, 1991.
4. Parodi JC, Palmaz JC, Barone HD: Transfemoral intraluminal graft implantation for abdominal aortic aneurysms. Ann Vasc Surg 5:491–496, 1991.
5. Harris PL, Buth J, Miahle C, et al: The need for clinical trials of endovascular abdominal aortic stent-graft repair: The Eurostar project. J Endovasc Surg 4:491, 1997.
6. The Vascular Surgical Society of Great Britain and Ireland and the British Society of Interventional Radiology: Annual report on the registry of endovascular treatment of aortic aneurysms (RETA): 1997 and 1998.
7. White GH, Yu W, May J, et al: Endoleak as a complication of endoluminal grafting of abdominal aortic aneurysms. J Endovasc Surg 4:152, 1997.
8. Wain RA, Marin ML, Ohki T, et al: Endoleaks after endovascular graft treatment of aortic aneurysms: Classification, risk factors and outcome. J Vasc Surg 27:69, 1998.
9. Blum U, Voshage G, Beyersdorf F: Two centre German experience with aortic endografting. J Endovasc Surg 4:137, 1997.
10. Harris PL: Aneurysms of the abdominal aorta: Results of endoluminal repair. J Cardiovasc Surg 39(suppl):23, 1998.
11. Norgren L, Jernby B, Engellau L: Aortoenteric fistula caused by a ruptured stent-graft: A case report. J Endovasc Surg 5:269, 1998.
12. Harris PL, Brennan J, Martin J, et al: Longitudinal shrinkage following endovascular aneurysm repair: A source of intermediate and late complications. J Endovasc Surg 6:4, 1999.
13. Lumsden AB, Allen RC, Chaikof EL: Delayed rupture of aortic aneurysms following endovascular stent grafting. Am J Surg 170:174, 1995.
14. Schurink GWH, Aarts NJM, Wilde J, et al: Endoleakage after stent-graft treatment of abdominal aortic aneurysm: Implications on pressure and imaging—an in vitro study. J Vasc Surg 28:234, 1998.
15. Faries PL, Sanchez LA, Marin ML, et al: An experimental model for the acute and chronic evaluation on intra-aneurysmal pressure. J Endovasc Surg 4:290, 1997.
16. Woodburn KR, May J, White GH: Endoluminal aortic aneurysm surgery. Br J Surg 85:435–443, 1998.
17. Yusuf SW, Baker DM, Chuter TAM, et al: Transfemoral endoluminal repair of abdominal aortic aneurysm with bifurcated graft. Lancet 344:650–651, 1994.
18. Armon MP, Yusuf SW, Lateif K, et al: The anatomical suitability of abdominal aortic aneurysms for endovascular repair. Br J Surg 84:178–180, 1997.
19. Yusuf SW, Whitaker SC, Chuter TAM, et al: Early results of endovascular abdominal aortic aneurysm repair with aorto uni-iliac graft and femoro-femoral bypass. J Vasc Surg 25:165–172, 1997.
20. MacSweeney STR, Lawrence-Brown MM, Hartley D, Sineuarine K: The Zenith™ (Perth) system. In SW Yusuf, M Marin, K Ivancev, BR Hopkinson (eds): Operative Atlas of Endovascular Aneurysm Surgery. Oxford, ISIS Medical Media (In press).
21. Armon MP, Yusuf SW, Whitaker SC, et al: Influence of abdominal aortic aneurysm size on the feasibility of endovascular repair. J Endovasc Surg 4:279–283, 1997.
22. Baxendale B, Baker DM, Hutchinson A, et al: Haemodynamic and metabolic changes during endovascular stent insertion for repair of infra-renal aortic aneurysms. Br J Anaesth 77:581–585, 1996.
23. Baker DM, Wenham PW: Renal damage. In Hopkinson BR, Yusuf SW, Whitaker SC, Veith FJ (eds): Endovascular Surgery for Aortic Aneurysms. London, WB Saunders, 1997, p 254–263.
24. ElMarasy N, Yusuf SW, Lonsdale RJ, et al: Study on the effect of endovascular repair on colonic perfusion (abstract). J Endovasc Surg 3:95, 1996.
25. Thompson MM, Nasim A, Sayers RD, et al: Oxygen free radical and cytokine generation during endovascular and conventional aneurysm repair. Eur J Vasc Endovasc Surg 12:70–75, 1996.
26. Jones A, Cahill D, Gardham R: Outcome in patients with a large abdominal aortic aneurysm considered unfit for surgery. Br J Surg 85:1382–1384, 1998.
27. Greenhalgh RM: Prognosis of abdominal aortic aneurysm. BMJ 301:136, 1995.
28. Yusuf SW, Whitaker SC, Chuter TAM, et al: Emergency endovascular abdominal aortic aneurysm repair (letter). Lancet 344:1645, 1994.
29. Yusuf SW, Hopkinson BR: It is feasible to treat contained abdominal aortic aneurysm rupture by stent graft combination. In Greenhalgh RM (ed): Indications in Vascular and Endovascular Surgery. London, WB Saunders, 1998, pp 153–165.
30. Whitaker SC: Pre-operative imaging. In Hopkinson BR, Yusuf SW, Whitaker SC, Veith FJ (eds): Endovascular Surgery for

Aortic Aneurysms. London, WB Saunders, Company, 1997, pp 17–39.

31. Fillinger MF, Robbie PJ, McKenna MA, et al: The "virtual graft": Pre-operative simulation of endovascular grafts using spiral CT with interactive three-dimensional reconstructions (abstract). J Endovasc Surg 4(suppl 1):1–10, 1997.

32. Ernst CB: Current therapy of infrarenal aortic aneurysms. N Engl J Med 336:59, 1997.

33. Parodi JC, Palmaz JC, Barone HD: Transfemoral intraluminal graft implantation for abdominal aortic aneurysms. Ann Vasc Surg 5:491, 1991.

34. White GH, Yu W, May J, et al: A new nonstented balloon-expandable graft for straight or bifurcated endoluminal bypass. J Endovasc Surg 1:16, 1994.

35. May J, White GH, Yu W, et al: Endoluminal grafting of abdominal aortic aneurysms: Causes of failure and their prevention. J Endovasc Surg 1:44, 1994.

36. Dake M, Miller C, Semba CP, et al: Transluminal placement of endovascular stent-grafts for the treatment of descending thoracic aortic aneurysms. N Engl J Med 331:1729, 1994.

37. Parodi JC: Endovascular repair of abdominal aortic aneurysms and other arterial lesions. J Vasc Surg 21:549, 1995.

38. Chuter TAM, Risberg B, Hopkinson BR, et al: Clinical experience with a bifurcated endovascular graft for abdominal aortic aneurysms repair. J Vasc Surg 24:655, 1996.

39. Moore WS, Rutherford RB, for the EVT Investigators: Transfemoral endovascular repair of abdominal aortic aneurysm: Results of the North America EVT phase 1 trial. J Vasc Surg 23:543, 1996.

40. Balm R, Eikelboom BC, May J, et al: Early experience with transfemoral endovascular aneurysm management (TEAM) in the treatment of aortic aneurysms. Eur J Endovasc Surg 11:214, 1996.

41. Blum U, Voshage G, Lammer J, et al: Endoluminal treatment of infrarenal aortic aneurysms with stent-grafts. N Engl J Med 336:13, 1997.

42. Machan L, Fry P: Abdominal aortic aneurysm repair using the World Medical Talent prosthesis. Tech Vasc intervent Radiol 1:25, 1998.

43. Brewster DC, Geller SC, Kaufman JA, et al: Initial experience with endovascular aneurysm repair: Comparison of early results with outcome of conventional repair. J Vasc Surg 27:992, 1998.

44. Matsumara JS, Pearce WH, McCarthy WJ, et al: Reduction in aortic aneurysm size: Early results after endovascular graft placement. J Vasc Surg 25:113, 1997.

45. May J, White G, Yu W, et al: A prospective study of anatomico-pathological changes in abdominal aortic aneurysms following endoluminal repair: Is the aneurysmal process reversed? Eur J Vasc Endovasc Surg 12:11, 1996.

46. Alimi YS, Chakfe N, Rivoal E, et al: Rupture of an abdominal aortic aneurysm after endovascular graft placement and aneurysm size reduction. J Vasc Surg 28:178, 1998.

47. Torsello GB, Klenck E, Kasprzak B, Umscheid T: Rupture of abdominal aortic aneurysm previously treated by endovascular stentgraft. J Vasc Surg 28:184, 1998.

48. Matsumara JS, Moore WS, for the Endovascular Technologies Investigators: Clinical consequences of periprosthetic leak after endovascular repair of abdominal aortic aneurysms. J Vasc Surg 27:606, 1998.

49. Marty B, Sanchez LA, Ohki T, et al: Endoleak after endovascular graft repair of experimental aortic aneurysms: Does coil embolization with angiographic "seal" lower intraaneurysmal pressure? J Vasc Surg 27:454, 1998.

50. Killen DA, Reed WA, Gorton ME, et al: 25-Year trends in resection of abdominal aortic aneurysms. Ann Vasc Surg 12:436–444, 1998.

51. Dardik A, Burleyson GP, Bowman H, et al: Surgical repair of ruptured abdominal aortic aneurysms in the state of Maryland: Factors influencing outcome among 527 recent cases. J Vasc Surg 28:413–421, 1998.

52. May J, White GH, Yu W, et al: Focus on the proximal neck: The key to durability of endoluminal AAA repair. J Endovasc Surg 4(Suppl 1):I–27, 1997.

53. Gadowski GR, Pilcher DB, Ricci MA: Abdominal aortic aneurysm expansion rate: Effect of size and beta-adrenergic blockade. J Vasc Surg 19:727–731, 1994.

54. May J, White GH, Yu W, et al: Concurrent comparison of endoluminal repair versus no treatment for small abdominal aortic aneurysms. Eur J Vasc Endovasc Surg 13:472–476, 1997.

55. Johnston KW: Nonruptured abdominal aortic aneurysm: Six-year follow-up results from the multicentre prospective Canadian aneurysm study. Canadian Society for Vascular Surgery Aneurysm Study Group. J Vasc Surg 20:163–170, 1995.

56. Zarins CK, White RA, Schwarten D, et al: AneuRx stent graft versus open surgical repair of abdominal aortic aneurysms: Multicenter prospective clinical rial. J Vasc Surg 29:292–308, 1999.

57. Katz DJ, Stanley JC, Zelenock JB: Operative mortality rates for intact and ruptured abdominal aortic aneurysms in Michigan: An eleven-year statewide experience. J Vasc Surg 19:804–817, 1994.

58. May J, White GH, Waugh R, et al: Adverse effects after endoluminal repair of abdominal aortic aneurysms: A comparison during two successive periods of time. J Vasc Surg 29:32–39, 1999.

59. May J, White GH, Yu W, et al: Concurrent comparison of endoluminal versus open repair in the treatment of abdominal aortic aneurysms: Analysis of 303 patients by life table method. J Vasc Surg 27:213–221, 1998.

60. May J, White GH, Yu W, et al: Conversion from endoluminal to open repair of abdominal aortic aneurysms: A hazardous procedure. Eur J Vasc Endovasc Surg 14:4–11, 1997.

61. Johnston KW: Multicenter prospective study of nonruptured abdominal aortic aneurysm: Part II. Variables predicting morbidity and mortality. J Vasc Surg 9:437–447, 1989.

62. Syk I, Brunkwall J, Ivancev K, et al: Postoperative fever, bowel ischaemia and cytokine response to abdominal aortic aneurysm repair—A comparison between endovascular and open surgery. Eur J Vasc Endovasc Surg 15:398–405, 1998.

63. White GH, May J, Waugh RC, Yu W: Type I and type II endoleaks: A more useful classification for reporting results of endoluminal AAA repair. J Endovasc Surg 5:189–191, 1998.

64. White GH, May J, Waugh RC, et al: Type III and type IV endoleak: Toward a complete definition of blood flow in the sac after endoluminal AAA repair. J Endovasc Surg 5:305–309, 1998.

65. Malina M, Lanne T, Ivancev K, et al: Reduced pulsatile wall motion of abdominal aortic aneurysms after endovascular repair. J Vasc Surg 27:624–631, 1998.

66. May J, White GH, Yu W, et al: A prospective study of changes in morphology and dimensions of abdominal aortic aneurysms following endoluminal repair: A preliminary report. J Endovasc Surg 2:343–347, 1995.

67. Malina M, Ivancev K, Chuter TAM, et al: Changing aneurysmal morphology after endovascular grafting: Relation to leakage or persistent perfusion. J Endovasc Surg 4:23–30, 1997.

68. Broeders IAMJ, Blankensteijn JD, Gvakharia A, et al: The efficacy of transfemoral endovascular aneurysm management: A study on size changes of the abdominal aorta during mid-term follow-up. Eur J Vasc Endovasc Surg 14:84–90, 1997.

69. White GH, May J, Waugh R, et al: Shortening of endografts during deployment in endovascular AAA repair. J Endovasc Surg 6:4–10, 1999.

70. Umscheid T, Stelter WJ: Time-related alterations in shape, position and structure of self-expanding, modular aortic stent-grafts: A 4-year single-center follow-up. J Endovasc Surg 6:17–32, 1999.

71. White GH, May J, Waugh RC, et al: Secondary radiological interventions and endovascular graft revision procedures after AAA endografting (abstract). J Endovasc Surg 6:121, 1999.

Endovascular Repair of Thoracic and Dissecting Aneurysms and Aortic Coarctation

Endovascular Contributors: Stephen T. Kee, Michael D. Dake, and Alex J. Paddon *(Endovascular Treatment of Coarctation of the Aorta)*
Surgical Contributors: Jeffrey C. Milliken and Dan L. Serna

THORACIC AORTIC ANEURYSMS

Clinical Problem

Thoracic aortic aneurysm is a relatively uncommon life-threatening condition caused by weakness within the media of the vessel.[1] The damage of the medial elastic layer of the vessel is usually caused by atherosclerosis; aortic dissection, trauma, and infection are less likely etiologies.[2] Thoracic aneurysms are usually asymptomatic, appearing as an unsuspected mass on a chest radiograph. When symptoms do occur, they are usually caused by compression of adjacent structures, dissection, or rupture. Twenty percent of patients with thoracic aortic aneurysm have aneurysms elsewhere, frequently affecting the abdominal aorta.[3]

Rupture of a thoracic aneurysm is catastrophic and almost uniformly fatal. Studies of the natural history of patients with untreated thoracic aneurysms estimate mortality rates of 50% after 5 years, and 70% after 10 years.[4] The 5-year survival rate is lower than that reported for patients with untreated abdominal aneurysms. Actual rupture of the aneurysm is responsible for almost half of the mortality rate; other causes of fatality are usually related to coexisting medical disease, particularly hypertension and cardiovascular disease. The most frequent site of a thoracic aortic aneurysm is in the descending aorta, although isolated aneurysmal involvement of the ascending aorta or transverse arch, or extension of the disease into the thoracoabdominal aorta, is not uncommon.

Conventional therapy for treatment of patients with thoracic aortic aneurysm is surgical repair.[3] Descending aneurysms are usually approached by a left thoracotomy, with surgical resection of the aneurysm and replacement with a segment of prosthetic graft material. Operative repair is indicated if an aneurysm is larger than 5 or 6 cm in diameter, and particularly if serial imaging studies show progressive enlargement. Surgery is also indicated in cases of aortic regurgita-

tion, or acute chest or back pain. For a patient with an isolated descending thoracic aortic aneurysm distal to the left subclavian artery, surgical resection can often be performed without the need for extracorporeal circulation. Elective operations by dedicated cardiothoracic surgeons have a surgical mortality rate approaching 10 to 15%.[5] The operative morbidity rate approaches 10%, with a significant incidence of paraplegia (5 to 10%) because of interruption of the intercostal arteries. In emergent cases, the surgical mortality rate approaches 50%.

Endoluminal placement of endovascular stent grafts offers an alternative method of treatment that is potentially less invasive, less expensive, and less hazardous than that of standard operative repair. The concept of treating patients with aortic aneurysms transluminally via stent grafts was introduced by Dotter in 1969.[6] Subsequently, several animal experiments were reported for the treatment of patients with abdominal aortic aneurysms with use of stent grafts.[7, 8] The first clinical case of aortic aneurysm repair with a stent graft was reported by Parodi in 1991.[9] Since then, the clinical feasibility of endovascular grafting for the treatment of patients with abdominal aortic aneurysm, subclavian artery aneurysm, arteriovenous fistula, or femoral occlusive disease has been well documented in the literature. Since 1992, 121 patients have undergone thoracic aneurysm repair in our institution with use of stent grafts. Our initial results would suggest that stent grafting is a safe and effective technique, with excellent short-term results and reduced morbidity as well as mortality comparable with that of surgical repair (Figs. 32–1 and 32–2).[10]

Indications for Treatment

Patients with thoracic aortic aneurysms caused by arteriosclerosis, trauma, dissection, infection, or previous surgery have been treated with endovascular techniques.[11] Patients with aneurysms secondary to

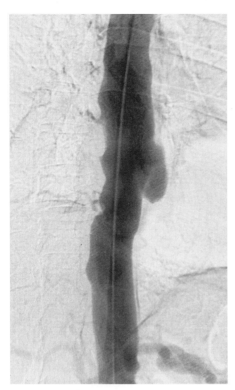

Figure 32–1. Descending thoracic aortogram showing a penetrating aortic ulcer with a pseudoaneurysm.

dissection will be discussed in a later section. All patients with aneurysms undergo preprocedural spiral computed tomography (CT) with three-dimensional reconstructions and thoracic aortography. The main anatomic considerations that need to be evaluated before placement of an endovascular device are the presence of adequate proximal and distal necks. The distance from the origin of the left subclavian artery to the proximal aspect of the aneurysm should be at least 2 cm. This distance allows adequate anchoring of the device and ensures that the stent graft is not inadvertently placed over the origin of the artery. If the aneurysm is adjacent to the left subclavian artery, a more favorable neck may be created by transposing the left subclavian artery onto the left common carotid artery before commencing the stent-graft procedure. To avoid branch vessel occlusion, the aneurysm should terminate between 2 and 3 cm proximal to the celiac axis. To limit exclusion of intercostal arteries, the overall length of the stent graft is kept to a minimum.

The diameters of the proximal and distal stent-graft necks are determined by spiral CT information. Overall stent-graft length is the result of a combination of CT reconstructions and thoracic aortography performed with use of a calibrated angiographic catheter.

While the thoracic aortogram is being recorded, the pelvic vasculature is also studied to evaluate the diameter and tortuosity of the vessel through which the stent graft will be delivered. Most thoracic aortic stent grafts require a sheath up to size 24-French (F) (8-mm) in internal diameter. In circumstances in which the diameter of the pelvic vasculature is insufficient to accommodate the required sheath, an alternative approach is required, such as a retroperitoneal iliac incision or aortic incision.

Selection of Devices for Treatment

In selecting a device to exclude a thoracic aortic aneurysm, a number of factors need to be taken into consideration. In addition to the diameter and overall length of the stent graft, the tortuosity of the thoracic aorta is also worthy of consideration. The initial thoracic aortic stent-graft work performed at Stanford University Hospital made use of modified Gianturco Z stents as the framework for the endoskeleton.[10]

Z stents are composed of 0.016-inch stainless steel wire, and each stent body is 2.5 cm in length, with variable diameters. The stent bodies are connected to each other with 2–0 polypropylene sutures, and the diameter of an individual stent can be adjusted by changing the length of the suture. The overall length is determined by the number of stent bodies sutured together, and the endoskeleton of Z stents supports the entire length of graft material. This acts as a frame

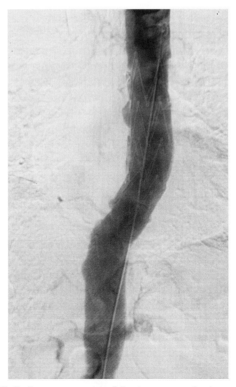

Figure 32–2. Repeat aortogram following stent-graft placement with exclusion of the aneurysm.

that prevents kinking, torsion, or collapse of the graft material. Although this design is innovative and provides a suitable means of exclusion of flow to most aneurysms, the Gianturco Z stents are relatively inflexible, and difficulty can be encountered when treating an aneurysm that involves a tortuous portion of the aorta. It is likely that more modern adaptations of the initial design will be more flexible. We do not put any anchoring devices, such as pins or hooks, on the stent-grafts but rely exclusively on the radial force and column strength of the stent structure to maintain the position of the device. Woven polyester is sutured to the stent at both ends, using multiple 5–0 polypropylene sutures. The entire device is gas-sterilized with an ethylene–oxide process before it is used.

Description of Technique

The stent-graft delivery system consists of four components: a teflon sheath with an external hemostatic valve, a tapered dilator, a loading cartridge, and a pusher mandrel. The size of the delivery sheath used for device introduction varies from a 20- to 24-F in outer diameter based on the required stent-graft dimension. The gradually tapered dilator and sheath are advanced over a stiff guide wire into the appropriate position proximal to the aneurysm. The stent graft is loaded into the delivery sheath via a cartridge, and the pusher mandrel is used to advance the stent graft from the cartridge to the sheath, and finally from the sheath to the thoracic aorta.

Stent-graft procedures are performed either in the surgical operating room (OR) or in an OR-compatible interventional radiology laboratory. General anesthesia is administered to the patient with endobronchial intubation. The patient is placed on the table in a shallow right decubitus position, and the thorax is prepped and draped as for a standard left thoracotomy. This is done to facilitate a rapid conversion to an open chest procedure, if necessary. The abdomen, pelvis, and groin of the patient are also draped for femoral, iliac, or retroperitoneal aortic access, depending on the preoperative pelvic arteriogram. The artery to be accessed, usually the right common femoral artery, is exposed by a surgical cutdown. After isolation of the artery, a standard needle puncture is performed, and a 5-F angiographic sheath is introduced. A 5-F pigtail catheter is introduced into the thoracic aorta to facilitate performance of an initial aortogram, which is obtained with the patient in a left anterior oblique position.

A high-quality fluoroscopic imaging system is essential for accurate placement of the stent graft. A modern portable C-arm unit may be used, but in the interventional radiology laboratory, a ceiling-mounted, high-resolution fluoroscopic unit with digi-

tal subtraction, playback, and roadmapping is required. The initial thoracic aortogram is replayed to identify the proximal and distal necks (Fig. 32–3). These are marked with external opaque markers or anatomic landmarks are used (road mapping) with guidance.

At this stage, the patient is aggressively anticoagulated with intravenous heparin (150 U per kg) to prevent ischemic complications in the limb that are associated with use of a large delivery sheath. The 5-F pigtail catheter is withdrawn over a super-stiff wire. An arteriotomy is performed, and the delivery sheath and guide wire assembly are introduced over the guide wire under fluoroscopic guidance. After successful manipulation of the sheath into a position proximal to the proximal neck of the aneurysm, the dilator and guide wire are withdrawn. The stent graft is introduced from the loading cartridge to the delivery sheath and advanced through the sheath by means of the pusher mandrel. The stent graft is manipulated until the device is at the proximal aspect of the sheath. The sheath is then withdrawn until the stent graft is in an appropriate position, bridging the superior and inferior necks. Before stent-graft deployment, the mean arterial blood pressure is lowered to between 50 and 60 mm Hg by administration of a sodium nitroprusside solution. This is given to reduce the risk of downstream migration caused by intra-aortic blood flow during deployment. When the stent-graft position is appropriate and the blood pressure is optimal, the stent graft is deployed by rapidly withdrawing the sheath while the pusher mandrel is held firmly in position. Immediately after stent-graft deployment, the nitroprusside infusion is discontinued to normalize the blood pressure.

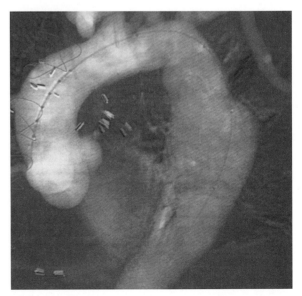

Figure 32–3. Arch aortogram revealing a 6-cm aneurysm of the descending thoracic aorta.

The pigtail catheter is introduced through the sheath to perform postdeployment aortography (Fig. 32–4). Whenever possible, any residual filling of the aneurysm through either the superior or the inferior neck is treated by placement of a second stent graft. If a perigraft leak persists, and is thought to be caused by poor apposition of the stent graft to the aortic wall, balloon dilatation of the stent graft can be considered. The sheath is removed and the arteriotomy is repaired, reversing the effects of systemic heparin by administration of protamine sulfate. For cases in which the pelvic vessels are of insufficient size to accommodate the sheath, the surgical component of the procedure is somewhat more extensive, with exposure of the retroperitoneal iliac artery or aorta to allow introduction of the stent graft; however, the stent-graft deployment is similar.

Postprocedural Monitoring

The patient is usually monitored in an intensive care unit for the first 24 hours after the procedure and transferred to a regular nursing unit the next day. Average time to discharge of our patients is approximately 3 days. No postprocedural anticoagulation is administered. Before discharge, all patients undergo a follow-up chest radiograph, a thoracic aortogram, and a contrast-enhanced spiral CT examination to evaluate the shape and position of the stent graft, the possibility of perigraft leak, and any residual patency of the aneurysm. Patients have repeat spiral CT examinations 6 months after stent-graft placement, and yearly thereafter.

Results

Since 1992, 121 patients with descending thoracic aortic aneurysm have been treated by stent-graft placement at Stanford University Hospital. The technical success rate for stent-graft deployment was 99% (120 of 121). In the one case of technical failure, stent-graft deployment was abandoned after injury occurred to the descending aorta during introduction of the delivery sheath. This was the only case that required immediate surgical conversion. There were 85 men and 36 women, and their ages ranged from 34 to 88 years (mean, 68.2 years). More than 50% of the patients were older than 70 years of age. The mean diameter of the aneurysms was 6.2 cm (range, 4 to 11 cm). A single stent graft was used in 68% of cases, whereas multiple stent grafts were used in 32%. Average stent-graft dimensions were 3.4 cm diameter (range, 2.4 cm to 4.5 cm) and 10.6 cm in length (range, 4.0 cm to 22.0 cm).

Primary successful aneurysmal thrombosis was obtained in 99 of 121 cases. In another 16 cases, thrombosis was achieved with use of an additional stent graft or coil embolization of a perigraft leak. The overall success rate for aneurysmal thrombosis was, therefore, 96% (115 of 121 cases).

Complications

Ten of the 121 patients died in the postoperative period (8%). The cause of death was respiratory failure in 3 patients, cerebral vascular accidents in 2, iliac arterial rupture in 1, aortic arch injury in 1, multiorgan failure in 1, cardiac arrest in 1, and cardiac perforation (related to another operative aortic repair under the same anesthesia) in 1. The majority of these deaths were related to the patients' significant preexisting medical comorbidities.

In four patients (3.2%), paraplegia occurred after stent-graft insertion. In all of these patients, repair of an abdominal aortic aneurysm was performed either before or simultaneously with stent-graft deployment. The interruption of a significant number of intercostals vessels with use of a thoracic aortic stent-graft, combined with interruption of multiple lumbar arteries during an abdominal–aortic aneurysm repair, was the likely cause of paraplegia in these patients. For this reason, we recommend that a time interval elapse between abdominal and thoracic aneurysm repair to allow establishment of collateral vessels. Four patients

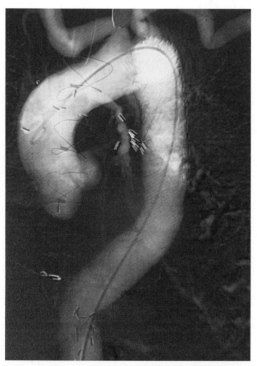

Figure 32–4. Aortogram performed following placement of a polytetrafluoroethylene (PTFE) covered Nitinol stent-graft, with exclusion of the aneurysm.

had a cerebral vascular accident. Two of these patients had simultaneous surgical procedures, including bypass of the left subclavian artery to the carotid artery in 1 patient and resection of a transverse aortic arch aneurysm in another. No cases of distal embolization or stent-graft infection were identified.

THORACIC AORTIC DISSECTIONS

Clinical Problem

Thoracic aortic dissection is the most common catastrophe involving the human aorta, It occurs two to three times more frequently than acute rupture of abdominal aortic aneurysm.[12] The condition affects approximately 5 to 10 patients per million population per year. If patients are untreated, there is a mortality rate of 90% after 3 months. Dissections have been described in the literature as far back as the second century AD, and a clear description of a double-lumen aorta appeared in the early years of the 19th century.[13] However, consistent and encouraging surgical results were not achieved until 1955, when DeBakey and associates introduced thoracic fenestration followed by grafting of the origin of the dissection.[14] Despite surgical advances, mortality remained high until Wheat and associates successfully introduced radical medical therapy in 1965, consisting of aggressive medical treatment of the underlying hypertension.[15] This allows stabilization of the dissection and is the mainstay of treatment for most patients who have dissections of the thoracic aorta commencing distal to the left subclavian artery. In these patients, aggressive interventions are reserved for cases in which medical treatment fails or associated complications develop.

Classification

CLINICAL CLASSIFICATIONS

Clinical classifications have been proposed to divide the disease into acute and chronic categories. A dissection is considered to be acute if it is less than 14 days old, with the time of initial dissection being defined as the onset of acute pain.[16] If a dissection is present for more than 14 days, it is classified as chronic. A chronic dissection is dependent on a sufficient re-entry tear at the distal end of the dissection allowing flow in a double-lumen aorta. The initial flap thickens with time, and a chronic dissection can either maintain two lumens of the aorta or can result in clotting of the false lumen with eventual fibrosis.

ANATOMIC DEFINITIONS

A number of anatomic definitions have been proposed, initially by DeBakey and associates, who described nine different dissection types according to the origin and extent of disease.[14] This definition was subsequently changed to include 3 types in 1965, and was further simplified by Daily and associates in 1970.[17] The current commonly used description divides aortic dissections into Stanford Type A, B. In type A (60 to 70%), the dissection involves the ascending aorta, and the primary intimal tear is usually in the ascending, or transverse, aorta. The critical factor is the involvement of the ascending arch by the dissecting flap, which can potentially cause insufficiency of the aortic valve, rupture into the pericardium, or both. Because of these potentially fatal complications, the current standard of care for acute type A dissection is immediate surgical repair after initial stabilization is a achieved. Associated operative mortality rates are between 5 and 30%.

In type B dissection (30 to 40%), the intimal tear usually arises distal to the origin of the left subclavian artery and extends distally. The ascending aorta is not involved. In these patients, surgical therapy is associated with mortality rates of up to 50%, and treatment is mainly directed at pharmacologically lowering the blood pressure. Surgery is reserved for type B patients with acute aortic rupture, expanding aneurysms, or end-organ ischemia. Despite aggressive medical therapy, mortality rates in patients with acute type B dissections approach 20%.

Etiology

Cystic Medial Necrosis. This condition occurs in young patients with Marfan syndrome if cystic degeneration of the media is present. Cystic medial necrosis also occurs in patients with Ehlers-Danlos syndrome.

Pregnancy. Fifty percent of dissections in women younger than 40 years of age occur during pregnancy.[18] Rupture commonly occurs in these patients during the third trimester or the first stage of labor. These dissections are usually type A, with the tear originating within 2 cm of the aortic valve. Associated cystic medial necrosis or congenital cardiovascular abnormalities, such as coarctation, may also be present.

Hypertension. Approximately 90% of patients with aortic dissection are either clinically hypertensive or have a history of hypertension. The condition occurs two to three times more commonly in hypertensive males and is most common in black patients. The patient is frequently a middle-aged black man with known hypertension who experiences sudden onset of excruciating, tearing back pain.[19]

Atherosclerosis. Most frequently, atherosclerosis is associated with dissection in elderly patients.[20] These patients develop a dissection secondary to an atherosclerotic penetrating ulcer (see Figs. 32–1 and 32–2), and they also commonly have underlying hypertension. The tear in the aorta usually occurs in a supradiaphragmatic location. This can result in a classic dissection, with a re-entry tear, or more commonly, a thrombosed dissection, otherwise termed an intramural hematoma.

Endocrine Disorders. These may lead to dissection through the development of hypertension, as with Cushing's disease or pheochromocytoma.

Congenital Cardiovascular Anomalies. Coarctation of the aorta, aortic stenosis with bicuspid valve, ductus arteriosus, atrial septal defect, tricuspid valve defect, or aortic hyperplasia may be associated with aortic dissection. In approximately 10% of patients with coarctation of the aorta, the cause of death is rupture of a dissecting aneurysm.[21]

Trauma. This may result in intimal rupture and dissecting hematoma, which is seen following a sudden deceleration injury, with resultant intimal tear of the descending thoracic aorta at the ligamentum arteriosum attachment. Dissection or aneurysm after an intimal tear caused by trauma may remain undetected for weeks or years.

Iatrogenic Causes. Limited or extensive dissection of the aorta may result from inadvertent intimal tear during percutaneous endovascular procedures. If these conditions are recognized, patients can usually be treated with placement of an endovascular stent. This condition is seen after extracorporeal circulation, with the intimal tear occurring secondary to the large catheters used during this process.[22]

Indications for Treatment

TYPE A DISSECTIONS

The current standard of care for treatment of patients with acute aortic dissection affecting the ascending aorta is still open surgical repair with replacement of the ascending aorta by a composite graft.[16] During the initial evaluation, patients with hypertension should receive medical treatment, and after stabilization, the patient should be placed on cardiopulmonary bypass, the aortic wall should be resected, and the ascending aorta should be replaced. If aortic valvular incompetence resulting from commissural detachment is present, the aortic valve should also be replaced. Surgical mortality rates approach 30%, with myocardial infarction being the most common cause of late death. In these cases, surgery is undertaken to prevent the catastrophic consequences of rupture of the aorta into the pericardium or development of severe aortic regurgitation.

TYPE B DISSECTIONS

Medical therapy for type B dissections has resulted in decreased mortality compared with that after surgery (50 vs. 80%).[15] Medical therapy involves aggressive treatment in a cardiovascular surgical intensive care unit using invasive monitoring. Pulmonary artery wedge pressures are obtained via a Swan-Ganz catheter, urinary output is tracked via a Foley catheter, and aggressive antihypertensive therapy is instituted. Treatment regimens now commonly include esmolol, sodium nitroprusside, or both. Relief of the severe, tearing pain usually indicates termination of the dissecting process and is probably the single most important clinical sign in the management of these patients. After initial stabilization, patients are evaluated to determine whether further intervention is required.

Intervention in the treatment of type B aortic dissection is indicated in a limited number of circumstances, such as the following:

1. Acute aortic rupture is associated with severe pain and hypotension. This condition requires urgent surgery and has a high operative mortality.
2. An enlarging false-lumen aneurysm usually occurs in a chronic setting. After initial stabilization, the patient develops progressive widening of the mediastinum that is visible on follow-up chest radiographs, or an enlargement of the false lumen, which appears on sequential CT scans.[23]
3. Branch artery involvement can involve the renal arteries, the mesenteric vessels, or the iliac arteries. Involvement of the renal arteries is suspected in cases with hypertension resistant to aggressive medical therapy or with deteriorating renal function. Mesenteric vessel involvement is suspected in patients who usually have postprandial abdominal pain. Iliac artery involvement is suspected in patients with changing femoral pulses. In the chronic setting, intermittent claudication is a sign of iliac artery involvement.
4. The other possible complication of an aortic dissection is the patient's development of paraplegia. This occurs as a result of involvement of the spinal arteries that originate from the intercostal or lumbar arteries. These arteries are affected by the dissection.

Selection of Devices for Treatment

The rapid advancements in stent development and stent-graft technology have raised hopes that endovascular techniques may be applied to treat patients with aortic dissection. The aim of the procedure would be to compress the false lumen and flap against the outer wall of the aorta, thereby restoring total flow to the true lumen and effectively reversing the dissection process. Alternatively, the stent graft could be used to cover the initial aortic tear, which usually occurs distal to the left subclavian artery, thereby resulting in decreased flow and thrombosis of the false lumen. The initial application of this technique was first attempted in a cadaver model, and since then, animal models have been successfully used to investigate this hypothesis.[24–26] In all animal studies, the initial tear was created distal to the origin of the left subclavian artery. Dissections in these models have been relatively acute, and the animal were usually treated within 3 weeks of creation of the dissections. Invariably, to prevent re-entry of blood flow through natural fenestrations into the false lumen below the site of the original tear, the animals required stenting of almost the entire thoracic aorta. Unfortunately, endovascular repair of thoracic aortic dissection has a number of complicating factors. Most important, each case has its unique anatomic considerations. An understanding of the relative size, location, and extent of the true and false lumens, as well as the orientation of the intimal flap, is crucial before treatment is begun. The false lumen often supplies flow to important structures, notably the mesenteric vessels, the renal vessels, or the lower extremities, and the consequences of obliterating the false lumen in such a patient by placement of either stents or a stent graft in the true lumen could be disastrous. Advances in the use of intravascular ultrasonography have supplemented CT and angiography and enhanced our understanding of the individual anatomy, allowing adequate visualization of the extent of the entire aortic flap and branch vessel involvement.[27] Patients usually undergo dynamic enhanced CT as the initial diagnostic test. CT is extremely helpful in deciphering a complex anatomy, because the orientation of the intimal flap and the relative rates of flow within the true and false lumens can be discerned from a well-performed spiral CT scan.[28] In our institution, aortography is reserved for cases in which endovascular treatment is deemed necessary from the standpoint of clinical evaluation and noninvasive studies. Aortography requires cannulation of both lumens, with intraluminal pressure monitoring, and endovascular ultrasonography.

Once the anatomy is understood and the relative flow to true and false lumens and distal branches is understood, intervention can be planned. If consideration of stenting or stent grafting of the thoracic aorta is undertaken, the site of the initial intimal tear is the most important consideration. This can be localized with use of aortography and intravascular ultrasonography, and the orientation of the intimal tear and its relation to the branch vessels, notably the left subclavian artery, can be defined. Assuming sufficient neck exists between the superior aspect of the intimal tear and the left subclavian artery, a stent graft can be placed to occlude the tear. We use covered Gianturco Z stents, in a similar fashion to that mentioned in treating patients with aortic aneurysms. The

device deployment system is identical and the mechanism of delivery similar.

After stent grafting of the initial intimal tear is performed, continued flow within the false lumen may be seen through fenestrations that exist in dissected aortic segments below the initial tear. In our experience, however, the decrease in flow through the primary entry tear is usually sufficient to reorient the flow to the true lumen, thereby maintaining perfusion of visceral, renal, and lower extremity vessels. As there is usually persistent flow to the false lumen, development of a false-lumen aneurysm is still possible, and patients are followed up with sequential CT scans.

Renal and mesenteric ischemia and infarction are major causes of morbidity and death in patients with acute dissection. When either or both renal or mesenteric circulation are compromised by acute dissection, significant sequelae occur. Renal ischemia is noted to occur in approximately 8% of patients who manifest type B dissection, and mesenteric ischemia occurs in 5%. Operative mortality rates for patients with type B dissection and renal or mesenteric ischemia approach 88%.[29, 30]

The appropriate management of compromised branch vessel perfusion is a complicated algorithm that varies on a case-to-case basis. Treatment usually involves placement of a stent within either a renal or mesenteric vessel to redirect flow to a vascular bed from one of the aortic lumens. Decreased perfusion to vascular beds can occur with either direct involvement of the vessel origin by the dissection or by compromised flow in the aortic lumen supplying that vessel. When the branch vessel is directly involved by the flap, treatment involves placement of a stent within that branch to adequately redirect flow. When flow to a vessel is compromised because of decreased aortic lumen flow, treatment requires redirection of flow to that aortic lumen by placing a stent or stent graft in the aorta and covering the primary tear.

Description of Technique

In these cases, anatomic detail needs to be optimized, and endovascular procedures are usually performed in the angiography suite. Following extensive diagnostic evaluation with true-lumen and false-lumen aortography, pressure measurements, and intravascular ultrasonographic evaluation, attention is directed to the clinical problem to be addressed. In cases with mild malperfusion of a single vascular bed and involvement of the lumen of that vessel by the dissection flap, the true lumen of the aorta is catheterized, and a wire is passed into the true lumen of the affected branch vessel. An endovascular stent, usually a balloon-expandable Palmaz stent, is placed in the ostial region of the involved renal or mesenteric artery, and flow is re-established via the true lumen.

PERCUTANEOUS BALLOON FENESTRATION

Percutaneous balloon fenestration of the dissecting septum is performed with use of either intravascular ultrasonography or fluoroscopic guidance. With either technique, percutaneous access is obtained to both true and false lumens (Fig. 32–5). Under fluoroscopic guidance, a large balloon angioplasty catheter (12 to 14 mm diameter) is advanced, usually into the false lumen, and inflated. Simultaneously, a long metal cannula is advanced into the other lumen (Fig. 32–6). This is positioned at the same level as the inflated angioplasty balloon and rotated until the balloon becomes indented by the cannula. A 21-gauge inner needle and a 5-F catheter is then advanced, and the intimal flap is punctured during needle placement into the angioplasty balloon. After puncture of the intimal flap, the 5-F catheter and angioplasty balloon are advanced, the needle is removed, and the guide wire is advanced through the intimal flap into the false lumen. A balloon catheter is advanced over the guide wire, and the fenestration is enlarged to 14 to 20 mm with use of a balloon catheter. Repeat arteriography is performed to assess successful redirection of the flow (Fig. 32–7).

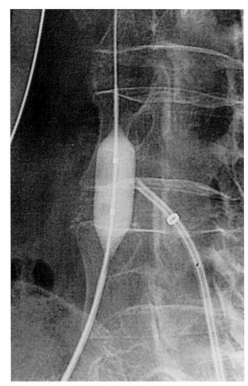

Figure 32–6. Fenestration of dissection flap. A large-diameter balloon is placed in the false lumen via the left iliac artery. A stiff cannula is advanced into the true lumen, and a needle is advanced across the flap. The fenestration is then dilated with an angioplasty balloon.

STENT GRAFT FOR FALSE-LUMEN ANEURYSMS

As previously described, a detailed evaluation is performed to assess the location of the initial intimal tear. The anatomy of patients with chronic type B dissections and false-lumen aneurysms is somewhat more complex than that of patients with atherosclerotic descending thoracic aortic aneurysm. The aim of treatment is to occlude flow into the false lumen through the initial tear, and, therefore, a stent graft that approximates the diameter of the true lumen is usually sufficient. Measurements are made based on data obtained from aortography, CT, intravascular ultrasonography, and a stent graft manufactured by Gianturco Z Stents, which is covered with woven polyester. The stent graft is introduced under fluoroscopic guidance through a large sheath. The device is advanced by a pushing mandrel. The stent graft is then deployed by withdrawing the sheath and holding the mandrel in position. A repeat angiographic evaluation is performed to assess the change in the flow to the false-lumen aneurysm. Often, after successful occlusion of the initial tear, residual flow is detected in the false lumen via natural fenestrations; however, the pressure within the false lumen should be sufficiently decreased to reduce the likelihood of aortic rupture. Patients are followed via sequential CT.

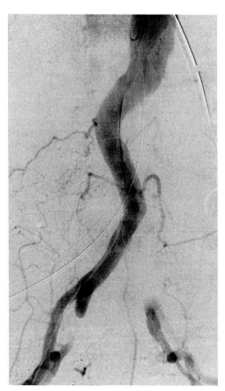

Figure 32–5. False lumen abdominal arteriogram in a 44-year-old male with a type B dissection. The dissection flap occludes flow to the left common iliac artery.

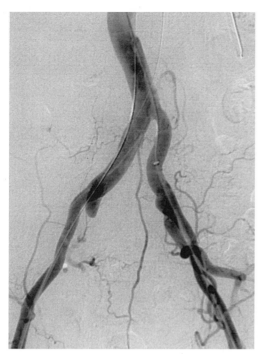

Figure 32–7. Postfenestration false-lumen arteriogram showing flow in both iliac arteries.

Results and Complications

Sixty patients have undergone vascular stenting, balloon fenestration, or both to treat end-organ ischemia. The procedures were technically successful in all cases. The 30-day mortality rate was 18%. Four patients died in the initial postprocedural period of profound metabolic acidosis secondary to multiorgan failure accompanied by mesenteric ischemia. It is likely that these patients had severe, irreversible bowel ischemia before the intervention. The surviving patients have experienced persistent clinical benefit. No patient has undergone surgery for chronic end-organ ischemia. Mean follow-up was 16 months (range, 3 to 48 months). Eleven patients have undergone stent-graft placement. In 6 of these cases, the device was placed to redirect the flow to the true lumen and increase end-organ flow. In 5 cases, the purpose was to direct flow away from a large false-lumen aneurysm.

DISCUSSION

Although technically involved, endovascular treatment of patients with thoracic aortic aneurysms is a relatively simple concept compared with treatment of patients with aortic dissections. In the case of aneurysmal disease, the decision to treat a patient requires a detailed understanding of the anatomy, and selection of an appropriately sized stent-graft device that can adequately exclude flow from the aneurysm. The device delivery system used in our initial study requires attention to detail and expertise in delivery technique; however, a number of simpler and lower profile devices are currently being developed or undergoing feasibility trials. These will allow safer and more accurate deployment, with a resultant decrease in procedure time and complications. Given our initial results, it appears that within the next decade, endovascular repair will become the procedure of choice for many patients with descending thoracic aortic aneurysms.

Treatment of patients with aortic dissections is considerably more complex. Endovascular treatment options can be considered to alleviate end-organ ischemia, and, in certain cases, decrease false-lumen flow, in an attempt to reduce the likelihood of false-lumen aneurysm formation and possible rupture (Figs. 32–8, 32–9, 32–10, and 32–11). With regard to treatment of ischemic complications of dissection, surgical options are severely limited. Patients undergoing aortic surgery for dissection who have preprocedural renal or mesenteric ischemia, have a mortality rate approaching 88%. It was in an effort to reduce this figure that the current program of aggressive evaluation and treatment of type B aortic dissections was undertaken. As can be seen from our results with placement of vascular stents in 60 patients, the mortality rate is considerably lower than that achieved with open surgery, and the treatment algorithm is now well established. In general, the interventionalist can play an important role in the treatment of the ischemic complications of dissection, with medical therapy remaining the mainstay of treatment for the majority of patients who have uncomplicated type B dissection.[31]

Because of other etiologies, treatment of chronic dissection with associated aneurysms is significantly more complicated that that of aneurysms. The aortic anatomy in these patients is unique, with complex geometric shapes dependent on the orientation of the intimal flap or flaps. The noncircular proximal and distal aortic necks make the likelihood of attaining a seal between the graft material and the aortic wall or dissection septum problematic. Stent grafts, regardless of their morphology, are likely to leave considerable gaps for blood flow at either neck, thereby allowing persistent flow into the aneurysm lumen. The possibility of false-lumen aneurysm rupture is unchanged. The most effective therapy for reducing the risk of false-lumen aneurysm rupture is open surgery. As an effective low-morbidity technique, use of the endovascular alternative appears unlikely in the near future.

ENDOVASCULAR TREATMENT OF COARCTATION OF THE AORTA

Coarctation of the aorta is a rare condition. It most commonly affects the aortic isthmus (95%) but rarely

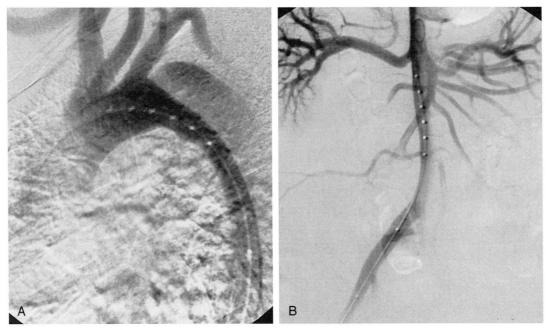

Figure 32-8. A, Thoracic aortogram of a type B dissection with flow in a narrow true lumen and filling of the false lumen through an intimal tear distal to the left subclavian artery. B, Abdominal aortogram with true-lumen compression and resultant absence of flow to the left common iliac artery.

the abdominal aorta, where it results in a mesenteric syndrome. A distinction in narrowing between adult type (distal to the ductus) and infantile type (proximal to the ductus) has been made, but perhaps a more useful method of classification is by the age of the patient. An infant usually has hypertension or demonstrates failure to thrive. The condition may also be detected by routine clinical examination. The coarctation may be associated with other congenital defects, including bicuspid aortic valve, ventriculo-

septal defect, or hypoplastic left heart syndrome. Treatment of an infant may be surgical or endovascular. The choice in part is determined by the presence of associated anomalies. If recoarctation occurs after surgical correction, balloon angioplasty remains an option for further treatment.

Follow-up of children treated by balloon angioplasty shows an appreciable rate of recoarctation, which has been reported as between 39[32] and 46%[33] in infants, whereas the recoarctation rate is lower in

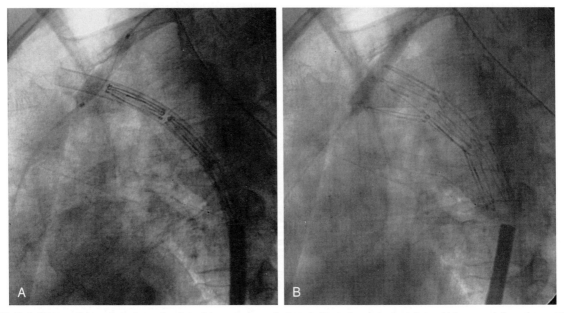

Figure 32-9. A, Stent graft in an introducer sheath in the aorta. An angioplasty balloon placed via the left brachial artery defines the position of the left subclavian artery. B, Deployed stent graft in position in the descending thoracic aorta.

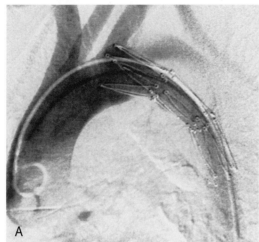

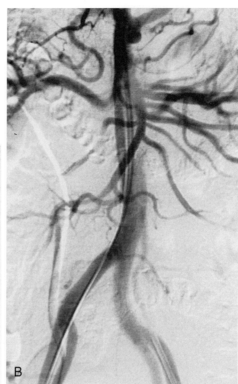

Figure 32–10. *A*, Aortogram obtained after stent-graft deployment shows redirection of flow to the true lumen, with minimal filling of the false lumen. *B*, Repeat abdominal aortogram with improved true-lumen flow and filling of the left common iliac artery.

older children. A lower restenosis rate of 18% has been seen after performance of angioplasty for recoarctation that has occured after previous surgical repair.[33] Recoarctation is especially common if there is associated hypoplasia of the transverse aortic arch.[34] Other complications include aneurysm formation at the angioplasty site in 5% of patients and femoral arterial damage in 14%.[32]

The use of stents in children has yet to be fully evaluated. The problem is that the stent requires sequential dilatation for the growing aorta. In animals, there is evidence that stents can be sequentially distended, but this has been demonstrated only in preliminary clinical studies in human subjects.[35]

Detection of aortic coarctation in the adult usually occurs if hypertension that is diagnosed during a routine physical examination fails to be controlled by standard treatment. It may be diagnosed as a result of chest radiograph findings, or the patient may manifest symptoms related to consequent ischemic heart disease or cardiac decompensation. An untreated patient is prone to develop cardiac and cerebrovascular complications secondary to the resultant hypertension. The aim of treatment is to reduce the patient's hypertension by relieving the pressure gradient across the coarctation.

Surgical treatment has been in use since 1944 and was the only available method of gradient reduction until the late 1980s. Since then, experience has grown in the use of balloon angioplasty, and more recently, evaluation of stent placement has also been reported.

Surgical treatment can be performed with use of endogenous or synthetic patch grafting or by excision of the coarctation site and end-to-end anastomosis. Early reported results were poor, but more recent work has shown effective reduction in blood pressure, with low complication rates.[36-39] Complication rates are shown in Table 32–1.

Balloon angioplasty has been in use since the late 1980s, and there is considerable experience described in the literature, with a wealth of short- and intermediate-term follow-up data available. Long-term follow-up data are more limited. One of the largest series available describes 43 patients.[40] There were no deaths in this series, with a 7% aneurysm formation rate and a 7% restenosis rate. Seventy-three percent of patients had normalization of blood pressure following angioplasty. The summated experience of four series[40-43] described a total of 136 patients who had improvement in blood pressure in 60 to 90% of cases. The observed complications in these four series are shown in Table 32–2.

The long-term significance of aneurysms at the

Table 32–1. Surgical Complication Rates

	(%)
Mortality	2.6–3.1
Paraplegia	0.5–1
Aneurysm	5.4
Residual stenosis	3

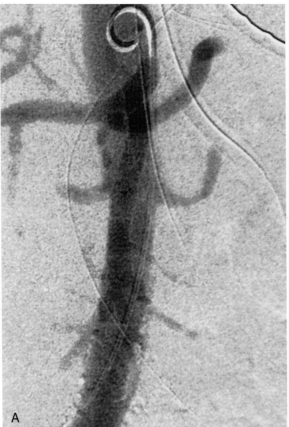

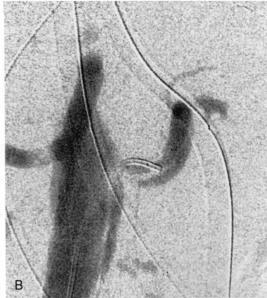

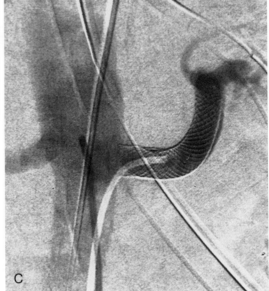

Figure 32–11. *A*, Carbon dioxide (CO_2) abdominal aortogram in a 56-year-old man with a type B dissection and renal failure. There is evidence of narrowing of the left renal artery. *B*, Selective CO_2 left renal arteriogram identifies involvement of the left renal artery by the dissection flap with subsequent stenosis of the true lumen. *C*, Contrast arteriogram of the left renal artery obtained after deployment of a stent demonstrates good flow within a normal-caliber vessel.

coarctation site is debatable. Experience with follow-up of 14 patients for a mean of 7.3 years suggests that small aneurysms at the dilatation site are likely to resolve over time and that later formation of such aneurysms does not occur.[44]

If the surgical and angioplasty complication rates are compared, it is clear that mortality is lower after

Table 32–2. Balloon Angioplasty Complication Rates

	(%)
Mortality	0.7
Aneurysm	3–10
Residual stenosis	7–26
Aortic dissection	0–10
Femoral arterial complications	2–7

performance of angioplasty, and that paraplegia, another serious complication of surgical treatment, is not seen in these balloon angioplasty series. Rates of aneurysm formation at the treated site are comparable for the two modalities, but the residual stenosis rate is higher after angioplasty. Aortic dissection related to overdilatation of the site is discussed later. This complication may require urgent surgical treatment. Femoral arterial complications, such as stenosis, thrombosis, and pseudoaneurysm formation result from the use of large-caliber sheaths that are required for the procedure. Such complications may be dealt with in many cases by endovascular means.

Data concerning the use of stents in adult coarctation are less available. Small series have described stent placement in patients with native and recurrent coarctation. Of these, the largest one suggests that results in the short and intermediate term are favorable compared with those of balloon angioplasty alone.[35] However, no long-term follow-up is yet available, especially regarding the long-term stability and structural integrity of stents at this site, and patient numbers are small.

With modern imaging methods, such as magnetic resonance imaging (MRI) and Duplex ultrasonography, it is possible to confirm the diagnosis and the severity of coarctation before performance of the definitive procedure. The presence of large collateral vessels closely applied to the coarctation site may make the likelihood of dissection greater. Similarly, excess tortuosity of the coarctation site results in interference with deployment of the balloon and may make dissection more likely. Total occlusion of the aorta results in inability to cross the coarctation.

These factors can be assessed by the noninvasive techniques that have been described but may require confirmation by angiography, with approach made from either the groin or the arm if severe aortic narrowing precludes easy catheter manipulation into the ascending aorta from below.

TECHNIQUE

The procedure is performed in the angiography suite under either general anesthesia or neuroleptanalgesia, depending on the patient. Ideally, thoracic surgical backup should be available on site, if required. After sterile preparation, the common femoral artery is punctured and a 7-F introducer sheath is placed. If the femoral artery is not palpable, this can be located with use of a hand-held Doppler probe. A shaped catheter, such as a right coronary catheter, is advanced to the level of the coarctation and with a steerable wire, the obstruction is gently probed until the orifice is located. The wire and catheter are then advanced into the ascending aorta. The steerable wire is removed, and a 260-cm stiff wire is inserted. The catheter is withdrawn and replaced by a 5-F marker pigtail catheter. At all times, from this point until completion of the procedure, either a catheter or wire is always positioned across the coarctation. Heparin 5000 units is given. Simultaneous pressures are now measured in the ascending aorta and at the femoral level via the sheath. This gives an accurate gradient (Fig. 32–12A). An angiogram is performed via the pigtail catheter (Fig. 32–13). Using the marker catheter for calibration, the width of the aorta immediately below the left subclavian artery is measured (Fig. 32–14). A balloon catheter 2 mm less than this diameter is selected for the dilatation in the hope that the slightly undersized balloon will not cause an aortic tear. With the long, stiff wire in place, an appropriately sized sheath is inserted into the femoral artery (usually 11-

or 12-F). The large balloon catheter (usually 18 to 24 mm) is advanced over the stiff wire into the coarctation site and inflated with dilute contrast. An indentation confirms its position in the coarctation (Fig. 32–15), and it can be fully inflated until the waist is abolished. The balloon is then thoroughly deflated and withdrawn through the sheath. The pigtail catheter is reinserted over the wire into the ascending aorta. Simultaneous pressures are again measured (see Fig. 12B), and if these show a gradient of less than 10 mm Hg, angiography is performed (Fig. 32–16). This serves to check that a good lumen has been obtained and that no significant aortic tear has occurred. If a satisfactory result is demonstrated, the pigtail is withdrawn over a wire, and both are removed. The large sheath is removed, and for at least 30 minutes, pressure is applied to the artery to obtain hemostasis. It is usually necessary to perform only a single balloon inflation to obtain a good result. If, however, a significant gradient remains, further dilatation, perhaps with a slightly larger balloon, may be required.

Aftercare and Follow-up

Because of the large size of the introducer sheath (11- or 12-F), the patient should be maintained on bed rest for 24 hours, lying flat for the first 6 hours. Blood pressure and heart rate should be continuously monitored during bed rest. The patient can be mobilized after this 24-hour period and should then have MRI and Duplex scans performed to obtain a postprocedure base line. The patient is usually discharged after 36 hours. After 1 month, the patient has clinical follow-up with MRI and Duplex scanning. This is repeated after 6 months and 1 year, after which, if all is well, no further follow-up is required. Ambulant blood pressure requires monitoring if the patient had been taking antihypertensive medication before angioplasty was performed.

Conclusion

Balloon angioplasty is an established, safe, and effective treatment for both children and adults who have thoracic aortic coarctation. Various technical considerations must be made in patient selection. Further evaluation is required to establish the niche for stenting in coarctation repair.

SURGICAL ALTERNATIVES TO ENDOVASCULAR TREATMENT

In 1956, Cooley and DeBakey reported the first successful replacement of the ascending aorta with a

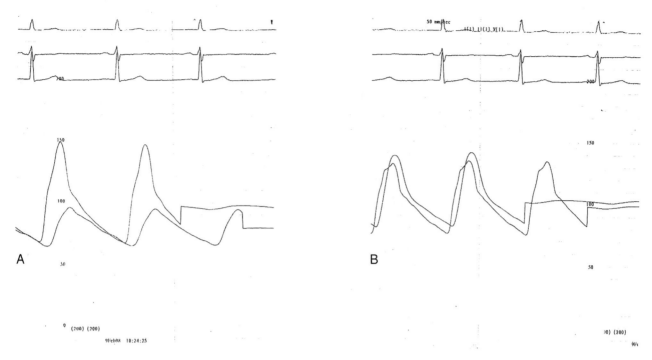

Figure 32–12. Measurement of gradients. A, Preangioplasty gradient of 50 mm Hg. B, Postangioplasty, the gradient has been reduced to 10 mm Hg.

prosthetic graft.[45] One year later, DeBakey and associates reported resection of a fusiform aneurysm of the aortic arch and replacement with a homograft.[46] Since these landmark reports, many advances have been made in the surgical techniques and postoperative care for treatment of patients with thoracic aortic disease. Although we have vast knowledge of the natural history of infrarenal aortic aneurysms, there exist considerably fewer data on the natural history of thoracic aortic aneurysms.[47] As noninvasive diagnostic tests for the thoracic aorta have been developed, our understanding of the natural history of thoracic aortic aneurysms has deepened. It is estimated that rupture of an existing thoracic aortic

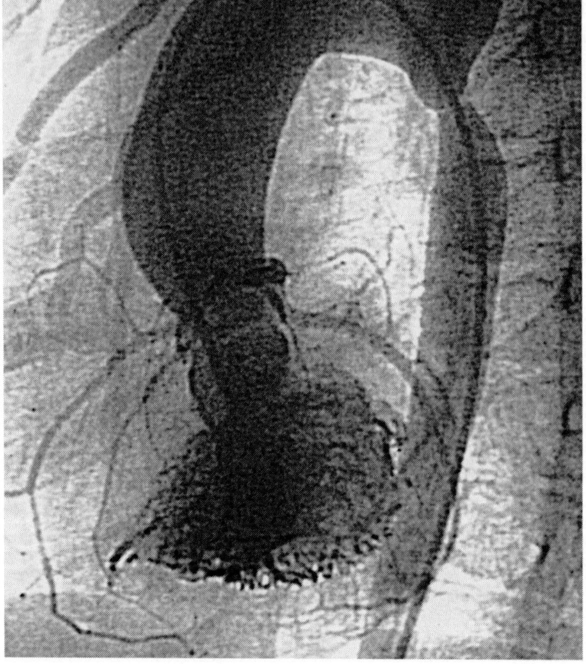

Figure 32–13. Preangioplasty angiogram showing the coarctation site.

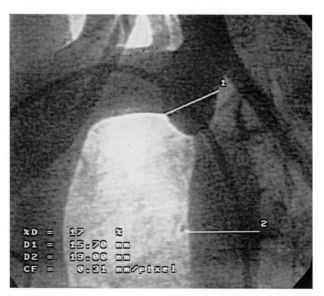

Figure 32–14. The aortic diameter just below the left subclavian artery origin is measured.

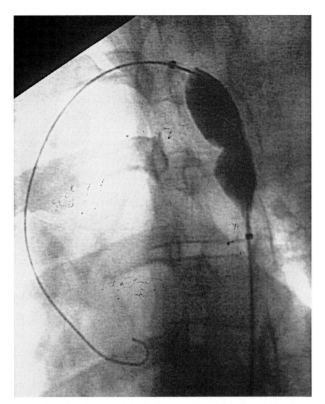

Figure 32–15. Waisting of the balloon at the coarctation site is demonstrated.

aneurysm causes death in approximately 42 to 70% of patients with this disease who do not undergo repair.[2, 4, 48] The natural history of all aneurysms includes the potential for progressive expansion and eventual rupture. The goal of surgical treatment of aneurysms and dissections of the thoracic aorta is to prevent rupture of the aneurysm and death, as well as to prevent complications associated with aortic aneurysm dissection. This includes alleviation of symptoms associated with progressive dissection or aneurysm enlargement.

Elective surgical replacement of a descending thoracic aneurysm should be undertaken if the aneurysm equals or exceeds 5 cm in diameter, or if the patient becomes symptomatic. Patients who have contraindications for surgery, such as those with severe pulmonary disease, must be considered individually. Patients with acute dissections originating distal to the subclavian artery (type B) are initially managed with medical therapy, which consists of β-blockers for controlling the force of left ventricular contraction as well as intravenous nitrates and/or angiotensin-converting enzyme (ACE) inhibitors for lowering systolic blood pressure. Urgent operative repair is indicated in dissections that demonstrate impending rupture (bloody pleural effusion, rapidly increasing size, or uncontrollable pain) or ischemia of vital organs or the extremities. Graft replacement of the involved aorta should also be considered in patients who develop

pseudoaneurysms and those who have severe atherosclerotic disease of the aorta and who suffer from repeated episodes of thromboembolic events to the lower extremities or abdominal viscera. Long-term survivors of aortic dissection may require late surgery if the false channel becomes aneurysmal. These patients are managed in the same way as those whose aneurysms have an atherosclerotic origin.

Many successful operative approaches have been developed to deal with problems of the descending aorta. No method is universally accepted, and all experienced surgeons generally have preferred techniques that are most comfortable for them and provide the best results. However, careful consideration must be given to safety, visualization, and limitation of cross-clamp time. For instance, a clamp-and-sew technique may provide outstanding results in simple traumatic aortic transection, but it would be far more hazardous to use in repair of a large thoracoabdominal aneurysm. Because some of these procedures are quite complex and time-intensive, it is useful to have methods to perfuse the abdominal viscera and the lower intercostal arteries during at least part of the procedure to prevent ischemic damage. Spinal cord ischemia, with resultant paresis or paralysis, remains one of the most devastating complications associated with these surgeries. For this reason, most surgeons

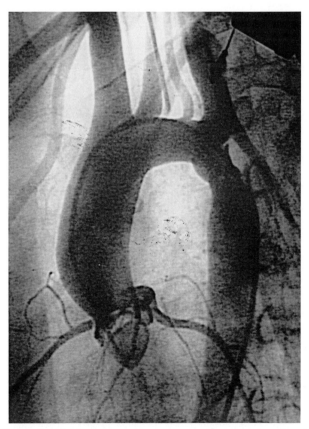

Figure 32–16. The postangioplasty angiogram shows a good result with no evidence of aortic tear.

make an effort to reimplant the intercostal arteries in the mid- and low-thoracic regions in an effort to preserve spinal cord blood flow. Some of the techniques of spinal cord protection used during repair of descending thoracic and thoracoabdominal aneurysms include cerebrospinal fluid drainage, profound hypothermia with circulatory arrest, intraoperative monitoring of somatosensory and motor-evoked potentials, preservation of critical intercostal and lumbar arteries, pharmacologic protection (e.g., steroids, free radical scavengers), maintenance of distal perfusion by means of a Gott shunt or left atrial-to-femoral artery partial bypass, and most recently, lower body exsanguination with the performance of open distal anastomosis.[49–53] Although none of the above methods has been shown conclusively to be superior to the others in reducing spinal cord injury, it is generally accepted that some attention must be paid to spinal cord protection during the more complex procedures.

Ischemic complications related to aortic cross-clamping, particularly spinal cord injury and renal failure, are responsible for the large share of morbidity after surgical replacement of the descending thoracic aorta.[53, 54] Reoperation increases the risk of postoperative neurologic injury.[55] The type and location of the disease in the aorta, as well as the urgency of the procedure, influence operative mortality. However, results have improved in centers that have experienced surgeons, and operative mortality rates between 5 and 15% for repair of thoracoabdominal aorta can be expected in elective cases.[49–53, 55, 56] Unfortunately, elective repair of the descending thoracic and thoracoabdominal aorta may still be associated with a 5 to 10% incidence of spinal cord injury,[57] depending on the location and complexity of the procedure. Reports on the incidence of renal failure in these cases range from 0 to 16%.[49–53, 55, 56]

REFERENCES

1. Lindsay J, DeBakey M, Beall A: Diagnosis and treatment of diseases of the aorta. In Schlant R, Alexander R (eds): The Heart. New York; McGraw-Hill, 1994.
2. Pressler V, McNamara J: Thoracic aortic aneurysm: Natural history and treatment. J Thorac Cardiovasc Surg 79:489–498, 1980.
3. DeBakey M, McCollum C, Graham J: Surgical treatment of aneurysms of the descending thoracic aorta: Long-term results in five hundred patients. J Cardiovasc Surg (Torino) 19:571–576, 1978.
4. Bickerstaff L, Pairolero P, Hollier L, et al: Thoracic aortic aneurysms: A population-based study. Surgery 92:1103–1108, 1982.
5. Moreno-Cabral C, Miller D, Mitchell R, et al: Degenerative and atherosclerotic aneurysms of the thoracic aorta: Determinants of early and late surgical outcome. J Thorac Cardiovasc Surg 88:1020–1032, 1984.
6. Dotter C: Transluminally placed coilspring endarterial tube grafts: Long-term patency in canine popliteal artery. Invest Radiol 4:329–332, 1969.
7. Laborde J, Parodi J, Clem M, et al: Intraluminal bypass of

8. Chuter T, Green R, Ouriel K, et al: Transfemoral endovascular aortic graft placement. J Vasc Surg 18:185–197, 1993.
9. Parodi J, Palmaz J, Barone H: Transfemoral intraluminal graft implantation for abdominal aortic aneurysms. Ann Vasc Surg 5:491–499, 1991.
10. Dake MD, Miller DC, Semba CP, et al: Transluminal placement of endovascular stent-grafts for the treatment of descending thoracic aortic aneurysms. N Engl J Med 331:1729–1734, 1994.
11. Semba C, Sakai T, Slonim S, et al: Mycotic aneurysms of the thoracic aorta: Repair with use of endovascular stent-grafts. J Vasc Intervent Radiol 9:33–40, 1998.
12. Wheat M, Palmer F: Dissecting aneurysms of the aorta. Curr Probl Surg 1–43, 1971.
13. Shekelton J: Healed dissecting aneurysm. Dublin Hosp Rec 3:231, 1822.
14. DeBakey M, Cooley D, Creech OJ: Surgical consideration of dissecting aneurysm of the aorta. Ann Surg 142:586–612, 1955.
15. Wheat MJ, Palmer RF, Bartley TD, et al: Treatment of dissecting aneurysms of the aorta without surgery. J Thorac Cardiovasc Surg 50:364–373, 1965.
16. Miller D, Stinson E, Oyer P, et al: Operative treatment of aortic dissections: Experience with 125 patients over a sixteen-year period. J Thorac Cardiovasc Surg 78:365–382, 1979.
17. Daily P, Trueblood H, Stinson E, et al: Management of acute aortic dissections. Ann Thorac Surg 10:237–247, 1970.
18. Pedowitz P, Perell A: Aneurysms complicated by pregnancy. 1. Aneurysms of the aorta and its major branches. Am J Obstet Gynecol 73:720–735, 1957.
19. Hirst A, Gore I: The etiology and pathology of aortic dissection. In Doroghazi R, Slater E (eds): Aortic dissection. New York, McGraw-Hill, 1983.
20. Lodwick G: Dissecting aneurysms of thoracic and abdominal aorta; report of 6 cases, with discussion of roentgenologic findings and pathologic changes. Am J Roentgenol 69:907–925, 1953.
21. Burchell H: Aortic dissection (dissecting hematoma; dissecting aneurysm of the aorta). Circulation 12:1068–1079, 1955.
22. Salama F, Blesovsky A: Complication of cannulation of the ascending aorta for open-heart surgery. Thorax 25:604–607, 1970.
23. Crawford E, Svensson L, Coselli J, et al: Aortic Dissection and dissecting aortic aneurysms. Ann Surg 208:254–273, 1988.
24. Charnsangavej C, Wallace S, Wright K, et al: Endovascular stent for use in aortic dissection: An in vitro experiment. Radiology 157:323–324, 1985.
25. Kato N, Hirano T, Takeda K, et al: Treatment of aortic dissections with a percutaneous intravascular endoprothesis: Comparison of covered and bare stents. J Vasc Intervent Radiol 5:805–812, 1994.
26. Moon MR, Dake MD, Pelc LR, et al: Intravascular stenting of acute experimental type B dissections. J Surg Res 54:381–388, 1993.
27. Pande A, Meier B, Fleisch M, et al: Intravascular ultrasound for diagnosis of aortic dissection. Am J Cardiol 67:662–663, 1991.
28. Sommer T, Fehske W, Holzknecht N, et al: Aortic dissection: A comparative study of diagnosis with spiral CT, multiplanar transesophageal echocardiography, and MR imaging [see comments]. Radiology 199:347–352, 1996.
29. Fann J, Sarris G, Mitchell R, et al: Treatment of patients with aortic dissection presenting with peripheral vascular complications. Ann Surg 212:705–713, 1990.
30. Miller D, Mitchell R, Oyer P, et al: Independent determinants of operative mortality for patients with aortic dissections. Circulation 70(3 pt 2):I153–164, 1984.
31. Wheat MJ: Current status of medical therapy of acute dissecting aneurysms of the aorta. World J Surg 4:563–569, 1980.
32. Rao PS, Galal O, Smith PA, et al: Five to Nine-year follow-up of balloon angioplasty of native aortic coarctation in infants and children. J Am Coll Cardiol 27:462–70, 1996.
33. Ino T, Nishimoto K, Kato H, et al: Balloon angioplasty for aortic coarctation—Report of a questionnaire survey by the Japanese Pediatric Interventional Cardiology Committee. Jpn Circ J 61:375–383, 1997.
34. Yetman AT, Nykanen D, McCrindle BW, et al: Balloon angio-

abdominal aortic aneurysm: Feasibility study. Radiology 184:185–190, 1992.

plasty of recurrent coarctation: A 12 year review. J Am Coll Cardiol 30:811–816, 1997.

35. Ebeid MR, Prieto LR, Latson LA: Use of balloon expandable stents for coarctation of the aorta: Initial results and intermediate term follow-up. J Am Coll Cardiol 30:1847–1852, 1997.

36. Bobby JJ, Emami JM, Farmer RDT, et al: Operative survival and 40-year follow-up of surgical repair of aortic coarctation. Br Heart J 65:271–276, 1991.

37. Kirklin JW, Barratt-Boyes BG (eds): Cardiac Surgery. New York, Churchill Livingstone, 1986, pp 1263–1327.

38. Peyton RB, Isom OW, Gaynor JW, et al: The aorta. *In* Sabiston DC, Jr, Spencer FC (eds): Surgery of the Chest, Vol II, 5th ed. Philadelphia, WB Saunders, 199, pp 1126–1221.

39. Knyshov GV, Sitar LL, Glagola MD, et al: Aortic aneurysm at the site of repair of coarctation of the aorta: A review of 48 patients. Ann Thorac Surg 61:935–939, 1996.

40. Fawzy ME, Sivanandam V, Galal O, et al: One- to ten-year follow-up of balloon angioplasty of native coarctation of the aorta in adolescents and adults. J Am Coll Cardiol 30:1542–1546, 1997.

41. Schrader R, Bussmann WD, Jacobi V, et al: Long-term effects of balloon coarctation angioplasty on arterial blood pressure in adolescent and adult patients. Cathet Cardiovasc Diagn 36:220–225, 1995.

42. Tyagi S, Arora R, Kaul UA, et al: Balloon angioplasty of native coarctation of the aorta in adolescents and young adults. Am Heart J 123:674–680, 1992.

43. Biswas PK, Mitra K, De S et al: Follow-up results of balloon angioplasty for native coarctation of aorta. Indian Heart J 48:673–676, 1996.

44. Dyet JF, Paddon AJ, Ettles DF, et al: Long-term follow up of balloon angioplasty for native adult aortic coarctation. Cardiovasc Intervent Radiol 21(suppl):S145, 1998.

45. Cooley DA, DeBakey ME: Resection of entire ascending aorta in fusiform aneurysm using cardiac bypass. JAMA 152:673–676, 1953.

46. DeBakey M, Crawford ES, Cooley DA, et al: Successful resection of a fusiform aneurysm of the aortic arch with replacement by homograft. Surg Gynecol Obstet 105:657–664, 1957.

47. Gillum RF: Epidemiology of aortic aneurysms in the United States. J Clin Epidemiol 48:1289–1298, 1995.

48. Perko MJ, Norgaard M, Herzog TM, et al: Unoperated aortic aneurysms: A survey of 170 patients. Ann Thorac Surg 59:1204–1209, 1995.

49. Verdant A, Cossette R, Page A, et al: Aneurysms of the descending thoracic aorta: Three hundred sixty-six consecutive cases resected without paraplegia. J Vasc Surg 21:385–90, 1995.

50. Borst HG, Jurmann M, Buhner B, et al: Risk of replacement of descending aorta with a standardized left heart bypass technique. J Thorac Cardiovasc Surg 107:126–133, 1994.

51. Schor JS, Yerlioglu ME, Galla JD, et al: Selective management of acute type B aortic dissection: Long-term follow-up. Ann Thorac Surg 61:1339–1341, 1996.

52. Hollier LH, Money SR, Naslund TC, et al: Risk of spinal cord dysfunction in patients undergoing thoracoabdominal aortic replacement. Am J Surg 164:210–214, 1992.

53. Crawford ES, Crawford JL, Safi HJ, et al: Thoracoabdominal aortic aneurysms: Preoperative and intraoperative factors determining immediate and long-term results of operations in 605 patients. J Vasc Surg 3:389–404, 1986.

54. Schepens MA, Defauw JJ, Hamerlijnck RP, et al: Surgical treatment of thoracoabdominal aortic aneurysms by simple cross-clamping. Risk factors and late results. J Thorac Cardiovasc Surg 107:134–142, 1994.

55. Scheinin SA, Cooley DA: Graft replacement of the descending thoracic aorta: Results of "open" distal anastomosis. Ann Thorac Surg 58:19–23, 1994.

56. Kouchoukos NT, Rokkas CK: Descending thoracic and thoracoabdominal aortic surgery for aneurysm or dissection: How do we minimize the risk of spinal cord injury? Semin Thorac Cardiovasc Surg 5:47–54, 1993.

57. Anagnostopoulos CE, Prabhakar MJ, Kittle CF. Aortic dissections and dissecting aneurysms. Am J Cardiol 30:263–73, 1972.

Chapter 33

Endovascular Repair of Iliac and Other Aneurysms

Endovascular Contributors: Henry W. Loose, John F. Dyet, Anthony A. Nicholson, and Duncan F. Ettles
Surgical Contributors: Geoffrey White, Takao Ohki, Frank J. Veith, and Arthur Stanton

BASIC CONCEPTS

An aneurysm can be defined as a bulging or dilatation of an artery associated with thinning of its wall. The main causes are atherosclerosis, infection, vasculitis, and injury. A false aneurysm is a contained rupture with a fibrous tissue wall that maintains its connection to the parent artery. Aneurysms usually are described as being either saccular or fusiform in shape.

The principal aim of treatment is to exclude the aneurysmal portion of artery from the general circulation to avoid the complications of rupture or embolization. This can be accomplished in five possible ways:

1. Simple occlusion of the artery both distally and proximally to the aneurysm as shown in Figures 33–1A–C. These show a mycotic aneurysm arising from the profunda femoris artery in a patient who had undergone removal of an infected hip prosthesis. In this case, it was possible to treat the aneurysm by sacrificing the artery. Embolization coils have been placed proximal and distal to the aneurysm neck.
2. By packing the aneurysmal sac with embolization coils. Figures 33–2A and 33–2B show an aneurysm of the left gastric artery that had bleed into the lesser sac. Treatment was embolization of all branches related to the aneurysm and filling the sac with coils. Although it may be possible to exclude an aneurysm by simply filling the sac with embolization coils, there have been instances in which the clot ball has later retracted away from the wall, allowing fresh filling of the cavity with subsequent rupture. Therefore, if possible, all feeders also should be embolized.
3. By occluding the neck of the aneurysm with a covered stent graft. Figure 33–3A shows a false aneurysm arising from the right subclavian artery and tracking down into the mediastinum. The an-

eurysm is iatrogenic in nature, caused by attempted central line placement. Treatment was by means of stent graft, as shown in Figure 33–3B.
4. By occluding the neck of the aneurysm by external pressure until thrombosis occurs within the aneurysm. (See discussion later.)
5. By causing thrombus formation within the aneurysm by direct injection of thrombin. (See discussion later.)

The subsequent sections in this chapter deal with specific methods of treating iliac and popliteal aneurysms, treatment of femoral pseudoaneurysms, and the use of stent grafts in traumatic arterial injury. Details of coil embolization are given in Chapter 25.

ILIAC ANEURYSMS

Demography

Iliac artery aneurysms most commonly affect the common iliac artery (70%) and the internal iliac artery (23%). The external iliac artery is involved infrequently. Aneurysms of the iliac arteries are bilateral in one quarter of cases and multiple in one third. It has been reported that 10 to 20% of patients with abdominal aortic aneurysms also have iliac aneurysms. Their occurrence in isolation is uncommon, accounting for less than 2% of all iliac aneurysms[1] and a prevalence of 8 to 30 per 100,000 in the population. Solitary aneurysms occur more commonly in men; the male:female ratio is 7:1.

Etiology

Iliac aneurysms have a diverse etiology, with degenerative, atherosclerotic aneurysms being most common. These aneurysms have a similar etiology to abdominal aortic aneurysms (AAAs), including an

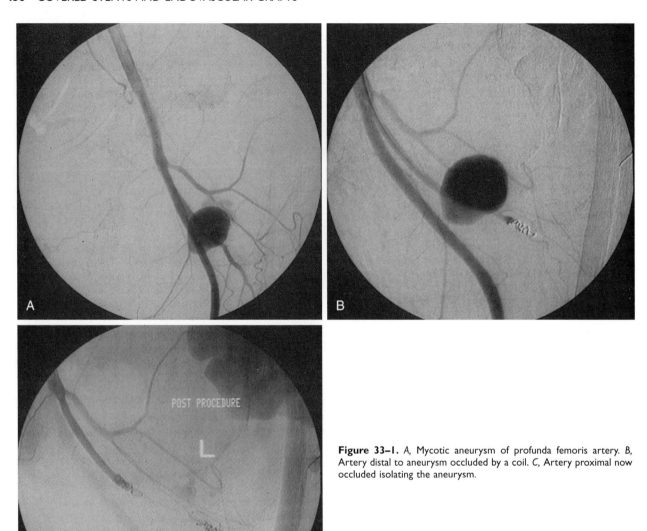

Figure 33–1. *A,* Mycotic aneurysm of profunda femoris artery. *B,* Artery distal to aneurysm occluded by a coil. *C,* Artery proximal now occluded isolating the aneurysm.

element of elastin degradation. Other causes include trauma and infections, occasionally related to percutaneous vascular procedures. False aneurysms are common, particularly anastomotic iliac aneurysms at the distal suture line of previously implanted aortoiliac grafts (Fig. 33–4). Other rare causes are Marfan's syndrome, Kawasaki disease, Takayasu's arteritis, Ehlers-Danlos syndrome, and cystic medial necrosis.

Symptoms and Signs

Physical examination reveals a palpable mass in 70% of patients with iliac aneurysms, this being palpable abdominally, rectally or vaginally. The mass is frequently tender. Hematuria or urosepsis may result from compression of the ureter at the pelvic brim or within the pelvis. Gastrointestinal bleeding may occur as a result of rupture into the rectosigmoid. Neurogenic pain may result from compression of branches of the lumbosacral plexus. About one quarter of solitary iliac aneurysms have rupture as their first sign of presentation. Alternatively, pain may be present by virtue of the mass effect of the aneurysm, especially if it lies in the true pelvis. More recently, asymptomatic aneurysms are being detected, particularly with the increasing use of ultrasonography, but also of computed tomography (CT) and magnetic resonance imaging (MRI), to investigate unrelated abdominal symptoms.

Isolated aneurysms of the internal iliac artery occur even less frequently, and because these are true pelvic aneurysms, abdominal physical examination is notoriously unreliable. Thus, rectal and vaginal exam-

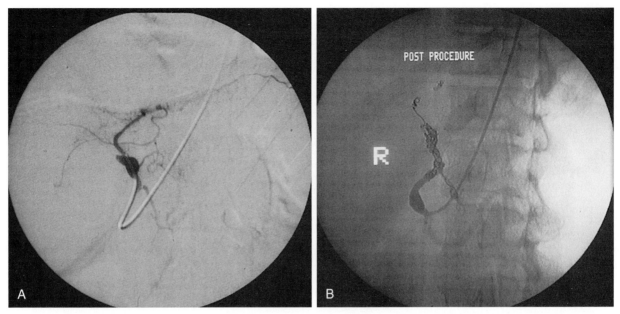

Figure 33–2. *A*, Aneurysm of left gastric artery. *B*, Result after embolization of feeders and packing the sac with coils.

ination is particularly important. Because these aneurysms are not detected at an early stage, when they are small, one third of patients present with rupture.

Investigation and Assessment

As with endovascular repair of AAAs, good-quality pretreatment imaging is essential. All patients should have helical CT and angiography performed. The maximum diameter and length of the aneurysmal segment should be determined, regardless of whether the internal iliac artery is involved. Careful assessment of the length and diameter of the normal artery

proximal and distal to the aneurysm is required to select the most appropriate endovascular device. Although CT is best for assessment of diameter (Fig. 33–5), an angiogram performed with a graduated catheter through the aneurysm gives a better indication of the length of the stent graft required and also the relationship of the internal iliac artery to the aneurysm sac (Fig. 33–6). Because good anchoring points are required for successful aneurysm exclusion, a proximal neck of at least 2 cm of normal artery is taken as ideal, with a similar distal neck. If the aneurysm arises at the aortic bifurcation, then the only form of endovascular repair possible is the use of a bifurcated aortic system.

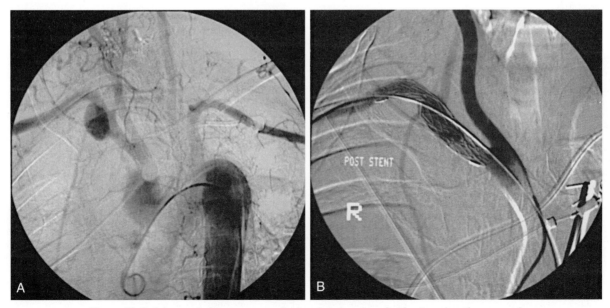

Figure 33–3. *A*, Iatrogenic false aneurysm of right subclavian artery. *B*, After insertion of a stent graft.

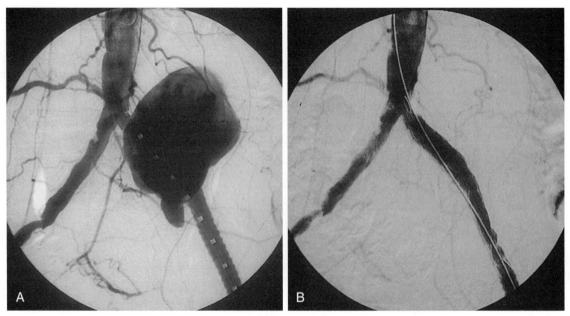

Figure 33–4. *A*, False aneurysm at upper anastomosis of an iliofemoral graft. *B*, Appearance after stent grafting.

Natural History

The natural history of untreated iliac aneurysms is not well defined. Aneurysms as small as 3 cm have been known to rupture.[2] The estimated expansion rate of iliac aneurysms is 4 mm/year (similar to that of infrarenal AAA). Operative intervention generally is recommended if the size is greater than 3 cm.

Complications of untreated iliac aneurysms primarily are related to rupture. This occurs most commonly into the retroperitoneum or peritoneal cavity, although rupture into the colon also has been described.

Operative Treatment

The details of operative technique depend on a variety of factors, the most important being the site of the

aneurysm(s), the presence of bilateral aneurysms, and whether the inferior mesenteric artery is patent to provide adequate flow to the pelvic organs. Operative intervention on iliac aneurysms may be very challenging because these aneurysms are usually large on presentation, because they are closely related and beneath the ureter, and especially because they are located in the pelvis, where limited space hinders exposure, especially in males.[3] Because of this, the mortality rate from elective repair of iliac aneurysms

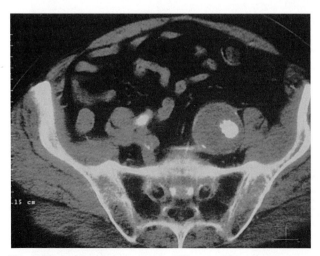

Figure 33–5. Computed tomography (CT) scan of iliac aneurysm immediately after stent insertion.

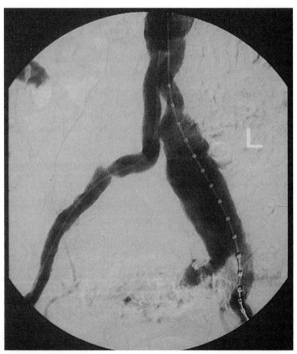

Figure 33–6. Aneurysm of the left common iliac artery involving the origin of the internal iliac. Graduated catheter in situ.

approaches 10%.[4] In addition, the problems associated with bilateral repair of iliac aneurysms carry a risk of pelvic and buttock ischemia if restitution of internal iliac flow is not maintained.

Open surgical treatment of common iliac aneurysms usually consists of control of blood flow by vascular clamping, opening into the aneurysm, and reconstitution of flow by graft inlay using a straight prosthetic graft (polytetrafluoroethylene [PTFE] or Dacron) anastomosed distally to the site of bifurcation of the common iliac artery. If the iliac aneurysm is associated with an AAA, then repair of both the aortic and iliac aneurysms is achieved with a bifurcated graft.

Aneurysms of the internal iliac artery are more difficult to reconstruct because of their position in the pelvis. Simple ligation at the origin of the internal iliac artery is not sufficient because there is major collateral flow crossing the pelvis from the contralateral side, which continues to perfuse the aneurysm with systemic pressure, resulting in continued growth. These aneurysms should be managed operatively by inflow control, opening the aneurysm, and oversewing the patent orifices of the branches of the artery. Temporary control of backflow from the branches may be achieved by the use of multiple balloon catheters. If both internal iliac arteries must be sacrificed, then efforts should be made to ensure that there is adequate pelvic perfusion by the inferior mesenteric artery. One of the most important complications that occurs in male patients is impotence, which may result from either neurogenic (division of the sympathetic plexus overlying the distal aorta and the proximal left common iliac artery) or vasculogenic causes (from ligation of both internal iliac aneurysms).

Endoluminal Repair

RATIONALE FOR ENDOVASCULAR REPAIR OF ILIAC ANEURYSMS

Although open surgical repair of iliac aneurysms has excellent long-term results, the operative procedure carries high morbidity and the perioperative mortality rate is similar to open repair of AAAs. There are particular technical problems associated with gaining proximal control, avoiding damage to the ureter and to the iliac veins, and treatment of the aneurysmal or diseased internal iliac artery. The operation usually requires an intraperitoneal approach, so that paralytic ileus or bowel obstruction may result. Repair of iliac artery aneurysms has been reported in several series.[5–8] Tube grafts of diameter ranging from 10 to 16 mm usually are used, and adjunctive coil embolization of the internal iliac artery often is required to prevent retrograde backflow into the aneurysm sac. The smaller-diameter grafts may be implanted by percutaneous technique.[8]

Conversely, endovascular repair can be achieved by percutaneous sheath access or by a small cut-down incision to the femoral artery, and to date has been associated with low rates of morbidity and mortality. In our vascular unit, the early excellent results and low incidence of severe complications has led to endovascular repair becoming the treatment of choice for most patients with iliac aneurysms, particularly those who have had previous aortic surgery or who have significant risk factors for open surgery.

ENDOVASCULAR DEVICES

Early reports of this procedure initially documented the use of homemade devices.[9] More recently, commercially manufactured systems have become available, and reports of their use have been documented.[7, 10, 11]

There currently are two devices that can be placed percutaneously via a 10-French sheath. These are the Boston Scientific Passager device and the Jomed covered stent. The Passager has a nitinol endoskeleton consisting of individual rings of zigzag nitinol wire sutured together to form a self-expanding stent. The stent then is covered by thin-walled Dacron, which is sutured intermittently onto the stent. The stent graft is delivered using a pusher to advance it through its own sheath. The Jomed stent graft consists of a tube of Dacron sandwiched between two stainless steel balloon-expandable stents. The stent graft has to be hand-crimped onto an appropriately sized balloon and then delivered via a 10-French sheath.

There are a number of other devices that can be used. These consist of the iliac limbs of modular AAA stent grafts. They are self-expanding stents covered either externally or internally with thin-walled Dacron. Most of these devices require a femoral arteriotomy for insertion.

Whichever device is chosen, good-quality imaging is mandatory. Angulation of the X-ray tube and intensifier in both medial-to-lateral and cranial-to-caudal directions is required to visualize the normal arterial neck proximal to the aneurysm to ensure accurate placement.

TECHNIQUES AND PATIENT SELECTION

For isolated iliac aneurysms, a proximal segment of relatively normal iliac artery is required for implantation and attachment of the proximal part of the graft. This proximal implant area or "attachment zone" should be at least 10 mm in length and free of mural thrombus. Severe angulation or tortuosity of the iliac segment and firm calcification of the arterial wall are negative factors that may lead to failure of the procedure. If there is no proximal iliac neck segment, the choice becomes one of use of a bifurcated aortic graft with extension iliac limbs used to exclude the iliac aneurysm, or conventional open repair.

Device selection depends on accurate imaging and precise measurement of the diameter of the iliac segment proximal and distal to the aneurysm. In most cases, a graft needs to bridge both the common and external iliac arteries; the size change from the common iliac to the external artery usually results in external compression and narrowing of the distal section of the graft.

The deployment and implantation techniques vary according to the individual device being used. Preprocedure on-table angiography may be done via an angiographic catheter introduced from the contralateral side, which also allows for progress images to be obtained during and immediately after the deployment.

Embolization of the internal iliac artery often is required as an adjunctive procedure to prevent persistent retrograde blood flow into the aneurysm sac. This usually is achieved by percutaneous metallic coil introduction, done at the time of the iliac endograft or some days before. In some cases, the orifice of the internal iliac is occluded by the iliac endograft itself so that embolization of this vessel is not necessary. When there is an aneurysm of the internal iliac artery itself, the primary branches must be embolized rather than the trunk. Before this embolization, it is important to know whether the opposite internal iliac is patent; otherwise, disabling buttock claudication may develop, and the patient must be warned of this possibility. In addition, if the inferior mesenteric artery is occluded, a single internal iliac artery may give the blood supply to the distal colon, and embolization of this vessel may cause ischemic colitis.

From the ipsilateral groin, the internal iliac artery is selectively catheterized—a Sos catheter or SIM 1 design is usually best for this. Either via this catheter or through a coaxially placed microcatheter, embolization coils are passed into the artery to occlude it (Fig. 33–7). A steerable hydrophilic wire then is used to negotiate the iliac system, through the aneurysm and into the aorta. It is probably advisable at this stage to advance a catheter into the aorta and exchange the steerable wire for an extra stiff one to give extra support. The appropriately sized sheath or delivery introducer then is advanced over the wire to a point above the proximal delivery site. Using fluoroscopic guidance and angiography, the stent graft is advanced through the delivery sheath such that its upper margin lies precisely where required. The stent graft then is delivered, taking care that it is not displaced during this maneuver.

After delivery, self-expanding stent grafts are best

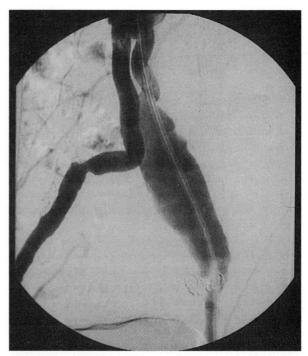

Figure 33–7. Same case as Figure 33–6; the internal iliac artery has been occluded with embolization coils.

ballooned throughout their length and particularly at their anchor sites to make sure they have fully expanded. If the aneurysm is long, it may be necessary to use more than one stent graft. If this is required, a good overlap should be ensured (at least 2 cm), or the stent grafts may dislocate as the aneurysm begins to shrink after successful exclusion. Once the graft is satisfactorily deployed, a completion angiogram is obtained to check for endoleaks. In such cases, additional balloon expansion or occasionally placement of an additional stent graft may be required.

Unless contraindicated, all patients having this procedure should begin low-dose aspirin 48 hours before the procedure and continue it for life. The procedure also should be covered by adequate heparinization. This regimen helps prevent early and late graft thrombosis. Follow-up of the patient should be by CT (Fig. 33–8), with a baseline examination before discharge, then at 3 and 6 months, and yearly thereafter (Fig. 33–9).

COMPLICATIONS

To date, the major problems encountered in endoluminal grafting of iliac artery aneurysms have been caused by difficult anatomy or inadequate graft design. Inadequate proximal "neck" segment or severe angulation of the common iliac artery results in endoleak and unsuccessful procedures in many cases. Ill-advised attempts to perform endoluminal graft repair of iliac aneurysms that do not have a proximal neck

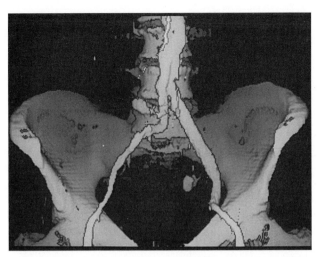

Figure 33–8. Completion CT. Same case as Figures 33–6 and 33–7.

or have a very dilated iliac segment result in failure to exclude the aneurysm; such cases are an indication for use of an aortoiliac or bifurcated aortic endovascular graft device.

Perforation or dissection injury of the iliac arterial wall can be caused by the introducer sheath in tortuous, calcified arteries. Severe angulation also can result in kinking and thrombosis of the implanted endograft.

Persistent retrograde perfusion and late expansion of an internal iliac artery aneurysm may result if the branches have not been occluded by embolic coils or other means. Stent graft misplacement may be corrected by placement of an additional stent or may result, as with device failure, in conversion to conventional surgical repair.

With commercially manufactured fully supported stent grafts, kinking is unlikely, but if it does occur, it can be corrected by insertion of an additional endovascular stent. In this instance, a balloon-expandable stent with high radial force is probably best. Graft thrombosis can be treated by thrombolysis followed by anticoagulation.

Late endoleaks remain the greatest potential problem, although it may be possible to treat these with additional stent graft placement. Persistent endoleaks put the aneurysm at risk of rupture, and if endovascular treatment is unsuccessful or not possible, then conventional surgical repair with explantation of the device or bypass must be carried out.

RESULTS

Our experience of endoluminal graft repair of iliac aneurysms is summarized in Table 33–1. We did our early cases with improvised balloon-expandable devices custom-made for each patient.[5] This allowed size adjustment of the graft for the individual anatomy, including graft tapering. The more recent experience has been with commercially manufactured self-expanding devices. Direct comparison of results is not valid because case selection included more challenging anatomies as experience increased. Graft thrombosis occurred in two patients because of external compression and kink of the graft lumen. Graft infection occurred in one patient who was treated with three percutaneously placed self-expanding grafts in a protracted case. The infection presented as an episode of bacterial endocarditis, and the source was confirmed to be the endoluminal graft after graft excision.

Perioperative mortality occurred in one patient (4%) in this series who suffered postoperative stroke several weeks after the implant procedure. This mor-

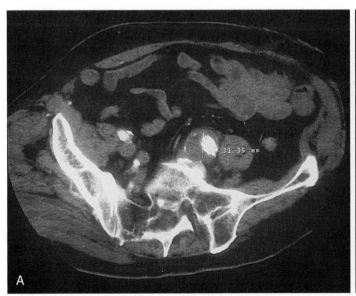
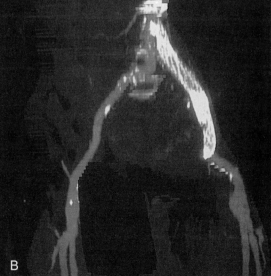

Figure 33–9. *A,* Transverse CT showing aneurysm shrinkage compared with Figure 33–5 at 2 years. *B,* Same case at 2 years.

Table 33–1. Endoluminal Repair of Iliac Aneurysms—Results

Device	No. of Cases	Endoleak	Thrombosis	Infection	Success
Balloon-expandable (White-Yu GAD Graft)	13	1	0	0	12 (92%)
Self-expanding (Passager, Talent, AneuRx, Wallgraft)	11	2	1	1	7 (64%)

tality rate compares favorably with open surgical repair.

To date, the largest published series is the French multicenter study.[7] Twenty-seven aneurysms were excluded using the Cragg Endopro 1 system. There was one death (4%) due to bleeding from the arterial puncture site, two device failures, and two endoleaks. There was one late graft thrombosis. In the series of Marin and colleagues,[6] three complications were reported in 11 patients—transient colonic ischemia, groin lymphocele, and a kinked graft. In the series of Razavi and associates[12] and Quinn and colleagues[13] there were no deaths and only one device failure in a total of 16 cases.

The long-term results of this treatment are not known because no series has yet reported beyond 12 months.

ANASTOMOTIC ANEURYSMS

Several clinical studies have reported good results for endograft placement for management of anastomotic aneurysms after aortic or aortoiliac graft procedures.[9–11] In many of these cases, a tube graft can be used, and the presence of the aortic graft provides an excellent proximal implant zone. These procedures can be done with a high degree of success, low morbidity, and short hospital stay.

POPLITEAL ANEURYSMS

Demography

Popliteal aneurysms account for 90% of all peripheral aneurysms. Males are more commonly affected, and in 50% of patients the popliteal aneurysms are bilateral.[14] The presence of a popliteal aneurysm is a good indicator of the presence of other aneurysms, with aortic, femoral, and iliac aneurysms having an increased incidence. This is especially so if bilateral popliteal aneurysms are present.

Etiology and Natural History

Popliteal aneurysms are most commonly caused by atherosclerosis or by trauma. They are most commonly fusiform in shape and may extend to involve a portion or all of the superficial femoral artery. This morphology usually is associated with atherosclerotic degeneration. Saccular aneurysms are less common and are usually false in nature, with most caused by trauma. These aneurysms usually are well localized to the midpopliteal level.

Of initially asymptomatic aneurysms, it is estimated that two thirds become symptomatic over a 5-year follow-up. Complications of popliteal aneurysms usually result in a significant risk for the involved limb. This forms the basis for early treatment of popliteal aneurysms because the natural history is one of continued obliteration of the runoff vessels and, ultimately, thrombosis of the aneurysm. This is more likely to occur if the popliteal aneurysm is greater than 2 cm in diameter. Patients who have their popliteal aneurysms repaired should be observed closely because a new peripheral aneurysm will develop in half these patients within 10 years.

Symptoms and Signs

The symptoms and signs of popliteal aneurysms depend on the complications produced. Embolization is the most common complication and results in occlusion of tibial vessels and distal ischemia. Patients usually have absent pulses in the foot and calf claudication. Thrombosis of the aneurysm is relatively common. Again, pedal pulses are absent, as is the popliteal pulse. However, a mass is palpable in the popliteal fossa. Rupture is a rare event, possibly because of the support afforded the popliteal artery by surrounding tissue. Nerve and vein compression may occur in the popliteal fossa, with resultant neurogenic pain in the distribution of the posterior tibial nerve or with deep vein thrombosis and edema.

Diagnosis

Diagnosis is best established by physical examination and duplex scanning. A high degree of suspicion is necessary because the presence of other peripheral aneurysms is a particularly important indicator. Duplex scanning is helpful in documenting size, extent, and the presence of mural thrombus within the aneurysms. Angiograms always are performed before operative or endovascular treatment because they are essential in procedure planning. Duplex scanning is an ideal way of follow-up or of monitoring aneurysm size in patients not undergoing intervention.

Operative Treatment

The indications for treatment of popliteal aneurysms are controversial. Aneurysm diameter greater than 2 cm and the presence of symptoms are the two main indications for treatment. The presence of symptoms or the recent onset of symptoms are known to be associated with a higher incidence of complications and limb loss compared with patients who are asymptomatic.[15]

Selection of operative technique depends on a variety of factors, including the etiology and morphology of the aneurysm and the presence of inflow and outflow vessels. Treatment consists of ligation above and below the aneurysm, with subsequent bypass to the distal popliteal artery or to a patent tibial vessel. The aneurysm is not excised because compressive symptoms are usually not present. The conduit of choice is the autogenous vein because the reconstruction is usually below the knee. The site of proximal ligation may be at the origin of the superficial femoral artery if this vessel is involved by diffuse aneurysmal disease. The popliteal artery usually is approached medially in this situation. However, a localized popliteal aneurysm is easily approachable via a posterior approach. In this scenario, saccular aneurysms may be treated by lateral repair or interposition grafting. Thrombolytic therapy may be beneficial in the initial management of thrombosed popliteal aneurysms. Thrombolysis before surgical intervention decreases the amputation rate by restoring flow to the popliteal artery and recanalizing the tibial runoff vessels. However, the volume of thrombus in the popliteal artery is problematic and may require prolonged use of lytic therapy.

Long-term graft patency rates of 90% at 5 years are common after elective operative intervention for popliteal aneurysms. However, results are less favorable in patients who present with limb-threatening ischemia, with 5-year patency rates reduced to approximately 40%.

Endovascular Repair of Popliteal Aneurysms

Successful exclusion of popliteal aneurysms by endoluminal stent grafts has been reported from several sources.[5, 16–19] The procedure may be performed by percutaneous access sheath or by cutdown to the femoral artery. It appears, however, that thrombosis occurs in a high percentage of cases within the first 6 to 12 months of follow-up. This has been our experience, and for this reason, we currently do not favor endoluminal repair for aneurysms at this site, except for patients at significantly high risk for conventional open repair. Devices implanted within the popliteal artery are subject to frequent flexion, with the potential for stent breakage, kinking, or compression.

FEMORAL PSEUDOANEURYSMS

Previously, false aneurysm formation at the puncture site after cardiac or peripheral catheterization was regarded as a relatively rare occurrence. There is little doubt that over the past few years, this complication has increased in frequency, particularly in relation to interventional cardiologic procedures. This has occurred for two reasons: first, the larger French systems used for coronary angioplasty and coronary atherectomy carry a small but significant increase in puncture site complications; and second, the more aggressive anticoagulant and antiplatelet therapies used in conjunction with coronary artery stenting predispose these patients to postprocedural bleeding and hematoma formation. Early reports concerning puncture site pseudoaneurysm formation suggested that this complication was predisposed to by low femoral puncture.[20] This is often the case, but practical experience from ultrasound examinations in such patients demonstrates that pseudoaneurysms can arise after both low and high femoral punctures. The use of mechanical hemostatic devices and careless attention to hemostasis are, in the authors' experience, further possible contributory factors in the increased incidence of femoral artery pseudoaneurysms.

The typical presenting features of a pulsatile and painful groin swelling allow clinical diagnosis in most cases, which is confirmed easily by duplex ultrasound. Usually, the patient is aware of the pseudoaneurysm within 24 hours of catheterization, but later presentations of up to 1 week sometimes are seen. Almost always there is a history of significant postprocedural bleeding or groin hematoma.

Conservative management may be all that is needed, and some small false aneurysms undergo spontaneous thrombosis. More commonly, patients are referred for radiologic intervention to provide symptomatic relief and avoid the rare but potentially catastrophic complication of false aneurysm rupture. Treatment options include ultrasound-guided compression, percutaneous injection of fibrin adhesive or thrombin, and coil embolization.

Ultrasound-Guided Compression

This simple technique was first described by Fellmeth and colleagues.[21] Ultrasound examination with color flow Doppler is used to confirm the presence of the false aneurysm and determine its size and the position and orientation of the puncture site. It is not uncommon to find lateral or low-positioned puncture sites, but equally common is the appearance of a calcified and diseased vessel that may be less likely to have the ability to exhibit the mural response that contributes to hemostasis. The degree of thrombosis within the sac also can be assessed by ultrasound. In those cases in which there is already a large amount of thrombus and a small flow within the aneurysms, it may be reasonable to manage the patient conservatively and repeat the scan within 2 to 3 days to determine whether there has been spontaneous thrombosis.

TECHNIQUE

The technique of ultrasound-guided compression uses the ultrasound probe to image the vessel and false aneurysm and to act as the compression device. In most cases, local infiltration using 1% lignocaine is helpful in allowing the patient to tolerate the procedure. In some patients, intravenous sedation or analgesia may be required because of the considerable discomfort that may be experienced during compression. Having established the position and orientation of the track between the vessel and false aneurysm, the transducer is applied firmly to the site until color flow within the pseudoaneurysm is abolished. Often, the compression needed will be sufficient to also abolish flow within the common femoral artery. A series of compressions then is performed, starting with 10 minutes of compression and increasing incrementally to 30 minutes. Check examinations can be made immediately once the pressure has been removed. As well as showing residual flow within the aneurysm, the degree of thrombus formation also can be documented. It is always a mistake to release pressure too soon, but the procedure can be very tiring for the operator. Success is confirmed by cessation of color flow within the pseudoaneurysm on release of compression and the presence of thrombus within the aneurysm. A check ultrasound examination before hospital discharge to confirm continued success is useful. One approach that may avoid prolonged manual compression involves the use of an external compression device (Femostop) to abolish flow within the false aneurysm.[22] If the diaphragm of the compression device is filled with water rather than air, it is possible to image the common femoral artery through the water-filled chamber and confirm effective compression. Ultrasound-guided compression of common femoral false aneurysm currently is regarded as the treatment of choice in managing this complication and has an initial high success rate ranging between 76% and 97%.[21, 23, 24] When the false aneurysms is

small and can be compressed against bone, strenuous efforts should be made to treat the false aneurysms by this means before proceeding to other alternatives. For the patient, this sometimes can mean more than one visit to the ultrasound department on consecutive days for attempted compression. After successful treatment, there is a recurrence rate of up to 20%, and continued anticoagulation is associated with a lower success rate.

Coil Embolization

If there is an identifiable vessel feeding the false aneurysm and this vessel can be sacrificed without compromise of other structures, then embolization of the feeding vessel can be performed via a contralateral arterial approach (Fig. 33–10). An alternative technique is to place coils directly into the false aneurysm percutaneously, thereby inducing thrombosis.[25] Close packing of coils may be needed to abolish flow, and the technique leaves a permanent mass lesion that can give rise to discomfort beneath the skin. Covered stents have been used successfully to exclude femoropopliteal aneurysms,[26, 27] but these are not ideally suited to treatment of puncture site aneurysms because of the proximity to the hip joint and potential for stent break-up with repeated flexion.

Percutaneous Injection of Thrombin or Fibrin Adhesive

Percutaneous puncture and injection of thrombin for the treatment of aneurysms was described by Cope and Zeit in 1986,[28] and transluminal catheter delivery of thrombin has been described in treatment of a profunda femoris pseudoaneurysm.[29] The use of bovine thrombin in this way has not been associated with significant adverse reactions, but there is a potential for allergic reactions. Fibrin was noted to function as an adhesive many years ago,[30] and clot adhesives are used in surgery to repair cerebrospinal fluid (CSF) leaks and seal vascular anastomoses, for hemostasis after hepatic tumour resection, and in dental surgery to promote hemostasis in patients taking anticoagulants.[31–34] Commercially produced fibrin adhesive (Beriplast) is presented in two vials that can be injected simultaneously or sequentially into the false aneurysm. The vials contain fibrinogen concentrate, factor VIII, aprotinin, calcium chloride, and thrombin. Production from identifiable sources is essential to avoid any possibility of transmission of human immunodeficiency virus (HIV) or bovine spongiform encephalopathy (BSE). In vitro thromboelastogram studies have confirmed rapid clot formation with a measurable strength greater than natural clot in the

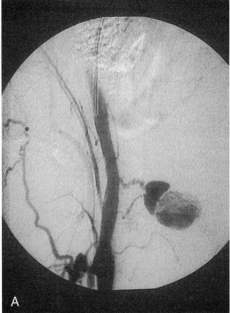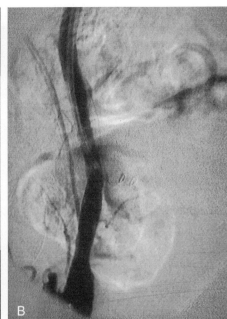

Figure 33–10. *A,* False aneurysm arising from the inferior epigastric artery in a patient who had undergone previous antegrade femoral puncture. Ultrasound-guided compression was unsuccessful. *B,* Using a contralateral approach, a single embolization coil was positioned in the feeding vessel with complete cessation of flow.

same individual, particularly those receiving anticoagulation.[35]

TECHNIQUE

Preliminary angiography, usually from a contralateral approach, confirms the position of the false aneurysm and its neck. An appropriately sized angioplasty balloon is placed across the aneurysm neck and inflated. Balloon occlusion both abolishes flow in the false aneurysm and prevents possible distal embolization. After cessation of flow within the aneurysm has been confirmed by ultrasound, the aneurysm cavity is punctured using a 21-gauge needle under local anaesthetic. If necessary, the angioplasty balloon can be deflated to confirm correct positioning. Two to 3 ml of blood then is injected through the needle until the patient feels distension. The reason for this is as follows: although angiography usually demonstrates a single aneurysm cavity, ultrasound often reveals one or more loculi containing soft thrombus. These loculi must be filled before injection of the coagulant.

The fibrin adhesive is injected in small aliquots through the 21-gauge needle, and the formation of thrombus is monitored by repeated ultrasound examination. The angioplasty balloon is deflated after 20 minutes, and angiography is performed to confirm complete cessation of flow. Check ultrasound is performed at 24 hours.

The foot should be observed during the procedure if the balloon has been inflated in the common femoral artery. This artery may require a larger balloon than first anticipated to occlude flow because pseudoaneurysms often are situated at the common femoral bifurcation (Fig. 33–11). Figure 33–12 shows

the technique used in a aneurysm of the tibioperoneal trunk. Although most operators prefer to perform this technique with an occluding balloon, direct injection and thrombin injection of femoral false aneurysms has been described without balloon protection.[35, 36] In this technique, careful ultrasound monitoring is used to confirm the relationship of the tip of a small percutaneously placed catheter or needle to the aneurysm neck. With the catheter tip adjusted to point away from the neck, thrombin is injected until there is cessation of flow. Clearly, the potential risk with this approach is of thrombus propagation or embolization back into the femoral artery. However, in the small reported series, there are no reported embolic episodes.[35, 36]

ENDOVASCULAR STENTS IN THE MANAGEMENT OF ARTERIAL TRAUMA

Over the past 20 years, there has been an increase in the incidence of acute arterial injuries. This has been the result of an increase in the numbers of road traffic accidents, a rise in civilian violent crime, and the development in medicine of procedures complicated by iatrogenic arterial injuries. Penetrating arterial trauma may cause exsanguination, arterial occlusion, or the formation of pseudoaneurysms and arteriovenous fistulas. The 20th century has seen enough war for there to be an extensive literature on the surgical management of such injuries.[37, 38] All agree that speed in diagnosis and treatment is essential. Surgical repair may be complicated by inaccessibility, particularly in the thorax, abdomen, and pelvis. In addition, hematomas, pseudoaneurysms, and arteriovenous fistulas

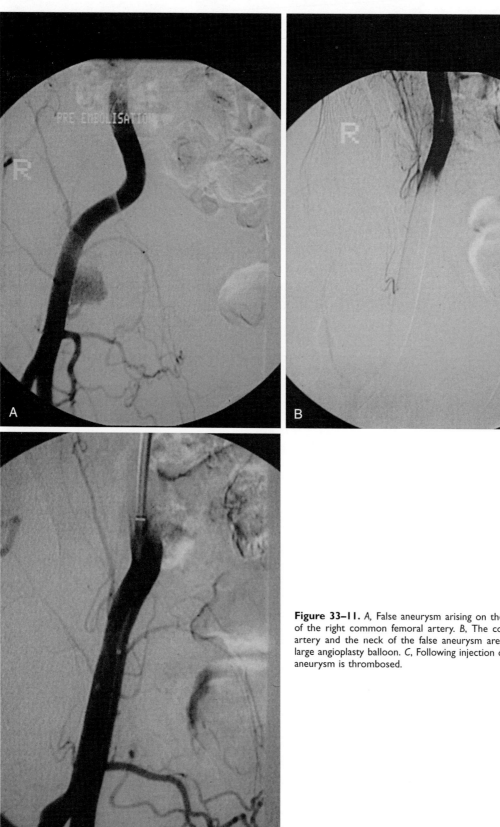

Figure 33–11. *A,* False aneurysm arising on the medial aspect of the right common femoral artery. *B,* The common femoral artery and the neck of the false aneurysm are occluded by a large angioplasty balloon. *C,* Following injection of thrombin the aneurysm is thrombosed.

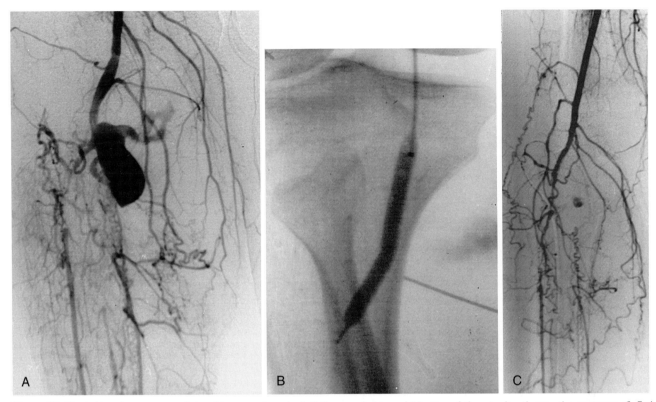

Figure 33–12. *A,* Mycotic aneurysm of the tibioperoneal trunk. *B,* Balloon occlusion and injection of thromin directly into the aneurysm. *C,* End result—the aneurysm no longer fills.

may distort anatomy and increase venous pressure, leading to significant surgical blood loss.

Embolization, described in Chapter 24, is the treatment of choice for such trauma in which small arteries are damaged, particularly when these can be sacrificed. However, in large arteries, in which continued forward flow is essential for more distal viability, stent grafts offer a useful alternative. These devices offer endovascular repair of arterial injury from sites remote to the area of trauma. They have extended significantly the potential of endovascular therapy for vascular trauma and have been used in circumstances in which coil embolization was deemed inappropriate. Although most cases that have been treated with stent grafts have been hemodynamically stable, in some instances, they have been used to treat life-threatening acute hemorrhage.[39] Devices used have been predominantly a combination of a Palmaz stent and an expanded PTFE graft (Fig. 33–13). Because the traumatized field often is contaminated, the use of autologous vein covering a Palmaz stent also has been reported (Fig. 33–14*A*).[40, 41] The different types of stent grafts that have been reported are summarized in Table 33–2 and are shown in Figure 33–14.

The lesion characteristics, site of arterial access, technical success rate, and the outcome of stent grafts in the treatment of vascular trauma are summarized in Table 33–3. These results have been encouraging, with a high technical success rate (94–100%) and a

complication rate of 0 to 7% (see Table 33–4), especially when one considers the difficulties that could be encountered in treating these lesions by a direct surgical repair. In addition, the minimal invasiveness and the potential for cost-effectiveness of such endovascular techniques are apparent from the short length of stay (3.3–5.3 days) in patients so treated (see Table 33–2). Because these devices mainly were inserted in nonatherosclerotic, central vessels of a large caliber, patency has been impressive, ranging from 85 to 100%, depending on location, with a mean follow-up of 16 months. One of the largest world experiences with stent grafts for arterial trauma has been at the Montefiore Medical Center in New York (Table 33–4).

The Montefiore Experience

TECHNIQUE AND DEVICES

At Montefiore Medical Center, the Palmaz stent in combination with a thin-walled PTFE graft covering has been the main device used to perform arterial repairs of pseudoaneurysms and arteriovenous fistulas. Depending on the length of the lesion, either a single stent device or a doubly stented device has been used (see Fig. 33–13). The stents vary between 2 to 3 cm in length (Palmaz P-204, 294, 308) and are

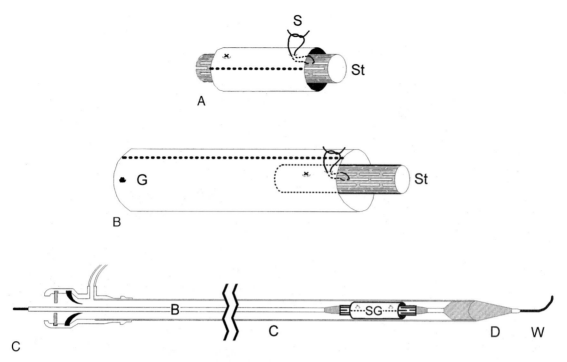

Figure 33–13. *A,* Schematic drawing of a single stent endovascular stented graft or covered stent. A segment of polytetrafluoroethylene (PTFE) is attached to a Palmaz stent (st) using two 5-0 Prolene "U" stitches (s). *B,* Schematic drawing of a double stent endovascular stented graft. The proximal stent (st) is sutured to the distal end of the graft as described in *A.* In addition, the distal end of the graft is marked with gold markers (G) for visualization under fluoroscope. The second (distal) stent is delivered and deployed separately after proximal stent deployment. *C,* The stent graft (SG) is mounted on an angioplasty balloon (B) and placed into a sheath (C) before insertion. Note the presence of a dilator tip (D) at the end of the balloon catheter, which provides a smooth taper within the catheter (W = guide wire). (Reprinted with permission from Ohki T, Veith FJ, Marin ML, et al: Endovascular approaches to vascular injuries. Semin Vasc Surg 10:272–285, 1997.)

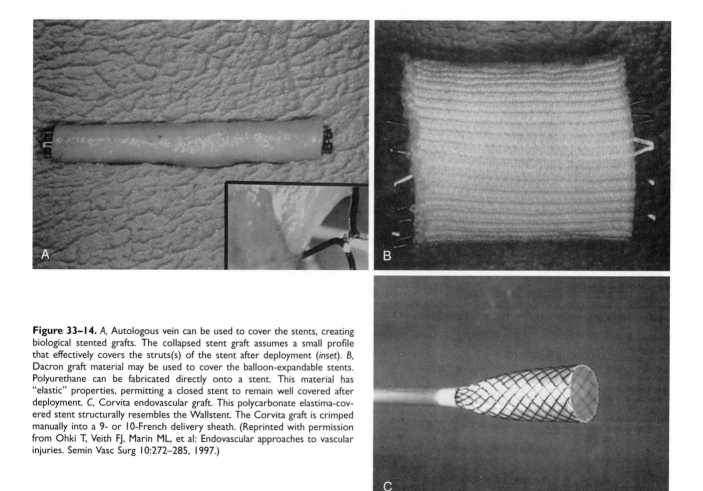

Figure 33–14. *A,* Autologous vein can be used to cover the stents, creating biological stented grafts. The collapsed stent graft assumes a small profile that effectively covers the struts(s) of the stent after deployment (*inset*). *B,* Dacron graft material may be used to cover the balloon-expandable stents. Polyurethane can be fabricated directly onto a stent. This material has "elastic" properties, permitting a closed stent to remain well covered after deployment. *C,* Corvita endovascular graft. This polycarbonate elastima-covered stent structurally resembles the Wallstent. The Corvita graft is crimped manually into a 9- or 10-French delivery sheath. (Reprinted with permission from Ohki T, Veith FJ, Marin ML, et al: Endovascular approaches to vascular injuries. Semin Vasc Surg 10:272–285, 1997.)

Table 33–2. Endovascular Grafts for Arterial Trauma

Type	Combination of Palmaz Stent and Various Grafts				Cragg Endopro	Corvita Graft
Stent	Palmaz stent				Nitinol	Self-expanding braided stent
Graft material	PTFE	Dacron	Vein	Silicone	Ultrathin woven polyester fabric	Polycarbonate urethane
Arterial access	1 or 2	2	2	1 or 2	2	2
Reference	11–18, 24	12	14, 19	15, 20	21	12, 22

PTFE = polytetrafluoroethylene.
1 = Open arteriotomy; 2 = percutaneous.
Reprinted in part from Ohki T, Marin ML, Veith FJ: Use of endovascular grafts to treat non-aneurysmal arterial disease. Ann Vasc Surg 11:200–205, 1997.

fixed inside 6-mm Goretex grafts by two "U" stitches. The stent grafts then are mounted on a balloon angioplasty catheter that has a tapered dilator tip firmly attached to its end. The entire device is contained within a 12-French delivery system for over-the-wire insertion either percutaneously or through an open arteriotomy.

An alternative device used has been the Corvita stent graft, which is fabricated from a self-expanding stent of braided wire. The stent is covered with polycarbonate elastimer fibers (Fig. 33–14C). The stent graft may be cut to the desired length in the operating room, using a wire-cutting scissors, and then loaded into a specially designed delivery sheath. This sheath has a central "pusher" catheter that is used for maintaining the graft in position while the outer sheath is being retrieved.

RESULTS

All procedures but one have been performed in the operating room under fluoroscopic and intravascular ultrasonographic control. One Corvita graft was in-

serted in the angiography room. A total of 17 stent grafts or covered stents have been used to treat 17 patients with traumatic arterial lesions (see Table 33–3). Seven injuries occurred as a result of gunshot wounds and one as a result of a knife wound. There were four iatrogenic catheterization injuries, and three as a result of arterial graft disruptions possibly associated with infection. In addition, two iatrogenic arterial injuries, the result of lumbar disc surgery and gynecologic surgery, were treated.

All injuries except one were associated with an adjacent pseudoaneurysm. In five instances, the arterial injury formed a fistula to an injured adjacent vein (Fig. 33–15A–D). Associated injuries were present in eight patients with arterial trauma (see Table 33–3). Most procedures were performed under either local or epidural anesthetic. Procedural complications were limited to one distal embolus, which was treated with suction embolectomy, and one wound hematoma, which resolved without further intervention. Graft patency rate was 100% with no early or late graft occlusions (mean follow-up 30 months [range 6–46 months]). One patient with a left axillary–subclavian

Table 33–3. Characteristics of Lesion and Outcome by Location of Injury

Location of Trauma	Axillary–Subclavian Artery	Aorta or Iliac Artery	Femoral Artery
No. of Cases	18	15	5
Cause of Injury	Bullet: 55%; catheterization: 28%; others: 17%	Surgical: 36%; catheterization: 18%; bullet: 9%; others: 36%	Bullet: 60%; catheterization: 40%
Presence of Pseudoaneurysm	61%	67%	80%
Presence of AV Fistula	44%	73%	40%
Arterial Access	Brachial arteriotomy: 39%	Femoral arteriotomy: 64%	Femoral arteriotomy: 80%
	Brachial percutaneous: 39%	Femoral percutaneous: 36%	Femoral percutaneous: 20%
	Femoral percutaneous: 22%		
Technical Success Rate	94% (17/18)*	100%	100%
Complication: Minor	0%	7%	0%
Major	6%†	7%§	0%
Mean Length of Stay	3.3 d	4 d	5.3 d
Mean Follow-Up	18 m	10.5 m	17.4 m
Primary Patency	85%‡	100%	100%
References	11, 12, 14, 16, 17, 20, 22, 24	11, 12, 14, 15, 18, 21, 23	11, 12, 14, 19

*One failure due to misdiagnosis.
†Brachial artery injury during device insertion.
‡Two failures due to stent deformity.
§Distal embolization requiring thrombectomy.
Reprinted with permission from Ohki T, Marin ML, Veith FJ: Use of endovascular grafts to treat non-aneurysmal arterial disease. Ann Vasc Surg 11:200–205, 1997.

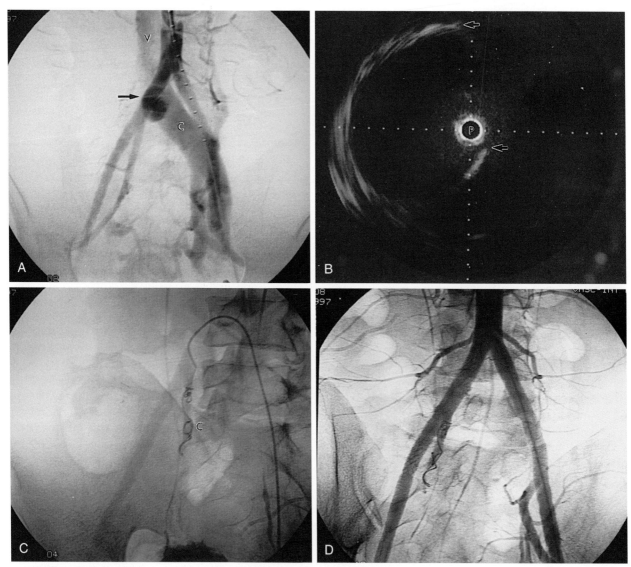

Figure 33–15. *A,* Preinterventional angiogram of an iatrogenic arteriovenous fistula (AVF) involving the right common iliac artery due to lumbar disc surgery. The left common iliac vein (C) and the inferior vena cava (V) are visualized by the contrast flowing through the AVF (*arrow*). However, the exact location of the AVF relative to the internal iliac artery and the precise size of the fistula are not clearly shown. *B,* Intravascular ultrasound (IVUS) image taken at the time of angiography. The amount of substance loss and the location (by identifying the location of the probe, P, of the IVUS under fluoroscopy) are well demonstrated (arrows denote the extent of the fistula). *C,* Coil embolization of the right internal iliac artery. Because the location of the fistula was 0.5 cm from the origin of the internal iliac artery measured by the technique described previously, the internal iliac artery was embolized with embolization coils (C) at the time of angiogram. *D,* Completion angiogram. A Corvita graft (10 × 6 cm) was used to repair the AVF. Note the preservation of iliac flow and the obliteration of the AVF. (Reprinted with permission from Ohki T, Veith FJ, Marin ML, et al: Diagnostic and therapeutic strategies for vascular injuries. *In:* Baert AL (ed): Medical Radiology—Diagnostic Imaging and Radiation Oncology. Heidelberg, Springer-Verlag, 1997, pp 235–243.)

stent graft developed compression of the stent at 12 months. This was treated with balloon angioplasty. This problem recurred 3 months later, and no intervention was required. This device has not thrombosed with follow-up over 3 years. In another patient, stenosis developed at either end of his stent graft (Corvita). This was treated percutaneously with additional balloon dilatation and stent insertion.

Other Experience and Examples

As with so many other endovascular techniques currently used, arterial repair after trauma was first thought of by Dotter in 1969.[42] The initial experience was with "homemade" devices, which were mainly Palmaz or Gianturco stents covered with PTFE or Dacron, although as described previously, the use of autologous vein to cover a stent still can be useful.

However, there are now commercially made stent grafts that use polyurethane as a covering that have the advantage of being available, sterile, off the shelf in a range of sizes, increasing the speed and ease of the procedure. Such a device is the Corvita stent graft currently being developed by the Schneider Company. This is essentially a Wallstent with a woven polyurethane covering. The advantage of this system

Table 33–4. Endovascular Grafts for Traumatic Arterial Injuries: Montefiore Experience

Sex/Age (yr)	Mechanism of Injury	Vessel(s) Involved	PA	AVF	Anesthetic	Associated Injuries	Injury to Repair Time Interval	Stent-Graft Length (cm)	Access	Hospital Stay (d)	Patency (mo)	Complications
F/80	Catheterization	RASA	No	No	Local	None	2 d	4†	Right brachial artery	2	1	—
M/21	Surgical trauma	RCIA LCIV	Yes	Yes	Local	None	4 wk	6†	RCFA percutaneous	4	6	—
M/22	Bullet	LSFA	Yes	No	Local	Soft tissue injury; left DVT	12 h	3	LSFA arteriotomy	6	9*	—
F/85	Surgical trauma	RCIA	Yes	Yes	Local	None	8 yr	5†	LCFA percutaneous	4	11	Distal emboli‡
M/49	Catheterization	RCIA	Yes	Yes	Epidural	None	18 mo	5	RCFA arteriotomy	5	11	Wound hematoma
M/68	Iliac graft disruption	LCIA	Yes	No	Epidural	None	1 mo	9	LCFA arteriotomy	5	9	—
M/66	Aortic graft disruption	Aorta	Yes	No	Epidural	None	1 wk	10	LCFA arteriotomy	5	18	—
M/76	Aortic disruption	Aorta	Yes	No	Epidural	None	3 d	7	LCFA arteriotomy	7	20	—
M/18	Bullet	RASA	Yes	No	Local	None	6 h	3	Right brachial artery	3	21	—
M/22	Bullet	RASA	Yes	No	Local	Hemothorax	3 h	3	Right brachial artery	6	21	—
M/18	Bullet	RSA	Yes	Yes	Local	Hemothorax	48 h	3	Right brachial artery	4	30	—
F/78	Catheterization	RSA	Yes	No	Local	Hemothcrax	24 h	3	Right brachial arteriotomy	8 wk§	37	—
M/78	Catheterization	LCIA	Yes	No	Epidural	None	4 mo	2	LCFA arteriotomy	2	37	—
M/35	Bullet	RASA	Yes	No	Local	Brachial plexus	3 wk	3	Right brachial arteriotomy	4	38	—
M/24	Knife	LASA	Yes	No	General	Pneumothorax; hemcthorax	4 h	3	Left brachial arteriotomy	7	42	Stent compression
M/28	Bullet	RSFA	Yes	No	Local	Left open femur fracture	12 h	3	RSFA arteriotomy	9	45	—
M/20	Bullet	LSFA LSFV	Yes	Yes	General	Soft tissue buttock	36 h	3	LSFA percutaneous	5	47	—

*Died 2 months postprocedure (homicide).
†Corvita stent graft.
‡Treated with catheter suction thrombectomy.
§Hospitalized for multiple medical problems.

is the relatively small sheath size required (8 French for an 8-mm diameter graft), long delivery system, and the fact that it can be cut with scissors to a desired length. The advantage of this is shown in Figure 33–16A–C, in which trauma resulted in the development of a pseudoaneurysm and occlusion at the subclavian artery origin in a 68-year-old woman. The patient had an ischemic arm, and CT had shown that the aneurysm was increasing in size. The device, inserted via the right common femoral artery, could be inserted and removed repeatedly, cutting it each time until it fit perfectly, allowing the vertebral artery to remain uncovered and patent. Unfortunately, because of production problems, the device is not yet available, but the Wallgraft, made by the same company, is.

Other devices include the Passager and the JoMed. The former is a self-expanding nitinol stent and the latter a balloon-mounted stainless steel stent, both with polyurethane covering. Figure 33–17A–C shows the use of the Passager stent graft in a 60-year-old patient who suffered trauma to the root of his neck. The left common carotid artery was damaged, and a pseudoaneurysm developed. This caused respiratory compromise, and the patient developed a right-sided motor weakness. Because he was almost 2 m tall, the delivery system on the Passager would not reach, and therefore the device was inserted successfully from a high left common carotid cut down. The patient thus was saved a thoracotomy that otherwise might have been necessary and is still alive and well with a patent carotid artery on duplex at 5 years.

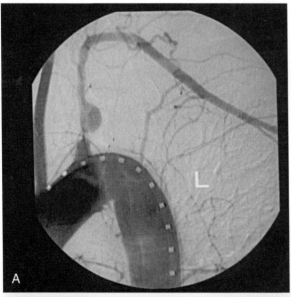

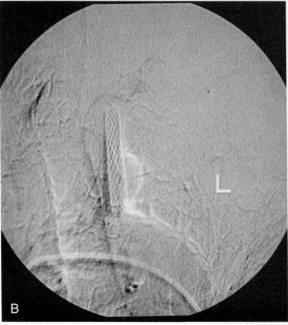

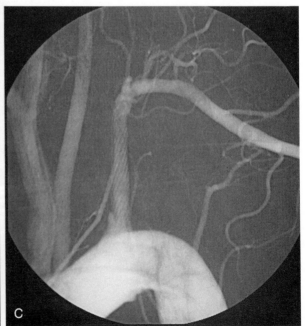

Figure 33–16. *A*, Traumatic false aneurysm at the left subclavian artery origin. *B*, Corvita stent graft in position. *C*, Patent left subclavian artery and occlusion of the pseudoaneurysm with a Corvita stent graft.

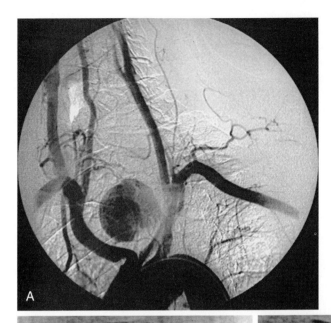

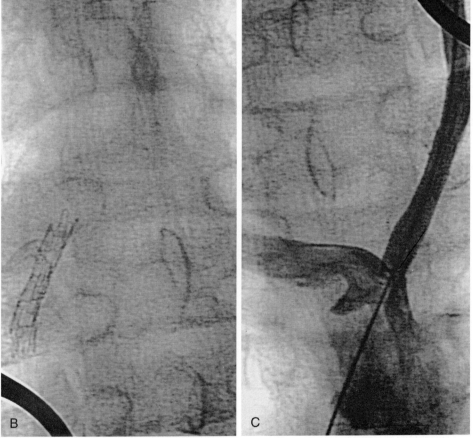

Figure 33–17. *A,* Traumatic false aneurysm at the origin of the left common carotid artery. *B,* Passager stent graft in position. *C,* Exclusion of the pseudoaneurysm with a Passager stent graft inserted via a high left common carotid arteriotomy.

Summary

Despite the potential disadvantages of using prosthetic materials that could stimulate intimal hyperplasia in traumatized arteries, the advantages of a minimally invasive procedure with reduced blood loss under local anesthetic from remote sites, rather than crossing body cavities, make endovascular techniques for arterial repair in trauma important tools. This is especially true in critically ill patients and in multiple-trauma cases. Stent grafts are important tools in the treatment of vascular trauma and should be included in the armamentarium of the vascular interventionist.

REFERENCES

1. Lowry S, Kraft R: Isolated aneurysms of the iliac artery. Arch Surg 113:1289–1293, 1978.
2. Brankwall J, Hauksson N, Bengtsson H, et al: Solitary aneurysm of the iliac artery system: An estimate of their frequency of occurance. J Vasc Surg 10:381–384, 1989.
3. Krupski WC, Selzman CH, Floridia R, et al: Contemporary management of isolated iliac aneurysms. J Vasc Surg 28:1–11, 1998.
4. Richardson JW, Greenfield LJ: Natural history and management of iliac aneurysms. J Vasc Surg 8:165–171, 1988.
5. White GII, Yu W, May J, et al: Three-year experience with the White-YU endovascular GAD graft for transluminal repair of aortic and iliac aneurysms. J Endovasc Surg 4:124–136, 1997.
6. Marin R, Veith FJ, Lyon RT, et al: Transfemoral endovascular repair of iliac artery aneurysms. Am J Surg 170:179–182, 1995.
7. Cardon JM, Cardon A, Joyeux A, et al: Endovascular repair of iliac artery aneurysms with endosystem 1: A multicentric French study. J Cardiovasc Surg 37(Suppl 1):45–50, 1996.
8. Dorros G, Cohn JM, Jaff MR: Percutaneous endovascular stent graft repair of iliac artery aneurysms. J Endovasc Surg 4:370–375, 1997.
9. Yuan JG, Marin ML, Veith FJ, et al: Endovascular grafts for non-infected aortoiliac anastomotic aneurysms. J Vasc Surg 26:210–221, 1997.
10. May J, White GH, Yu W, et al: Endoluminal repair: A better option for the treatment of complex false aneurysms. Aust N Z J Surg 68:29–34, 1998.
11. White RA, Donayre CE, Walot I, et al: Endoluminal graft exclusion of a proximal para-anastomotic pseudoaneurysm following aortobifemoral bypass. J Endovasc Surg 4:88–94, 1997.
12. Razavi MK, Dake MD, Semba CP, et al: Percutaneous endoluminal placement of stent grafts for the treatment of isolated iliac artery aneurysms. Radiology 197:801–804, 1995.
13. Quinn SF, Sheley RC, Semonsen KG, et al: Endovascular stents covered with pre-expanded Polytetra fluoroethylene for treatment of iliac artery aneurysms and fistulas. J Vasc Intervent Radiol 8:1057–1063, 1997.
14. Wychulis AR, Spittell JA Jr, Wallace RB: Popliteal aneurysms. Surgery 68:942, 1970.
15. Szilagyi DE, Schwartz RL, Reddy DJ: Popliteal arterial aneurysms. Arch Surg 116:724, 1981.
16. Dorffner R, Winkelbauer F, Kettenbach J, et al: Successful exclusion of a large femoropopliteal aneurysm with a coated nitinol stent. Cardiovasc Intervent Radiol 19:117–119, 1996.
17. Rousseau H, Gieskes L, Joffre F, et al: Percutaneous treatment of peripheral aneurysms with Cragg Endopro system. J Vasc Intervent Radiol 7:35–39, 1996.
18. Marcade JP: Stent graft for popliteal aneurysms: Six cases with Cragg Endo-Pro system 1 Mintec. J Cardiovasc Surg 37:41–44, 1996.
19. Criado E, Marston WA, Ligush J, et al: Endovascular repair of peripheral aneurysms, pseudoaneurysms, and arteriovenous fistulas. Ann Vasc Surg 11:256–263, 1997.
20. Rapoport S, Sniderman KW, Morse SS, et al: Pseudoaneurysm: A complication of faulty technique of femoral arterial puncture. Radiology 154:529–530, 1985.
21. Fellmeth BD, Roberts AC, Bookstein JJ, et al: Postangiographic femoral artery injuries: Non-surgical repair with US-guided compression. Radiology 178:671–675, 1991.
22. McGlinchey I, Baxter GM: Technical report: An alternative mechanical technique of pseudoaneurysm compression therapy. Clin Radiol 52:621–624, 1997.
23. Kazmers A, Meeker C, Nofz K, et al: Nonoperative therapy for postcatheterisation femoral artery pseudoaneurysms. Am Surg 63:199–204, 1997.
24. Chaterjee T, Do DD, Kaufmann U, et al: Ultrasound guided compression repair for treatment of femoral artery pseudoaneurysm: Acute and follow-up results. Cathet Cardiovasc Diagn 38:335–340, 1996.
25. Murray A, Buckenham T, Belli AM: Direct puncture coil embolisation of iatrogenic pseudoaneurysms. J Intervent Radiol 9:183–186, 1994.
26. Manns RA, Duffield RGM: Case report: Intravascular stenting across a false aneurysm of the popliteal artery. Clin Radiol 52:151–153, 1997.
27. Dorffner R, Winklebauer F, Kettenbach J, et al: Successful exclusion of a large femoropopliteal aneurysm with a covered nitinol stent. Cardiovasc Intervent Radiol 19:117–119, 1996.
28. Cope C, Zeit R: Coagulation of aneurysms by direct percutaneous thrombin injection. AJR Am J Roentgenol 147:383–387, 1986.
29. Walker TG, Geller SC, Brewster DC: Transcatheter occlusion of a profunda femoral artery pseudoaneurysm using thrombin. AJR Am J Roentgenol 149:185–186, 1987.
30. Young JZ, Medawar PB: Fibrin suture of peripheral nerves. Lancet 275:126–132, 1940.
31. Bergel S: Uber wirkungen des firins. Dtsch Med Wochenschr 35:633, 1909.
32. Tawes RL, Sydorak GR, Du Vall TB: Autologous fibrin glue: The last step in operative haemostasis. Am J Surg 168:120–122, 1994.
33. Lee KC, Park SK, Lee KS: Neurosurgical application of fibrin adhesive. Yonsei Med J 32:53–57, 1991.
34. Rodriguez-Fuchs CA, Bezares RF, Celebrin L, et al: Safe minor surgery in patients taking anticoagulants. Sangre (Barc) 38:239–241, 1993.
35. Liau C-S, Ho F-M, Chen M-F, et al: Treatment of iatrogenic femoral artery pseudoaneurysm with percutaneous thrombin injection. J Vasc Surg 26:18–23, 1997.
36. Kang SS, Labropoulos N, Mansour M, et al: Percutaneous guided thrombin injection: A new method for treating postcatheterisation femoral pseudoaneurysms J Vasc Surg 27:1032–1038, 1998.
37. Jahnke EJ, Seeley SF: Acute vascular injuries in the Korean War: An analysis of 77 consecutive cases. Ann Surg 138:158–177, 1953.
38. Perry MO, Thal ER, Shires ET: Management of arterial injuries. Ann Surg 173:403–408, 1971.
39. Patel AV, Marin ML, Veith FJ, et al: Endovascular graft repair of penetrating subclavian artery injuries. J Endovasc Surg 3:382–388, 1996.
40. Parodi JC: Endovascular repair of abdominal aortic aneurysms and other arterial lesions. J Vasc Surg 21:549–557, 1995.
41. Dorros G, Joseph G: Closure of a popliteal arteriovenous fistula using autologous vein-covered Palmaz stent. J Endovasc Surg 2:177–181, 1995.
42. Dotter CT: Transluminally placed coilspring endarterial tube-grafts: Long term patency in canine popliteal arteries. Invest Radiol 4:329–332, 1969.

The Future of
Endovascular Therapy

Chapter 34

Future Developments in
Endovascular Therapy

Endovascular Contributor: Lindsay Machan
Surgical Contributor: Thomas J. Fogarty

Until recently, a chapter on this topic would deal only with technical innovations that most interventional radiologists were lucky enough to introduce into clinical practice with relative ease. Technological advances still occur, largely refinements or new applications of existing devices, but no chapter on the future of endovascular interventions would be complete without discussion of the social, political, and economic factors that affect the daily practice of interventional medicine. These issues, which will have as much effect as technical innovation on the future of endovascular intervention, are discussed before speculation about new procedures.

FACTORS AFFECTING CHANGE IN ENDOVASCULAR MEDICINE

Advances in medical technology, including endovascular devices, influence changes in health-care delivery. Patient demographics and expectations and government and administrative priorities influence their distribution and application. There are several factors presently affecting the development and application of minimally invasive therapies that appear likely to have an even greater impact in the future.

Patients

Patients naturally wish to avoid any procedures, in particular those that involve open surgery, and find minimally invasive therapies appealing. They are more aggressive at seeking out therapeutic options for their own illnesses and have easy access to an unprecedented amount of medical information. Information regarding new procedures currently is considered news. For example, the *New England Journal of Medicine* routinely releases its articles to the lay press the day before publication. There is detailed information on the Internet on virtually any medical subject, including endovascular procedures. This medium not

only is a powerful tool for patient education, but through chat rooms patients can share their experiences. Any health provider group that does not anticipate, appreciate, and accommodate the power of an educated patient base will suffer.

In 1998, 37% of the US population was older than 45 years of age; in 2010 it is estimated to be 41% (Fig. 34–1). This aging trend will be more pronounced in European countries, which have lower birth and immigration rates. There not only will be more people in the demographic group most predisposed to atherosclerosis, but these patients will tolerate less interruption of their lifestyle by poor health and will wish to stay active throughout their lives. These factors would appear to increase the demand for endovascular treatments.

Paying Agencies

Increasing patient and physician demand, a population predisposed to vascular disease by aging, and the relatively high initial materials costs of catheter-based technologies have caused both government and private insurers to note with alarm the increasing number of endovascular procedures. These occur at a time when "evidence-based medicine" has become a mantra among the administration of these organizations. The ultimate application of these procedures in each jurisdiction will depend to a large extent on the ability of endovascular practitioners to prove their efficacy and cost-effectiveness in comparison to other therapies. It is contingent on all endovascular therapists to maintain credible databases using physiologic and clinical outcomes including quality of life and cost-effectiveness, reported using standardized outcome markers.[1] In the evolving climate of health-care delivery, those procedures for which this information is not available may not be performed at all, or those groups who cannot demonstrate these data for their own procedures may be restricted from performing them.[2]

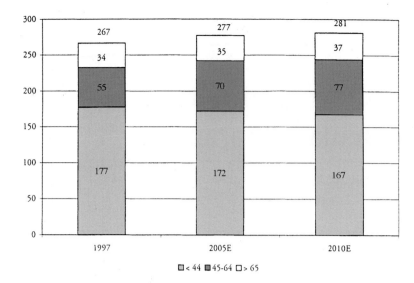

Figure 34–1. Changing demographics in the population of the United States. Source: US Census Bureau. x axis = US population in millions.

□ < 44 ■ 45-64 □ > 65

Turf Disputes

In 1997, industry data on peripheral angioplasty balloon sales revealed that 71% of balloon catheters were purchased by radiologists, 15% by cardiologists, and 14% by surgeons.[3] These ratios undoubtedly are changing, and who will perform these procedures in the future is currently a subject for debate and contest. Endovascular therapies currently account for 15% of all peripheral vascular procedures, and in the future this percentage may increase to as high as 40%[4, 5]; thus, it is not surprising that vascular surgeons wish to participate. In addition, many operations can be improved by endovascular adjuncts such as fluoroscopically assisted thromboembolectomy.[6] Performing these procedures will improve the vascular surgeons' facility and familiarity with endovascular techniques. In some instances, this only will serve to increase awareness of the procedures and thus cooperation with their interventional radiologic colleagues, but increasingly, vascular surgeons will want to perform at least some portion of endovascular interventions themselves.

Cardiologists increasingly see themselves as providers of care of vascular disease outside the heart.[7] There are approximately 2000 interventional cardiologists trained in the United States each year,[8] compared with approximately 225 to 250 from accredited interventional radiology fellowships[9] and 98 for vascular surgery.[10] This far exceeds the number of physicians required to perform cardiac endovascular procedures, and thus cardiologists currently perform increasing numbers of peripheral endovascular procedures in the United States. Depending on the outcome of ensuing turf battles, a possible consequence of this in some centers may be a shift in practice composition for interventional radiologists to a larger proportion of embolization and nonvascular procedures and less emphasis on vascular recanalization.

In some hospitals, the response to these developments has been development of closer liaisons between two of the three interested specialities or even formation of "endovascular groups."[11] Such an arrangement allows the optimal application of the skills of each specialist to the patient but works satisfactorily only if a good collaborative relationship exists.

Even when a formal liaison is not established, two factors are pushing the various specialities together. As endovascular procedures become more complex, they require separate skill sets for the same procedure. For example, the treatment of abdominal aortic aneurysms with endovascular stent grafts requires open incisions to allow passage of the large sheaths, a skill not possessed by most radiologists, and advanced angiographic skills, including advanced catheter manipulations and embolization, skills not possessed by most vascular surgeons. This is a closer working relationship than most are used to. When the devices eventually are reduced in size, the cutdowns no longer will be required, but a procedural relationship will have been established.

Procedures that require collaborating specialists and the evolution of combined procedures, such as operative angioplasty at the time of bypass graft insertion, have resulted in development of procedure rooms with various combinations of operating room (OR) level sterility and lighting, angiography with full digital capabilities, ultrasound, computed tomography (CT) (including CT fluoroscopy), or open-field magnetic resonance imaging (MRI). How these are paid for and where these are physically situated have further implications to the local practice of endovascular medicine.

These factors have led to the contemplation of a separate specialty of endovascular medicine with its own training and accreditation system. This combination of interventional radiologists, vascular surgeons, cardiologists, and vascular medicine specialists would diminish turf battles and might provide a more conducive working atmosphere for interventional radiologists, who increasingly find that the demands of a patient care practice bear little resemblance to those of their radiologic colleagues.

Noninvasive Imaging Techniques

Duplex ultrasound, CT angiography (CTA), and especially magnetic resonance angiography (MRA) have improved enormously and currently can provide vascular images of acceptable quality and accuracy without the disadvantages of invasive angiography. For example, duplex ultrasound has decreased markedly the need for angiography before carotid endarterectomy.[12] Limited accessibility to technologies such as MRI limits their application, but with time and increasing patient and physician education, the number of purely diagnostic arteriograms will diminish. As a result, the daily mix of cases on the typical angiographic schedule will become more complex as more patients will be sent with a view to intervention. The catheter skills currently acquired by radiology trainees are developed mostly at the time of diagnostic angiography; this source of training material can be expected to largely disappear in the future. This will result in the need to resort to training radiology residents on angiography simulators or to have them exposed to more complex interventions as their initial exposure to guide wire and catheter technique.[13]

Nonoperative Treatment of Vascular Disease

Risk factor modification is generally unpopular with patients but is very popular with paying agencies and may be legislated in some controlled practice situations before any intervention. Programs that include exercise, smoking cessation, control of hypertension and hyperlipidemia, and aggressive therapy of diabetes will be instituted increasingly.[14–17] These will be supervised exercise and lifestyle modification programs that have shown benefit in comparison to unsupervised programs that have not.[18] Drug treatments for claudication, including prostaglandin E$_1$,[19] L-carnitine,[20] and a phosphodiesterase inhibitor, cilostazol,[21] are promising in early investigations and will be evaluated further alone or in combination with lifestyle modification.

Recent advances in genetic engineering have led to therapeutic angioneogenesis.[22–24] When fibroblast growth factor (FGF) or vascular endothelial growth factor (VEGF), produced using recombinant gene technology, is delivered by intramuscular injection into ischemic tissues, marked increase in collateral blood vessels and blood flow develops (Fig. 34–2). This technology will be used initially in patients with rest pain to promote local vascularization and to accelerate ischemic wound healing, and ultimately it also will be used in conjunction with or in place of endovascular or operative procedures for claudication.

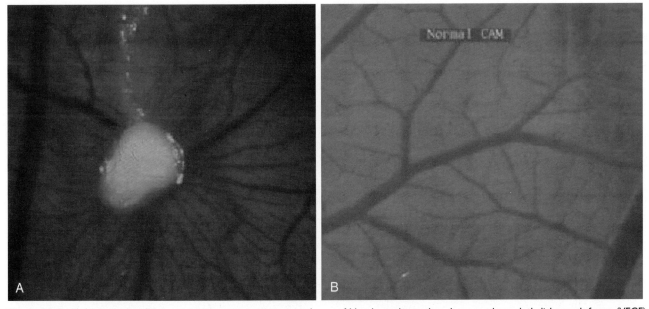

Figure 34–2. Angioneogenesis. Discs secreting agents containing stimulators of blood vessel growth such as vascular endothelial growth factor (VEGF) or fibroblast growth factor (FGF) cause new blood vessels to grow in an irregular fashion (A) compared with the normal arborization pattern of unstimulated blood vessels (B).

ENDOVASCULAR STENT GRAFTS

Concern remains for the long-term outcome of endovascular stent grafts as therapy for abdominal aortic aneurysms (AAAs). The durability of existing devices is unknown, and component failure has occurred, which has led to device revision.[25] Persistence of late-onset endoleak is associated with aneurysm expansion.[26, 27] A single-center comparison between endoluminal and open AAA repair found that postoperative survival was similar between the two groups but survival with a functioning prosthesis without endoleak was significantly higher after open AAA repair.[28] Although there is a rush to improve the ease of use of these devices, clearly there are more basic questions that must be addressed. Nevertheless, changes in endovascular stent graft technology will occur in three spheres: improvement in existing technology, increase in the number of patients for whom the technology is appropriate, and expansion of indications for endovascular stenting.

Improvements in Stent Graft Technology

The principal focus will be development of devices that can be delivered percutaneously. Smaller sheaths imply thinner fabric on the device, but the fabric must be as strong and durable as surgically inserted grafts (Fig. 34–3). Endovascular AAA repair is unlikely to become exclusively percutaneous if it is to be applied to as broad a spectrum of aneurysm morphology as possible, but we will see the development of devices of small size with more flexible delivery systems. The stent grafts themselves will be malleable and capable of repositioning or retrieval after insertion.

Extension of Aneurysm Morphology Suitable for Endovascular Grafting

Present designs require that the proximal neck be 15 mm in length and the distal neck 10 mm, resulting in approximately 30 to 50% of patients with suitable anatomy for endograft insertion.[29, 30] In addition to smaller introduction sheaths that allow traversal of tortuous iliac arteries, devices to accommodate larger diameter necks, and modification to allow treatment of shorter necks, more radical modifications will include the design of stent graft branches that accommodate renal arteries, photodynamically activated adhesives to enhance fixation to the arterial wall (Fig. 34–4), and biologic stent grafts designed by tissue engineering.

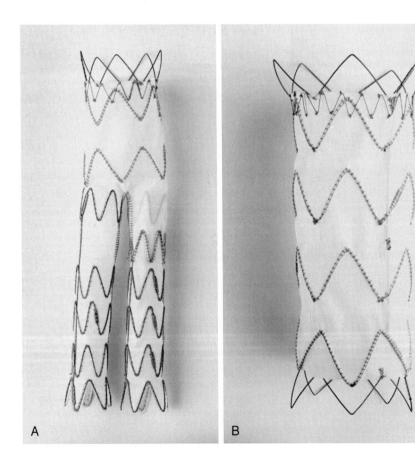

A

B

Figure 34–3. *A* and *B*, Low-profile stent graft. Stent graft constructed using extrathin fabric providing superior tensile strength will allow percutaneous stent-graft insertion in some patients. (Courtesy of World Medical Manufacturing Ltd., Sunrise, FL.)

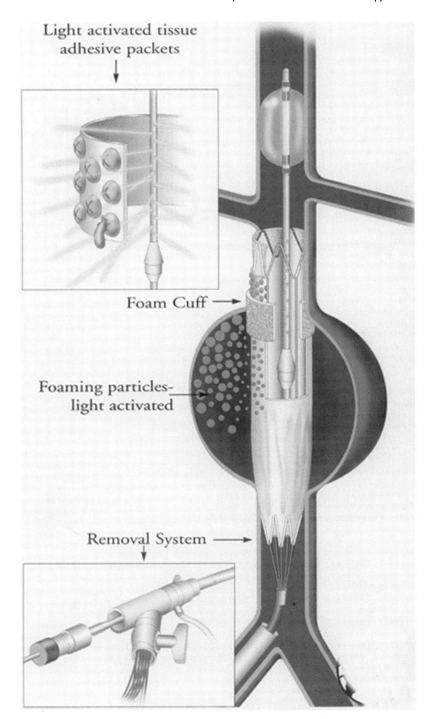

Light activated tissue adhesive packets

Foam Cuff →

Foaming particles–
light activated

Removal System →

Figure 34–4. Enhancement of stent-graft adhesion to blood vessel wall. A light-activated adhesive applied to the outer surface of the stent-graft material becomes active when exposed to ultraviolet light.

Application of Stent Grafts to a Wider Spectrum of Disease

In arteries, stent grafts will be used more frequently for aortic trauma and dissections, in aneurysms other than those of the abdominal or thoracic aorta, and for occlusive disease and trauma in the periphery. In the venous system, we can contemplate increased use in transjugular intrahepatic portosystemic shunt (TIPS) and for the prevention of intimal hyperplasia after treatment of occlusions. Creation of extra-anatomic conduits, such as tunneled arterial bypass channels and dialysis fistulas, is being investigated actively. The use of stent grafts in emergent situations implies maintenance of an inventory in the hospital. Because of the variations in anatomy that must be accommodated, devices that are adjustable in length and diameter will be developed or the costs and volume of devices required will restrict their use in emergencies.

RESTENOSIS

Restenosis is defined as the chronic recurrence of a stenosis after an initially successful treatment and is the major shortcoming of endovascular procedures for vascular occlusive disease. Despite advances in mechanical techniques of revascularization, recurrent stenoses develop in up to 100% of peripheral vascular lesions, depending on the patient's clinical status,[31] and within 6 months in 30 to 60% of successfully treated coronary lesions.[32] For endovascular treatments to gain even wider application, this problem must be resolved, and this will be the principal area of research in endovascular treatment of stenoses and occlusions in the near future. Efforts will be directed to the application of pharmacologic therapies or radiation to treat or prevent restenosis.

Pathology of Restenosis

Restenosis, actually a type of wound healing, has two components: arterial wall remodeling and neointimal hyperplasia. Neointimal hyperplasia is multifactorial and is essentially the arterial response to injury.[33] Literally any vascular manipulation, including angioplasty, stent insertion, or creation of a surgical anastomosis, initiates to some degree the same biologic healing response. Platelets and other cells aggregate in the region of vascular injury and secrete signaling substances called cytokines that cause normally quiescent vascular smooth muscle cells to migrate to the area of injury and secrete the extracellular proteinaceous matrix, which is the largest component of the lesion (Fig. 34–5). This creation of a reparative scar also may narrow the vascular lumen.

Pharmacotherapy for Restenosis

Prevention of restenosis with drugs is an attractive idea that is not yet applicable to clinical practice.

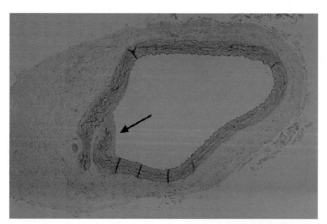

Figure 34–5. Restenosis after arterial injury. The lesion is largely acellular proteinaceous material.

These therapies are directed against one or more of the steps in the biologic process.[34] Many agents have been shown to reduce neointimal hyperplasia in animal models but have not been effective in human use.[35–38] More than 50 trials of systemic pharmacotherapy to reduce restenosis in humans have been attempted and failed.

Therefore, the focus of investigation will be on devices that allow application of drugs or biologically active molecules directly onto the surface, into the matrix, or around the lesion to be treated. There are several potential advantages to local drug delivery. Very high concentrations of drugs can be achieved at the required site, even of agents that may be degraded when administered systemically. By concentrating the drug at the target site, adverse systemic effects can be avoided. If the drug is delivered in a slow-release polymer, prolonged administration of the drug can be achieved. Drug delivery schemes can be divided into those in which the drug is delivered intraluminally, intraluminally/intramurally, or into the perivascular space.

INTRALUMINAL DRUG DELIVERY

The most common method of intraluminal drug delivery is the drug-eluting stent (Figs. 34–6 and 34–7). These can be conventional stents coated with a polymer from which drugs are slowly delivered, or a stent in which the tines themselves are made of a drug-eluting polymer ("resorbable stents"). In the latter instance, as the stent dissolves, the drug is released. Appropriate slow-release polymers for coating of conventional stents or for composition of resorbable stents include polyurethane, polygalactic acid (PGLA), polylactic acid (PLA), and polycaprolactone (PCL), among others. Promising stent coatings include paclitaxel, a broad-spectrum chemotherapeutic agent[39] (see Fig. 36–6), and dexamethasone.[40]

INTRAMURAL DRUG DELIVERY

Various devices can be used to deliver medication directly onto the surface of or into the vessel wall.[41, 42] These either are dedicated drug delivery devices used separately after angioplasty or stent insertion or devices that can deliver medication at the time of angioplasty. The former include infusion catheters that allow drugs to diffuse into the wall without occluding distal flow[43] (Fig. 34–8) and double-balloon catheters that isolate the treatment segment, allowing medication to be instilled onto the surface of the isolated segment via a central lumen.

Devices capable of drug delivery at the time of angioplasty are said to produce no additional arterial trauma because drug delivery occurs simultaneously with lesion dilatation. These include sweating bal-

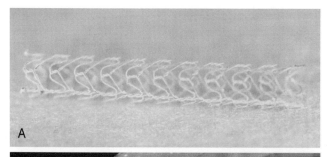

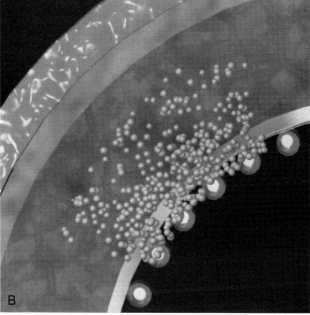

Figure 34–6. *A,* Drug-eluting stent. The coating is less than 100 microns thick. *B,* Drug released from a slow-release polymer on the stent tine diffuses into the arterial wall.

loons that extrude drugs from a chamber between an inner conventional angioplasty balloon and an outer fenestrated balloon (Fig. 34–9) or drug infusion sleeve. Alternatively, an angioplasty balloon can be coated with a thin layer of hydrophilic polyacrylic acid polymer (hydrogel) that can absorb drugs or biologically active substances. Once loaded, the hydrogel containing the drug is pressed onto the arterial wall during balloon inflation (Fig. 34–10). Finally, an angioplasty balloon can be manufactured with rows of tiny delivery nipples on its surface. After inflation of the balloon, the nipples penetrate the vessel wall, and through independent drug delivery ports, controlled amounts of various substances can be infiltrated into the vessel wall.[44]

All catheter-based designs suffer the limitations of small administered volumes, limited duration of administration, poor efficiency of delivery, and washout of drug through the vasa vasorum, and it seems unlikely that these will be used as commonly as drug-eluting stents.

PERIVASCULAR DRUG DELIVERY

Perivascular drug delivery is a logical approach to prevention of restenosis. The most active vascular smooth muscle cells in the restenosis process appear to reside normally in the periadventitial region. Drug application can occur without endoluminal manipulations, and there is less constraint of the amount of polymer that can be applied. The initial and most frequent example of perivascular drug application will be wraps placed at the time of open surgery, such as graft anastomosis (Fig. 34–11), but drugs also could be applied percutaneously via endovascular catheters with transmural injection ports under imaging guidance or injected directly into the pericardial sac. Drugs that will be used in perivascular drug delivery include heparin, nitrous oxide potentiators, and paclitaxel.[45, 46]

Radiation Therapy

Radiation can prevent restenosis by inhibiting vascular smooth muscle cell proliferation and migration.[47] Brachytherapy is the delivery of a low dose of radiation by inserting a radioactive source adjacent to the area to be treated (Fig. 34–12). Preliminary studies have been performed largely in the coronary circulation and undoubtedly will be applied to the peripheral circulation. The two predominant modes of delivery of vascular radiation are by temporary insertion of radioactive guide wire or seeds[48, 49] or by insertion of a permanent radioactive stent.[50] Based on current trials, it appears that bolus treatment with a removable radioactive device will be most effective and most commonly used. For example, gamma radiation with iridium 192 wire after coronary stenting prospectively compared with placebo in the Scripps Coronary Radiation to Inhibit Proliferation Poststenting (SCRIPPS) trial reduced angiographic restenosis from 54% of placebo-treated patients to 17% after irradiation.[49] Both gamma and beta emitters are being evaluated, and which one ultimately will be used will depend as much on local radioisotope regulatory requirements as efficacy.

Drug treatments for restenosis allow the possibility of longer treatment times (because they can be loaded into slow-release polymers), and drug-coated stents or sweating balloons do not add additional complexity to the procedure because the drug is delivered by the primary treatment device. Brachytherapy requires an additional manipulation after the initial therapy to insert a centering device to ensure that the dose is evenly distributed circumferentially, and in many catheter laboratories, there are problems with handling radiopharmaceuticals, which normally are

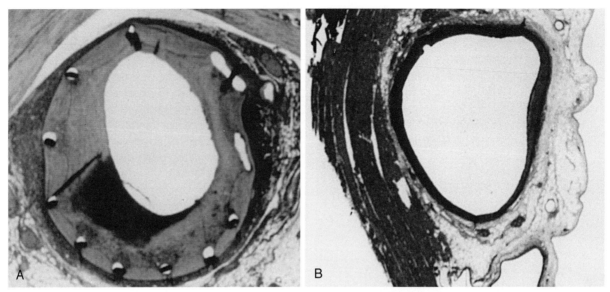

Figure 34–7. Effect of a drug-eluting stent on restenosis. *A,* Uncoated stent 4 weeks after insertion into the pig coronary artery results in significant arterial wall thickening (restenosis). *B,* Paclitaxel-coated stent at the same interval has caused no mural thickening. A small impression from a stent tine is noted.

restricted to the nuclear medicine or radiotherapy department, risk of staff exposure, and in some cases, storage of devices with limited half-lives. The endovascular therapist of the future will have a wide range of easy-to-use devices available for the treatment or prevention of restenosis, perhaps dispensing drugs for some applications and radiation for others.

SUMMARY

An ancient Chinese curse was "may you live in interesting times." Whether one feels blessed or cursed to be an endovascular therapist may depend on how well he or she negotiates the interesting political times ahead of us, but the practice of endovascular medicine undoubtedly will remain fascinating and continually evolving.

THE SURGICAL PERSPECTIVE

Endovascular interventions can be classified roughly into two distinct time frames—a 30-year period from 1930 to 1960 that constitutes the *diagnostic* era, fol-

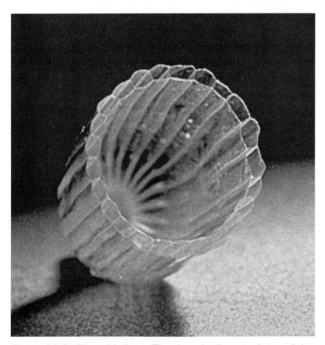

Figure 34–8. Channel balloon. The channels allow circulation of drug against and diffusion into the arterial wall without obstruction of blood flow.

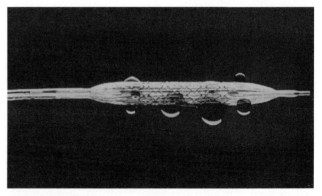

Figure 34–9. Sweating balloon. Inflation of the angioplasty balloon at the catheter tip results in extrusion of drug from a space between the balloon and a fenestrated outer sleeve.

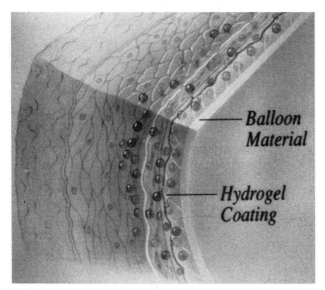

Figure 34–10. Coating of hydrogel on the luminal surface of an artery left after inflation of a hydrogel-coated angioplasty balloon against the arterial wall. The coating can serve as a barrier ("endoluminal paving") or to deliver drugs active against thrombosis or restenosis.

lowed by a *therapeutic endovascular* period that essentially began in the early 1960s and continues into the present. Catheter-based therapeutic modalities originated with the embolectomy catheter, developed in the late 1950s and used clinically in the early 1960s. The therapeutic advantage of this endovascular device was the reduction of high mortality and morbidity rates associated with acute embolic occlusion at that time. Amputations were reduced dramatically, and a new method for treating vascular disease using remote access, rather than a direct approach, was introduced.

Forays into the uncharted world of endovascular interventions were controversial. New ideas rarely are embraced immediately, and this was especially true when nonstandard surgical instrumentation was presented to a traditional vascular community in the 1960s. The foreign concept of treating vascular lesions via remote introduction of a device mounted on a catheter platform seriously deviated from the surgeons' typical approach; thus, it not only had to be proven safe and effective but also required an alteration to surgeons' prejudgment mindsets to gain acceptance. The original article describing the catheter balloon embolectomy procedure was rejected by three major peer-reviewed journals before it was accepted by the *Journal of Surgery, Gynaecology and Obstetrics* and published in an abbreviated form under the section "Surgeon at Work." Eventually, catheter-mediated treatments were accepted and the technological deviation, which began with the balloon catheter introduced in the 1960s, created a subsequent revolution that has burgeoned into a subspecialty over the past 5 to 10 years.

Once the endovascular platform was proven to be efficacious and the technique deemed safe by the surgical community, other devices followed using the catheter mainframe construction. The slow acceptance of endovascular concepts since the initial embolectomy catheter introduction for therapeutic applications retarded its rapid development within the vascular surgical community. Now that these techniques have been evaluated more thoroughly, a plethora of devices have been developed. Many of these "new surgical instruments" currently are standard treatment modalities in the field of endovascular technology.

We have come a long way in the past 30 years. The technologic advances made in the medical/surgical arena have been influenced heavily by social, economic, political, educational, relational, governmental, and other sciences. These external factors will continue to play a major role in directing the development of future technologies that will be made available to our speciality.

As a clinician and inventor, I see a clear trend toward an escalation of endoluminal technology. It fits the model for technologic success; it is simple, is relatively easy to understand and learn, and is minimally invasive and consequently less traumatic to the patient both physically and emotionally. It is proving to be clinically and economically effective and is "doable," primarily because of the enabling visualization and computerization that accompanies its use.

Statistics relating to this endovascular growth movement have been pointed out in many recent papers and were presented succinctly by Frank Veith in his discussion of this topic during the 1995 E. Stanley Crawford Critical Issues Forum. Both Dr. Veith and I were in agreement that "within the next 5 to 10 years fully 50 to 75% of standard vascular surgeries could potentially be performed via endovascular routes." This was considered to be a staggering number at the time but served as a blatant "wake-up call" for vascular surgeons to become involved in these different, revolutionary, but inevitably viable, surgical techniques.

I would further reaffirm and update those figures for the *next* 5 years, with a prediction that 50 to 75% of AAAs and 75 to 90% of descending thoracic aortic aneurysms will be treated with endovascular implants. In addition, carotid treatment options will be expanded. The current routine practice of balloon angioplasty for treating renal, peripheral, and coronary arteries by vascular surgeons and interventional radiologists gave rise to the possibility of also using this technique for carotid stenosis. Initial reports described mixed efficacy for this highly controversial procedure. Also, ethical concerns regarding the rationale for subjecting patients to this potentially dangerous treatment in the face of safe and effective tradi-

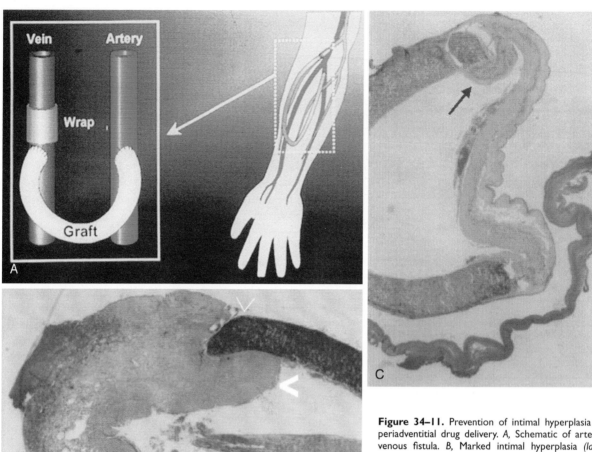

Figure 34–11. Prevention of intimal hyperplasia by periadventitial drug delivery. *A,* Schematic of arterial venous fistula. *B,* Marked intimal hyperplasia *(large arrow)* and untreated venous anastomosis with polytetrafluoroethylene (PTFE) graft *(small arrow). C,* Minor focal area of intimal hyperplasia after a perivascular wrap of paclitaxel was applied.

tional approaches has created heated arguments and has polarized the surgical community. Despite these early impediments to development (the balloon embolectomy catheter initially was not enthusiastically adopted either), it is anticipated that by the year 2004, approximately 20 to 30% of all carotid stenoses will be handled effectively by using a combination of endovascular angioplasty and stenting rather than surgical endarterectomy.

For technologic advances to be achieved, new methodologies must be given the opportunity to be explored and refined. The biggest deterrent to the success of invention and technology is one's inability to learn from the mistakes that inevitably are made during the process of development.

The information age also has allowed us to rapidly share data and disseminate results and outcomes that will significantly reduce the time line to product acceptance and promote significant appropriate product adaptations. In a similar manner, legislation recently enacted limiting materials manufacturers' liability for products used in the medical arena should

ensure availability of improved synthetic biomaterials, leading to device enhancements. Local drug delivery concepts also will be applied to all fields of surgery.

What does the future hold? One thing is certain—vascular surgeons will *not* be conducting "business as usual." "Cutting and sewing" is, and will continue to be, replaced by alternate methods of performing procedures. The simple incision made with a surgical scalpel now can be achieved using lasers or ultrasound, or vascular access may be gained via percutaneous puncture. In a similar way, standard surgical suturing has been supplanted by clips, staples, bioglues, sealants, plugs, and pressurized implants such as stents and stent grafts. The capability to remotely visualize intraluminal surfaces, coupled with the ability to manipulate pathology using a whole range of new drugs and miniaturized instrumentation, creates the necessity to develop new skills to effect these refined operations.

One rather significant change will be the combining of diagnostics and therapeutics into one proce-

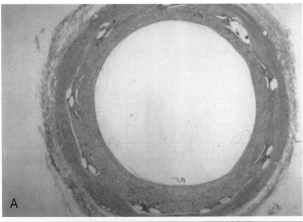

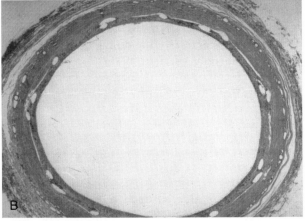

Figure 34–12. Prevention of restenosis by radiation. *A,* Porcine femoral artery 6 weeks after stent insertion demonstrating significant intimal hyperplasia overgrowing the stent tines. *B,* Opposite femoral artery in same animal. 5.2 rads of gamma radiation delivered by iridium wire at the time of stent insertion resulted in significantly less intimal hyperplasia.

dure. This already is being employed by cardiologists in their cardiac catheterization interventions with excellent success. The move toward less invasive treatments is dramatic. It is apparent in every area of medicine. To a large extent, the minimally invasive mandate is being driven by economic concerns. Less invasive technology, when used appropriately, saves money, and with the shift to a managed health-care mentality the *business* of treating disease is acutely aware of the bottom line. This shift in power and decision making from physician to insurance provider and corporate controller equates to economy-based therapy using only treatment modalities that reduce costs. However, organizations that will be successful in this area understand that it is short-sighted to reject a new treatment based solely on a higher actual cost of a device or treatment and thus will be forced to consider the larger "net economic impact" surrounding a new technology to realize overall cost savings. That net economic impact is composed of a variety of factors, including procedure time, supply cost, recovery time, decreased costs influencing increased utilization, labor costs, surveillance, hospital stay, after care, and pain and suffering.

Vascular surgery, specifically the subspeciality of endovascular surgery, has not evolved in a vacuum. As previously mentioned, technologies from other medical-surgical speciality forums have been and will continue to be adapted, borrowed, enhanced, modified, and tested to determine their applicability for treating *vascular* disease. Because of this relationship, we must necessarily then closely observe what is occurring in our allied "sister" specialities to understand *why* and *what* will ultimately impact the vascular specialists' future. For example, angioplasty, first used for cardiac applications, has found acceptance as treatment for peripheral lesions and has potential for utility in the carotid conduit, perhaps when combined with adjunctive stenting. Laparoscopic techniques developed to reduce the trauma of large incisions and extensive surgical interventions in general surgery have been modified to allow extravascular performance of minimally invasive perforator vein ligation with direct visualization achieved by using remote optical camera systems. The incredible advances made in the field of visualization have changed forever the course and direction of medical-surgical interventions. In addition, computer reconstruction of virtually every part of the body permits highly accurate diagnosis of disease in its early stages rather than discovering anatomic changes or abnormalities at the macroscopic level, when treatments may or may not be effective based on the extent of the disease progression. The techniques and operative options that surgeons currently have at their disposal to treat vascular disease have expanded. These include precise elimination of the offending lesion not only by excision (now possible as minimally invasive superfine "surgeries" performed remotely through a distant access arteriotomy, venotomy, or percutaneous puncture) but by ablation (via radiofrequency, radiation, laser, ultrasound, and thermal modalities), pulverization, and instillation of therapeutic agents.

As I have alluded to over the past 5 years, the main technologic advances all will involve minimalization of surgical procedures with specific significant influences taking place in the areas of combining diagnostics and treatments in the same device, access site management, implant development, and control of the healing response.

In concert with this less intrusive instrument development, the field of robotics for medical applications has surfaced as a promising futuristic therapy. Since the introduction of robotic endoscopic master–slave manipulator devices in the late 1980s, high interest has been generated in the entire field of telemanipulator technology. The three major aims of using these surgical robotics in the field of operative medicine are (1) to replace human manpower, (2) to enhance surgical precision, and (3) to expand manipulative capabilities within a limited endoscopic environment. Physicians will be assisted in their robotic surgery by performing procedures at an input terminal that controls steerable endoscopic instruments, some of which actually will be equipped with tactile sensors providing information regarding pressure and tension exerted on the operative tissue or conduit. Although limitations to visualization of the entire operative field present challenges to this technology, these impediments likely will be overcome as enabling technologies improve, but robots replacing surgeons will not be realized anytime soon. Our specialty and other surgical specialities involved in the performance of fine operative interventions should benefit greatly with access to this space-age technology.

The following is a partial list of forces impacting the future development of endovascular and minimally invasive technologies:

- Surgeons' attitudes toward endovascular and less invasive alternatives
- Multispeciality team approaches
- Speciality competition
- Economic impact of managed care oversight
- Computerization affecting sharing of information
- Remote proctoring of new, advanced, or complicated operative techniques
- Teaching of techniques via satellite interactive operative interventions
- Computer-driven miniaturization of devices, robotic refinements to reduce gross motorized movements to minute motions, permitting superfine surgeries never before possible
- Redefining "what's possible" in the realm of surgical intervention
- Access to biomaterials that will expand the applications of implants
- Increased emphasis on outcomes as judged by patients.

We will see increased use of modular, "customized" devices to fit individual patient anatomy, improved methods to assist closure of interventional incisions and puncture sites and aid in healing, radiation therapies and implant coatings to inhibit restenosis after "surgery," and steriotactic localization for precise excision of target lesions—and all will conform to the minimally invasive, low-cost model of the future.

Concurrently, improvements in medical care have contributed to increasing the life expectancy of our patients, producing an aged population who are subject to developing attendant diseases of the elderly. Although we have improved technologies and drugs to deter or defeat cardiovascular diseases and logically would expect to see a decline of these disease entities, the sheer numbers of elderly patients produce an inverse relationship in which vascular and cardiovascular cases are steadily increasing. This situation will only continue to become more pronounced with time.

With the advent of endovascular techniques came the intrusion of other specialists into the field of vascular treatment. In many cases, the *need* to perform surgical incisions was diminished by the introduction of catheter techniques, and consequently, interventional radiologists and cardiologists could percutaneously access the offending vascular lesion. In this way, the accessibility of endovascular technologies served to broaden the number of specialists treating vascular disease entities. The multispecialty treatment approach will only escalate in the coming years. In addition, vascular surgeons themselves contribute to this competitive situation by not readily adopting the newer treatment alternatives, choosing instead to retain their standard and comfortable "cutting and sewing" techniques. This steadfast clinging to traditional treatment models and procedures consequently has fostered the movement of a significant percentage of our business to encroaching specialists who are eager to tap into the growing vascular market. Only if we choose to break from our traditions and accept the concept of alternative, less invasive treatments, will we benefit from the technologic advances that we have at our disposal. Without vision, specialities perish.

In addition to these attitudinal encumbrances, there is another concern relating to our educational system that must be addressed as we forge into the future with this new technology. Academic centers must rethink their educational goals and revamp outdated programs to produce competent future physicians. They should design educational programs that formally address the technologic innovations that are inherent to our practice.

We have come a long way since balloon embolectomy catheters. New technologies are reshaping the way that we treat vascular disease, and the changes are good. They must be evaluated and either adopted or rejected judiciously. Finally, they must be used with skill in appropriate situations and accepted for the benefits that they ultimately will provide to our vascular patients.

REFERENCES

1. Jordan WD Jr, Roye GD, Fisher WS, et al: A cost comparison of balloon angioplasty and stenting versus endarterectomy for the treatment of carotid artery stenosis. J Vasc Surg 27:16–22, 1998.
2. Sacks D, Marinelli DL, Martin LG, et al: General principles for

evaluation of new interventional technologies and devices. J Vasc Intervent Radiol 8:133–149, 1997.

3. Katzen BT: Endovascular stent grafts: The beginning of the future, or the beginning of the end? J Vasc Intervent Radiol 7:469–476, 1996.

4. Veith FJ, Sanchez LA, Ohki T: Should vascular surgeons perform endovascular procedures and how can they acquire the skills to do so? Semin Vasc Surg 10:191–196, 1997.

5. Veith FJ, Marin ML: Impact of endovascular technology on the practice of vascular surgery. Am J Surg 172:100–104, 1996.

6. Parsons RE, Marin ML, Veith FJ, et al: Fluoroscopically assisted thromboembolectomy: An improved method of treating acute occlusions. Ann Vasc Surg 10:201–210, 1996.

7. DeMaria AN: Peripheral vascular disease and the cardiovascular specialists. J Am Coll Cardiol 12:869–870, 1988.

8. American College of Cardiology: Direct communication.

9. Society of Cardiovascular and Interventional Radiology: Direct communication.

10. Society of Vascular Surgery: Direct communication.

11. Veith FJ: Turf issues: How do we resolve them and optimize patient selection for intervention and ultimately patient care? J Vasc Surg 28:370–372, 1998.

12. Chaw K-T: Does carotid duplex imaging render angiography redundant before carotid endarterectomy? Br J Radiol 70:235–238, 1997.

13. Nemcek AA: Vascular and interventional radiology training: What should it be? Semin Intervent Radiol 12:228–232, 1995.

14. Hirrsch AT, Treat-Jacobson D, Lando HA, Hatsukami DK: The role of tobacco cessation, antiplatelet and lipid-lowering therapies in the treatment of peripheral arterial disease. Vasc Med 2:243–251, 1997.

15. Blankenhorn DH, Azen SP, Crawford DW, et al: Effects of colestipol-niacin therapy on human femoral atherosclerosis. Circulation 83:438–447, 1991.

16. Lamarche B, Lewis GF: Atherosclerosis prevention for the next decade: Risk assessment beyond low density lipoprotein cholesterol. Can J Cardiol 14:841–851, 1998.

17. Orchard TJ, Strandness DE, Cavenagh PR, et al: Assessment of peripheral vascular disease in diabetes: Report and recommendations of an international workshop. Circulation 88:819–828, 1993.

18. Regensteiner JG, Meyer TJ, Krupski WC, et al: Hospital vs home-based exercise rehabilitation for patients with peripheral arterial occlusive disease. Angiography 48:291–300, 1997.

19. Diehm C, Balzer K, Bisler H, et al: Efficacy of a new prostaglandin E1 regimen in out-patients with severe intermittent claudication: Results of a multicenter placebo-controlled double-blind trial. J Vasc Surg 25:537–544, 1997.

20. Brevetti G, Perna S, Sabba C, et al: Effect of propionyl-L-carnitine on quality of life in intermittent claudication. Am J Cardiol 79:777–780, 1997.

21. Dawson DL, Cutlet BS, Meissner MH, Strandness DE: Cilostazol has beneficial effects in treatment of intermittent claudication: Results from a multicenter, randomized, prospective, double-blind trial. Circulation 98:678–686, 1998.

22. Isner JM, Walsh K, Symes J, et al: Arterial gene therapy for therapeutic angiogenesis in patients with peripheral artery disease. Circulation 91:2687–2692, 1995.

23. Mack CA, Magovern CJ, Budenbender KT, et al: Salvage angiogenesis induced by adenovirus-mediated gene transfer of vascular endothelial growth factor protects against ischemic vascular occlusion. J Vasc Surg 27:699–709, 1998.

24. Dzau VJ, Gibbons GH, Mann M, Braun-Dullaeus R: Future horizons in cardiovascular molecular therapeutics. Am J Cardiol 80:331–391, 1997.

25. Moore WS, Rutherford RB, for the EVT Investigators: Transfemoral endovascular repair of abdominal aortic aneurysm: Results of the North American EVT phase 1 trial. J Vasc Surg 23:543–553, 1996.

26. Lloyd WE, Paty PSK, Darling RC, et al: Results of 1000 consecutive elective abdominal aortic repairs. Cardiovasc Surg 4:724–726, 1996.

27. Chuter TAM, Wendt G, Hopkinson BR, et al: European experience with a system for bifurcated stent graft insertion. J Endovasc Surg 4:13–22, 1997.

28. May J, White GH, Yu W, et al: Concurrent comparison of endoluminal versus open repair in the treatment of abdominal aortic aneurysms: Analysis of 303 patients by life table method. J Vasc Surg 27:213–220, 1998.

29. Armon MP, Yusuf W, Latief K, et al: Anatomical suitability of abdominal aortic aneurysms for endovascular repair. Br J Surg 84:178–180, 1997.

30. Blum U, Voshage G, Lammer J, et al: Endoluminal stent grafts for infrarenal abdominal aortic aneurysms. N Engl J Med 336:13–20, 1997.

31. Coffman J: Intermittent claudication: Be conservative. N Engl J Med 325:577–578, 1991.

32. Popma JJ, Califf RM, Topol EJ: Clinical trials of restenosis after angioplasty. Circulation 84:1426–1436, 1991.

33. Waller BF, Pinkerton CA, Orr CM, et al: Restenosis 1 to 24 months after clinically successful coronary balloon angioplasty: A necropsy study of 20 patients. J Am Coll Cardiol 17:58B–70B, 1991.

34. Schwartz RS: Pathophysiology of restenosis: Interaction of thrombosis, hyperplasia, and/or remodelling. Am J Cardiol 71:14E–17E, 1998.

35. Powell JS, Muller RKM, Baumgartner HR: Suppression of the vascular response to injury: The role of angiotensin-converting enzyme inhibitors. J Am Coll Cardiol 17:137B–142B, 1991.

36. Multicenter European Research Trial with Cilazapril after Angioplasty to Prevent Transluminal Coronary Obstruction and Restenosis (MERCATOR) Study Group: Does the new angiotensin converting enzyme inhibitor cilazapril prevent restenosis after percutaneous transluminal coronary angioplasty? Results of the MERCATOR study: A multicenter, randomized, double-blind placebo-controlled trial. Circulation 86:100–110, 1992.

37. Currier JW, Pow TK, Haudenschild CC, et al: Low molecular weight heparin (enoxaparin) reduces restenosis after iliac angioplasty in the hypercholesterolemic rabbit. J Am Coll Cardiol 17:118B–125B, 1991.

38. Faxon D, Spiro T, Minor S, et al: Enoxaparin, a low molecular weight heparin, in the prevention of restenosis after angioplasty: Results of a double blind randomized trial (Abstract). J Am Coll Cardiol 19:258A, 1992.

39. Heldman A, Cheng L, Heller P, et al: Paclitaxel applied directly to stents inhibits neointimal growth in a porcine coronary artery model of restenosis. Presented at the Annual Meeting of the American Heart Association, Washington, DC, 1997.

40. Strecker EP, Gabelmann A, Boos I, et al: Drug releasing stents for the prevention of intimal hyperplasia after stent implantation—An experimental study. Cardiovasc Intervent Radiol 20(suppl 1):S88, 1997.

41. Wolinsky H, Thung SN: Use of a perforated balloon catheter to deliver concentrated heparin into the wall of the normal canine artery. J Am Coll Cardiol 15:475–481, 1990.

42. Bailey SR: Local drug delivery: Current applications. Prog Cardiovasc Dis 40:183–204, 1997.

43. Boudghene FP, Lagarde V, Makita Y, et al: A leaktight pressure-driven site-specific drug delivery device. Radiology 209(P suppl):184, 1998.

44. Barath P, Popov A, Michiels R: Nipple balloon catheter. Semin Intervent Cardiol 1:43, 1996.

45. Edelman ER, Adams DH, Kamovsky MJ: Effect of controlled adventitial heparin delivery on smooth muscle proliferation following endothelial injury. Proc Natl Acad Sci USA 87:3773–3777, 1990.

46. Machan L, Signore P, Bromley P, et al: Prevention of neointimal hyperplasia by periadventitial taxol. Cardiovasc Intervent Radiol 20(suppl 1):S87, 1997.

47. Fischell TA, Kharma BK, Fischell DR, et al: Low-dose, β-particle emission from stent wire results in complete, localized inhibition of smooth muscle cell proliferation. Circulation 90:2956–2963, 1994.

48. Teirstein PS, Massullo V, Jani S, et al: Catheter-based radiotherapy to inhibit restenosis after coronary stenting. N Engl J Med 336:1697–1703, 1997.

49. Verin V, Urban Popowski Y, et al: Feasibility of intracoronary beta-irradiation to reduce restenosis after balloon angioplasty. Circulation 95:1138–1144, 1998.

50. Laird JR, Carter AJ, Kufs W, et al: Inhibition of neointimal proliferation with a beta particle emitting stent. Circulation 93:529–536, 1996.

Index

Note: Page numbers in *italics* indicate figures; those with a t indicate tables.

ISBN 0-443-06541-1

9 780443 065415

90038